T0280536

SECOND EDITION

ANALYSIS AND APPLICATION OF ANALOG ELECTRONIC CIRCUITS TO BIOMEDICAL INSTRUMENTATION

Biomedical Engineering Series

Michael R. Neuman, Series Editor

Published Titles

Electromagnetic Analysis and Design in Magnetic Resonance Imaging, Jianming Jin

Endogenous and Exogenous Regulation and Control of Physiological Systems, Robert B. Northrop

Artificial Neural Networks in Cancer Diagnosis, Prognosis, and Treatment, Raouf N.G. Naguib and Gajanan V. Sherbet

Medical Image Registration, Joseph V. Hajnal, Derek Hill, and David J. Hawkes

Introduction to Dynamic Modeling of Neuro-Sensory Systems, Robert B. Northrop

Noninvasive Instrumentation and Measurement in Medical Diagnosis, Robert B. Northrop

Handbook of Neuroprosthetic Methods, Warren E. Finn and Peter G. LoPresti

Angiography and Plaque Imaging: Advanced Segmentation Techniques, Jasjit S. Suri and Swamy Laxminarayan

Biomedical Image Analysis, Rangaraj M. Rangayyan

Foot and Ankle Motion Analysis: Clinical Treatment and Technology, Gerald F. Harris, Peter A. Smith, Richard M. Marks

Introduction to Molecular Biology, Genomics and Proteomic for Biomedical Engineers, Robert B. Northrop and Anne N. Connor

Signals and Systems Analysis in Biomedical Engineering, Second Edition, Robert B. Northrop

An Introduction to Biomaterials, Second Edition Jeffrey O. Hollinger

Analysis and Application of Analog Electronic Circuits to Biomedical Instrumentation, Second Edition, Robert B. Northrop

SECOND EDITION

ANALYSIS AND APPLICATION OF ANALOG ELECTRONIC CIRCUITS TO BIOMEDICAL INSTRUMENTATION

ROBERT B. NORTHROP

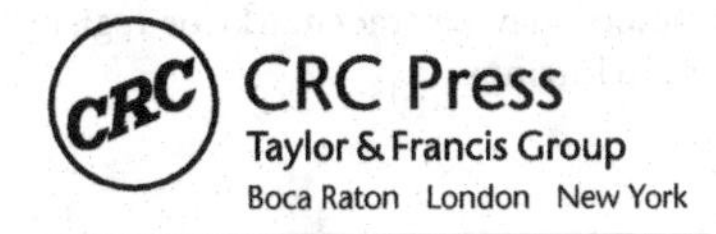

CRC Press is an imprint of the
Taylor & Francis Group, an **informa** business

CRC Press
Taylor & Francis Group
6000 Broken Sound Parkway NW, Suite 300
Boca Raton, FL 33487-2742

First issued in paperback 2017

Version Date: 20120120

ISBN 13: 978-1-4398-6669-6 (hbk)
ISBN 13: 978-1-138-07305-0 (pbk)

Visit the Taylor & Francis Web site at
http://www.taylorandfrancis.com

and the CRC Press Web site at
http://www.crcpress.com

Contents

List of Figures

Preface

READER BACKGROUND

This text is intended for use in a classroom course on Analysis and Application of Analog Electronic Circuits to Biomedical Instrumentation taken by junior or senior undergraduate students specializing in biomedical engineering. It focuses on the electronic components and subsystems that make up the diverse instruments that are used in biomedical instrumentation. It will also serve as a reference book for biophysics and medical students interested in the topics. Readers are assumed to have had introductory, core courses up to the junior level in engineering mathematics, including complex algebra, calculus, and introductory differential equations. They also should have taken a college physics course containing electricity and magnetism. As a result of taking these courses, readers should be familiar with systems block diagrams, the concepts of frequency response and transfer functions, and should be able to solve simple, linear, ordinary differential equations, and do basic manipulations in linear algebra. It is also important to have an understanding of the working principles of the various basic solid-state devices (diodes, bipolar junction transistors, and field-effect transistors) used in electronic circuits with biomedical applications.

RATIONALE

The interdisciplinary field of biomedical engineering is demanding in that it requires its followers to know and master not only certain engineering skills (electronics, materials, mechanical, and photonic) but also a diversity of material in the biological sciences (anatomy, biochemistry, molecular biology, genomics, physiology, etc.). This text was written to aid undergraduate biomedical engineering students by helping them to understand the basic analog electronic circuits used in signal conditioning in biomedical instrumentation. Because many bioelectric signals are in the microvolt range, noise from electrodes, amplifiers, and the environment is often significant compared to the signal level. This text introduces the basic mathematical tools used to describe noise and how it propagates through linear systems. It also describes at a basic level how signal-to-noise ratios can be improved by signal averaging and linear filtering.

Bandwidths associated with endogenous (natural) biomedical signals range from DC (e.g., hormone concentrations or DC potentials on the body surface) to hundreds of kilohertz (bat ultrasound). Exogenous signals associated with certain noninvasive imaging modalities (e.g., ultrasound, MRI) can reach into the 10s of MHz.

Throughout the text, op amps are shown to be the keystone of modern, analog signal conditioning system design. This text illustrates how op amps can be used to build instrumentation amplifiers, isolation amplifiers, active filters, and many other systems and subsystems used in biomedical instrumentation.

The text was written based both on the author's experience in teaching EE 204 Electronic Devices and Circuits, EE 240 Electronic Circuits and Applications, and EE 370 Biomedical Instrumentation I for more than 35 years in the Electrical & Computer Engineering Department at the University of Connecticut, and on his personal research in biomedical instrumentation.

DESCRIPTION OF THE CHAPTERS IN *ANALYSIS AND APPLICATION OF ANALOG ELECTRONIC CIRCUITS TO BIOMEDICAL ENGINEERING, 2ND EDITION*

This book is organized into 15 chapters, plus an Index, a Glossary, and a Bibliography and a Recommended Reading section. Extensive chapter examples are given based on electronic circuit problems in biomedical engineering. The chapter contents are summarized as follows:

In **Chapter 1, *Sources and Properties of Biomedical Signals,*** the sources of bioelectric phenomena in nerves and muscles are described. The general characteristics of biomedical signals are set forth and the general properties of physiological systems, including nonlinearity and nonstationarity are examined.

In **Chapter 2, *Properties and Models of Semiconductor Devices Used in Analog Electronic Systems,*** the mid- and high-frequency models used for analysis of *pn* junction diodes, BJTs, and FETs in electronic circuits are described. The high-frequency behavior of basic one- and two-transistor amplifiers is treated, and the Miller effect is introduced. This chapter also describes the properties of photodiodes, photoconductors, LEDs, and laser diodes.

In **Chapter 3, *Differential Amplifier,*** the important analog electronic circuit architecture is analyzed for both BJT and FET DAs. Mid- and high-frequency behavior is treated, as well as the factors that lead to a desirable high common-mode rejection ratio. DAs are shown to be essential subcircuits in all op amps, comparators, and instrumentation amplifiers.

In **Chapter 4, *General Properties of Electronic, Single-Loop Feedback Systems,*** the four basic kinds of electronic feedback (± voltage feedback and ± current feedback) are introduced, and how they affect linear amplifier performance is described.

The important topics of ***Feedback, Frequency Response, and Amplifier Stability*** are treated in **Chapter 5.** Bode plots and the root locus technique are presented as design tools and means of predicting closed-loop system stability. The effects of negative voltage and current feedback, and positive voltage feedback on an amplifier's gain, bandwidth, and input and output impedance are described. The design of certain "linear" oscillators is treated.

In **Chapter 6, *Operational Amplifiers and Comparators,*** first the properties of the ideal op amp are examined and then how its model can be used in quick, pencil-and-paper circuit analysis of various op amp circuits.

Circuit models for various types of practical op amps are described, including current feedback op amps. Gain-bandwidth products are shown to differ for different op amp types and circuits. Analog voltage comparators are introduced, and practical circuit examples are given. The final subsection illustrates some applications of op amps in biomedical instrumentation.

In **Chapter 7, *Introduction to Analog Active Filters,*** three major, easy-to-design-with architectures for op amp–based active filters are illustrated. These include the Sallen & Key quadratic AF, the one- and two-loop biquad AF, and the GIC-based AF. Voltage and digitally tunable AF designs are also described and examples given.

AF applications are discussed.

In **Chapter 8, *Instrumentation and Medical Isolation Amplifiers,*** the general properties of instrumentation amplifiers (IAs), and some of the circuit architectures used in their design are described. Medical isolation amplifiers (MIAs) are shown to be necessary to protect patients from electrical shock hazard during bioelectric measurements. All MIAs provide extreme galvanic isolation between the patient and the monitoring station. We illustrate several MIA architectures, including a novel direct sensing system, which uses the giant magnetoresistive effect. Also described are the current safety standards for MIAs.

In **Chapter 9,** ***Noise and the Design of Low-Noise Signal Conditioning Systems for Biomedical Applications,*** descriptors of random noise such as the probability density function, the auto- and cross-correlation functions, and the auto- and cross-power density spectra are introduced and their properties discussed. Sources of random noise in active and passive components are presented, and we show how noise propagates statistically through LTI filters. Noise factor, noise figure, and signal-to-noise ratio are shown to be useful measures of a signal conditioning system's noisiness. Noise in cascaded amplifier stages, DAs, and feedback amplifiers are treated. Examples of noise-limited signal resolution calculations are given. Factors affecting the design of low-noise amplifiers and a list of low-noise amplifiers are presented.

In **Chapter 10,** ***Digital Interfaces*** are described. Aliasing is described mathematically, and the sampling theorem is derived. Analog-to-digital and digital-to-analog converters are described. Hold circuits and quantization noise are also treated.

In **Chapter 11,** ***Modulation and Demodulation of Bioelectric Signals,*** the basics of modulation schemes used in instrumentation and biotelemetry systems is illustrated. AM, single-sideband AM (SSBAM), double-sideband suppressed carrier (DSBSC) AM, angle modulation including phase and frequency modulation (FM), narrow-band FM, delta modulation, and integral pulse frequency modulation (IPFM) systems are analyzed, as well as means for their demodulation.

In an all-new **Chapter 12,** we cover the important topic of ***Power Amplifiers and Their Applications in Biomedicine.*** Power op amps, the use of transformers for load impedance matching, and switched, class D PAs are described. IC series voltage regulators are also covered.

In a new **Chapter 13,** ***Wireless Patient Monitoring,*** WPM systems are described, including system architecture, UHF oscillators, antennas, modulators, and power sources. The issue of patient privacy is considered. WPM is shown to prevent patient microshock.

In a new **Chapter 14,** ***RFID Tags, GPS Tags, and Ultrasonic Tags Used in Ecological Research,*** the new technologies of RFID tags and their applications are explored. RFID tag circuit architecture, fractal antennas, and power sources are described. The use of GPS-based ID tags in animal ecological studies is described, and the design of ultrasonic tags to ID and track individual fish is presented.

In **Chapter 15,** ***Examples of Special Analog Circuits and Systems used in Biomedical Instrumentation,*** we describe and analyze certain circuits and systems important in biomedical and other branches of instrumentation. These include the phase-sensitive rectifier, phase detector circuits, voltage- and current-controlled oscillators, including VFCs and VPCs, phase-locked loops and applications, true RMS converters, and IC thermometers. Three examples of complicated biomedical measurement systems developed by the author are presented.

FEATURES

Some of the Unique Contents of This Text Are as Follows:

- **Chapter 2** describes the properties of photonic sensors and emitters, including PIN and avalanche photodiodes, and photoconductors. Signal conditioning circuits for these sensors are given and analyzed. Also in **Section 2.6** the properties of LEDs and laser diodes are described, as well as the circuits required to power them.
- **Chapter 8** gives a thorough treatment of the design of instrumentation amplifiers and medical isolation amplifiers. Also described in detail are current safety standards for MIAs.
- A comprehensive treatment of noise in analog signal conditioning systems, and the design of low-noise amplifiers are given in **Chapter 9**.

- **Chapter 10** on digital interfaces examines the designs of many types of ADCs and DACs and introduces *aliasing* and *quantization noise* as possible costs for going to and/or from analog or digital domains.
- **Chapter 11** considers the modulation and demodulation of biomedical signals. The use of phase-locked loops to generate or demodulate angle-modulated signals, including phase- and frequency-modulation, as well as AM and DSBSCM signals is described.
- A new **Chapter 12** describes analog power amplifier "building blocks," including the use of power op amps and class D (switched) PAs. The design and properties of series DC voltage regulators are also described.
- Wireless patient monitoring is described in a new **Chapter 13**. Wi-Fi and Bluetooth communications protocols are described.
- **Chapter 14** is a new chapter on RFID tags and their uses in biomedicine. Also introduced is a unique section on compact, broadband, fractal antennas. GPS tags are also described, as well as ultrasonic tags used in aquatic and marine ecological research.
- **Chapter 15** covers examples of certain special analog electronic circuits and systems used in biomedical instrumentation. In it we describe phase-sensitive rectifiers, phase detector circuits, VCOs and CCOs, phase-locked loops and their many applications, true RMS converter ICs, IC thermometers, and three examples of biomedical instrument systems using many of the special ICs introduced in this text.
- Home problems that accompany each chapter (except Chapters 1, 8, 14, and 15) stress biomedical electronic applications.
- There is an extensive **Bibliography, Index,** and **Glossary** (new).

Robert B. Northrop
Chaplin, Connecticut

Author

Robert B. Northrop, PhD, majored in electrical engineering at MIT, graduating with a bachelor's degree in 1956. At the University of Connecticut, he received a master's degree in systems engineering in EE in 1958. As a result of a long-standing interest in physiological systems, he entered a PhD program at UCONN in physiology, doing research on the neuromuscular physiology of molluscan catch muscles. He received his PhD degree in 1964.

In 1963, he joined the UCONN EE Department as a lecturer and was hired as an assistant professor of electrical engineering in 1964. In collaboration with his PhD advisor, Dr. Edward G. Boettiger, he secured a 5-year training grant in 1965 from NIGMS (NIH), and started one of the first, interdisciplinary, biomedical engineering graduate training programs in New England. UCONN currently awards MS and PhD degrees in this field of study, as well as BS degrees in engineering under the BME area of concentration.

Throughout his career, Dr. Northrop's research interests have been broad and interdisciplinary and have been centered on biomedical engineering and physiology. He has done sponsored research (by the AFOSR) on the neurophysiology of insect compound eye vision and devised theoretical models for visual neural signal processing. He also did sponsored research on electrofishing and developed, in collaboration with Northeast Utilities, effective working systems for fish guidance and control in hydroelectric plant waterways on the Connecticut River at Holyoke, Massachusetts, using underwater electric fields.

Still another area of his research (funded by NIH) has been in the design and simulation of nonlinear, adaptive, digital controllers to regulate *in vivo* drug concentrations or physiological parameters, such as pain, blood pressure, or blood glucose in diabetics. An outgrowth of this research led to his development of mathematical models for the dynamics of the human immune system, which were used to investigate theoretical therapies for autoimmune diseases, cancer, and HIV infection.

Biomedical instrumentation has also been an active research area for Dr. Northrop and his graduate students: An NIH grant supported studies on the use of the ocular pulse to detect obstructions in the carotid arteries. Minute pulsations of the cornea from arterial circulation in the eyeball were sensed using a no-touch, phase-locked, ultrasound technique. Ocular pulse waveforms were shown to be related to cerebral blood flow in rabbits and humans.

More recently, Dr. Northrop addressed the problem of noninvasive blood glucose measurement for diabetics. Starting with a Phase I SBIR grant, he developed a means of estimating blood glucose by reflecting a beam of polarized light off the front surface of the lens of the eye, and measuring the very small optical rotation resulting from glucose in the aqueous humor, which in turn is proportional to blood glucose. As an offshoot of techniques developed in micropolarimetry, he developed a magnetic sample chamber for glucose measurement in biotechnology applications. The water solvent was used as the Faraday optical medium.

He has written eleven textbooks: *Analog Electronic Circuits* (1990); *Introduction to Instrumentation and Measurements* (1st and 2nd editions) (1997 and 2005); *Endogenous and Exogenous Regulation and Control of Physiological Systems* (2000); *Dynamic Modeling of Neuro-Sensory Systems* (2001); *Signals and Systems Analysis in Biomedical Engineering* (1st and 2nd editions.) (2003 and 2010); *Noninvasive Instrumentation and Measurements in Medical Diagnosis* (2002); *Analysis and Application of Analog Electronic Circuits in Biomedical Engineering* (2004); and

Introduction to Molecular Biology, Genomics & Proteomics for Biomedical Engineers (with Anne N. Connor) (2009); *Introduction to Complexity and Complex Systems* (2011).

His current research interests include complex systems, catastrophe theory, and sustainability.

Dr. Northrop was on the Electrical & Systems Engineering faculty at UCONN until his retirement in June, 1997. Throughout this time, he was director of the Biomedical Engineering Graduate Program. As emeritus professor, he still teaches graduate courses in biomedical engineering and writes texts.

1 Sources and Properties of Biomedical Signals

1.1 INTRODUCTION

Before describing and analyzing the electronic circuits, amplifiers, and filters required to condition the signals found in clinical medicine, biomedical research, and physiology, it is appropriate to describe the sources and properties of these signals (i.e., their bandwidths, amplitude distributions, and noisiness). Broadly speaking, biomedical signals can be subdivided into two major classes: (1) *Endogenous signals,* which arise from natural physiological processes and which are measured within or on the surface of living creatures (examples include electrocardiogram (ECG), electroencephalogram (EEG), respiratory rate, temperature, blood pressure, blood glucose). (2) *Exogenous signals* that are applied from without (generally noninvasively) to measure internal structures and physiological parameters. These include, but are not limited to, *ultrasound* (imaging and Doppler), *X-rays (CAT scans),* and *monochromatic light* (such as the two wavelengths used in transcutaneous pulse oximeters, excitation of fluorescence from fluorophore-tagged cells and molecules stimulated with blue or near UV light, optical coherence tomography (OCT), laser Doppler velocimetry (LDV) used to measure blood velocity, and the strong magnetic fields used in magnetic resonance imaging (MRI)). For many other examples of exogenous signals refer to Northrop (2002).

In the following section, the properties of *endogenous bioelectric signals* used in medical diagnosis, care, and research are examined.

1.2 SOURCES OF ENDOGENOUS BIOELECTRIC SIGNALS

The sources of nearly all bioelectric signals are transient changes in the *transmembrane potential* observed in all living cells. In particular, bioelectric signals arise from the time-varying transmembrane potentials seen in nerve cells (neuron action potentials and generator potentials) and in muscle cells, including the heart and smooth muscles. The electrochemical basis for transmembrane potentials in living cells lies in several phenomena: First, cell membranes are *semipermeable.* That is, they have different transmembrane conductances and permeabilities for different ions and molecules (e.g., Na^+, K^+, Ca^{++}, Cl^-, glucose, and proteins). Second, cell membranes contain "ion pumps" driven by metabolic energy (e.g., ATP). The ion pumps actively transport ions and molecules across cell membranes against energy barriers set up by the transmembrane potential and/or concentration gradients between the inside and outside of the cell. In the steady state, there is a continual leakage of ions into a cell (e.g., Na^+), out of a cell (e.g., K^+), and ongoing ion pumping to restore the steady-state concentrations. In the widely studied squid giant axons, the steady-state *internal* concentrations are as follows: $[Na^+]_i = 50$ mM, $[K^+]_i = 400$ mM, and $[Cl^-]_i = 52$ mM. The steady-state *external* concentrations (in extracellular fluid) are as follows: $[Na^+]_e = 440$ mM, $[K^+]_e = 20$ mM, $[Cl^-]_e = 560$ mM, and $[A^-]_i = 385$ mM (Kandel et al. 1991). $[A^-]$ is the equivalent concentration of large, impermeable protein anions in the cytosol. Ion concentration data exist for the neurons and muscles of a variety of invertebrate and vertebrate species (Kandel et al. 1991; Katz 1966; West 1985).

The steady-state transmembrane potential can be modeled by the *Goldman–Hodgkin–Katz equation* (Guyton 1991):

$$V_{mo} = -\frac{RT}{F}\ln\left\{\frac{[Na^+]_i P_{Na^+} + [K^+]_i P_{K^+} + [Cl^-]_i P_{Cl^-}}{[Na^+]_e P_{Na^+} + [K^+]_e P_{K^+} + [Cl^-]_e P_{Cl^-}}\right\} \tag{1.1}$$

where T is the Kelvin temperature, R is the MKS gas constant (8.314 J/(mol K)), F is the Faraday number, 96,500 Cb/mol, and P_X is the permeability for ion species X.

The resting transmembrane potential of neurons, V_{mo}, varies with species, neuron type, ionic environment, and temperature. It can range from ca. 60 to 90 mV, inside negative with respect to outside. Muscle cells also have transmembrane potentials, ca. $80 < V_{mo} < 95$ mV, inside negative, for human muscles.

1.3 NERVE ACTION POTENTIALS

Nerve action potentials (APs) are, in general, the result of transient changes in specific ionic conductances and permeabilities induced in the nerve cell membrane electrically or chemically by neurotransmitters. In excitable neuron membranes, an *increase* in cell membrane sodium permeability leads to a *depolarization* of the transmembrane potential (i.e., sodium ions flow rapidly into the neuron's cytoplasm down a concentration gradient and electric field). The inrush of Na^+ through the membrane causes the normally negative transmembrane voltage V_m to go positive, which is a *depolarization.* When the excitable nerve transmembrane voltage reaches a *depolarization threshold*, which is on the order of a few millivolts more positive than the resting potential, the permeability events that lead to a propagating action potential or nerve spike begin to occur. First, there is a further, "all-or-nothing," large transient increase in sodium permeability causing a strong transient inrush of Na^+ ions. This Na^+ inrush causes a large, rapid depolarization so that V_m actually goes positive by 10s of mV, generally in less than a millisecond. Immediately, permeability to K^+ ions also increases, but at a slower rate, which causes an outward potassium ion current density, J_{K^+}, causing V_m to decrease from its positive peak to its negative resting value after a slight, transient undershoot (hyperpolarization). The total duration of the nerve action potential spike, including recovery to the SS V_m, is on the order of 2.5–3 ms. Once initiated, an action potential propagates down a neuron's axon at a velocity that depends on a number of physical and chemical factors, including the diameter of the axon. One of the earliest mathematical models for nerve impulse generation was given by Hodgkin and Huxley (1952). The H-H model now appears to be somewhat oversimplified with its description of a single type of potassium channel, but is still valid, and is a useful model to demonstrate the dynamics of nerve impulse generation. Figure 1.1 illustrates the result of a computer simulation of the H-H model using Simnon™ (Northrop 2001). Shown is the transmembrane voltage, $V_m(t)$, and the time-varying conductances for Na^+ and K^+. Readers interested in pursuing the molecular and ionic details of neurophysiology should consult the texts by Kandel et al. (1991), West (1985), Guyton (1991), and Northrop (2001).

Most neurons in the vertebrate central nervous system (CNS) are too small to directly record their transmembrane potentials with glass micropipette electrodes. However, their action potentials can be recorded over long periods of time with extracellular, metal microelectrodes whose uninsulated tips are in the neuropile within several micrometers of axons or cell bodies. Action potentials from peripheral nerve bundles can be recorded with simple platinum hook electrodes, saline-filled suction electrodes, or saline-wetted wick electrodes coupled to silver/silver chloride electrodes. All extracellular recording techniques suffer from the problem that the electrodes pick up nerve spikes from active, adjacent, or neighboring neurons. This neural background noise is added to the desired unit's signal and, unfortunately, has the same bandwidth as the

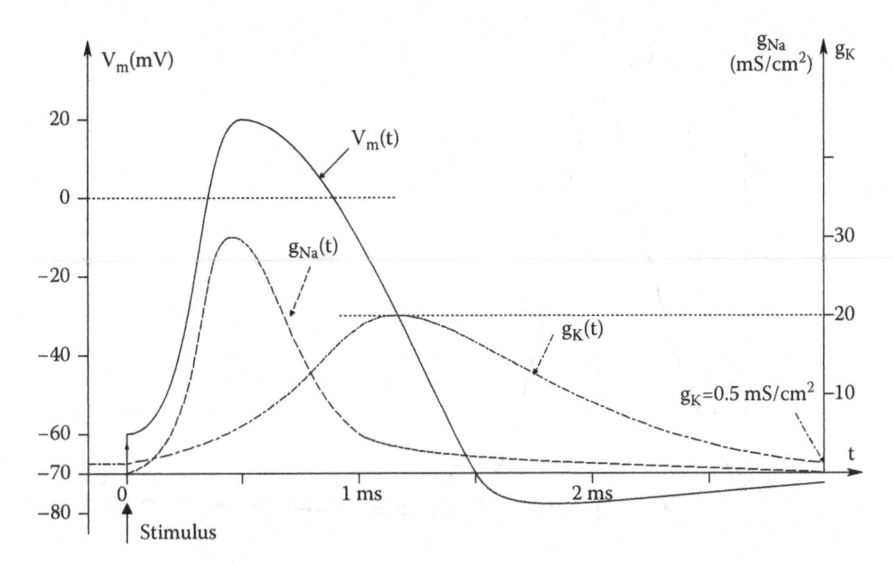

FIGURE 1.1 Results of a Simnon™ simulation of the Hodgkin–Huxley 1952 mathematical model for nerve action potential generation (Northrop, R.B., *Introduction to Dynamic Modeling of Neuro-Sensory Systems*. CRC Press, Boca Raton, FL, 2001.) Traces shown: $v_m(t)$ (transmembrane potential) in mV. $g_K(t, v_m)$ in mS/cm^2. $g_{Na}(t, v_m)$ in mS/cm^2. Time in ms.

desired unit's spikes. In dissected peripheral nerve fibers, it may be possible to isolate single axons with hook, suction, or wick electrodes, greatly improving the recording signal-to-noise ratio (SNR).

Because the nerve action potential is a traveling wave, it can be shown that an external electrode in close proximity to the outside surface of an axon (the second, (reference), (−) electrode is located remotely from the axon) will respond to the passage of the AP with an electric potential waveform that has in effect, the shape of the *second derivative* of the transmembrane spike waveform (Plonsey 1969), as shown in Figure 1.2. (The intracellular AP, V_m, is to scale, but its derivatives are not to scale.) The triphasic (second derivative) waveform of the AP recorded at a point near the axon comes from the fact that the AP is traveling along the axon with velocity, v. As the AP approaches the electrode, a weak, net *outward* J_{K^+} causes a low positive voltage peak. When the AP has moved opposite the electrode, the electrode responds to the strong *inward* flow of J_{Na} with a large negative voltage peak. Then, as the AP passes the electrode, its potential again goes positive from the net *outward* J_{K^+} in the recovery phase of the AP.

In the author's experience, using fine platinum–iridium extracellular microelectrodes (which were glass insulated down to 6–12 μm of their conical tips), we were able to record from single units in insect optic lobes and protocerebrum, and in frog tectum, with major spike amplitudes ranging from −50 to −500 μV. Midband gain for signal conditioning was 10^4, and signal conditioning bandwidth was typically 100 to 3000 Hz (Northrop and Guignon 1970).

Nerve APs recorded through the neuron membrane (in the cell body, base of dendrites, or axon) using glass micropipette electrodes can be ca. 100 mV or more, peak-to-peak. A capacity-neutralized, electrometer head stage used to couple the high resistance microelectrode generally has a gain of 2 or 3; the second stage may have gain from 5 to 30, so the overall gain can range from 10 to 90. Bandwidth is generally from dc to 3–5 kHz. The direct coupling is required because we are generally interested in the neuron's resting potential, V_{mo}, or slow changes in V_m caused by incoming excitatory or inhibitory signals. If we are not interested in V_{mo}, then it is technically simpler and less noisy to use *extracellular microelectrodes* and band-pass filtering (e.g., 100 Hz to 3 kHz). More amplifier gain will be required with external electrodes, however.

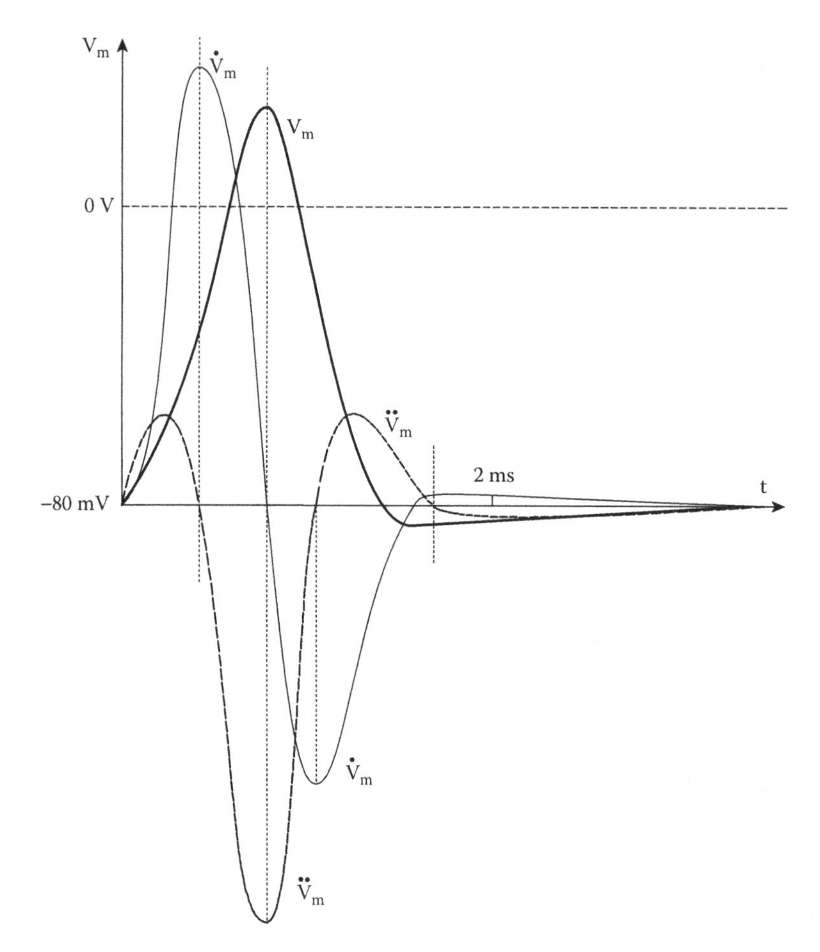

FIGURE 1.2 A nerve action potential and its first and second time derivatives (derivatives not to scale).

1.4 MUSCLE ACTION POTENTIALS

1.4.1 Introduction

An important bioelectric signal that has diagnostic significance for many neuromuscular diseases is the *electromyogram* (EMG), which can be recorded from the skin surface with electrodes identical to those used for electrocardiography, although in some cases, the electrodes have smaller areas than those used for ECG (<1 mm^2). To record from single motor units (SMUs), or even individual muscle fibers (several of which comprise a SMU), needle electrodes that pierce the skin into the body of a superficial muscle can also be used. (This semi-invasive method obviously requires sterile technique.) EMG recording is used to diagnose some causes of muscle weakness or paralysis, muscle or motor problems such as tremor or twitching, motor nerve damage from injury or osteoarthritis, and pathologies affecting motor end plates (myoneural junctions).

1.4.2 The Origin of EMGs

There are three types of muscle in the body, viz, striated, cardiac, and smooth. Striated muscle in mammals can be further subdivided into *fast* and *slow muscles* (Guyton 1991). Fast muscles are used for fast movements; they include, for example, the two gastrocnemii, laryngeal muscles, the extraocular muscles. Slow muscles are used for postural control against gravity; they include the soleus, abdominal muscles, back muscles, neck muscles, and so on. EMG recording is generally carried out on both slow and fast skeletal muscles. It can also be done on less superficial muscles such as the extraocular muscles that move the eyeballs, the eyelid muscles, and the muscles that work the larynx.

A particular striated muscle is innervated by a group of *motor neurons* that have origin at a certain level in the spinal cord. In the spinal cord, motor neurons receive excitatory and inhibitory inputs from motor control neurons from the CNS, as well as excitatory and inhibitory inputs from local feedback neurons from muscle spindles (responding to muscle length x and dx/dt) and Golgi tendon organs (responding to muscle tension) and Renshaw feedback cells (Guyton 1991; Northrop 2000).

Individual motor neuron axons controlling the contraction of a particular striated muscle innervate small groups of muscle fibers in the muscle called an SMU. Many SMUs comprise the entire muscle. The synaptic connections between the terminal branches of a single motor neuron axon and its SMU fibers are called *motor end plates* (MEPs). MEPs are chemical synapses in which the neurotransmitter, *acetylcholine* (ACh), is released presynaptically and then diffuses across the synaptic cleft or gap to ACh receptors on the subsynaptic membrane. When a motor neuron action potential arrives at an MEP, it triggers the exocytocis or emptying of about 300 presynaptic vesicles containing ACh. (There are ca. 3×10^5 vesicles in the terminals of a single MEP; each vesicle is about 40 nm diameter.) Some 10^7 to 5×10^8 molecules of ACh are needed to trigger a muscle action potential (Katz 1966). The ACh diffuses across the 20 to 30 nm synaptic cleft in ca. 0.5 ms, where some ACh molecules combine with receptor sites on the protein subunits forming the subsynaptic, sodium ion-gating channels. Five, high-molecular-weight protein subunits form each ion channel. ACh binding to the protein subunits triggers a dilation of the channel to ca. 0.65 nm. The dilated channels allow Na^+ ions to pass inward; however, Cl^- is repelled by the fixed negative charges on the mouth of the channel. Thus, the subsynaptic membrane is depolarized by the inward J_{Na} (i.e., its transmembrane potential goes positive from the ca. −85 mV resting potential), triggering a *muscle action potential.* The local subsynaptic, transmembrane potential can go to as much as +50 mV, forming an *end-plate potential* (EPP) spike fused to the muscle action potential it triggers, having a duration of ca. 8 ms, much longer than a nerve action potential.

The ACh in the cleft and bound to the receptors is rapidly broken down (hydrolyzed) by the enzyme *cholinesterase* resident in the cleft, and its molecular components are recycled. A small amount of ACh also escapes the cleft by diffusion and is also hydrolyzed.

Once the postsynaptic membrane under the MEP depolarizes in a superthreshold EPP spike, a *muscle action potential* is generated that propagates along the surface membrane of the muscle fiber, the *sarcolemma.* It is the muscle action potential that triggers muscle fiber contraction and force generation. Typical muscle action potentials recorded intracellularly at the MEP and at a point 2 mm from the initiating MEP are shown in Figure 1.3. A human skeletal muscle fiber action potential typically propagates at 3 to 5 m/s; its duration is 2 to 15 ms, depending on the muscle, and it swings from a resting value of ca. −85 mV to a peak of ca. +30 mV. At the skin surface, it appears as a triphasic spike of 20 to 2000 μV peak amplitude (Guyton 1991).

To ensure that all of the deep contractile apparatus in the center of the muscle fiber is stimulated to contract at the same time and with equal strength, many transverse, radially directed tubules penetrate into the center of the fiber along its length. These *T-tubules* are open to the extracellular fluid space, as is the surface of the fiber, and they are connected to the surface membrane at both ends. The T-tubules conduct the muscle action potential into the interior of the fiber in many locations along its length.

Running longitudinally around the outside of the contractile myofibrils that make up the fiber are networks of tubules called the *sarcoplasmic reticulum* (SR). Note that the terminal *cisternae* of the SR butt against the membrane of the T-tubes. When the muscle action potential penetrates along the T-tubes, the depolarization triggers the *cisternae* to release calcium ions into the space surrounding the myofibrils' contractile proteins. The Ca^{++} binds to the protein *troponin C,* which

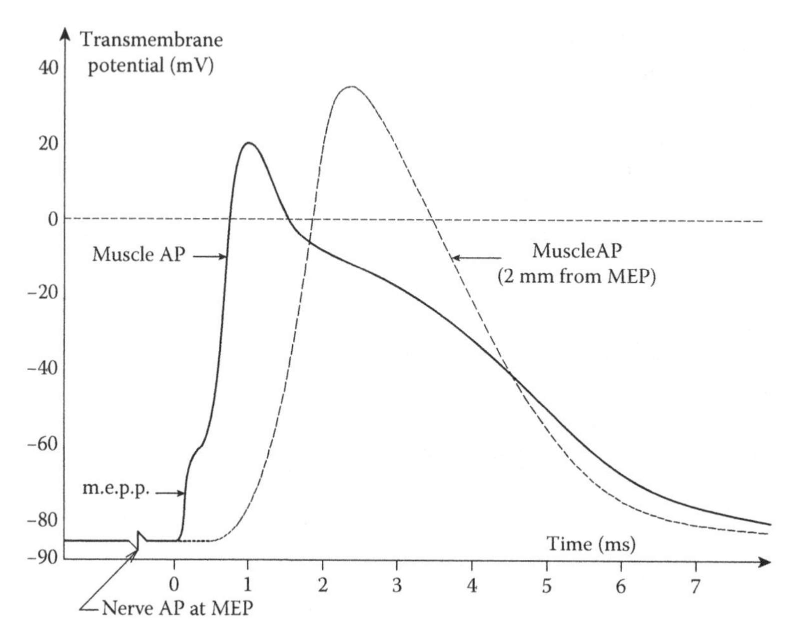

FIGURE 1.3 A typical single-fiber muscle action potential recorded intracellularly at the motor end plate and 2 mm along the fiber.

triggers contraction by the actin and myosin proteins. (We will not go into the molecular biophysics of the actual contraction process here.)

A synchronous stimulation of all of the motor neurons innervating a muscle produces what is called a *muscle twitch*; i.e., the tension initially falls to a slight amount, then rises abruptly, and then falls more slowly to zero again. Sustained muscle contraction is caused by a steady (average) rate of (asynchronous) motoneuron firing. When the firing ceases, the muscle relaxes.

Muscle relaxation is actually an *active process.* Metabolically driven calcium ion pumps located in the membranes of the SR's longitudinal tubules actively transfer Ca^{++} from outside the tubules to back inside the SR system. It is the lack of Ca^{++} in proximity to the protein *troponin C* that allows relaxation to occur. In resting muscle, the calcium ion concentration, $[Ca^{++}]$, is about 10^{-7} M in the myofibrillar fluid (Guyton 1991). In a twitch, $[Ca^{++}]$ rises to ca. 2×10^{-5} M, and in a tetanic stimulation, $[Ca^{++}]$ is about 2×10^{-4} M. It takes about 50 ms for the Ca^{++} released by a single motor nerve impulse to be taken up by the SR pumps to restore the resting $[Ca^{++}]$ level.

Just as in the case of the sodium pumps in nerve cell membrane, the muscles' Ca^{++} pumps require metabolic energy to operate; *adenosine triphoshate* (ATP) is cleaved to the diphosphate form to release the energy needed to drive the Ca^{++} pumps. The pumps can concentrate the Ca^{++} to ca. 10^{-3} M inside the SR. Inside the SR tubules and *cisternae,* the Ca^{++} is stored in readily available ionic form, and also as a protein chelate, bound to a protein, *calsequestrin.*

So far, we have described the events associated with a single, striated muscle fiber. As noted earlier, small groups of fibers innervated by a single motoneuron fiber are called an SMU. In muscles used for fine actions, such as those operating the fingers or tongue, there are fewer muscle fibers in a motor unit, or equivalently, more motoneuron fibers per total number of muscle fibers. For example, the laryngeal muscles used for speech have only two or three fibers per SMU, while large muscles used for gross motions, such as the gastrocnemius, can have several hundred fibers per SMU (Guyton 1991).

To make fine movements, only a few motoneurons fire out of the total number innervating the muscle, and these do not fire synchronously. Their firing phases are made random in order to produce smooth contraction. At maximum tetanic stimulation, the mean frequency on the motoneurons is higher, but the phases are still random to reduce the duty cycle of individual SMUs. It is this asynchronicity that makes strong EMGs look like noise on a CRT display.

1.4.3 EMG Amplifiers

The amplifiers used for *clinical* EMG recording must meet the same stringent specifications for low leakage currents as do ECG, EEG, and other amplifiers used to measure human body potentials (see Chapter 8). EMG amplifier gains are typically ×1000, and their bandwidths reflect the transient nature of the SMU action potentials. An EMG amplifier is generally reactively coupled with low- and high-frequency –3 dB frequencies of 100 Hz and 3 kHz, respectively. With an amplifier having variable low and high (–3 dB) frequencies, one generally starts with a wide pass bandwidth, for example, 50 Hz to 10 kHz, and gradually restricts it until individual EMG spikes just begin to round up and change shape. Such an ad hoc–adjusted bandwidth will give a better output SNR than one that is too wide or too narrow.

EMGs can be viewed in the *time domain* (most useful when single fibers or SMUs are being recorded), in the *frequency domain* (the fast Fourier transform (FFT) is taken from an entire, sampled, surface-recorded EMG burst under standard conditions), or in the *joint time-frequency* (JTF) *domain* (cf. Section 3.2.3 in Northrop 2002). In the latter case, the JTF display shows the frequencies in the EMG burst as a function of time. In general, a higher frequency content in the JTF display indicates that more SMUs are being activated at a higher rate (Hannaford and Lehman, 1986). JTF analysis can show how agonist–antagonist muscle pairs are controlled to do a specific motor task.

Still another way to characterize EMG activity in the time domain is to pass the EMG through a *true RMS* (TRMS) conversion circuit, such as an AD637 IC. The output of the TRMS circuit is a smoothed, positive voltage proportional to the square-root of the time average of the input signal squared, $x^2(t)$. The time averaging is done by a single time constant, low-pass filter. For another time domain display modality, the EMG signal can be full-wave rectified and low-pass filtered to smooth it.

1.5 ELECTROCARDIOGRAM

1.5.1 Introduction

One of the most important electrophysiological measurements in medical diagnosis and patient care is that of the electrocardiogram (ECG or EKG). Because the heart is an organ essentially made of muscle, every time it contracts during the cardiac pumping cycle, it generates a spatiotemporal electric field which is coupled through the anatomically complicated volume conductor of the thorax and abdomen to the skin where a spatiotemporal potential difference can be measured. The amplitude and waveshape of the normal ECG depends on where the measuring electrode pair is located on the skin surface.

Before electronic amplification was invented, Willem Einthoven measured the ECG in 1901 using a magnetic *string galvanometer.* The galvanometer was connected to the patient by two wires connected to two carbon rods immersed in two jars of saline solution in which the patient placed either two hands or a hand and a leg (Northrop 2002). With the advent of electronic amplification in 1928, it was quickly discovered that many interesting features of the ECG could be revealed by use of different electrode placements (e.g., AV leads, precordial leads, and the Frank vector cardiography lead system) (cf. Chapters 10, 11, and 12 in Guyton 1991, Section 4.6 in Webster, 1992, Section 4.4 in Northrop 2002).

Figure 1.4 illustrates schematically the important pacemaker, cardiac muscle and conduction bundle transmembrane potentials in the normal human heart, and their relation to the classic, Lead III ECG wave. Note that following atrial contraction, excitation is conducted to the AV node, then to the ventricles by a complex network of specialized muscle cells forming the *conduction bundle*

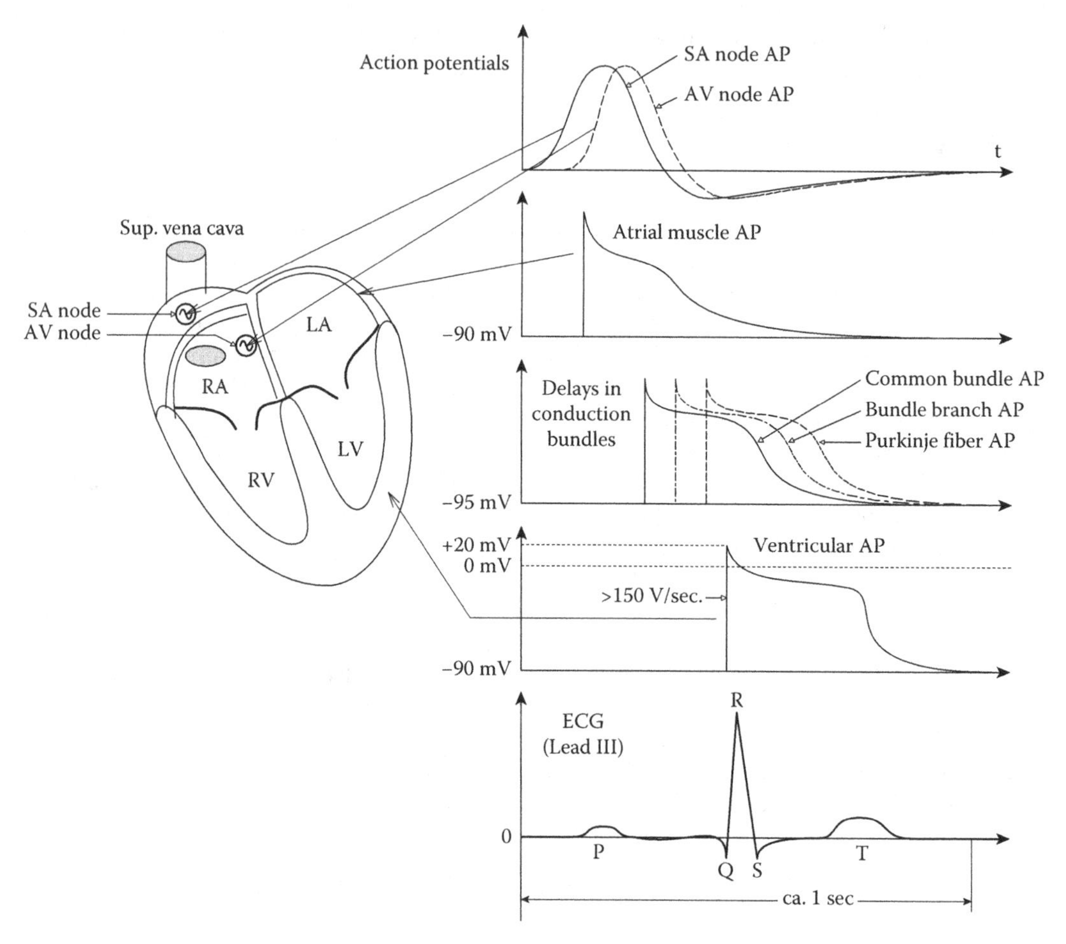

FIGURE 1.4 Schematic cut-away of a mammalian heart showing the SA and AV node pacemakers, also intracellular action potentials from different locations in the heart. Bottom trace is a typical Lead III skin surface-recorded ECG waveform.

system. Propagation delay through the bundles and *Purkinje fibers* allows the ventricles to contract *after* the atrial contraction has had time to fill them with blood. The QRS spike in the ECG is associated with the rapid rate of depolarization of ventricular muscle just preceding its contraction. The P-wave is caused by atrial depolarization, and the T-wave is associated with ventricular muscle repolarization.

1.5.2 ECG Amplifiers

Wherever recorded, the ECG QRS spike can range from 400 μV to 2.5 mV peak. Its amplitude depends on the recording site and the patient's body type. Thus, the gain required for ECG amplification is ca. 10^3. ECG amplifiers are reactively coupled (r-c) with standardized −3 dB corner frequencies at 0.05 and 100 Hz. If ECG bandwidth were not standardized, ECG interpretation would be difficult and confusing. Most ECG amplifiers allow the operator to switch in a 60 Hz notch filter to attenuate 60 Hz interference which can appears at the output in spite of differential amplification. The notch filter causes little distortion of the raw ECG output signal.

A further, important requirement of all ECG amplifiers is that they have *galvanic isolation* (see Chapter 8 in this text). Galvanic isolation is required to protect the patient from electroshock accidents. Galvanic isolation places a very high impedance between the patient, the ECG electrodes, and ECG amplifier input ground, and the ECG amplifier output and output ground. This limits any current which might flow through the patient to single microamps if the patient accidentally makes contact with the power mains while connected to the ECG system and is otherwise not grounded. Other biopotential amplifiers used in a clinical or research setting with humans, such as for measurement of EEG, EMG, ERG, ECoG, etc., must also have medically rated galvanic isolation.

1.6 OTHER BIOPOTENTIALS

1.6.1 INTRODUCTION

Many other biopotentials are measured for research and clinical purposes. These include the EEG, the *electroretinogram* (ERG), the *electrooculogram* (EOG), and the *electrocochleogram* (ECoG) (Northrop 2002). All of these signals are low amplitude (100s of μV peak) and contain primarily low frequencies (0.01–100 Hz).

1.6.2 *EEGs*

The EEG is used to diagnose brain injuries and brain tumors noninvasively, as well as in neuropsychology research.

EEGs are generally recorded from the scalp, which means the underlying, cortical brain electrical activity must pass through the *pia* and *dura mater* membranes, cerebrospinal fluid, the skull, and the scalp. Considerable attenuation and spatial averaging occurs because of these anatomical structures relative to the electrical activity which can also be recorded directly from the brain's surface with wick electrodes. The largest EEG potentials recorded on the scalp are ca. 150 μV pk. In an attempt to localize sites of EEG activity on the surface of the brain, multiple electrode EEG recordings are made from the scalp. The standard 10–20 EEG electrode array uses 19 electrodes, and some electrode arrays used in brain research use 128 electrodes (Northrop 2002).

EEGs have traditionally been divided into four frequency bands: *Delta waves* have the largest amplitudes and lowest frequencies (≤3.5 Hz); they occur in adults in deep sleep. *Theta waves* are large-amplitude low-frequency voltages (3.5–7.5 Hz). Theta waves are seen in sleep in adults and in prepubescent children. The spectrum of *alpha waves* lies between 7.5 and 13 Hz, and their amplitudes range from 20 to 200 μV. Alpha waves are recorded from adults who are conscious but relaxed with the eyes closed. Alpha activity disappears when the eyes are open and the subject focuses on a task. Alpha waves are best recorded from posterior lateral portions of the scalp. *Beta waves* are defined for frequencies from 13 to 50 Hz, and they are most easily found in the parietal and frontal regions of the scalp. Beta waves are subdivided into types I and II. Type I beta disappears during intense mental activity, while type II beta waves appear (Webster 1992).

EEG amplifiers must work with low-frequency and low-amplitude signals; consequently, they must be low noise types with low 1/f noise spectrums. EEG amplifiers can be reactively coupled; their −3 dB frequencies should be about 0.2 and 100 Hz. Amplifier midband gain needs to be on the order of 10^4 to 10^5.

EEG measurement also includes evoked cortical potentials used in experimental brain research. A patient is presented with a periodic stimulus, which can be auditory (a click or tone), visual (a flash of light, or a tachistoscopically presented picture), tactile (a pin prick), or some other transient sensory modality. Following each stimulus, there is a transient EEG response added to the ongoing EEG activity. Very often this evoked response cannot be seen with the naked eye on a monitor. Because the passband of the evoked response is the same as the interfering or masking EEG activity, linear filtering does not help in extracting transient. Thus, *signal averaging* must be used to bring forth the desired evoked transient from the unrelated, accompanying noise (Northrop 2002, 2010). Evoked transient electrical response can be recovered by averaging even when the input SNR to the averager is as low as −60 dB.

1.6.3 Other Body Surface Potentials

The EOG, ERG, and ECoG are all transient, low-amplitude, and low-bandwidth potentials recorded for diagnostic and research purposes (Northrop 2002). Each transient waveform is generally accompanied by unwanted, uncorrelated noise from EMGs and from the electrodes. The EOG is the largest of these three potentials, having a peak on the order of single millivolt. Thus, an ECG amplifier can be used with a 0.05 to 100 Hz, –3 dB bandwidth, and gain of 10^3. Signal averaging is generally not required.

The ERG, on the other hand, has a peak amplitude on the order of hundreds of microvolts, and accompanying noise make signal averaging expeditious. The ERG preamplifier generally has a bandpass of 0.3–300 Hz, a gain between 10^3 and 10^4, and an input impedance of at least 10 MΩ.

The ECoG is the lowest amplitude transient, having a peak of only ca. 6 μV, and waveform features of <1 μV. Signal averaging must be used to resolve the ECoG evoked transient. The signal conditioning amplifier has a midband gain of 10^4, and –3 dB frequencies at 5 Hz and 3 kHz. The ECoG amplifier band-pass is defined by 12 dB/octave (two-pole) filters.

1.6.4 Discussion

From the descriptions above, one sees that the frequency content of endogenous signals from the body range from near dc to about 3 kHz. They are all accompanied by noise which means that linear filtering to improve the SNR_{in} can often help. Some signals such as ECoG and evoked brain cortical transients require signal averaging for meaningful resolution. Endogenous signal peak amplitudes range from over 100 mV for nerve and muscle transmembrane potentials recorded with glass micropipette electrodes, to less than a microvolt for evoked cortical transients recorded on the scalp.

1.7 ELECTRICAL PROPERTIES OF BIOELECTRODES

To record biopotentials, we need an *interface* between the electron-conducting copper wires connected to signal conditioning amplifiers, and the ion-conducting, "wet" environment of living animals. Bioelectrodes form this interface. There are many kinds of bioelectrodes, some better than others in terms of low noise and ease of use. Early ECG electrodes were nondisposable, nickel–silver plated copper, or stainless steel disks hard-wired to the amplifier input leads. Although a conductive gel was used between the electrodes and skin, this type of electrode had inherently high low-frequency noise due to the complex redox reactions taking place at the metal electrode surfaces. Still, acceptable ECG and EMG signals could be recorded. Present practice in measuring ECG and EMG signals from the skin surface is to use disposable sticky patch electrodes. Patch electrodes use a silver|silver chloride (Ag|AgCl) interface to a conductive gel containing Na^+, K^+, and Cl^- ions. The gel makes direct, wet contact with the skin. Adhesive for the skin is found in a plastic ring surrounding the electrolyte and AgCl. The copper wire makes contact with the Ag metal backing of the electrode, generally with a snap connector. More recently, skin electrodes have used Ag|AgCl deposited in a thin layer on a ca. 2.5 cm square of thin plastic film. The conductive gel and adhesive are combined in a layer all over the AgCl film. Contact with this inexpensive, disposable electrode is made with a miniature metal alligator clip on one raised corner.

Silver chloride is used with skin patch electrodes and many other types because the dc half-cell potential of the Ag|AgCl electrode depends on the logarithm of the concentration of chloride ions (Webster 1992). Because the AgCl is in direct contact with the coupling gel which has a high concentration of Cl^- ions, the dc half-cell potential of the electrode remains fairly stable, and has a low impedance, hence low thermal noise.

Figure 1.5 illustrates the electrical characteristics of a pair of Ag|AgCl electrodes facing each other. The impedance, $|2\,\mathbf{Z}_{el}(f)|$, measured as a function of frequency, suggests that each electrode can be modeled by a parallel R-C circuit in series with a resistance. Analysis of the impedance

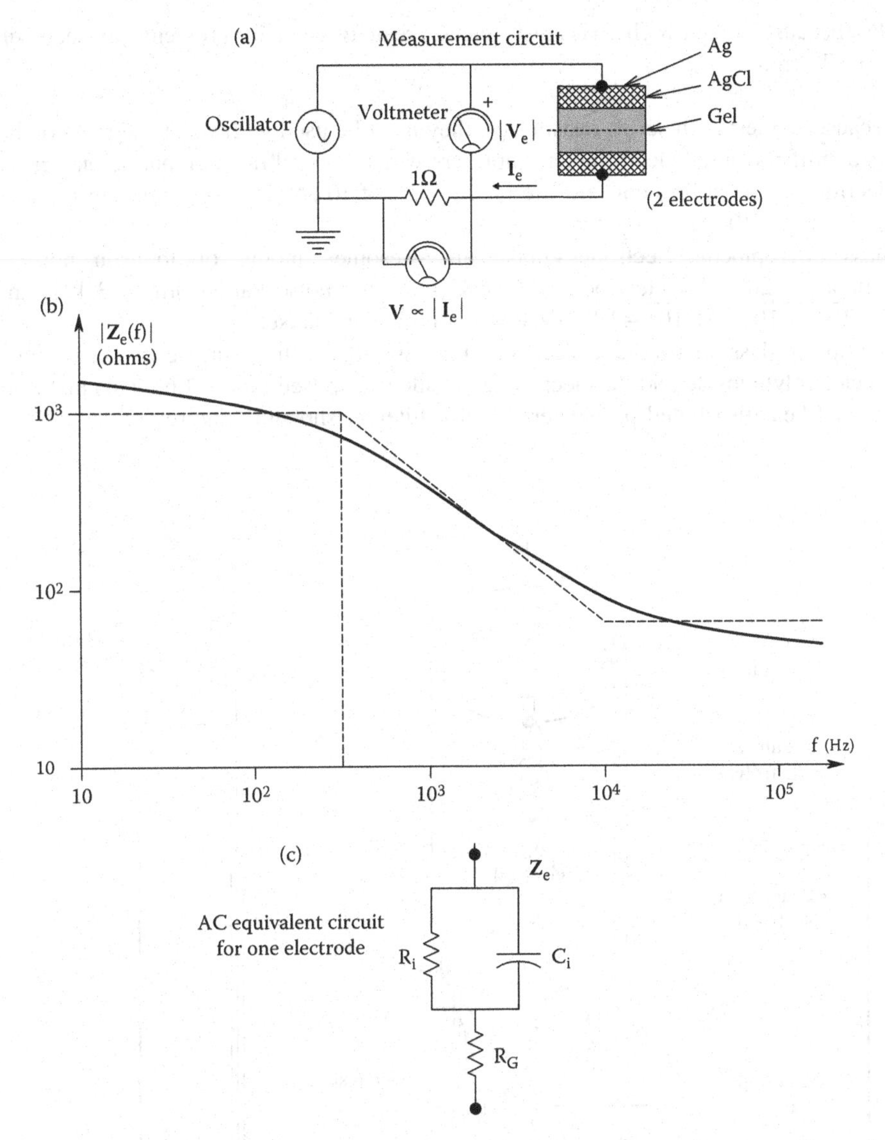

FIGURE 1.5 (a) Impedance magnitude measurement circuit for a pair of face-to-face, silver–silver chloride skin surface electrodes. (b) Typical impedance magnitude for the pair of electrodes in series. (c) Linear equivalent circuit for one electrode.

magnitude in this figure tells us that $R_G = 65\ \Omega$, $R_i = 1935\ \Omega$, and $C_i = 0.274\ \mu F$ for one electrode. The skin itself also adds a parallel R-C circuit to the electrode's equivalent circuit.

In general, it is desirable for the electrode $|\mathbf{Z}_{el}|$ to be as small as possible. Both resistors in the electrode model make thermal (white) noise. At low frequencies where the capacitive reactance is >>1935 Ω, one electrode's root noise spectrum is $\sqrt{4kT\ 2000} = 5.76\ \text{nVrms}/\sqrt{\text{Hz}}$, the same order of magnitude as an amplifier's equivalent short-circuit input noise voltage. If the gel dries out during prolonged use, the $|\mathbf{Z}_{el}|$ will rise, as will the thermal white noise from its larger real part.

Another type of electrode used in neurophysiological research is the saline-filled, glass micropipette electrode used for recording transmembrane potentials in neurons and muscle fibers. Because the tips of these electrodes are drawn down to diameters of a fraction of a micrometer before filling, their resistances when filled can range from ca. 20 MΩ to 10^3 MΩ, depending on the tip geometry, the filling medium, and the surround medium in which the tip is placed. Glass micropipette electrodes, because of their high series resistances, create three major problems not seen with other types of bioelectrodes:

1. Because of their high series resistances, they must be used with special signal conditioning amplifiers called electrometer amplifiers which have ultralow, input dc bias currents. Electrometer input bias currents are in the order of 10 fA (10^{-14} A), and their input resistances are ca. 10^{15} Ω.
2. Glass micropipette electrodes make an awesome amount of Johnson noise. For example, a 200 MΩ electrode at 300°K, having a noise bandwidth of 3 kHz makes $\sqrt{4kT \times 2 \times 10^8 \times 3 \times 10^3} \cong 100$ μV RMS of broadband noise.
3. The tips of glass micropipette electrodes have significant distributed capacitance between the electrolyte inside and the electrolyte outside the tip (see Figure 1.6). This makes them behave like a distributed-parameter low-pass filter, as shown in Figure 1.7a.

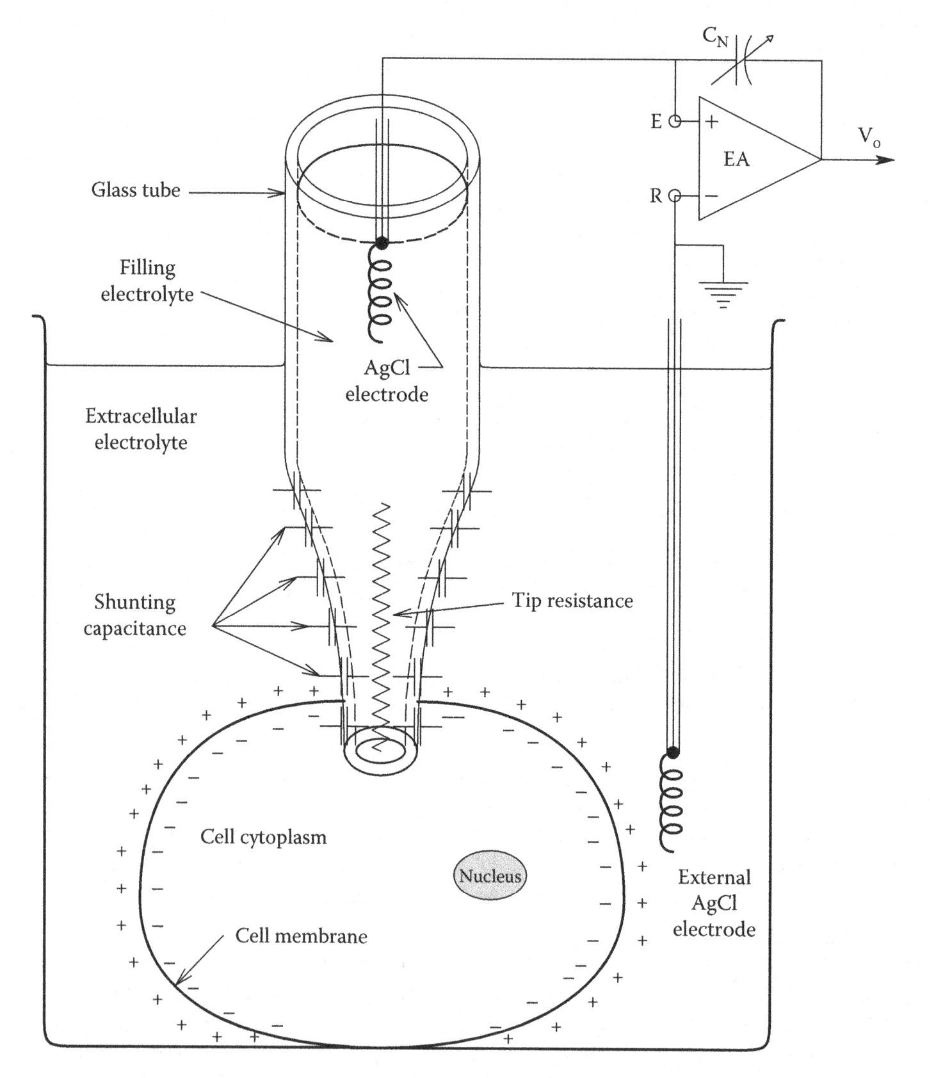

FIGURE 1.6 Schematic cross section (not to scale) of an electrolyte-filled, glass micropipette electrode inserted into the cytoplasm of a cell. Ag|AgCl electrodes are used to interface recording wires (generally Cu) with the electrolytes.

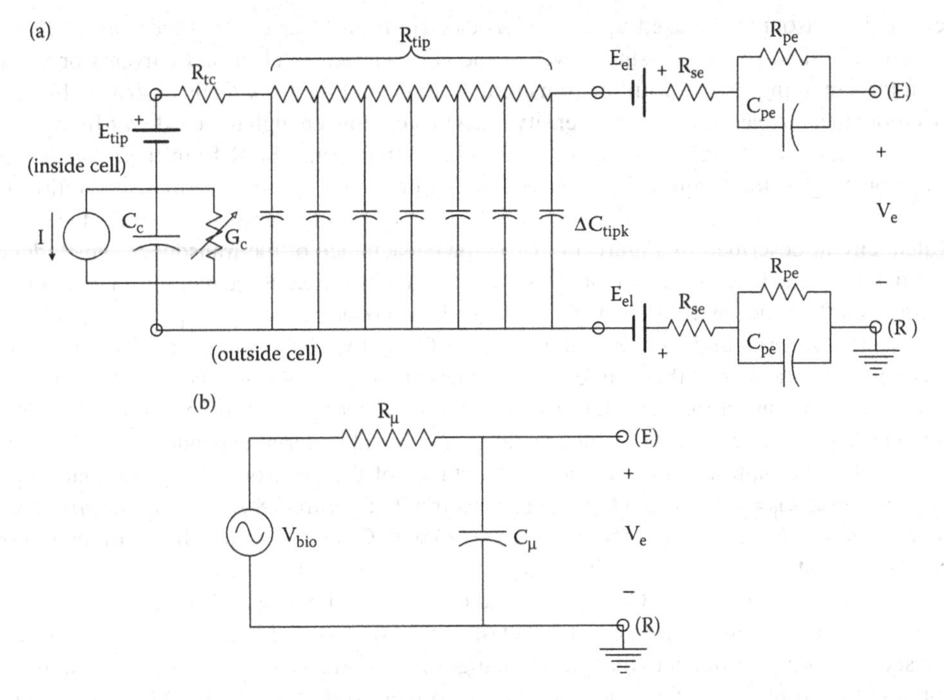

FIGURE 1.7 (a) Equivalent circuit of an intracellular glass microelectrode in a cell, including the equivalent circuits of the Ag|AgCl electrodes. Note the dc half-cell potentials of the electrodes and at the microelectrode's tip. The tip of the microelectrode is modeled by a lumped-parameter, nonuniform, R-C transmission line. (b) For practical purposes, the ac equivalent circuit of the glass micropipette electrode is generally reduced to a simple R-C low-pass filter.

Figure 1.7a also illustrates the equivalent circuits of the Ag|AgCl coupling electrodes, the cell membrane, and the microelectrode tip spreading resistance and tip EMF. The distributed resistance of the internal electrolyte in the tip, R_{tip}, plus the tip spreading resistance, R_{tc}, plus the cell membrane's resistance, $1/G_c$, are orders of magnitude larger than the impedances associated with the AgCl coupling electrodes. Thus, they can lumped together as a single R_μ, and the distributed tip capacitance can be represented by a single, lumped, C_μ in the simplified, R-C LPF of Figure 1.7b. V_{bio} is the bioelectric EMF across the cell membrane in the vicinity of the microelectrode tip. The break frequency of the B circuit is simply $f_b = 1/(2\pi R_\mu C_\mu)$ Hz. Typical values of circuit parameters are $R_\mu \cong 2 \times 10^8\ \Omega$, $C_\mu \cong 1 \times 10^{-12}$ F. Thus, $f_b \cong 796$ Hz. This is too low a break frequency to faithfully reproduce a nerve action potential, which requires a dc to 3 kHz bandwidth. To obtain the desired bandwidth, *capacitance neutralization* is used (capacitance neutralization is described in Section 4.5.2 of this text). As shown in Section 9.8.4, capacitance neutralization itself adds excess noise to the amplifier output.

1.8 EXOGENOUS BIOELECTRIC SIGNALS

We have seen from the above sections that *endogenous bioelectric signals* are invariably small, ranging from a single microvolt to over one-hundred millivolts. Their bandwidths range from dc to perhaps 10 kHz at the most. Signals such as ECG and EEG require ca. 0.1 to ca. 100 Hz. Exogenous signals, on the other hand, can involve modalities such as ultrasound which can use frequencies from hundreds of kilohertz to 10s of MHz, depending on the application. Ultrasound can be *continuous-wave* (CW) sinusoidal, sinusoidal pulses, or wavelets. It is not our purpose here to discuss the details of how ultrasound is generated, received, or processed but rather to comment on the frequencies and signal levels of the received ultrasound.

Reflected ultrasound is picked up by a piezoelectric transducer or transducer array that converts the mechanical sound pressure waves at the skin surface to electrical currents or voltages. Concern for damaging tissues with the transmitted ultrasound intensity (cells destroyed by heating or cavitation) means that input sound intensity must be kept low enough to be safe for living tissues, organs, fetuses, etc., yet high enough to give a good output signal SNR from the reflected sound energy impinging on the receiving transducer. Many ultrasound transducers are used at ultrasound frequencies below their mechanical resonance. In this region of operation, the transducer has an equivalent circuit described by Figure 1.8. C_x is the capacitance of the transducer, which depends on the thickness, the dielectric constant of its material, and the area of the metal film electrodes; C_x is generally on the order of 100s of pF. G_x is the leakage conductance of the piezomaterial. It, too, depends on the material and its dimensions. Expect G_x on the order of 10^{-13} S. The coaxial cable connecting the transducer to the charge amplifier has some shunt capacitance, C_c, which depends on cable length and insulating material. It will be on the order of ca. 30 pF/m. Similarly, the cable has some leakage conductance, G_c, which again is length and material dependent; G_c will be about 10^{-11} S. Finally, the input conductance and capacitance of the electrometer operational amplifier (op amp) are about $G_i = 10^{-14}$ S, and $C_i = 3$ pF. The circuit of Figure 1.8 is a *charge amplifier,* which effectively replaces $(C_x + C_c + C_i)$ and $(G_x + G_c + G_i)$ with C_F and G_F in parallel with the transducer's Norton current source. Thus, the low-frequency behavior of the system is not set by the poorly defined $(C_x + C_c + C_i)$ and $(G_x + G_c + G_i)$ but rather by the designer-specified components, G_F and C_F. (Analysis of the circuit is carried out in detail in Section 6.6 of this text.) Note that the Norton current source i_x is proportional to the rate-of-change of the ultrasound pressure waves impingent on the bottom of the transducer. The constant d has the dimensions of Coulombs/Newton. The charge

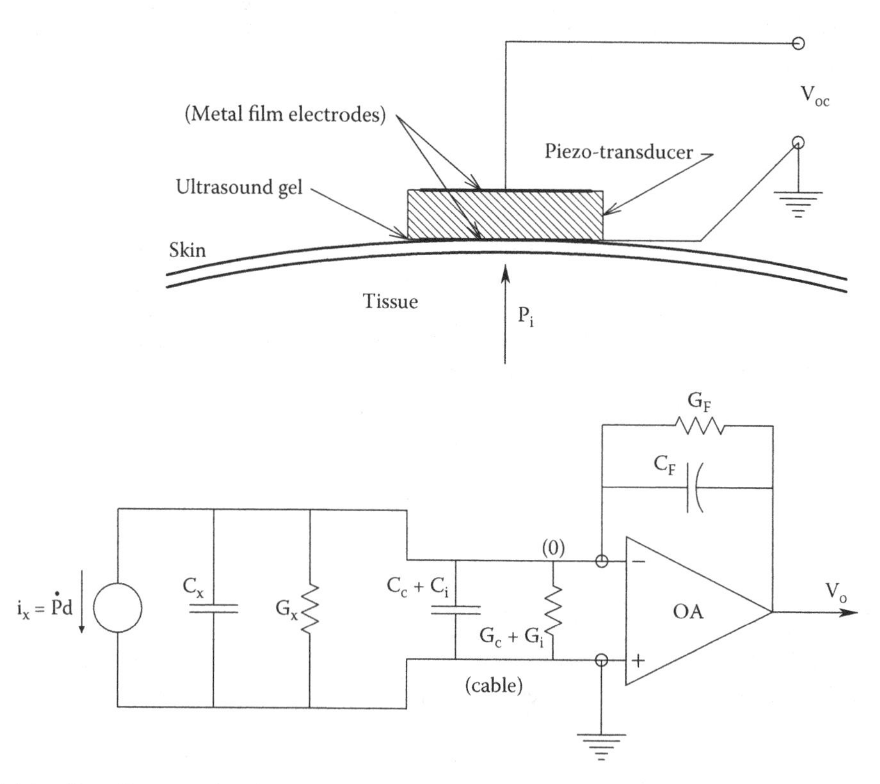

FIGURE 1.8 *Top:* Cross-sectional schematic of a piezoelectric transducer on the skin surface. The gel is used for acoustic impedance matching to improve acoustic signal capture efficiency. P_i is the sound pressure of the signal being sensed. *Bottom:* Equivalent circuit of the piezosensor and a charge amplifier. See text for analysis.

displaced inside the transducer is given by $q = d F$. The Norton current is simply, $i_x \equiv q = Fd = PAd$. When the op amp is assumed to be ideal, then the summing junction is at 0 V, and by Ohm's law, the op amp's output voltage is

$$V_o = \frac{d\,A\,s\,P(s)}{s\,C_F + G_F} \tag{1.2}$$

Written as a transfer function, this is

$$\frac{V_o}{P}(s) = \frac{d\,A\,s\,R_F}{s\,C_F R_F + 1} \tag{1.3}$$

At midfrequencies, the gain is

$$\frac{V_o}{P}(s) = \frac{dA}{C_F} \text{ Volt/Pascal} \tag{1.4}$$

The area A is in m^2. The pressure sensitivity parameter d varies considerably between piezomaterials and also depends on the direction of cut in natural crystals such as quartz, Rochelle salt, and ammonium dihydrogen phosphate. For example, d for X-cut quartz crystals is 2.25×10^{-12} Cb/N, d for barium titanate is ca. 160×10^{-12} Cb/N.

Now consider the midfrequency output of the charge amplifier when using a *lead–zirconate–titanate* (LZT) transducer having $d = 140 \times 10^{-12}$ Cb/N, given a sound pressure of 1 dyne/cm^2 = 0.1 Pa, $A = 1\text{ cm}^2 = 10^{-4}\text{ m}^2$, and $C_F = 100$ pF.

$$V_o = \frac{PAd}{C_F} = \frac{0.1 \times 10^{-4} \times 10^{-12}}{100 \times 10^{-12}} = 14\mu V \tag{1.5}$$

Thus, one sees that received voltage levels in piezoelectric ultrasonic sensors are very low. Considerable low-noise amplification is required, and bandpass filtering is necessary to improve SNR. Not included in the analysis above is the high-frequency response of the charge amplifier which is certainly important when conditioning low-level ultrasonic signals in the range of megahertz. (See Section 6.6.2 for high-frequency analysis of the charge amplifier.)

1.9 CHAPTER SUMMARY

In this chapter, attention has been drawn to the fact that endogenous biomedical signals, whether they be electrical such as the ECG or EEG, or physical quantities such as blood pressure or temperature, vary relatively slowly; their signal bandwidths are generally from dc to several hundred hertz and, in the case of nerve spikes or EMGs, may require up to 2–4 kHz at the high end. All bioelectric signals are noisy, that is, they are recorded in the company of broadband noise arising from nearby physiological sources and, in many cases (e.g., the EEG, ERG, EOG, and ECoG), are in the microvolt range where they must compete with amplifier noise. In the case of the skin-surface EMG, the recorded signals are the spatiotemporal summation of many thousand individual sources underlying the electrodes, i.e., many muscle fibers asynchronously generating action potentials as they contract to do mechanical work. In the case of the scalp-recorded EEG, many millions of cortical neurons signal by either spiking or by slow depolarization as the brain works, generating a spatiotemporally summed potential between pairs of scalp electrodes. On the other hand, the electrical activity from the heart is spatially localized, and the synchronous spread of depolarization of cardiac muscle during the cardiac cycle generates a relatively strong signal on the skin surface, in spite of the large volume conductor volume through which the ECG electric field must spread. Figure 1.9 illustrates the

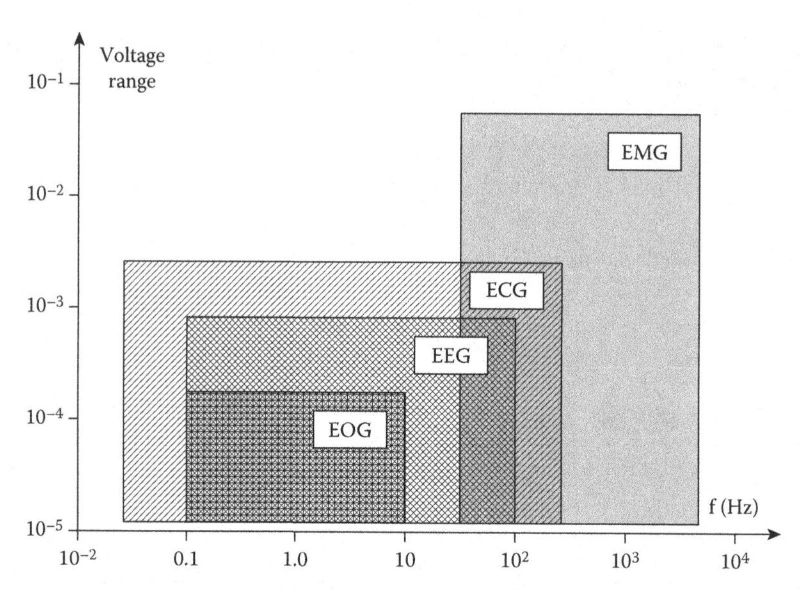

FIGURE 1.9 Approximate RMS spectra of four classes of bioelectric signals. Peak expected RMS signal is plotted versus extreme range of frequencies characterizing the signal.

approximate extreme ranges of peak signal amplitudes and the approximate range of frequencies that is required to condition EOG, EEG, ECG, and EMG signals. Note that the waveforms that contain spikes or sharp peak transients (ECG and EMG) require a higher bandwidth to characterize.

Exogenous biomedical instrumentation signals such as diagnostic and Doppler ultrasound and signals from MRI systems were shown to require bandwidths into the 10s of MHz, and higher. Amplifiers required for conditioning such exogenous signals must have high gain-bandwidth products (f_T), and high slew rates (η), as well as low noise.

2 Properties and Models of Semiconductor Devices Used in Analog Electronic Systems

2.1 INTRODUCTION

The properties and characteristics of the semiconductor components used in *analog integrated circuits* (AICs) and discrete circuits are described in this chapter. These include the various types of *diodes, bipolar junction transistors* (BJTs), and various kinds of *field-effect transistors* (FETs). As a biomedical engineer, you probably will never be called upon to design circuits with or use discrete transistors, with the possible exception of power transistors. Instead, modern analog electronic systems use integrated circuits. To appreciate the behavior and limitations of ICs, it is necessary to understand the fundamental behavior of its (internal) semiconductor components. (The actual design of ICs is beyond the scope of this text.) One of the most ubiquitous and useful analog ICs you will encounter is the *operational amplifier* (op amp); op amps are used in many signal conditioning applications, including *differential amplifiers, instrumentation amplifiers, active filters, true RMS converters, precision rectifiers, track-and-hold circuits,* etc. Other commonly encountered ICs in biomedical engineering are *DC voltage regulators, DC-to-DC converters, temperature sensors, phase-lock loops* (PLLs), *synchronous rectifiers (demodulators), analog multipliers, medical isolation amplifiers, analog-to-digital converters* (ADCs), *digital-to-analog converters* (DACs), *power amplifiers,* etc.

Specifically, in the following sections, the salient circuit characteristics of *pn* junction diodes, light-emitting diodes (LEDs), laser diodes (LADs), *npn* and *pnp* small-signal BJTs, junction field-effect transistors (JFETs), *n*- and *p*-MOSFETs will be examined. Both large-signal and mid- and high-frequency small-signal models will be considered. The mid- and high-frequency behavior of IC "building blocks," which use two transistors, will also be analyzed.

2.2 *PN* JUNCTION DIODES

2.2.1 INTRODUCTION

There are several uses for *pn* junction diodes as discrete components and in ICs. As standalone components, *power diodes* are used to rectify AC to produce DC in power supplies. They are also used with inductive components such as relay coils, motor coils, deflection coils, and loudspeaker windings to clamp high-voltage, inductive voltage switching transients (Ldi/dt) to prevent them from destroying the switching transistors. Small, discrete, *pn* diodes are also used in op amp *precision rectifier circuits, peak detectors, synchronous demodulators, sample-and-hold circuits,* and *logarithmic* and *exponential amplifiers.* Diodes are used in IC designs for *temperature compensation,* to make *current mirrors,* and for *DC-level shifting* (in the avalanche mode) (Millman 1979).

2.2.2 *PN* DIODE'S VOLT–AMPERE CURVE

Figure 2.1c illustrates the static volt–ampere curve of a typical, silicon, *pn signal diode* (as opposed to power rectifier diode). Note that there are three major regions in the curve: the *forward conduction region* in the first quadrant, the *blocking region* in the third quadrant, and the *avalanche breakdown (or zener) region*, also in the third quadrant. The volt–ampere behavior of a diode's forward and blocking regions can be approximated with the well-known, approximate, mathematical model:

$$i_D = I_{rs}\,[\exp(v_D/\eta V_T) - 1] \tag{2.1}$$

where v_D is the DC voltage across the diode, $V_T \equiv kT/q$, where T is the Kelvin temperature of the junction, q is the electron charge magnitude (1.6×10^{-19} Cb), k is *Boltzmann's constant* (1.38×10^{-23} J/K), and η is a "bugger factor" between 1 and 2 used to fit the diode curve to experimental data ($\eta \cong 2$ for silicon diodes). I_{rs} is the *reverse saturation current* (on the order of μA for signal diodes). I_{rs} is a strong, increasing function of temperature, and is non-negative. At 25°C, $V_T = 0.0257$ V.

The crudeness of the model can be appreciated in the blocking region where the exponential argument is large and negative, so $i_D \cong -I_{rs}$. In reality, there is a strong ohmic (leakage) component to the reverse i_D, so the approximation, $i_D \cong -I_{rs} + v_D/\rho_r$, is more realistic for $v_D < 0$. ρ_r has the dimensions of resistance (ohms).

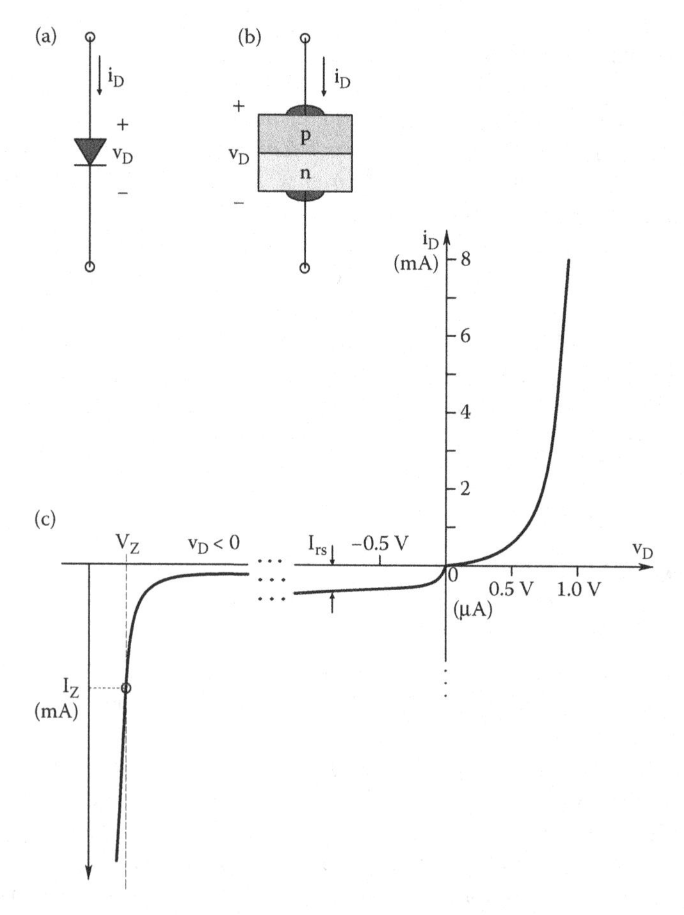

FIGURE 2.1 (a) *pn* junction diode symbol. (b) "Layer cake" model cross-section of a silicon *pn* junction diode. (c) Typical I-V curve for a small-signal, Si diode, showing avalanche (zener) breakdown at reverse bias $v_D = -V_Z$.

Avalanche occurs under reverse-biased conditions when minority carriers conducting the reverse i_D gain enough kinetic energy by accelerating in the strong electric field, and then collide with the substrate atoms' electrons, creating new electron/hole pairs. These new carriers, in turn, are accelerated in the high **E**-field and cause still more carriers to be formed. This avalanche process can be modeled by the empirical equation

$$i_D \cong \frac{-I_{rs}}{1-|(v_D/V_Z)^n|} \tag{2.2}$$

where the exponent n can range from 3 to 6, and v_D lies between 0 and V_Z. Depending on how the *pn* junction is doped (the density of donor atoms in the n material and acceptor atoms in the p-stuff), V_z can range from ca. 3.2 V to over 100 V.

Diodes operated in their avalanche regions can be used as *voltage sources or references,* and for DC voltage level shifting. Figure 2.2 illustrates an avalanche DC voltage source circuit. The tantalum filter capacitor is used to lower the source impedance of the avalanche supply at high frequencies. From Ohm's law we have,

$$I_L = V_Z/R_L \tag{2.3}$$

$$I_S = I_L + I_Z \tag{2.4}$$

$$R_S = (V_S - V_Z)/I_S = \frac{(V_S - V_Z)}{I_Z + V_Z/R_L} \tag{2.5}$$

Every avalanche (*aka zener*) diode has a preferred operating point (V_Z, I_Z) given by the manufacturer where its dynamic impedance is low and its power dissipation is safe. Thus, in Equation 2.5, V_Z and I_Z are known, and R_L is known (or I_L at V_Z), enabling one to find the required series R_S. The required power dissipated in R_S is simply $P_{Rs} = (V_S - V_Z)^2/R_S = I_S^2 R_S$ watts.

Excluding the avalanche region, for simplicity, one can often model the DC characteristics of a *pn* junction diode by an *ideal diode* (ID) model, shown in Figure 2.3a. For the ID, $i_D = 0$ for $v_D < 0$, and $v_D = 0$ for $i_D > 0$. In Figure 2.3b, by adding a reverse-biasing voltage source, V_F, the model diode volt–ampere curve is shifted to the right by V_F. The model is made yet more realistic by adding the series resistance, R_F, in the conduction path, as shown in Figure 2.3c. In Figure 2.3d, a leakage conductance is added in parallel with the model of C in order to model reverse diode leakage.

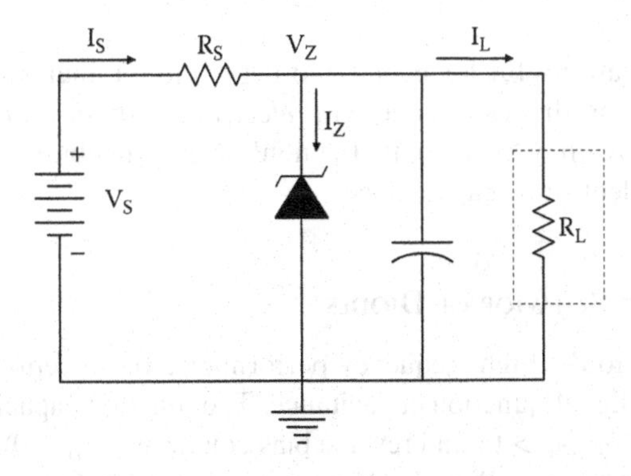

FIGURE 2.2 Use of an avalanche (zener) diode as a DC voltage source for R_L. The diode's zener resistance is neglected.

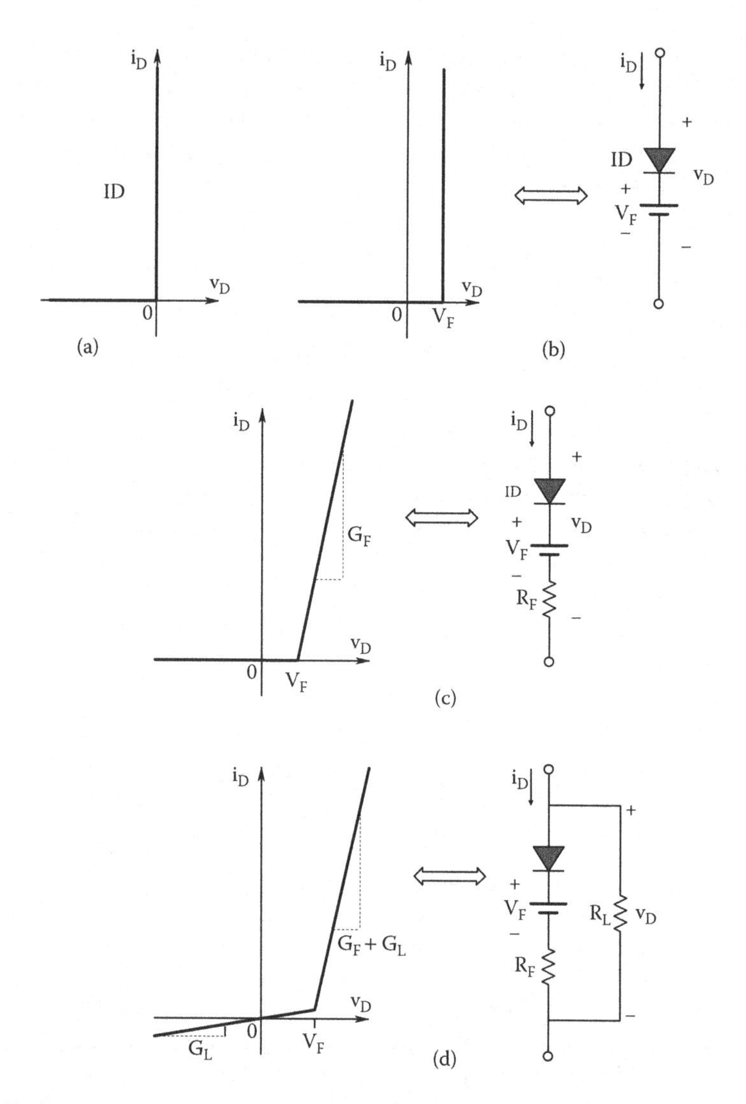

FIGURE 2.3 Various I-V models for junction diodes, excluding avalanche behavior. (a) The ideal diode. (b) Ideal diode in series with fixed forward voltage drop. (c) Ideal diode in series with fixed forward voltage drop and forward resistance. (d) Ideal diode in series with fixed forward voltage drop and forward resistance, and reverse leakage conductance, G_L.

The ID and its variations are useful for pencil-and-paper circuit analysis. Detailed simulation of electronic circuits containing diodes is done with *electronic circuit analysis programs* (ECAPs) such as PSPICE and *MicroCap,* which handle the nonlinearity algebraically, as well as computing the diode's voltage-dependent shunt capacitance.

2.2.3 High-Frequency Behavior of Diodes

A fundamental limitation to the high-frequency performance of *pn* semiconductor diodes is their voltage-dependent, small-signal, junction capacitance. The junction capacitance mechanism is different for forward conduction ($v_D > 0$) and reverse bias conditions ($v_D < 0$).

It was noted earlier that when a diode is DC reverse-biased, a very small (nA) *reverse leakage current* flows, part of which is due to the thermal (random) generation of hole/electron pairs in the *depletion region* of the device. The depletion region is a volume around the junction in both the *p*- and *n*-doped semiconductor sides that is free of mobile carriers (holes and electrons, respectively). The electric field from the negative v_D causes the carriers to move away from the junction, creating what is essentially a layer of charge-free, intrinsic semiconductor around the junction. The more negative the v_D is, the stronger the electric field and the larger the depletion region. The charge-free depletion region behaves like a leaky dielectric in a parallel-plate capacitor. The capacitor's "plates" are the dense, conductive, semicon region where majority carriers still exist and conductivity is high. Recall that the capacitance of a simple parallel-plate capacitor is given by

$$C = \frac{A\kappa\,\varepsilon_o}{d} \text{ Farads} \quad (2.6)$$

where κ is the dielectric constant of silicon, A is the area of the diode junction in m^2, and d is the effective "plate" separation in m.

Note that the effective plate separation d *increases* as v_D goes more negative and the electric field increases at the junction. Thus, C_d *decreases* as v_D goes more negative and is maximum at $v_D = 0$. Diode depletion capacitance can be modeled by the function

$$C_d(v_D) = \frac{C_d(0)}{(1 - v_D/\psi_o)^n} \text{ Farads, for } v_D < 0 \quad (2.7)$$

where $C_d(0)$ is the value of the depletion capacitance at $v_D = 0$, ψ_o is the contact potential of the *pn* junction determined by the carrier doping densities at the junction, and their gradients. ψ_o ranges from 0.2 to 0.9 V and is in the neighborhood of 0.75 V at room temperature for a typical silicon small-signal diode. The exponent **n** ranges from 0.33 to 3, depending on the doping profile near the *pn* junction; $\mathbf{n} = 0.5$ for an abrupt (symmetrical step) junction. For depletion, $v_D < 0$ in Equation 2.7. Note that as v_D goes positive and approaches ψ_o, C_d approaches ∞.

Clearly, Equation 2.7 is intended to model diode capacitance for $-V_Z < v_D < 0$. Typical values for $C_d(0)$ are in the range of 10s of pF. A typical reverse-biased, *pn* diode's junction capacitance vs. v_D is shown in Figure 2.4. Diodes that are intended to operate in the reverse-biased mode as

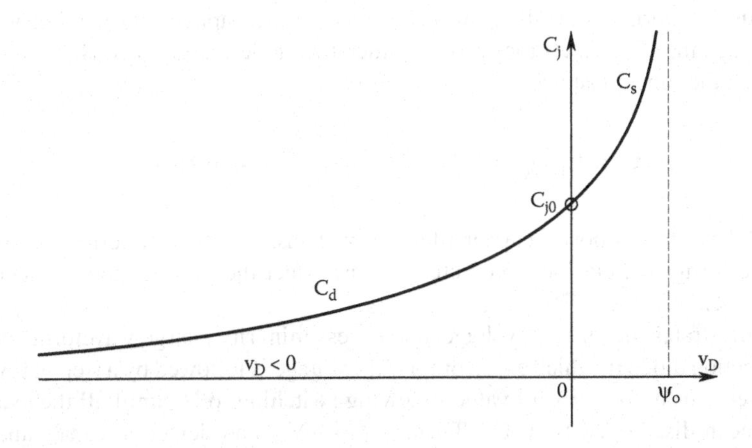

FIGURE 2.4 How the equivalent junction capacitance of a *pn* diode varies with v_D. C_d is mostly depletion capacitance (see Text), and C_s is due to stored minority carriers associated with forward conduction. C_{j0} is on the order of 10 pf.

voltage-variable capacitors are called varactor diodes. A detailed analysis of *pn* junction behavior can be found in the venerable texts by Millman (1979), Yang (1988), or Gray and Meyer (1984).

A forward-biased diode's *pn* junction is characterized by a large, current-dependent, *diffusion* or *charge storage capacitance,* which involves an entirely different mechanism from depletion capacitance. Under *forward bias conditions,* minority carriers are injected across the junction, where they quickly recombine. That is, electrons are injected into the *p*-side from the *n*-side, and holes are injected into the *n*-side from the *p*-side. The mean lifetime of electrons in the *p*-side is τ_n and of holes in the *n*-side, τ_p. These injected minority carriers represent a stored charge, Q_s, around the junction. By definition, the *small-signal diffusion capacitance* can be written for a symmetrical junction where $\tau = \tau_p = \tau_n$:

$$C_D = \frac{dQ_s}{dv_D} = \frac{\tau d\, i_D}{d\, v_D} = \tau g_d = \frac{\tau\, i_{DQ}}{\eta\, V_T} = \frac{\tau\, I_{rs} \exp(v_{DQ}/V_T)}{\eta V_T} \text{ Farads for } v_D > 0 \tag{2.8}$$

where g_d is the small-signal conductance of the forward-biased diode at its *DC operating* (Q) *point*; $g_d \equiv \partial i_D/\partial v_D$ at Q; i.e., $g_d = d[I_{rs} \exp(v_D/\eta V_T)]/dv_D|_Q = I_{rs} \exp(v_{DQ}/\eta V_T)/(\eta V_T) = i_{DQ}/\eta V_T$ Siemens.

If the diode junction doping is asymmetrical, it can be shown (Nanavati 1975) that the diffusion capacitance is given by

$$C_D = \frac{1}{\eta V_T}(I_{DnQ}\tau_n + I_{DpQ}\tau_p) \text{ Farads} \tag{2.9}$$

In Equation 2.9, the diode forward current is broken into the electron and hole injection currents.

For example, calculate the diffusion capacitance of a silicon diode with a symmetrically doped step junction at 300°K, forward-biased with $i_{DQ} = 10$ mA. Let $\tau = 1$ μs, $\eta = 2$,

$$C_D = \frac{1\text{ E-}6 \times 1\text{ E-}2}{2 \times 0.026} = 0.192\ \mu\text{F} \tag{2.10}$$

This is a relatively enormous small-signal capacitance which appears in parallel with the diode model. The capacitance C_D affects the speed at which the diode can turn off. However, the forward-biased diode has the time constant

$$\tau_d = C_D/g_d = 1.92\text{ E-}7/(1\text{ E-}2/(2 \times 0.026)) \cong 1\ \mu\text{s} \tag{2.11}$$

τ_d is basically the mean minority carrier lifetime, τ. Thus, C_D has little effect on midfrequency, small-signal performance, but the stored charge does affect the time to stop conducting when v_D goes step negative.

Figure 2.5 illustrates the current, voltage, and excess minority charge waveforms in the *n*-material for a *pn* junction diode in which a step of forward voltage is followed by a step of reverse voltage. Note that V_D remains at the forward value following switching to V_R until all the excess minority carriers have been discharged from C_D. Then, $V_D \rightarrow -V_R$, and depletion capacitance dominates the junction behavior. The storage time is on the order of nanoseconds for most small-signal, Si, *pn* diodes.

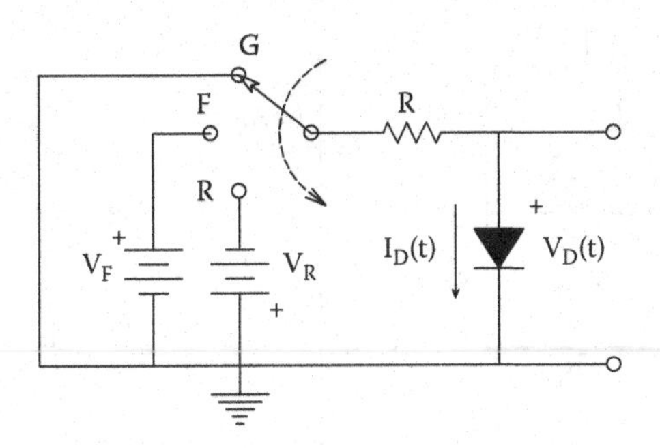

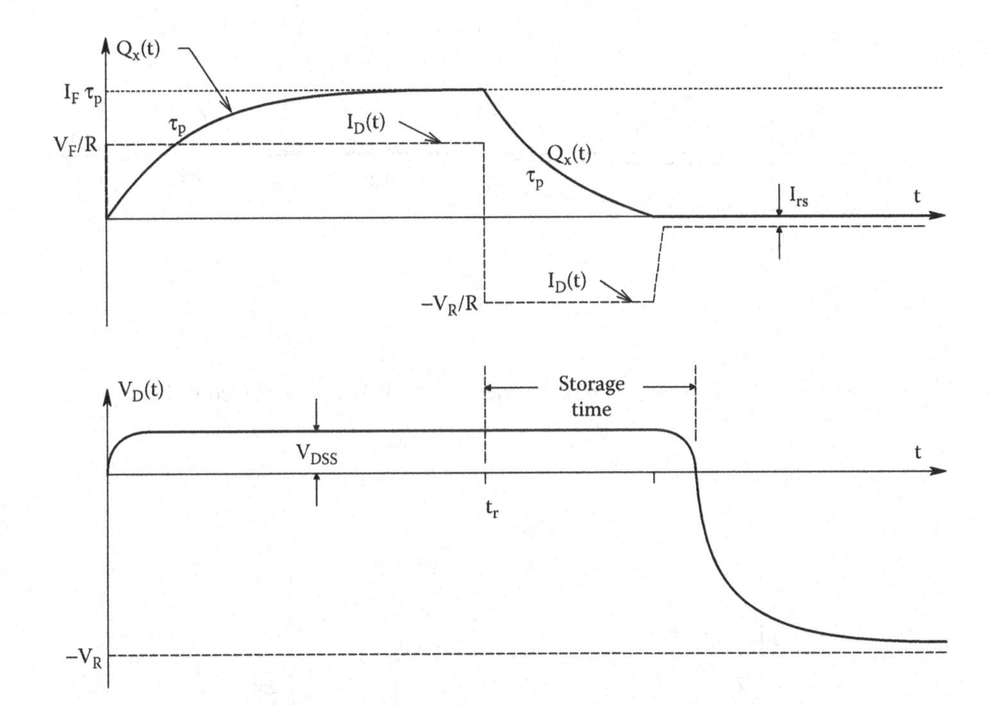

FIGURE 2.5 Schematic showing the effect of switching a diode from $v_D = 0$, $i_D = 0$, to forward conduction. With V_F applied, v_D quickly rises to the steady-state forward drop, $v_{DSS} \cong 0.7$ V, and the XS minority carriers build up to a charge, Q_x. When the applied voltage is switched to $-V_R$, a finite time is required for Q_x to be dissipated before the diode can block current. During this *storage time,* v_D remains at v_{DSS}.

2.2.4 Schottky Diodes

The *Schottky barrier diode* (SBD), also called a "hot carrier diode," consists of a rectifying, *metal–insulator–semiconductor* (MIS) junction. SBDs actually predate *pn* junction diodes by about 50 years. The first AM detectors in early crystal set radios were "cat's whisker" diodes, where a fine lead (Pb) wire made contact with a metallic mineral crystal, such as galena, silicon, or germanium. Such cat's whisker detectors were in fact, primitive SBDs. Because their rectifier characteristics were not reproducible, cat's whisker SBDs were only suited for early radio experimenters, and were replaced by *pn* junction diodes in the 1950s. What makes a modern SBD different from an ordinary, ohmic, metal–semiconductor connection is the presence of a very thin insulating, interfacial oxide layer from 0.5 to 1.5 nm thick between the metal and the semiconductor. Figure 2.6 shows the static I-V characteristics of a *pn* diode and an SBD. Note that the SBD has a lower cut-in voltage (ca. 0.3 V) than the *pn* diode (ca. 0.55 V)

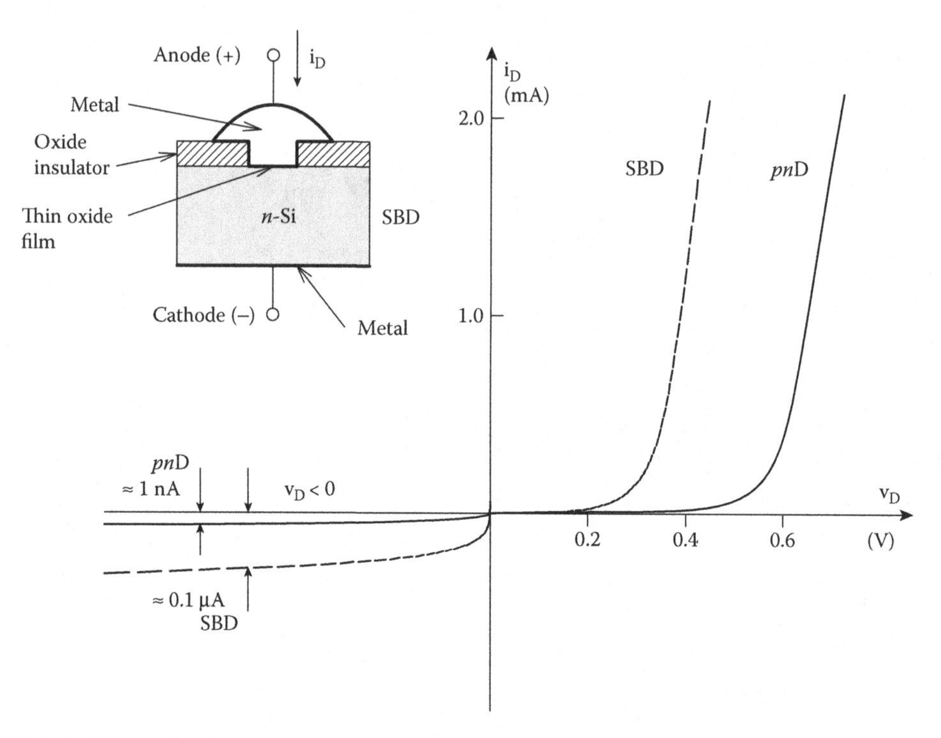

FIGURE 2.6 The static I-V curves of a Schottky barrier diode (SBD) and a *pn* junction diode.

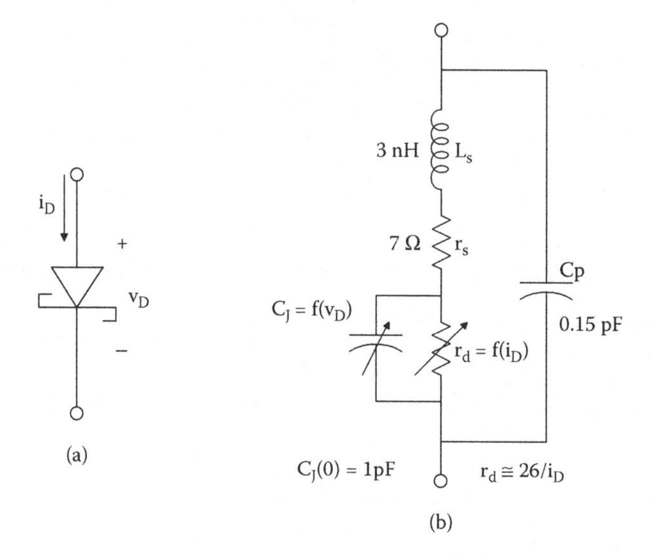

FIGURE 2.7 (a) Symbol for SDB (do not confuse it with that for the zener diode). (b) High-frequency equivalent circuit for an SBD.

and also has about 1000 times the reverse leakage current (0.1 μA vs. 1 nA) which does not saturate. A schematic cross-section of an SBD (after Boylstead and Nashelsky 1987) is shown in the figure.

The SBD is a majority carrier device; a *pn* diode is a minority carrier device. In order for a *pn* diode to block reverse current, the stored minority carriers must be swept out of the junction by the reverse electric field. This discharging limits the turn-off time to microseconds. On the other hand, the SBD has no minority carrier storage and can switch off in 10s of ns, meaning the SBD can rectify currents in the 100s of MHz. Figure 2.7 shows a high-frequency SSM for

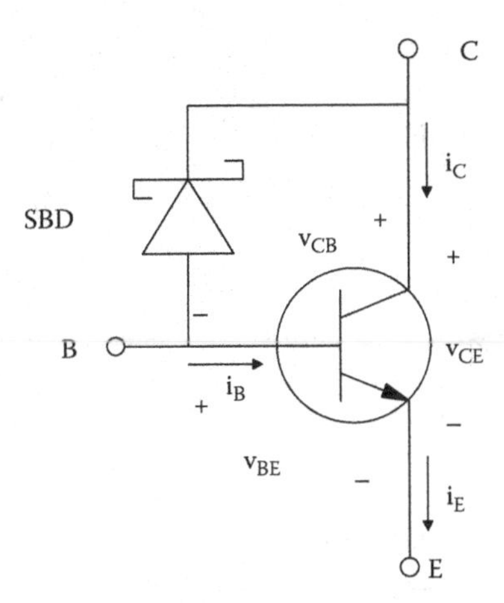

FIGURE 2.8 Use of an SBD to make a *Schottky transistor.* The SBD prevents excess stored charge in the BJT's C-B junction.

the SBD when conducting. Note that both the SS forward resistance, r_d, and the junction capacitance, C_J, are dependent on i_D and v_D, respectively. Hewlett–Packard hot carrier diodes of the 5082-2300 series have reverse currents of ca. 50–100 nA @ $v_D = -10$ V, and $C_J = 0.3$ pF @ $v_D = -10$ V.

Besides high-frequency rectification and detection, SBDs can be used to speed up transistor switching in logic gates. Figure 2.8 illustrates an SBD placed in parallel with the *pn* base-to-collector diode in an NPN BJT. In normal linear operation, the C-B junction is reverse-biased. When the transistor is *saturated*, both the B-E and the C-B junctions are forward-biased. Without the SBD, there is large minority charge storage in the C-B junction. With the SBD, much of the excess base current will flow through the SBD, preventing large excess charge storage in the C-B junction, allowing the BJT to turn-off much more quickly (Yang 1988). SBD thin film technology is also used in the fabrication of certain MOS transistors (Nanavati 1975).

2.3 MIDFREQUENCY MODELS FOR BJT BEHAVIOR

2.3.1 Introduction

Most BJTs found on ICs are silicon *pnp* or *npn*. (Other fabrication materials exist such as gallium arsenide and will not be treated here.) A heuristic view of BJTs is shown by the "layer cake" models shown in Figure 2.9b. BJTs are generally viewed as current-controlled current sources in their "linear" operating regions. As in the case of *pn* diodes, the large-signal, DC behavior of these three terminal devices will first be examined. Figure 2.9c illustrates typical volt–ampere curves for a small-signal (as opposed to power), *npn* BJT.

For purposes of DC biasing and crude circuit calculations on paper, one can represent an *npn* BJT in its *active region* by the simple circuit shown in Figure 2.10a. The voltage drop of the forward-biased B-E junction is represented by V_{BEQ}, on the order of 0.6 V. The DC collector current is approximated by the *current-controlled current source* (CCCS) with gain β_o. β_o is the transistor's nominal (forward) DC current gain. In Figure 2.10b, the DC model for the saturated transistor is illustrated. Saturation occurs for $i_B > i_C/\beta_o$, i.e., for high base currents. In saturation, both the B-E *and* C-B junctions are forward-biased, producing a V_{CEsat} that can range from ca. 0.2 to 0.8 V for high collector currents. The collector–emitter saturation curve can be approximated by the simple Thevenin circuit as shown: $r_{csat} = \partial v_{CE}/\partial i_C$ at the operating point on the saturation curve and V_{CEsat} is used to make the model fit the published curves.

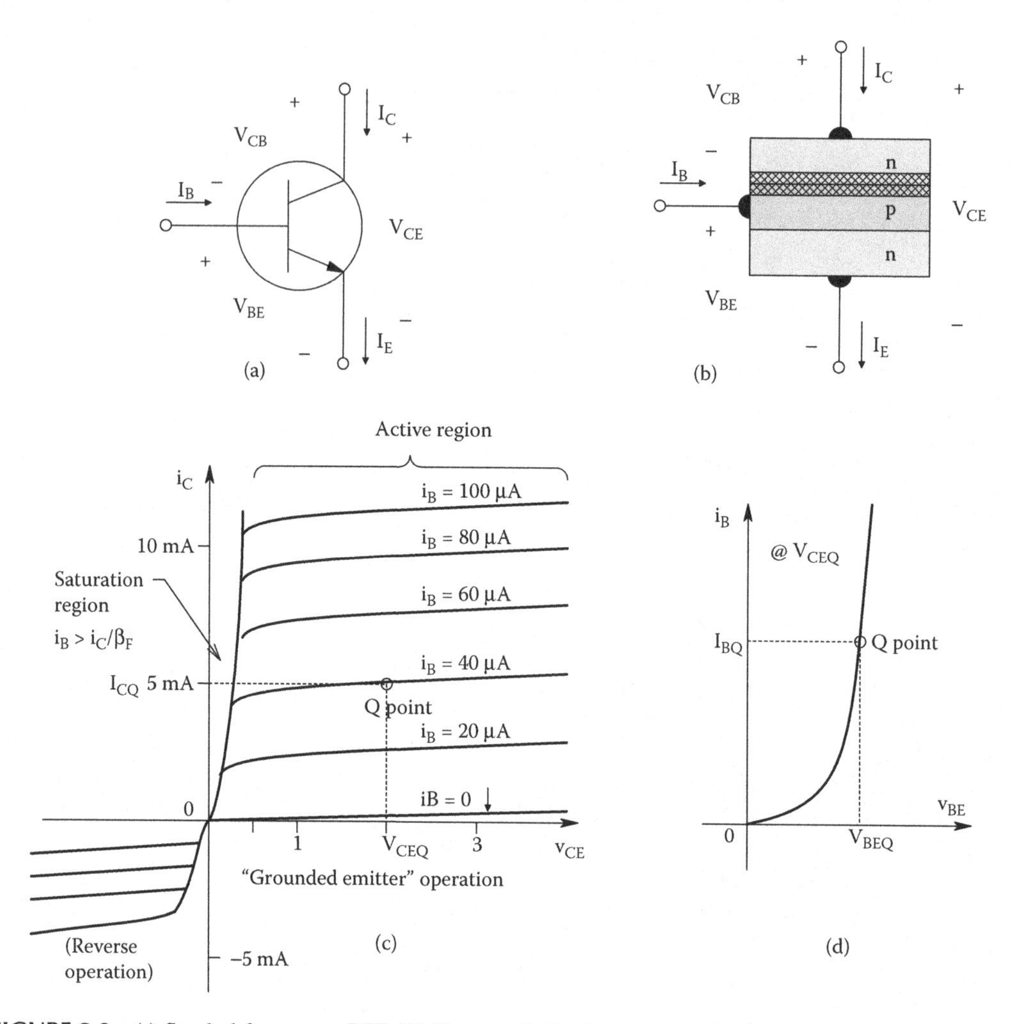

FIGURE 2.9 (a) Symbol for an *npn* BJT. (b) "Layer cake" cross-section of a forward-biased *npn* BJT. The cross-hatched layer represents the depletion region of the normally reverse-biased C-B junction. (c) Collector-base I-V curves as a function of i_B for the *npn* BJT. (d) Base-emitter I-V curve at constant V_{CEQ}. The B-E junction is normally forward biased.

When a *pnp* BJT's large-signal behavior is considered, the actual DC currents *leave* the base and collector nodes and *enter* the emitter node. Consequently, in the $i_C = f(v_{CE}, i_B)$ and $i_B = g(v_{BE}, v_{CE})$ curves shown in Figure 2.11, all currents and voltages are taken as *negative* (with respect to the directions and signs of the *npn* BJT). Figure 2.10c and d illustrate the DC biasing models for a *pnp* BJT. Note that the sign of the CCCS is not changed; a negative I_B times a positive β yields a negative I_C, as intended.

Figure 2.12 illustrates how the DC biasing model of Figure 2.10a is used to set an *npn* transistor's operating point in its active region. *As an example,* find the required base-biasing resistor, R_B, given the transistor's β_o, and the desired quiescent operating point (Q-point at I_{CQ}, V_{CEQ}) for the device; also find the necessary R_C and R_E, given V_{CC} and the requirement that $V_{CEQ} = V_{CC}/2$, and $V_E = 0.5$ V. Define the parameters: $V_{CC} \equiv 12$ V, at the Q-point $V_{CEQ} \equiv 6$ V, and the desired $I_{CQ} \equiv 1$ mA, $\beta_o \equiv 80$, and $V_{BEQ} \equiv 0.5$ V. It is known that $V_C = V_E + V_{CEQ} = 6.5$ V, thus the voltage across R_C is 5.5 V. From Ohm's law, $R_C = .5k/0.001 = 5.5$ kΩ. Further, $I_{BQ} = I_{CQ}/\beta_o = 0.001/80 = 12.5$ μA, $V_B = V_{BEQ} + V_E = 1$ V, so $R_B = (12 - 1)/12.5 = 880$ kΩ. Note that the emitter current is $I_E = (\beta + 1) I_B = I_C(1 + 1/\beta)$. So, $R_E = 0.5k/(1 + 1/80) = 494$ Ω.

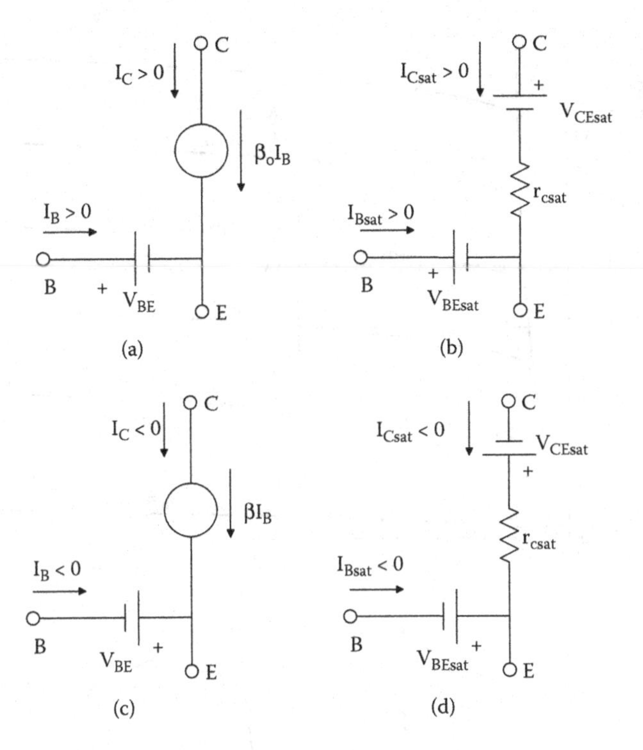

FIGURE 2.10 (a) Simple DC biasing model for an *npn* BJT in its forward linear operating region. See text for examples. (b) DC biasing model for an *npn* BJT in forward saturation. (c) and (d): Same as (a) and (b) for a *pnp* BJT.

2.3.2 Midfrequency Small-Signal Models for BJTs

To find the voltage amplification factor or gain of a simple *npn* BJT amplifier, a *two-port, midfrequency, small-signal model* (MFSSM) for the transistor is used. The MFSSM also allows one to calculate the amplifier's input and output resistances. The most common MFSSM for BJTs is called the *common-emitter (C-E) h-parameter model,* shown in Figure 2.13. The two-input *h*-parameters define a Thevenin input circuit between the base and emitter, and the output *h*-parameter pair defines a Norton equivalent circuit between the collector and emitter. The input resistance, h_{ie}, is derived operationally from the slope of the nonlinear $I_B = f(V_{BE}, V_{CE})$ curves at the Q-point, as shown in Figure 2.11. That is,

$$h_{ie} = \frac{\Delta\, v_{BE}}{\Delta\, i_B}\Big|_{Q,\, Vce\, =\, const.} \text{ Ohms} \tag{2.12}$$

h_{re} is the gain of a *voltage-controlled voltage source* (VCVS), which models how the base voltage is modulated by changes in v_{CE}. In other terms, h_{re} is the *open-circuit reverse transfer voltage gain:*

$$h_{re} = \frac{\Delta v_{BE}}{\Delta v_{CE}}\Big|_{Q,\, iB\, =\, const.} \tag{2.13}$$

For most pencil-and-paper transistor gain calculations using the C-E SMFSSM, h_{re} is set to zero because (a) it has a second-order contribution to calculations and (b) it simplifies calculations.

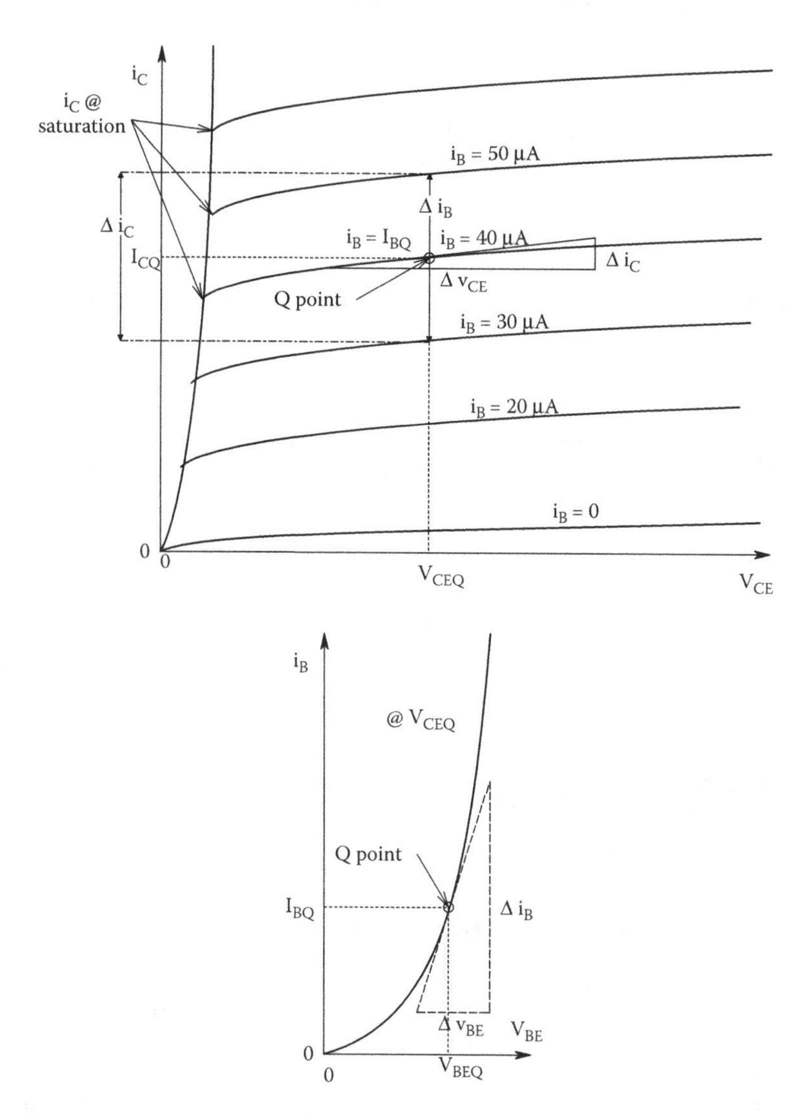

FIGURE 2.11 *Top:* A large-scale plot of a typical BJT's i_C vs. v_{CE} curves. The Q-point is the transistor's quiescent operating point. The small-signal conductance looking into the collector-emitter nodes is approximated by: $g_o = \Delta i_C/\Delta v_{CE}$ Siemens. The small-signal collector current gain is $\beta = \Delta i_C/\Delta i_B$. *Bottom:* The i_B vs. v_{BE} curve at the Q-point. The small-signal resistance looking into the BJT's base is $r_b = \Delta v_{BE}/\Delta i_B$ Ω.

In the collector-base Norton model, h_{oe} is the *output conductance* that results from the $i_C = f(v_{CE}, i_B)$ curves having a finite upward slope. From Figure 2.11, it is seen that h_{oe} is given by

$$h_{oe} = \left.\frac{\Delta\, i_C}{\Delta\, v_{CE}}\right|_{Q,\ iB\ =\ const.} \quad \text{Siemens} \tag{2.14}$$

Finally, the *forward, current-controlled current source gain*, h_{fe}, is found to be

$$h_{fe} = \left.\frac{\Delta\, i_C}{\Delta\, i_B}\right|_{Q,\ Vce\ =\ const.} \tag{2.15}$$

h_{fe} is also called the transistor's β.

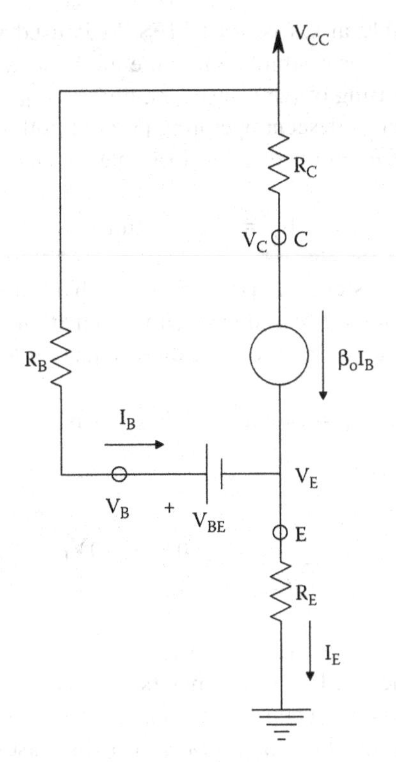

FIGURE 2.12 Model for DC biasing of an *npn* BJT having collector, base, and emitter resistors. See text for analysis.

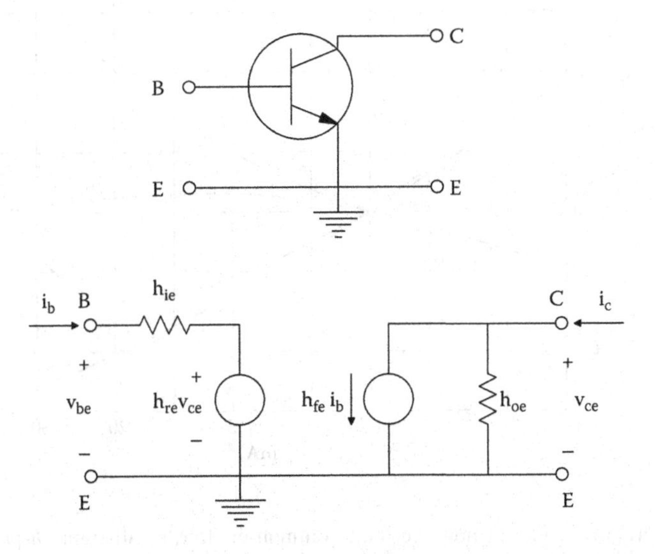

FIGURE 2.13 *Top:* An *npn* BJT viewed as a two-port circuit. *Bottom:* The linear, common-emitter, two-port, small-signal, *h*-parameter model for the BJT operating around some Q-point in its linear region. Note that the input circuit is a Thevenin model; the output is a Norton model.

One question which invariably arises is what MFSSM is used when a grounded emitter *pnp* transistor is considered. The answer is simple; the same model as for an *npn* BJT. Whether a BJT is *npn* or *pnp* affects the DC biasing of the transistors, *not their gains and small-signal input and output impedances.* However, the quiescent operating point of both *pnp* and *npn* transistors affects the numerical values of the C-E *h*-parameters. For example, h_{re} can be approximated by

$$h_{ie} = r_x + r_\pi \text{ ohm} \tag{2.16}$$

where r_x = the base spreading resistance, a fixed resistor with a range of 15 to 150 Ω, and $r\pi$ = the dynamic, SS resistance of the forward-biased base-emitter junction.

The value of $r\pi$ can be estimated from the basic diode equation for the B-E junction

$$I_B = I_{bs} \exp(V_{BEQ}/\eta V_T) \text{ Amps} \tag{2.17}$$

The resistance $r\pi$ is given by

$$r_\pi = \frac{1}{g_\pi} \cong \frac{1}{\partial i_B/\partial v_{BE}} = \frac{\eta V_T}{I_{BQ}} = \frac{\eta V_T h_{fe}}{I_{CQ}} \text{ ohms} \tag{2.18}$$

For a silicon BJT with $I_{BQ} = 5 \times 10^{-5}$ A, $r_\pi = 1.04$ kΩ.

Figure 2.14 illustrates how the four C-E *h*-parameters vary with I_C/I_{CQ} at constant V_{CEQ}. Note that the forward current gain, h_{fe}, is the most constant with I_C/I_{CQ}. The collector–emitter Norton conductance, h_{oe}, increases monotonically with I_C/I_{CQ} because as I_C increases, the $I_C = f(V_{CE}, I_B)$ curves tip upward. h_{ie} decreases monotonically with increasing I_C, as predicted by Equation 2.18. All four h_{xe} parameters increase with temperature.

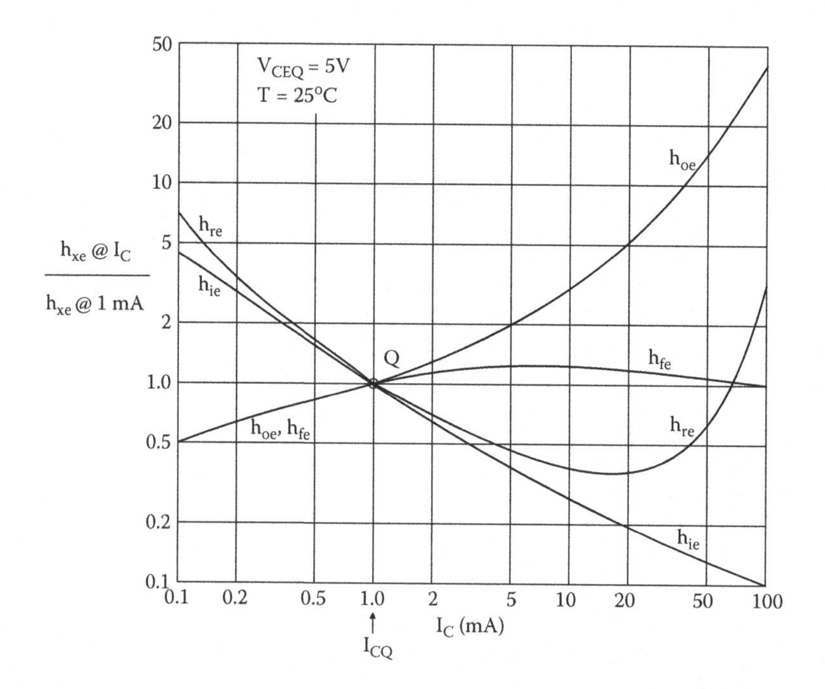

FIGURE 2.14 A normalized plot of how the four, common-emitter, small-signal *h*-parameters vary with collector current at constant V_{CEQ}. Note that the output conductance, h_{oe}, increases markedly with increasing collector current, while the input resistance, h_{ie}, decreases linearly. (Note that the same sort of plot can be made of normalized, C-E *h*-parameters vs. at constant I_{CQ}.)

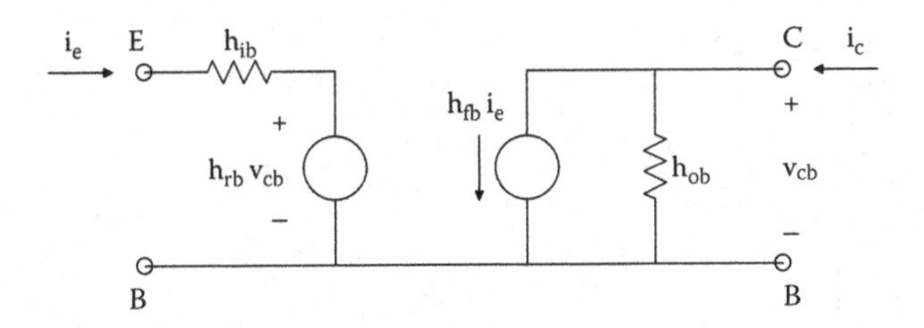

FIGURE 2.15 The common-base, *h*-parameter SSM for *npn* and *pnp* BJTs. Using linear algebra, it is possible to express any set of 4, linear, 2-port parameters in terms of any others (Northrop 1990).

Another MFSSM used to analyze transistor amplifier behavior on paper is the *grounded-base,* (G-B) *h-parameter model,* shown in Figure 2.15. Clearly, this G-B MFSSM is useful in analyzing grounded-base, BJT amplifiers. But as will be seen, the same results can be obtained using the more common, grounded-emitter, *h*-parameter MFSSM. The G-B *h*-parameters are found experimentally from

$$h_{ib} = \frac{\Delta v_{EB}}{\Delta i_E}\Big|_{Q,\ vCB\,=\,const.} \text{ Ohms} \tag{2.19a}$$

$$h_{rb} = \frac{\Delta v_{EB}}{\Delta v_{CB}}\Big|_{Q,\ ie\,=\,const} \tag{2.19b}$$

$$h_{fb} = \frac{\Delta i_C}{\Delta i_E}\Big|_{Q,\ vCB\,=\,const.} \tag{2.19c}$$

$$h_{ob} = \frac{\Delta i_C}{\Delta v_{CB}}\Big|_{Q,\ iE\,=\,const.} \text{ Siemens} \tag{2.19d}$$

Most manufacturers of discrete BJTs *do not* give G-B *h*-parameters in their specification data sheets.

2.3.3 Amplifiers Using One BJT

Three basic amplifier configurations can be made with one BJT: The *grounded-emitter,* the *emitter-follower (grounded collector),* and the *grounded base amplifier.* These three configurations are described and analyzed in the following section.

In the first example, methods to use the C-E, *h*-parameter, MFSSM to find expressions for the voltage gain, K_V, and the input and output resistances of a grounded-emitter amplifier are illustrated. Figure 2.16a illustrates a basic grounded-emitter amplifier driven through a coupling capacitor, C_c, by a small AC signal, v_s. In the MFSSM amplifier model, only small-signal variations around the BJT's operating (Q) point are considered; hence, all DC voltage sources are set to zero and replaced with short circuits to ground. Figure 2.16b illustrates the complete amplifier model ($h_{re} = 0$ has been set to 0 for simplicity). The SS output voltage is, by inspection,

$$v_o = \frac{-h_{fe} i_b}{G_c + h_{oe}} \tag{2.20}$$

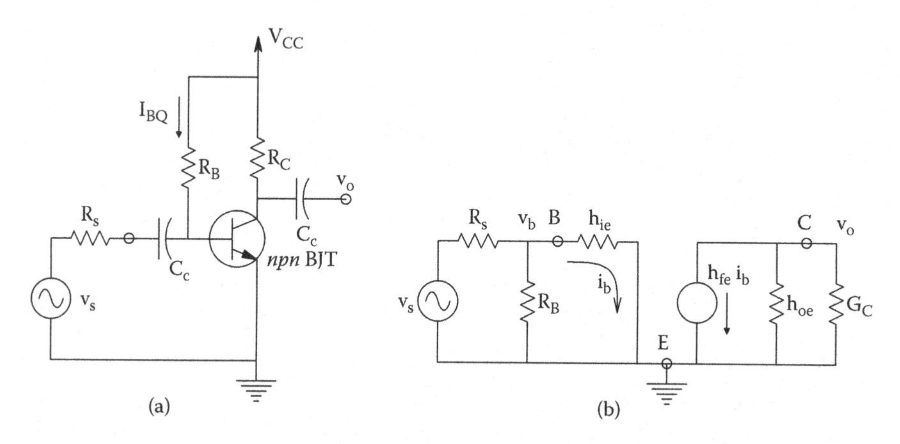

FIGURE 2.16 (a) Schematic of a simple, capacitively coupled, grounded emitter BJT amplifier. (b) Linear, midfrequency, small-signal model (MFSSM) of the grounded-emitter amplifier. Note at midfrequencies, capacitors are treated as short-circuits, and DC source voltages are small-signal grounds. The midfrequency gain, v_o/v_s, can be found from the model; see Text.

The base current is given by Ohm's law, assuming negligible SS current flows in R_B ($R_B >> h_{ie}$):

$$i_b \cong \frac{v_s}{R_s + h_{ie}} \tag{2.21}$$

Thus, the amplifier's SS voltage gain is found by substituting Equation 2.21 into Equation 2.20:

$$\frac{v_o}{v_s} = \frac{-h_{fe}R_C}{(h_{oe}R_C + 1)(R_s + h_{ie})} = K_v \tag{2.22}$$

By inspection, its SS input resistance is $R_{in} \cong R_s + h_{ie}$, and its (Thevenin) output resistance is $R_{out} = 1/(h_{oe} + G_C)$.

In the second example, a BJT emitter-follower amplifier is shown in Figure 2.17. Figure 2.17b illustrates the MFSSM for the emitter follower. To find an expression for the EF gain, the node equations for the v_b and v_o nodes are written as

$$v_b[G_s + G_B + g_{ie}] - v_o[g_{ie}] = v_sG_s \tag{2.23a}$$

$$-v_b g_{ie} + v_o[G_E + h_{oe} + g_{ie}] - h_{fe}i_b = 0 \tag{2.23b}$$

where $g_{ie} = 1/h_{ie}$, and $i_b = (v_b - v_o)g_{ie}$.

When the expression for i_b is substituted in Equation 2.23b, one obtains

$$-v_b[g_{ie}(1 + h_{fe})] + v_o[G_E + h_{oe} + gv_{ie}(1 + h_{fe})] = 0 \tag{2.24}$$

Now Equations 2.23a and 2.24 are solved using Cramer's rule, yielding the small-signal voltage gain:

$$\frac{v_o}{v_s} = \frac{G_sg_{ie}(1 + h_{fe})}{(G_s + G_B)[G_E + h_{oe} + g_{ie}(1 + h_{fe})] + g_{ie}(G_E + h_{oe})} = K_v \tag{2.25}$$

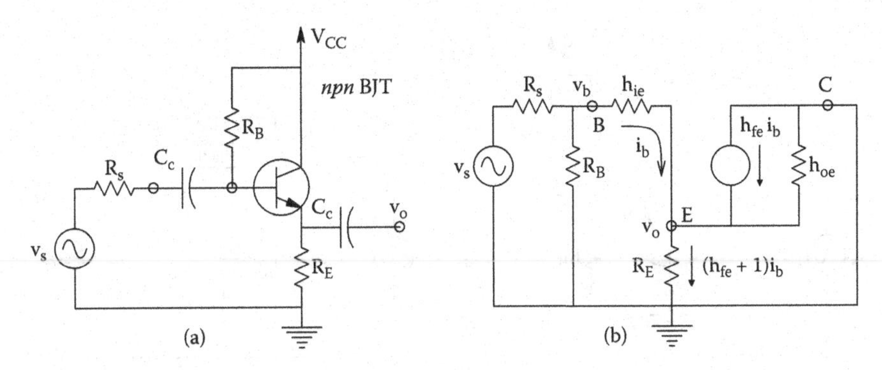

FIGURE 2.17 (a) Schematic of a simple, capacitively coupled, emitter follower amplifier. (b) MFSSM of the EF amplifier.

This rather unwieldy expression can be simplified if the a priori knowledge that usually $G_E >> h_{oe}$, and $G_s >> G_B$ is applied. The numerator and denominator of Equation 2.25 are also multiplied by $h_{ie}\ R_E\ R_s$. After some algebra, the simplified EF voltage gain is found to be

$$K_v \cong \frac{R_E(1+h_{fe})}{R_E(1+h_{fe})+h_{ie}+R_s} \tag{2.26}$$

Note that K_v for the EF is positive (noninverting) and slightly less than 1. The question arises, what then is the point of an amplifier with less than unity gain? The answer lies in the EF's high input impedance and low output impedance. The EF is used to buffer sources and drive coaxial cables and transmission lines with low characteristic impedances. It is easy to show that the EF's input impedance at the v_b node is simply R_B in parallel with $[h_{ie} + R_E\ (1 + h_{fe})]$ (h_{oe} is neglected). The Thevenin output impedance can be found for the linear MFSSM by taking the ratio of the open circuit voltage (OCV) to its short-circuit current (SCC). The OCV is simply $v_s\ K_V$

$$v_{oc} \cong \frac{v_s R_E(1+h_{fe})}{R_E(1+h_{fe})+h_{ie}+R_s} \tag{2.27}$$

The SCC is simply $i_{bsc}(1 + h_{fe})$. When the output is short-circuited, $v_o = 0$ and $i_{bsc} = v_s/(R_s + h_{ie})$. Thus, R_{out} is

$$R_{out} = \frac{\dfrac{v_s\ R_E(1+h_{fe})}{R_E(1+h_{fe})+h_{ie}+R_s}}{\dfrac{v_s(1+h_{fe})}{(R_s+h_{ie})}} \qquad \frac{R_E\dfrac{(R_s+h_{ie})}{(1+h_{fe})}}{\dfrac{(R_s+h_{ie})}{(R_s+h_{ie})}+R_E} \tag{2.28}$$

From Equation 2.28, it is seen that R_{out} is basically the emitter resistor R_E in parallel with the SS resistance seen looking up the emitter, $(R_s + h_{ie})/(R_s + h_{ie})$. In general, R_{out} is on the order of 10 to 30 Ω.

The third, single BJT circuit of interest is the grounded-base amplifier, shown in Figure 2.18. Again, to find the GB amp's gain, the node equations on the v_e and v_o nodes are written as

$$v_e[G_s + g_{ie} + h_{oe}] - v_o h_{oe} - h_{fe} i_b = v_s G_s \tag{2.29a}$$

$$-v_e h_{oe} + v_o[h_{oe} + G_C] + h_{fe} i_b = 0 \tag{2.29b}$$

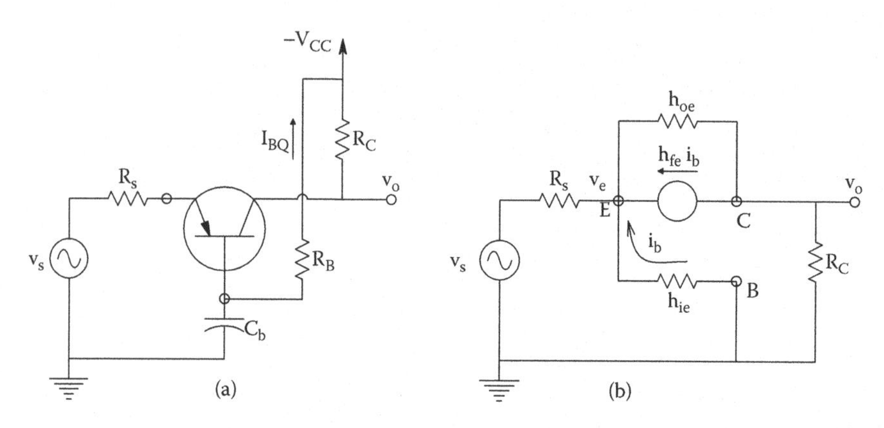

FIGURE 2.18 (a) Schematic of a simple, capacitively coupled, grounded-base amplifier. (b) MFSSM of the GB amplifier.

Now substitute $i_b = -v_e g_{ie}$ into the equations above to get the final form for the node equations:

$$v_e[G_s + h_{oe} + g_{ie}(1 + h_{fe})] - v_o[h_{oe}] = v_s G_s \tag{2.30a}$$

$$-v_e[h_{oe} + h_{fe}g_{ie}] + v_o[h_{oe} + G_C] = 0 \tag{2.30b}$$

These equations are also solved using Cramer's rule. After some algebra, the G-B amplifier's gain is obtained:

$$K_v = \frac{R_C[h_{fe} + h_{oe}h_{ie}]}{R_C[h_{oe}(h_{ie} + R_s)] + R_s[1 + h_{fe} + h_{oe}h_{ie}] + h_{ie}} \tag{2.31}$$

It is instructive to substitute typical numerical values into Equation 2.31 and evaluate the gain. Let $R_C = 5$ k, $h_{ie} = 1$ k, $h_{fe} = 100$, $R_s = 100$, and $h_{oe} = 10^{-5}$ S. Thus, $K_v = 44.8$. Note that the gain is noninverting. From the numerical evaluation, we find that certain terms in Equation 2.31 are small compared with others (i.e., $h_{oe} \to 0$), which leads to the approximation

$$K_v \cong \frac{R_C h_{fe}}{R_s(1 + h_{fe}) + h_{ie}} \tag{2.32}$$

Next, expressions for R_{in} and R_{out} for the GB amplifier will be found: R_{in} is the resistance the Thevenin source (v_s, R_s) "sees" looking into the emitter of the GB amplifier. Assume $h_{oe} \to 0$. The resistance looking into the emitter is approximately

$$R_{inem} \cong \frac{v_e}{i_e} = \frac{v_e}{-i_b(h_{fe} + 1)} = \frac{v_e}{-(-v_e/h_{ie})(h_{fe} + 1)} = \frac{h_{ie}}{(h_{fe} + 1)} \tag{2.33}$$

To get a feeling for the size of R_{in}, substitute realistic circuit parameter values in Equation 2.33. Let $R_C = 5000\ \Omega$, $R_s = 100\ \Omega$, $h_{fe} = 100$, $h_{oe} = 10^{-5}$ S, and $h_{ie} = 1000\ \Omega$. Thus, $R_{inem} = 9.9\ \Omega$.

The *output resistance* is the Thevenin resistance seen looking into the collector node with R_C attached. If we set $h_{oe} \to 0$ again, $R_{out} \cong R_C$, by inspection.

2.3.4 Simple Amplifiers Using Two Transistors at Midfrequencies

Figure 2.19 illustrates four common 2-BJT amplifier architectures. An *npn* Darlington pair is shown in Figure 2.19a. Darlington pairs can also use *pnp* BJTs. Darlington pairs are often used as power amplifiers, either in the emitter-follower architecture or as grounded-base amplifiers. The circuit of Figure 2.19b is called a *feedback pair;* it *is not* a Darlington. It, too, is often used as a power amplifier in the EF or GE modes. It will be analyzed below. Figure 2.19c is an EF-GB pair, used for small-signal, high-frequency amplification. Figure 2.19d is called a *cascode pair;* it, too, is often used as a small-signal, high-frequency amplifier.

In the first example, find an expression for the mid-frequency, small-signal voltage gain, and input and output resistances for a grounded-emitter Darlington amplifier. The amplifier circuit and its MFSS, C-E *h*-parameter model, are shown in Figure 2.20. To simplify analysis, we assume $R_B \to \infty$, $h_{oe1} \to 0$, and $h_{oe2} \to 0$. From Ohm' law, $i_{b1} = (v_s - v_{b2})/(R_s + h_{ie1})$, $i_{b2} = v_{b2}/h_{ie2}$. Now the node equations for the v_{b2} and the v_o nodes are written as

$$v_{b2}[1/h_{ie2} + 1/(R_s + h_{ie1})] - h_{fe1} i_{b1} = v_s/(R_s + h_{ie1}) \tag{2.34a}$$

$$v_o[G_C] + h_{fe1} i_{b1} + h_{fe2} i_{b2} = 0 \tag{2.34b}$$

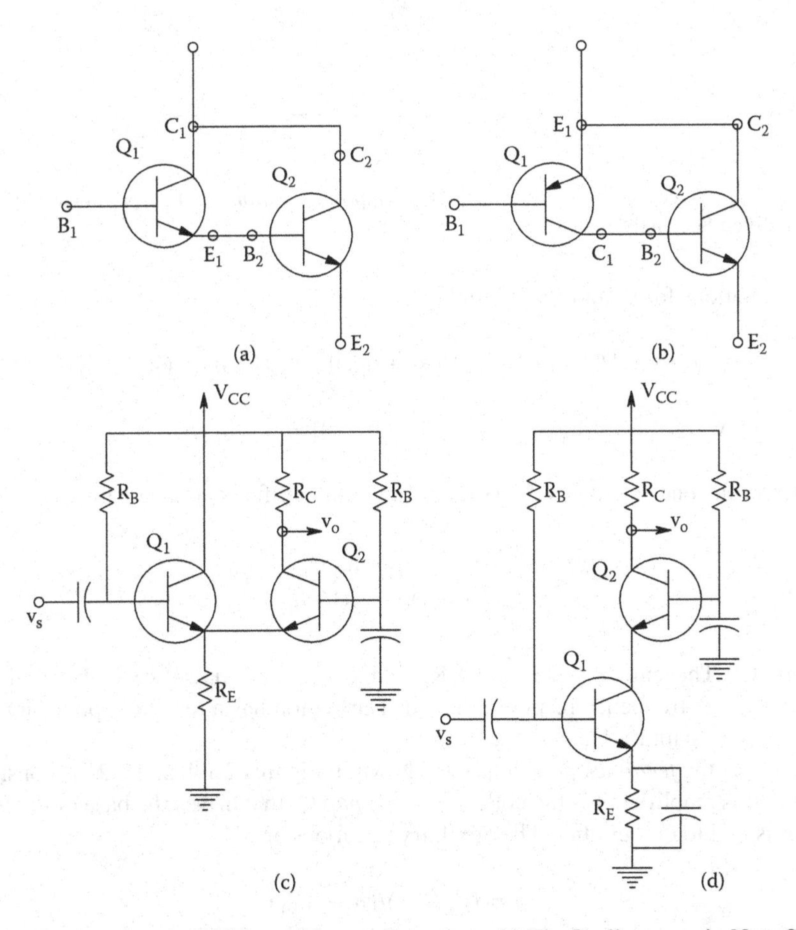

FIGURE 2.19 Four, common, 2-BJT amplifier configurations: (a) The Darlington pair. Note Q_1's emitter is connected directly to Q_2's base. (b) The feedback pair. The collector of the *pnp* Q_1 is coupled directly to the *npn* Q_2's base. (c) The emitter-follower-grounded-base (EF-GB) BJT pair. (d) The *cascode pair.*

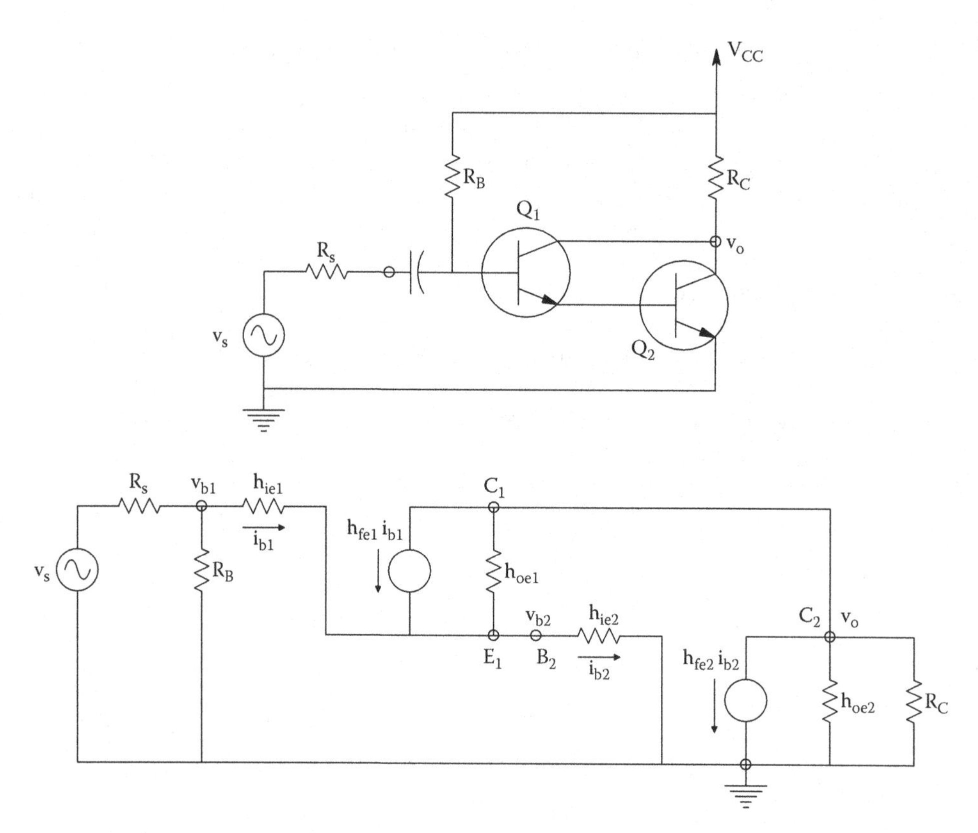

FIGURE 2.20 *Top:* A common-emitter Darlington amplifier. *Bottom:* C-E *h*-parameter MFSSM of the Darlington amplifier. See analysis in Text.

Substitute the relations for i_{b1} and i_{b2} and find

$$v_o[0] + v_{b2}[1/h_{ie2} + (1 + h_{fe1})/(R_s + h_{ie1})] = v_s[(1 + h_{fe1})/(R_s + h_{ie1}] \tag{2.35a}$$

$$v_o[G_C] + v_{b2}[h_{fe2}/h_{ie2} - h_{fe1}/(R_s + h_{ie1})] = -v_s h_{fe1}/(R_s + h_{ie1}) \tag{2.35b}$$

Using Cramer's rule, one calculates the G-E Darlington amplifier's voltage gain:

$$\frac{v_o}{v_s} \cong -\frac{R_C(1 + h_{fe1} + h_{fe1}h_{fe2})}{(R_s + h_{ie1}) + h_{ie2}(1 + h_{fe1})} = K_v \tag{2.36}$$

By inspection, the Thevenin $R_{out} \cong R_C$, and $R_{in} \cong h_{ie1} + (1 + h_{fe1})h_{ie2}$. As will be seen in the section on BJT amplifier frequency response, the GE Darlington has a relatively poor high-frequency response, trading off gain for bandwidth.

In this example, the *feedback pair* amplifier shown in Figures 2.19b and 2.21 is considered.

Note that in this amplifier, it is the collector of the *pnp* Q_1 that drives the base of the *npn* Q_2, and Q_2's collector is tied to Q_1's emitter. The auxiliary equations are

$$i_{b1} = (v_s - v_o)/(R_s + h_{ie1}) \tag{2.37a}$$

$$i_{b2} = v_{b2}/h_{ie2} \tag{2.37b}$$

Again, for mathematical convenience, the approximations: $h_{oe1} \to 0$, $h_{oe2} \to 0$ are used, and the node equations for v_o and v_{b2} are

$$v_o[G_C + 1/(R_s + h_{ie1})] + h_{fe2}i_{b2} - h_{fe1}i_{b1} = v_s/(R_s + h_{ie1}) \tag{2.38a}$$

$$v_{b2}[1/h_{ie1}] + h_{fe1}i_{b1} = 0 \tag{2.38b}$$

Now substitute the auxiliary relations for i_{b1} and i_{b2} into Equations 2.38a and b.

$$v_o[G_C + \frac{1 + h_{fe1}}{R_s + h_{ie1}}] + v_{b2}[h_{fe2}/h_{ie2}] = v_s \frac{1 + h_{fe1}}{R_s + h_{ie1}} \tag{2.39a}$$

$$-v_o \frac{h_{fe1}}{R_s + h_{ie1}} + v_{b2}[1/h_{ie2}] = -\frac{v_s}{R_s + h_{ie1}} \tag{2.39b}$$

The Equations 2.39a and b are solved by Cramer's rule to find K_v.

$$\Delta = (1/h_{ie1})[G_C + \frac{1 + h_{fe1}}{R_s + h_{ie1}}] + \frac{h_{fe1}h_{fe2}}{h_{ie2}(R_s + h_{ie1})} \tag{2.40}$$

$$\Delta v_o = \frac{(1 + h_{fe1})h_{ie2} + h_{fe2}h_{ie1}}{h_{ie1}h_{ie2}(R_s + h_{ie1})} \tag{2.41}$$

Thus, the voltage gain is

$$\frac{v_o}{v_s} \cong \frac{R_C[(1 + h_{fe1} + h_{fe2}h_{fe1}]}{R_C[(1 + h_{fe1} + h_{fe1}h_{fe2}] + (R_s + h_{ie1})} = K_v \tag{2.42}$$

If "typical" numerical values are used: $R_s + h_{ie1} = 1050\ \Omega$, $h_{fe1} = 100$, $h_{fe2} = 20$, and $R_C = 5000\ \Omega$, then $K_v = 0.999895$. It appears that the feedback pair amplifier of Figure 2.21 behaves like a super emitter-follower with (almost) unity gain.

Next, R_{in} and R_{out} of the FBP amplifier are examined. To find R_{out}, the open-circuit voltage/short-circuit current method will be used. The OCV approximated by $v_s \cong v_{oc}$ because of the near unity gain of the amplifier. The short-circuit current at the C_2-E_1 node is

$$i_{sc} = (1 + h_{fe1})i_{b1} - h_{fe2}\, i_{b2} \tag{2.43}$$

With the output short-circuited, $v_o = 0$ and $i_{b1} = v_s/(R_s + h_{ie1})$. Neglecting h_{oe1}, i_{b2} can be written as

$$i_{b2} = -h_{fe1}i_{b1} = -h_{fe1}v_s/(R_s + h_{ie1}) \tag{2.44}$$

Thus,

$$i_{sc} = (1 + h_{fe1})v_s/(R_s + h_{ie1}) + h_{fe2}h_{fe1}v_s/(R_s + h_{ie1}) \tag{2.45}$$

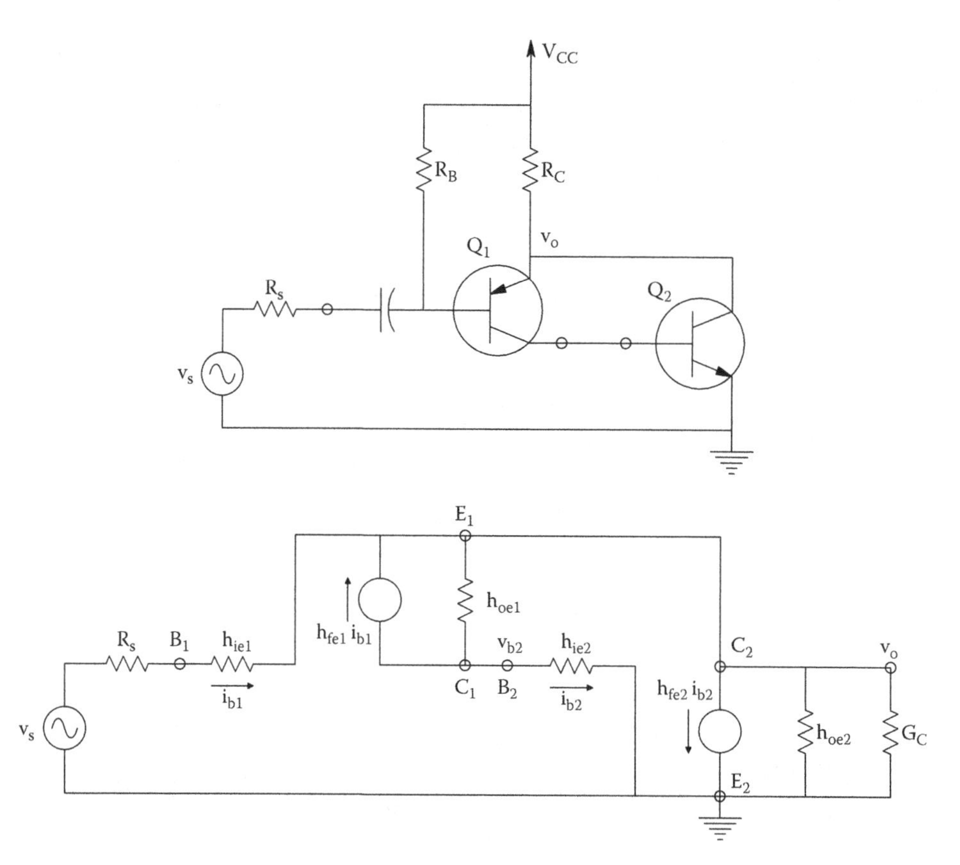

FIGURE 2.21 *Top:* Feedback pair amplifier with load resistor, R_C, attached to common Q_1 emitter + Q_2 collector. *Bottom:* MFSSM of the feedback pair amplifier above. The analysis in Text shows this circuit behaves like a "super" emitter-follower.

Clearly, $R_{out} = v_{oc}/i_{sc}$, and R_{out} is approximated by

$$R_{out} \cong \frac{R_s + h_{ie1}}{1 + h_{fe1} + h_{fe1}h_{fe2}} \tag{2.46}$$

If the numbers used above are substituted, $R_{out} = 0.5\ \Omega$, significantly smaller than a single BJT's emitter follower. R_{in} looking into the B_1 node is just v_s/i_{b1}. That is,

$$R_{in} = v_s h_{ie1}/(v_s - v_o) = h_{ie1}/(1 - v_o/v_s) = \frac{h_{ie1}}{1 - \dfrac{R_C[1 + h_{fe1} + h_{fe1}h_{fe2}]}{R_C[1 + h_{fe1} + h_{fe1}h_{fe2}] + h_{ie1}}}$$

$$\downarrow$$

$$R_{in} = R_C[1 + h_{fe1} + h_{fe2}] + h_{ie1} \tag{2.47}$$

$R_{in} \cong 10.51\ \text{M}\Omega$, using the parameters above.

Next, the behavior of the feedback pair amplifier is examined when the load resistor is connected to E2, and C2-E1 is connected to V_{cc}. The circuit is shown in Figure 2.22. It is not necessary to solve

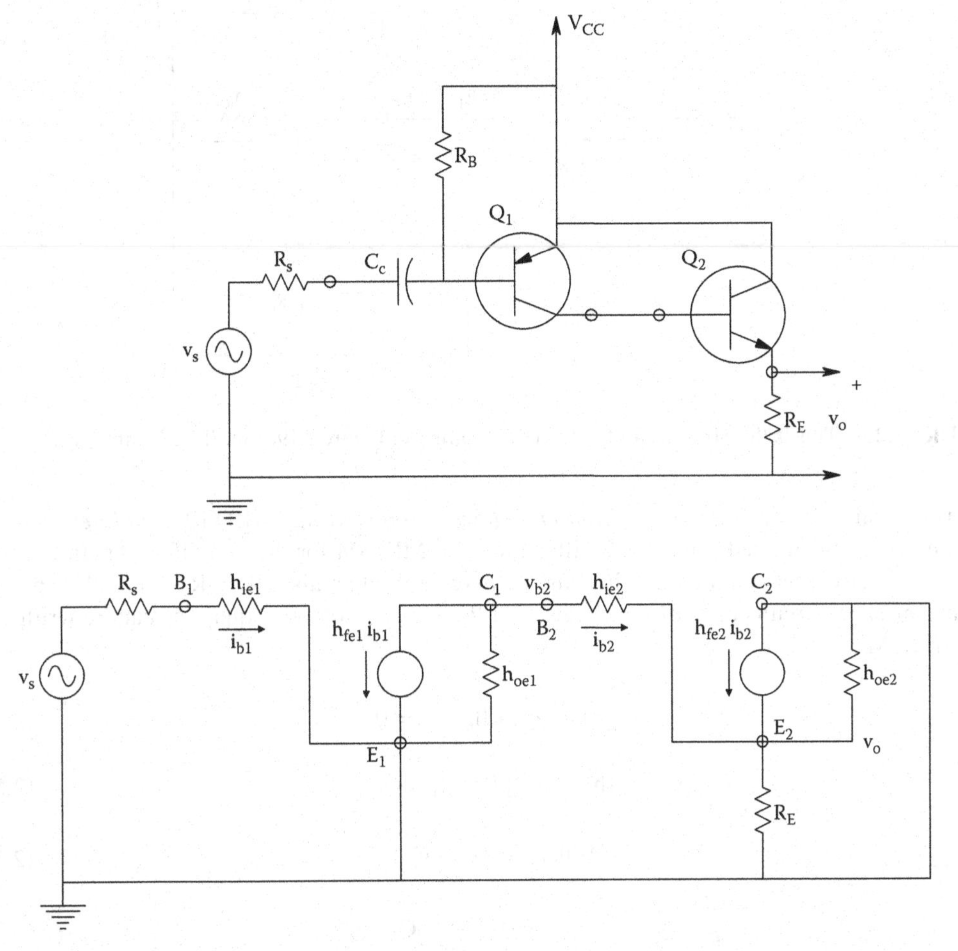

FIGURE 2.22 *Top:* Feedback pair amplifier with load resistor in Q_2's emitter. *Bottom:* MFSSM of the amplifier shown above. Analysis in text shows this amplifier has a high inverting midfrequency gain; it does not emulate an emitter-follower.

two simultaneous node equations to find K_v. By Ohm's law: $i_{b1} = v_s/(R_s + h_{ie1})$, and $i_{b2} = -i_{b1}h_{fe1}$. Now it is clear that

$$v_o = i_{b2}(1 + h_{fe2})R_E = -i_{b1}h_{fe1}(1 + h_{fe2})R_E = \frac{-v_s h_{fe1}(1 + h_{fe})R_E}{R_s + h_{ie1}} = v_{oOC}$$

Thus,

$$K_v = -\frac{R_E h_{fe1}(1 + h_{fe2})}{(R_s + h_{ie1})} \tag{2.49}$$

R_{in} for this amplifier is found by inspection: $R_{in} = h_{ie1}$. R_{out} is found by v_{oOC}/i_{oSC}:

$$R_{out} = \frac{\dfrac{-v_s h_{fe1}(1 + h_{fe2})R_E}{(R_s + h_{ie1})}}{\dfrac{-v_s h_{fe1}(1 + h_{fe2})}{(R_s + h_{ie1})}} \tag{2.50}$$

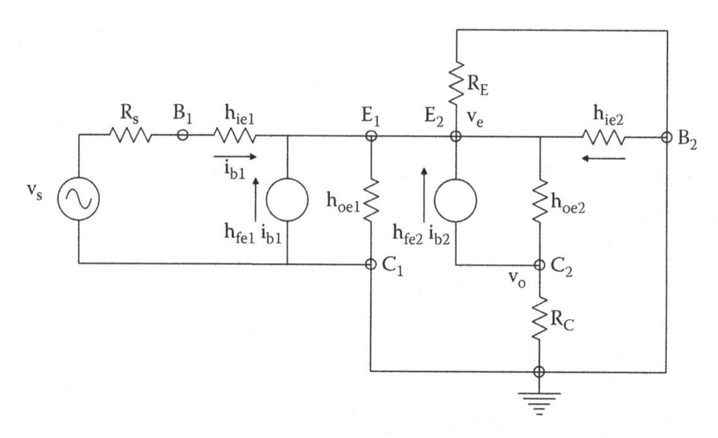

FIGURE 2.23 This is the MFSSM for the EF-GB amplifier of Figure 2.19c. See Text for analysis.

Next, the gain, R_{in} and R_{out} of the *emitter-follower-grounded base* (EFGB) *amplifier* shown in Figure 2.19c is examined. Figure 2.23 illustrates the MFSSM for this amplifier. Again, for algebraic simplicity, it is assumed that h_{oe1} and h_{oe2} are negligible; also, $R_1 = R_s + h_{ie1}$, all capacitors behave as short-circuits at midfrequencies, and $R_B \to \infty$. Two node equations can be written for the MFSSM:

$$v_o[G_C] + h_{fe2} i_{b2} = 0 \quad (2.51a)$$

$$v_e[G_E + 1/h_{ie2} + G_1] - h_{fe2} i_{b2} - h_{fe1} i_{b1} = v_s G_1 \quad (2.51b)$$

$$\text{Where, } i_{b2} = -v_e/h_{ie2} \quad (2.51c)$$

$$i_{b1} = (v_s - v_e)G_1 \quad (2.51d)$$

Substituting Equations 2.51c and 2.51d into the node equations, there results

$$v_o[G_C] - v_e[h_{fe2}/h_{ie2}] = 0 \quad (2.52a)$$

$$v_o[0] + v_e[G_E + (1 + h_{fe2})/h_{ie2} + G_1(1 + h_{fe1})] = v_s G_1 (1 + h_{fe1}) \quad (2.52b)$$

From Equation 2.52a and b, v_o and v_e can be found:

$$v_o = v_e R_C [h_{fe2}/h_{ie2}] \quad (2.53)$$

and

$$v_e = \frac{v_s G_1 (1 + h_{fe1})}{[G_E + (1 + h_{fe2})/h_{ie2} + G_1(1 + h_{fe1})]} \quad (2.54)$$

Now Equation 2.54 is substituted into Equation 2.53 to find K_v:

$$K_v = \frac{v_o}{v_s} = \frac{+R_C h_{fe2}(1 + h_{fe1})}{h_{ie2}(R_1/R_E) + R_1(1 + h_{fe2}) + h_{ie2}(1 + h_{fe1})} \quad (2.55)$$

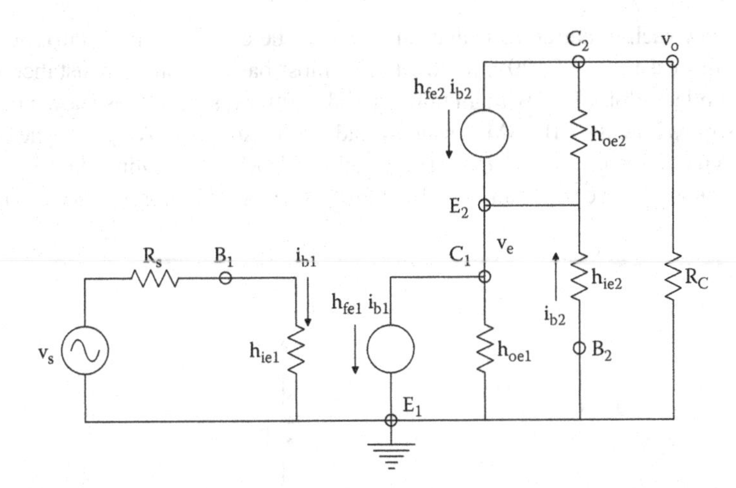

FIGURE 2.24 This is the MFSSM for the cascode amplifier of Figure 2.19d. See Text for analysis.

When the typical values: $R_C = 5000\ \Omega$, $R_1 = 1050\ \Omega$, $h_{fe1} = h_{fe2} = 100$, $h_{ie2} = 1000\ \Omega$, are substituted, one finds $K_v = +244$. Note that the EFGB amplifier is noninverting. The EFGB amplifier will be shown to have excellent high frequency response. It is left as an exercise for the reader to find expressions for the midfrequency R_{in} and R_{out} for this amplifier.

The final two-BJT amplifier stage to be analyzed using the CE MFSSM is the cascode amplifier, as shown in Figure 2.19d. The MFSSM for this amplifier is shown in Figure 2.24. Again, assume the capacitors behave as short-circuits at midfrequencies, $h_{oe1} = h_{oe2} = 0$, and $R_B \to \infty$. Clearly, $v_o = -h_{fe2} i_{b2} R_C$, $i_{b2} = -v_e/h_{ie2}$, so $v_o = v_e h_{fe2} R_C/h_{ie2}$, and $i_{b1} = v_s/R_1$. To find v_e, the node equation is written as

$$v_e[1/h_{ie2}] + h_{fe1} i_{b1} - h_{fe2} i_{b2} = 0 \tag{2.56}$$

Substituting for i_{b1} and i_{b2} into Equation 2.56, we find

$$v_e = \frac{-v_s h_{fe1} h_{ie2} G1}{1 + h_{fe2}} \tag{2.57}$$

Equation 2.57 is substituted into the equation for v_o above to find K_v.

$$K_v = \frac{v_o}{v_s} = \frac{-h_{fe1} R_C h_{fe2}}{R_1(1 + h_{fe2})} \approx \frac{-h_{fe1} R_C}{R_1} \tag{2.58}$$

By inspection, $R_{in} = R_1$, $R_{out} \cong R_C$. Like the EF-GB amplifier, the cascode amplifier is also has a defined high-frequency bandwidth. It also can be described as a GE-GB amplifier.

2.3.5 Use of Transistor Dynamic Loads to Improve Amplifier Performance

In many analog IC designs, including those with differential amplifiers, transistors and small transistor circuits are used to create small-signal, dynamic, high impedances that when used in amplifiers to replace conventional resistors, increase amplifier gain or differential amplifier common-mode rejection ratio. Figure 2.25 illustrates four BJT circuits that act as DC current sources or sinks having high, small-signal, Norton resistances. For example, if 2 mA DC flows through a potential difference of 5 V in an electronic circuit, a 2.5 kΩ resistor is needed. If a dynamic current source is used, the equivalent small-signal (Norton) resistance can range from 100 k to 10 M, depending on the circuit.

A good way to view such dynamic resistances in to treat the circuit as a DC current source in parallel with a Norton resistance of 100 k to 10 M. The most basic dynamic resistance is realized by looking into the collector of a BJT with an unbypassed emitter resistance, as shown in Figure 2.25a. Figure 2.26 illustrates how the MFSSM is used to find the resistance looking into the collector. Note that the base is bypassed to ground at signal frequencies. Clearly, from Ohm's law, $R_{incol} = v_t/i_t$. (v_t is a small-signal test source.) We begin analysis by finding an expression for $v_e = f(v_t)$. Writing the node equation

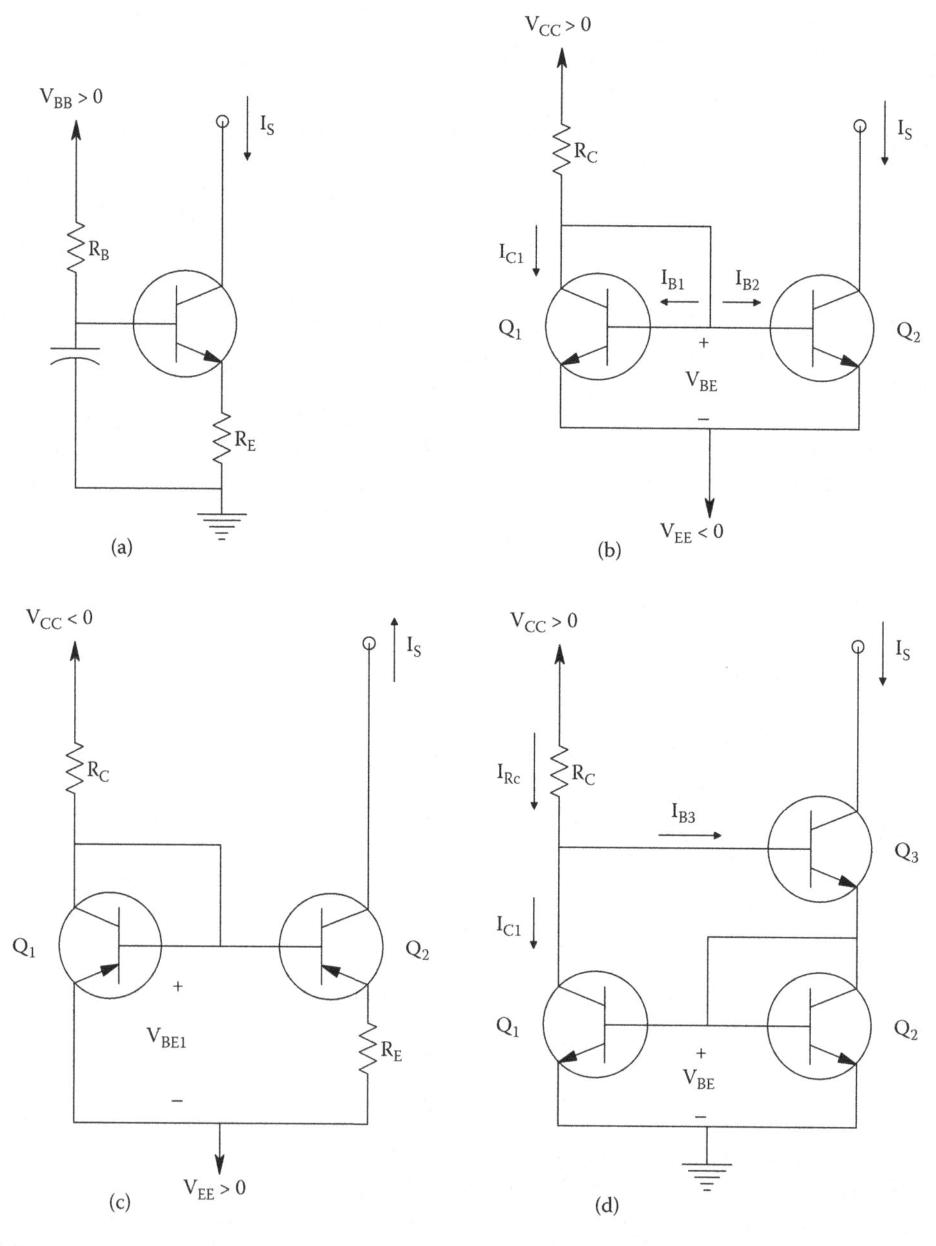

FIGURE 2.25 Four BJT circuits used for high-impedance current sources (and sinks) in the design of differential amplifiers and other analog ICs. They can serve as high-impedance active loads. (a) Collector of simple BJT with unbypassed emitter resistance. (b) Basic 2-BJT current sink (source). (c) Widlar current source. (*pnp* BJTs are used.) (d) Wilson current sink.

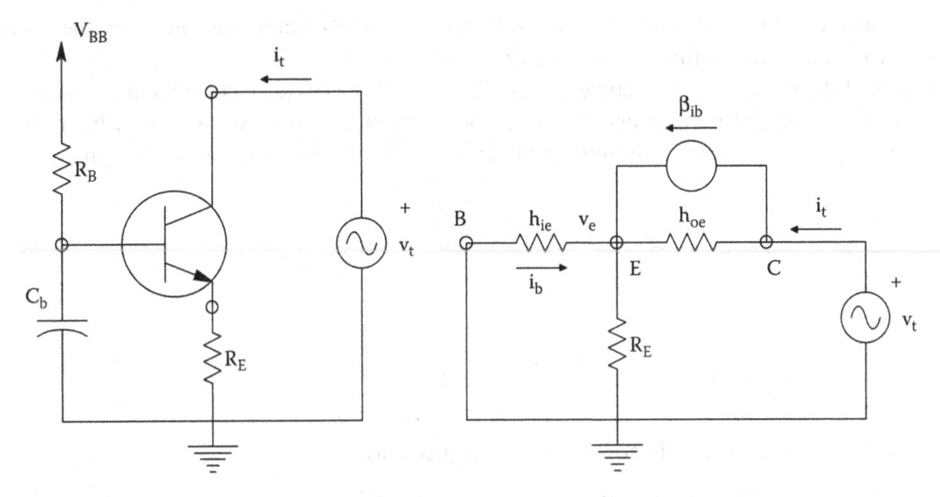

FIGURE 2.26 *Left:* Test circuit for calculating small-signal resistance looking into BJT's collector. An AC test source, v_t, is used, i_t is measured. *Right:* MFSSM of the test circuit used to calculate the expression for the small-signal resistance looking into collector.

$$v_e[(1/h_{ie}) + G_E + h_{oe}] - \beta\, i_b = v_t h_{oe} \tag{2.59a}$$

$$i_b = -v_e/h_{ie} \tag{2.59b}$$

$$v_e[(1/h_{ie})(1+\beta) + G_E + h_{oe}] = v_t h_{oe} \tag{2.59c}$$

Thus, v_e can be written as

$$v_e = \frac{v_t h_{oe}}{(1/h_{ie})(1+\beta) + G_E + h_{oe}} \tag{2.60}$$

The test current is

$$i_t = v_e[(1/h_{ie}) + G_E] \tag{2.61}$$

When Equation 2.60 is substituted into Equation 2.61, we can solve for R_{incol}:

$$R_{incol} = \frac{v_t}{i_t} = \frac{1 + \dfrac{\beta R_E + h_{oe}h_{ie}R_E}{R_E + h_{ie}}}{h_{oe}} \tag{2.62}$$

Looking into the collector of a BJT with no R_E, one sees a $R_{incol} \cong h_{oe}^{-1}\ \Omega$. To see how much R_E increases R_{incol}, let us substitute some typical parameter values into Equation 2.62: $R_E = 5k$, $h_{ie} = 1k$, $\beta = 100$, and $h_{oe} = 10^{-5}$ S. Crunching the numbers, $R_{incol} = 8.4\ M\Omega$. Note that the BJT's base was bypassed to ground in the development above. If the base *is not* bypassed, $h_{ie} \rightarrow h_{ie} + R_B$ in Equation 2.62, where R_B is the Thevenin resistance the base "sees looking out." The unbypassed base causes R_{incol} to decrease markedly, but it still remains above $1/h_{oe}$.

More sophisticated, high dynamic resistance, DC current sources are shown in Figures 2.25b–d. Figure 2.25b is the basic, two-BJT current sink; its dynamic input resistance is about 1/hoe Ω. c is the Widlar current source (note pnp BJTs are used). d is a Wilson current sink. Note that a collector–base junction in all three current source/active load circuits is short-circuited (Q_1 in

Figure 2.25b and c, Q_2 in d). The transistor with the shorted collector–base junction then behaves as a forward-biased, base-emitter diode junction.

Analysis of the basic, two-BJT current sink (Figure 2.25b) is made easy when it is assumed that Q_1 and Q_2 have identical parameters. Because both transistors have the same V_{BE}, their collector currents are equal, i.e., $I_{C1} = I_{C2}$. Summing currents at Q_1's collector, the node equation is

$$I_{Rc} - I_{C1} = 2I_{C1}/\beta \tag{2.63}$$

And thus,

$$I_{C1} = \frac{I_{Rc}}{1 + 2/\beta} = I_{C2} \tag{2.64}$$

If β is large (≥ 100), I_{C2} is nearly equal to the reference current:

$$I_{C2} \cong I_{Rc} = (V_{CC} - V_{BE})/R_C \tag{2.65}$$

Thus, R_C can be manipulated to obtain the desired quiescent DC current, I_{C2}. If V_{CE2} varies, there will be a small variation in the DC I_{CE2}. I_{CE2} can be expressed in terms of V_{BE2} and Q_2's *Early voltage* ($|V_x|$), which is used to model the upward tilt of the $I_{C2} = f(V_{BE2}, V_{CE2})$ curves. Gray and Meyer (1984) model I_{C2} by

$$I_{C2} = I_{CS}[\exp(V_{BE2}/V_T)](1 + V_{CE2}/|V_x|) \tag{2.66}$$

Now

$$\frac{\partial I_{C2}}{\partial V_{CE2}} = I_{CS}[\exp(V_{BE2}/V_T)](1/|V_x|) \tag{2.67}$$

So, the variation in I_{C2} is

$$\Delta I_{C2} = I_{CS}[\exp(V_{BE2}/V_T)](1/|V_x|)\Delta V_{CE2} \tag{2.68}$$

A very detailed treatment of the transistor current sources and active loads used in IC design beyond the scope of this text can be found in Chapter 4 of Gray and Meyer (1984) and in Ayers (2009). These authors show how certain active load designs can be used to reduce the overall, DC temperature coefficient (tempco) of certain amplifier stages, as well as to increase gain and CMRR.

2.4 MIDFREQUENCY MODELS FOR FIELD-EFFECT TRANSISTORS

2.4.1 INTRODUCTION

There are two basic types of field-effect transistor: The *junction field-effect transistor* (JFET), which can be further characterized as *n*- or *p*-channel, and the *metal-oxide semiconductor FET* (MOSFET) which can also be subdivided into *p*- and *n*-channel devices, and further distinguished by whether it operates by *enhancement* or *depletion* of charge carriers in the channel. Surprisingly, one midfrequency small-signal model describes the behavior of *all* types of FETs, although the DC biasing varies. MFSSMs for FETs use a voltage-controlled current source (transconductance) model in parallel with an output conductance to model the drain-to-source behavior.

In the following sections, the behavior of JFETs and the way they work as amplifiers will be examined.

2.4.2 JFETs at Midfrequencies

Figure 2.27 illustrates the symbols for n- and p-channel JFETs and the volt–ampere curves for an n-channel JFET. Note that the gate-to-channel *pn* junction is normally reverse-biased in a JFET, and the gate current is thus the reverse saturation current of this diode (I_{rs}), which is on the order of nA. In the n-channel JFET, all the currents and voltages are positive as written, with v_{GS} being negative. In the p-channel JFET, all the signs are reversed: That is, i_D and v_{DS} are negative, and v_{GS} is positive. The operating region of the JFET's (i_D, v_{DS}) curves is *ohmic* to the *left* of the I_{DB} line, and *saturated* to the *right* of the I_{DB} line.

Just as there is a mathematical model for *pn* junction diode current, there is also a mathematical approximation to JFET behavior *in the saturation region*. This is,

$$I_D = I_{DSS}(1 - V_{GS}/V_P)^2 \text{ for } V_{DS} > |V_{GS} + V_P| \text{ and } |V_{GS}| < |V_P| \quad (2.69)$$

In the ohmic region, I_D is modeled by

$$I_D = I_{DSS}[2(1 + V_{GS}/V_P)(V_{DS}/V_P) - (V_{DS}/V_P)^2] \text{ for } 0 < V_{DS} < |V_{GS} + V_P| \quad (2.70)$$

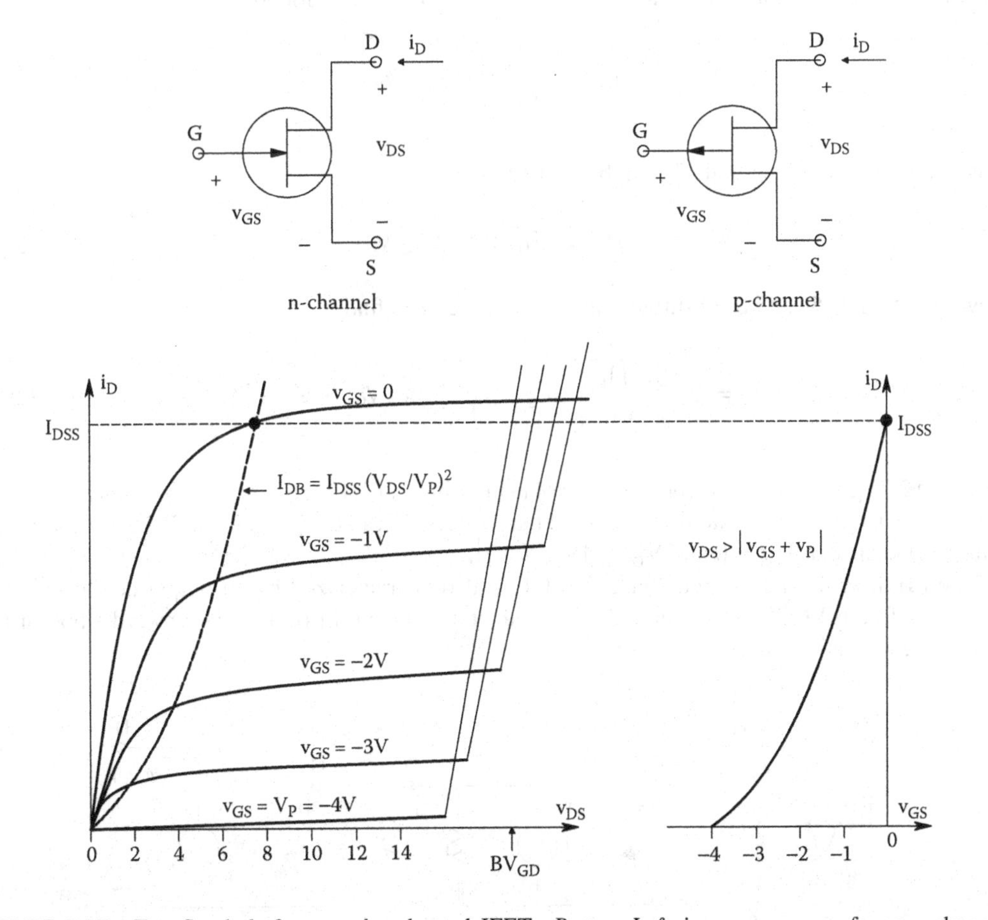

FIGURE 2.27 *Top:* Symbols for *n*- and *p*-channel JFETs. *Bottom Left:* i_D vs. v_{DS} curves for an *n*-channel JFET. Area to left of I_{DB} parabola has ohmic FET operation; area to right of I_{DB} line has saturated (channel) operation. *Bottom Right:* The i_D vs. v_{GS} curve for saturated operation [$v_{DS} > |v_{GS} + V_P|$]. The pinch-off voltage, $V_P = -4$ V in this example.

For $V_{GS} << V_P$,

$$I_D = I_{DSS}[2(1 + V_{GS}/V_P)(V_{DS}/V_P)] \quad (2.71)$$

where I_{DSS} is the drain current defined for $V_{GS} = 0$ and $V_{DS} > |V_{GS} + V_P|$. V_P is the *pinchoff voltage*, i.e., $V_P = V_{GS}$ where $I_D \to 0$, given $V_{DS} > |V_{GS} + V_P|$. In the ohmic region, the JFET behaves like a voltage-controlled conductance:

$$g_d = \frac{\partial i_D}{\partial v_{DS}}\Big|_{VGS} = I_{DSS}[2(1 + (V_{GS}/V_P)/V_P] \quad (2.72)$$

In the saturation region, both n- and p-channel JFETs have the same MFSSM, shown in Figure 2.28. The transconductance of the *voltage-controlled current source* (VCCS) is defined by

$$g_m = \frac{\partial i_D}{\partial v_{DS}}\Big|_{Q,\, vGS = \text{const.}} \quad (2.73)$$

By differentiating Equation 2.69, an algebraic expression for g_m is found:

$$g_m = \frac{2I_{DSS}}{|V_P|}(1 - V_{GS}/V_P) \quad (2.74)$$

Note from Equation 2.69 that $\sqrt{I_D}$ can be written as

$$\sqrt{I_D} = \sqrt{I_{DSS}}\,(1 - V_{GS}/V_P) \quad (2.75)$$

Now Equation 2.75 can be substituted into Equation 2.74 to find

$$g_m = \frac{2I_{DSS}}{|V_P|}\sqrt{\frac{I_{DQ}}{I_{DSS}}} = g_{mo}\sqrt{\frac{I_{DQ}}{I_{DSS}}} \quad \text{for } V_{DS} > |V_{GS} + V_P| \quad (2.76)$$

Equation 2.76 gives one an algebraic means of estimating a JFET's g_m in terms of its quiescent drain current (I_{DQ}) and the manufacturer-specified parameters, I_{DSS} and V_P. g_{mo} is the JFET's (maximum) transconductance at $V_{GS} = 0$ and $V_{DS} > |V_{GS} + V_P|$.

The MFSSM for a saturated-channel JFET is also characterized by an output conductance in parallel with the VCCS. This small-signal conductance is due in part to the upward slope of the $i_D = f(v_{GS}, v_{DS})$ curve family:

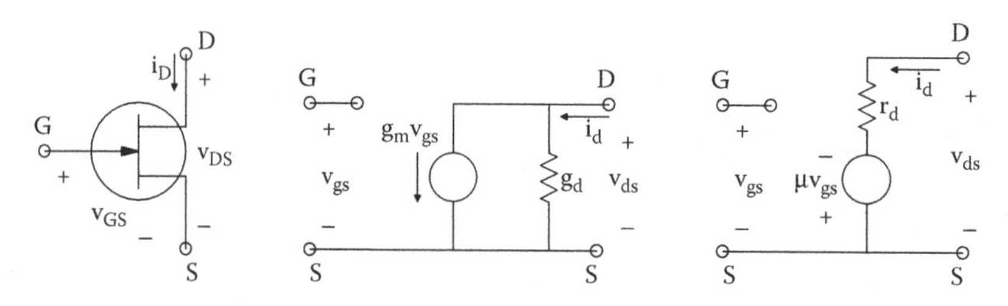

FIGURE 2.28 *Left:* Symbol for *n*-channel JFET. *Center:* Norton MFSSM for both *p*- and *n*-channel JFETs. *Right:* Thevenin MFSSM for all JFETs.

$$g_d = \frac{\partial i_D}{\partial v_{DS}}\Big|_{VGS} = \frac{\Delta I_D}{\Delta V_{DS}}\Big|_{Q,VGS=const.} \text{ Siemens} \tag{2.77}$$

To model the upward slope of the $i_D = f(v_{GS}, v_{DS})$ curve family, choose a voltage V_x such that

$$I_D \cong I_{DSS}(1 - V_{GS}/V_P)^2(1 - V_{DS}/V_x) \text{ for } V_{DS} > |V_{GS} + V_P| \text{ and } |V_{GS}| < |V_P| \tag{2.78}$$

Note that the intercept voltage V_x is typically 25 to 50 V in magnitude. V_x is negative and V_{DS} is positive for *n*-channel JFETs, and V_x is positive and V_{DS} is negative for *p*-channel JFETs. An algebraic expression for g_d can be found by differentiating Equation 2.78:

$$g_d = \frac{\partial I_D}{\partial V_{DS}}\Big|_Q = I_{DSS}(1 - V_{GS}/V_P)^2(-1/V_x) = -(I_{DQ}/V_x) > 0 \tag{2.79}$$

An estimate of V_x can be found by extrapolating the $i_D = f(v_{GS}, v_{DS})$ curves in the saturation region back to the negative V_{SD} axis, as shown in Figure 2.29.

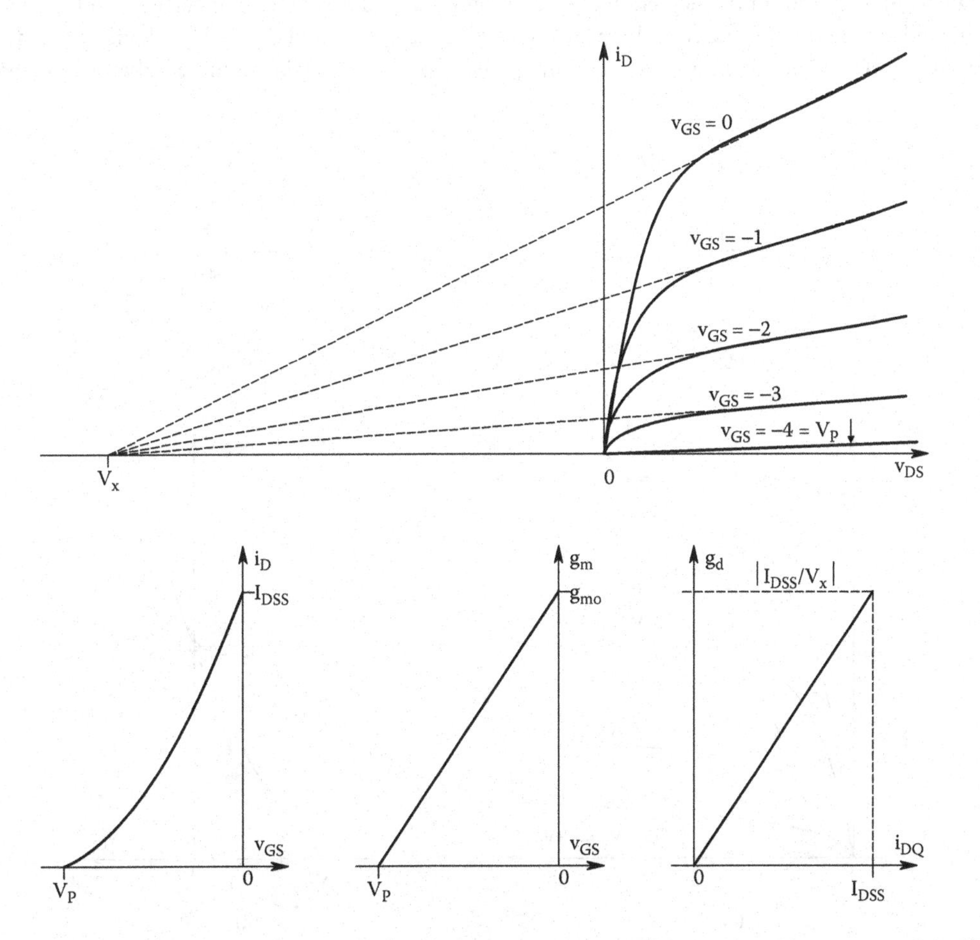

FIGURE 2.29 *Top:* Large-signal i_D vs. v_{DS} curves for an *n*-channel JFET showing the geometry of the FET equivalent of the BJT Early voltage, V_x. *Bottom, left to right:* Small-signal i_D vs. v_{GS} for a saturated channel. Small-signal g_m vs. v_{GS} for a saturated channel. Small-signal Norton drain conductance, g_d vs. i_D for a saturated channel.

The Norton drain-source model shown in Figure 2.28 can be made into a Thevenin model, where the series Thevenin resistance is just $r_d = 1/g_d$, and the open-circuit voltage is given by a VCVS, μv_{GS} (note the sign of the VCVS; *it is the same for both n- and p-channel JFETs*. The voltage gain, μ, is easily seen to be given by

$$\mu = g_m/g_d = g_{mo}\sqrt{(I_{DQ}/I_{DSS})}\left(|V_x/I_{DQ}| = \frac{g_{mo}|V_x|}{\sqrt{I_{DQ}I_{DSS}}}\right) \tag{2.80}$$

μ varies inversely with I_{DQ} in the saturation region of operation. Either the Norton or Thevenin model is valid. Most engineers use the Norton model because manufacturers generally provide V_P, I_{DSS} and g_{mo} for a given JFET.

2.4.3 MOSFET Behavior at Midfrequencies

MOSFETs are also known as *insulated gate field-effect transistors* (IgFETS). The gate electrode is insulated from the channel, hence gate leakage current is on the order of pA or less. Symbols for *n*-channel, *p*-channel and the $i_D = f(v_{GS}, v_{DS})$ curves for an *n-channel depletion MOSFET* are shown in Figure 2.30. In the depletion device, a lightly doped *p*-substrate underlies a lightly doped *n*-channel connecting two heavily doped n-regions for the source and drain. This device has a negative pinch-off voltage (V_P); however, $I_D = I_{DSS}$ when $V_{GS} = 0$, and the saturated channel conducts

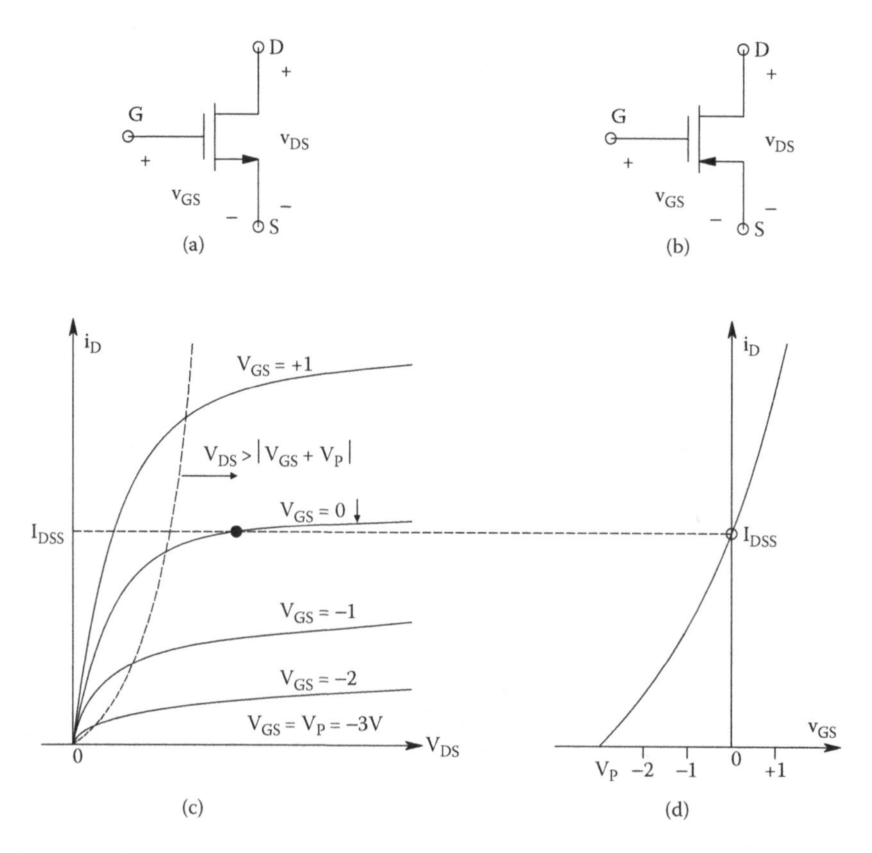

FIGURE 2.30 (a) Symbol for an *n*-channel MOSFET. (b) Symbol for a *p*-channel MOSFET. (c) The $i_D = f(v_{GS}, v_{DS})$ curves for an *n*-channel *depletion* MOSFET. (d) The $i_D = f(v_{GS})$ curve for a saturated-channel, *n*-channel *depletion* MOSFET.

heavily for $V_{GS} > 0$. Similar to the n-channel JFET, one can model the $i_D = f(v_{GS}, v_{DS})$ curves of the depletion *n*-channel MOSFET in the saturation region by

$$i_D = I_{DSS}[1-(v_{GS}/V_P)]^2 \text{ for } v_{DS} > |v_{GS} + V_P| > 0 \tag{2.81}$$

And *in the ohmic region*

$$i_D = I_{DSS}[2(1+(v_{GS}/V_P)(v_{DS}/V_P) - (v_{DS}/V_P)^2] \text{ for } 0 < v_{DS} < |v_{GS} + V_P| \tag{2.82}$$

When the $i_D = f(v_{GS}, v_{DS})$ curves of the *enhancement n-channel MOSFET*, shown in Figure 2.31, are considered it is seen that there is no I_{DSS} for this family of device. Channel cut-off occurs at a *threshold voltage*, $v_{GS} = V_T$, where i_D reaches some defined low value, e.g., 10 μA. The mathematical model for n-channel, enhancement MOSFET $i_D = f(v_{GS}, v_{DS})$ in the saturation region is

$$i_D = K(v_{GS} - V_T)^2 = K V_T^2(1 - v_{GS}/V_T)^2 \text{ for } 0 < |v_{GS} - V_T| < |v_{DS} \tag{2.83}$$

In the ohmic channel operating region, i_D is given by

$$i_D = K[2(v_{GS} - V_T)v_{DS} - v_{DS}^2] \text{ for } 0 < |v_{DS}| < |v_{GS} - V_T| \tag{2.84}$$

The line separating the saturated- and ohmic-channel regions is

$$I_{DB} = K V_{DS}^2 \tag{2.85}$$

p-channel MOSFETs have $i_D = f(v_{GS}, v_{DS})$ curves with the signs opposite those for *n*-channel devices. It is easy to see from Equation 2.73 which defines the small-signal transconductance and Equation 2.72 which defines the small-signal drain conductance, that all FETs (JFETs, MOSFETs, *n*-channel, *p*-channel, enhancement, depletion) have the same parsimonious MFSSM. This is a case of electronic serendipity.

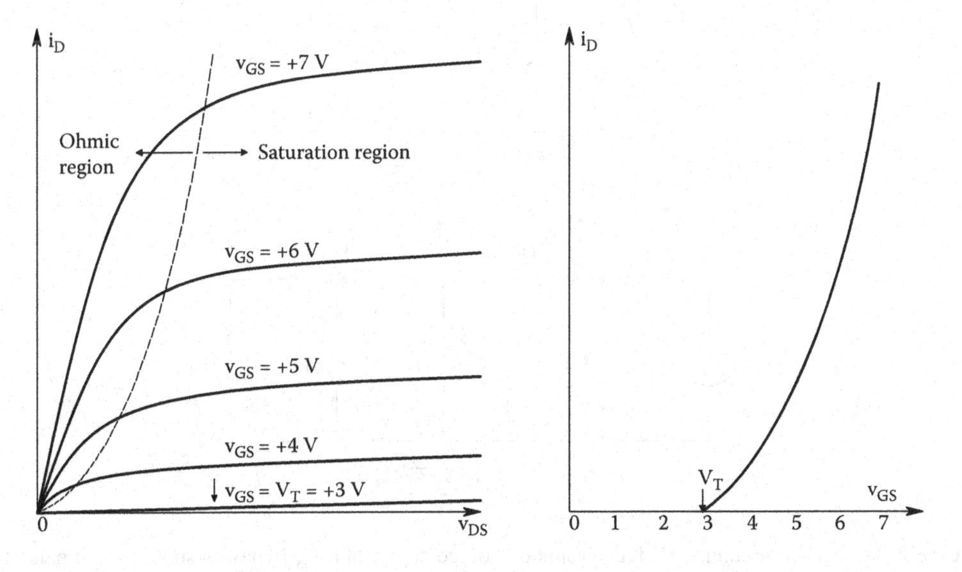

FIGURE 2.31 *Left:* The $i_D = f(v_{GS}, v_{DS})$ curves for an *n*-channel *enhancement* MOSFET. *Right:* The $i_D = f(v_{GS})$ curve for a saturated-channel, *n*-channel *enhancement* MOSFET.

2.4.4 Basic, Midfrequency, Single FET Amplifiers

Just as in the case of BJTs, there are so-called grounded source amplifiers, grounded gate amplifiers, and source-followers. The small-signal voltage gain of each if these amplifiers, as well as their input and output resistances will be found. First, examine a JFET grounded-source (G-S) amplifier, shown in Figure 2.32. At midfrequencies, treat the external coupling and bypass capacitors as short-circuits. Thus, the source is at small-signal ground, hence $v_s = 0$. The amplifier's midfrequency gain is found from the node equation:

$$v_o[G_D + g_d] = -g_m v_{gs} = -g_m v_1 \tag{2.86}$$

$$\downarrow$$

$$K_v = \frac{v_o}{v_1} = \frac{-g_m r_d R_D}{R_D + r_d} \tag{2.87}$$

From inspection of the MFSSM of the circuit, $R_{in} \to \infty$ and $R_{out} = R_D r_d/(R_D + r_d)$.

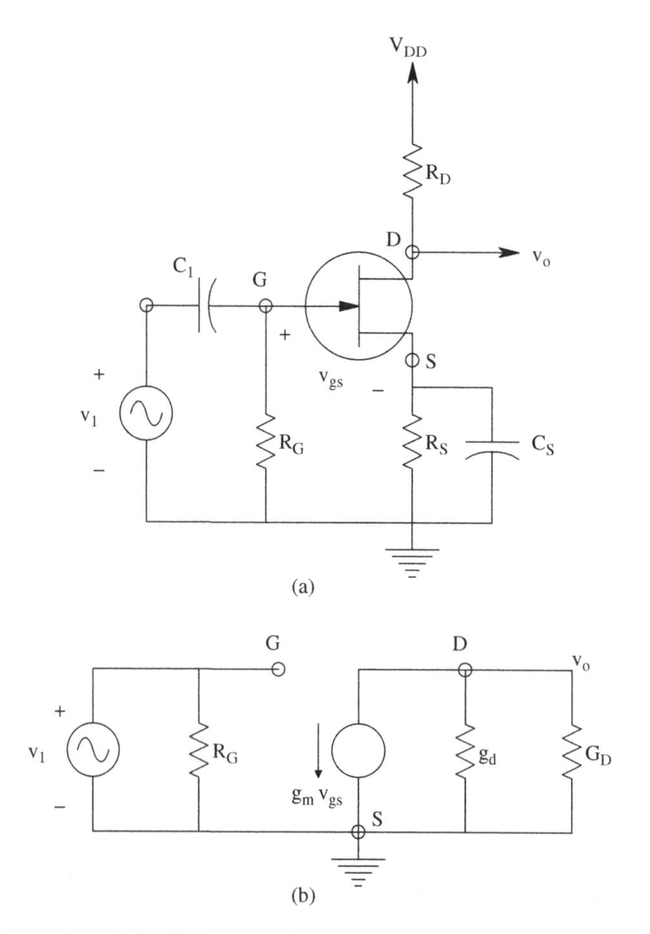

FIGURE 2.32 (a) An *n*-channel JFET "grounded source" amplifier. C_S bypasses small AC signals at the JFET's source to ground, making $v_s = 0$. (b) MFSSM of the amplifier. The same MFSSM would obtain if a *p*-channel JFET were used.

Next, consider an n-channel MOSFET grounded-gate amplifier at mid frequencies. The electrical circuit and its MFSSM are shown in Figure 2.33. Two node equations are written, one for the v_s node and the other for the drain (output) node.

$$v_s[G_S + g_d + g_m] - v_o[g_d] = v_1 G_S \tag{2.88a}$$

$$-v_s[g_d + g_m] + v_o[g_d + G_D] = 0 \tag{2.88b}$$

Using Cramer's rule, one finds

$$\Delta = G_S g_d + G_D[G_S + g_d + g_m] \tag{2.89}$$

$$\frac{v_s}{v_1} = \frac{R_D + r_d}{R_D + r_d + R_S(1 + g_m r_d)} \tag{2.90}$$

$$\frac{v_o}{v_1} = \frac{R_D(1 + g_m r_d)}{R_D + r_d + R_S(1 + g_m r_d)} = K_v \tag{2.91}$$

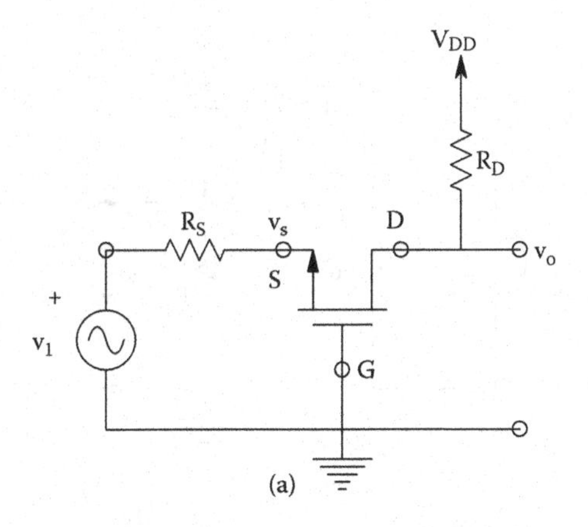

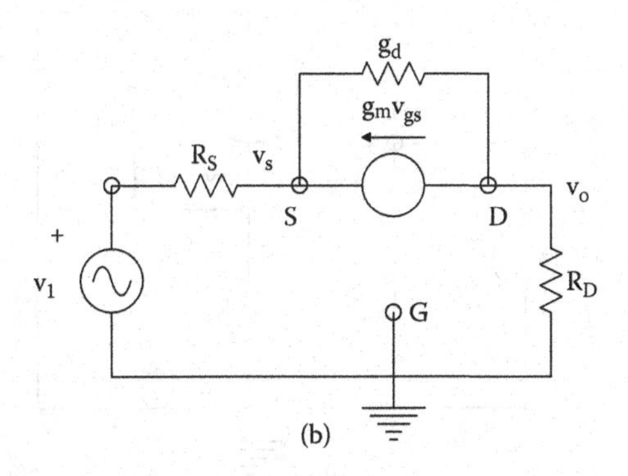

FIGURE 2.33 (a) An n-channel MOSFET grounded-gate amplifier. (b) MFSSM of the MOSFET G-G amplifier. See Text for analysis.

The input resistance, R_{in}, of the MOSFET GG-amplifier is found from

$$R_{in} = \frac{v_1}{i_s} = \frac{v_1 R_S}{v_1(1 - v_s/v_1)} = \frac{R_S}{1 - \dfrac{R_D + r_D}{R_D + r_d + R_S(1 + g_m r_d)}} = R_S + \frac{R_D + r_D}{(1 + g_m r_d)} \tag{2.92}$$

R_{out} is approximately R_D for the GG amplifier.

Finally, examine the MOSFET source-follower (S-F) amplifier at midfrequencies. The circuit and its MFSSM are shown in Figure 2.34. This an easy circuit to analyze because the drain is at small-signal (s-s) ground. The output node equation is

$$v_o[G_C + g_d + g_m] = g_m v_1 \tag{2.93}$$

Equation 2.93 leads to the S-F amplifier's gain

$$K_v = \frac{v_o}{v_1} = \frac{R_D g_m r_d}{r_d + R_D(1 + g_m r_d)} < 1 \tag{2.94}$$

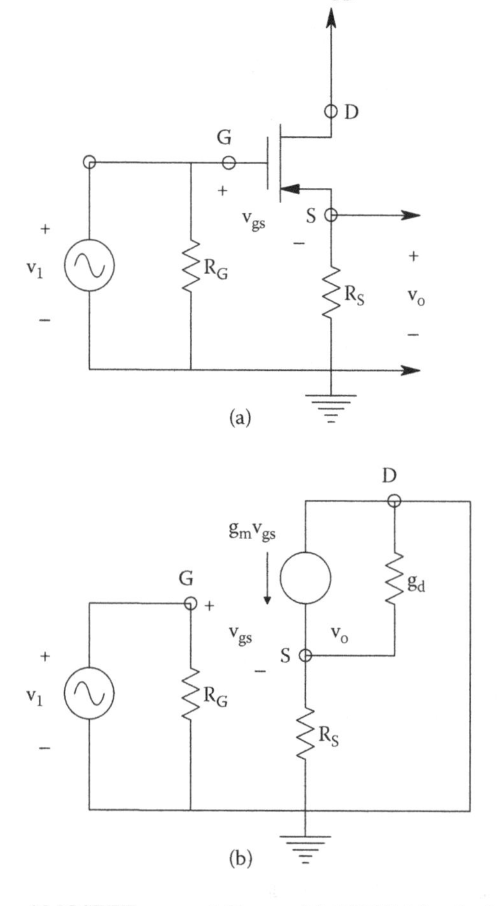

FIGURE 2.34 (a) A *p*-channel MOSFET source follower. (b) MFSSM for the MOSFET S-F.

By inspection, $R_{in} \rightarrow \infty$, And R_{out} can be found by v_{oc}/i_{sc}:

$$R_{out} = \frac{v_{oc}}{i_{sc}} = \frac{\dfrac{v_1 R_D g_m r_d}{r_d + R_D(1+g_m r_d)}}{g_m v_1} = \frac{R_D r_d/(1+g_m r_d)}{R_D + r_d/(1+g_m + r_d)} \tag{2.95}$$

Single FET amplifiers generally have higher R_{in}s, about the same R_{out}s, less gain, and more even harmonic distortion than equivalent BJT amplifiers.

2.4.5 Simple Amplifiers Using Two FETs at Midfrequencies

As seen in the case of BJTs, certain basic building blocks for analog ICs can be made from two transistors. Figure 2.35 illustrates four such circuits using field-effect transistors. Notably absent is the difference amplifier; because of its great importance in analog electronic circuits, the DA is treated separately in Chapter 3 of this text. Figure 2.35a illustrates a "Darlington" amplifier in which the input transistor is an n-channel MOSFET acting as a voltage-control-led current source

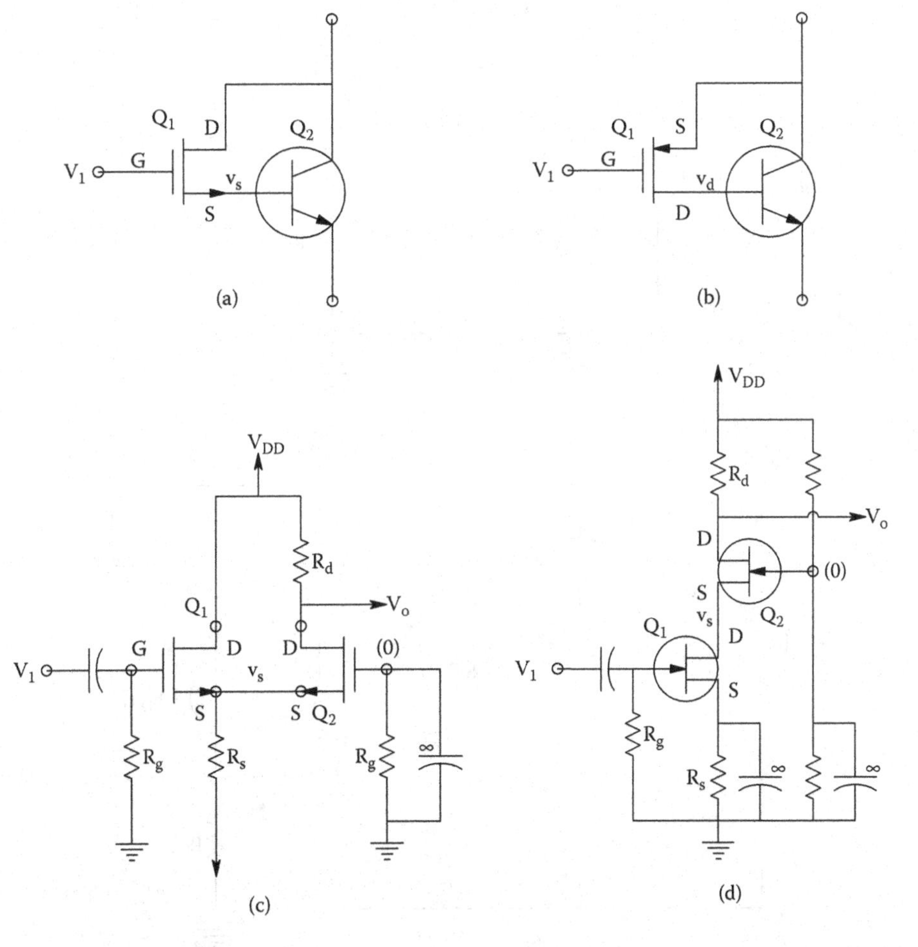

FIGURE 2.35 (a) An *n*-channel MOSFET/*npn* BJT "Darlington" configuration. (b) A *p*-channel MOSFET/*npn* BJT feedback pair configuration. (c) An *n*-channel MOSFET source-follower/grounded-gate amplifier. (d) An *n*-channel JFET cascode amplifier.

driving the base of a power *npn* BJT. Figure 2.35b shows the FET-BJT equivalent for the "feedback pair" power amplifier. Figure 2.35c illustrates a source-follower / grounded-gate high-frequency amplifier, and a FET–FET cascode amplifier is shown in Figure 2.35d.

First, examine the gain of the FET/BJT "Darlington" connected as an emitter-follower. This circuit and its MFSSM are shown in Figure 2.36. Analysis begins by writing the node equations for the v_s and v_o nodes: Note that $i_b = g_{ie}(v_s - v_o)$, $v_{gs} = v_1 - v_s$, $\mu = g_m r_d$, and $g_{ie} = 1/h_{ie}$:

$$v_s[g_d + g_{ie} + g_m] - v_o g_{ie} = v_1 g_m \tag{2.96a}$$

$$-v_s[g_{ie}(1 + h_{fe})] + v_o[g_{ie}(1 + h_{fe}) + G_E] = 0 \tag{2.96b}$$

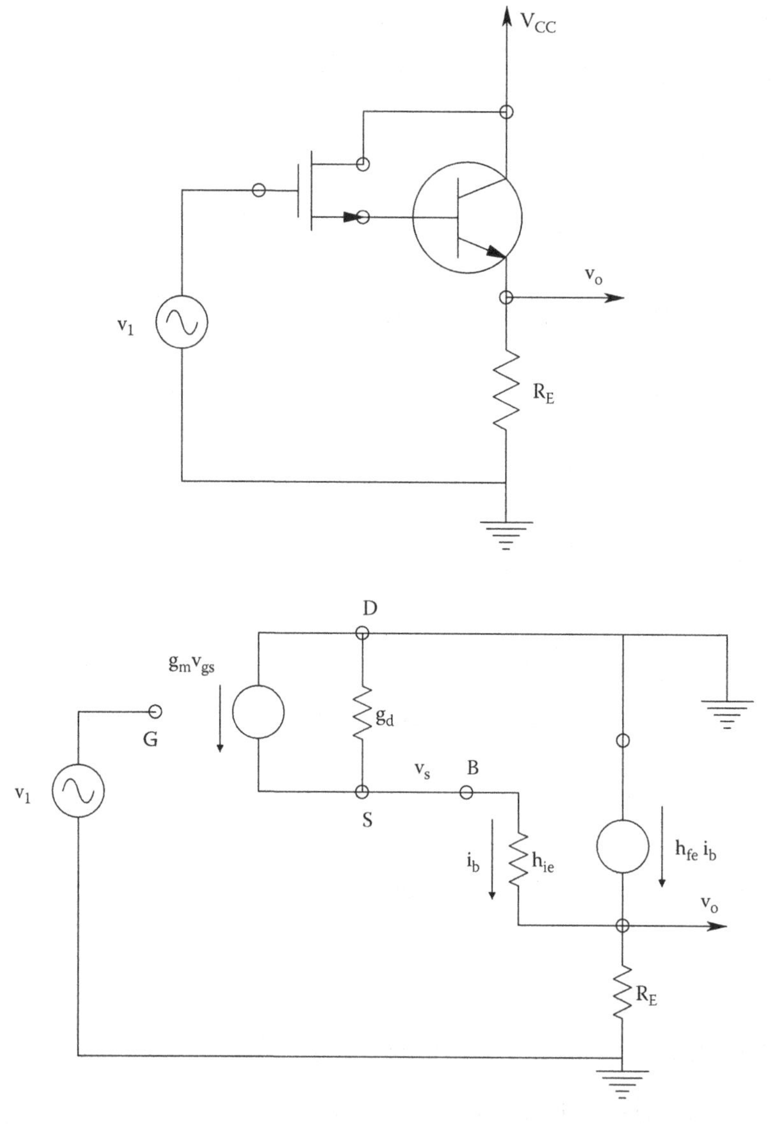

FIGURE 2.36 *Top:* A MOSFET/BJT "Darlington" connected as an emitter follower. *Bottom:* MFSSM of the Darlington EF. See analysis in Text.

Using Cramer's rule, one finds

$$\Delta = (g_d + g_m)g_{ie}(1 + h_{fe}) + G_E(g_d + g_{ie} + g_m) \tag{2.97}$$

$$\Delta v_o = v_1 g_m g_{ie}(1 + h_{fe}) \tag{2.98}$$

Solving for v_o/v_1, one finds

$$\frac{v_o}{v_1} = \frac{R_E(1 + h_{fe})\mu}{R_E(1 + h_{fe})(1 + \mu) + h_{ie}(1 + \mu) + r_d} \tag{2.99}$$

As expected, this voltage gain is <1. The amplifier's input resistance is extremely high, and the output resistance can be found by the open-circuit output voltage given by Equation 2.99 above, divided by the short-circuit output current which is simply $i_b(1 + h_{fe})$ for $v_o = 0$, ($R_{out} = OCV/SCC$). R_{out} is on the order of single ohms.

Next, find the gain for the FET/BJT feedback pair amplifier shown in Figure 2.35b. The node equations are

$$v_d[g_d + g_{ie}] - v_o[g_{ie}] = -v_1 g_m \tag{2.100a}$$

$$-v_d[g_{ie}(1 + h_{fe})] + v_o[G_E + g_{ie}(1 + h_{fe})] = 0 \tag{2.100b}$$

Using Cramer's rule one finds

$$\Delta = g_d[G_E + g_{ie}(1 + h_{fe})] + g_{ie}G_E \tag{2.101}$$

$$\Delta v_o = -v_1 g_m g_{ie}(1 + h_{fe}) \tag{2.102}$$

From which the midfrequency voltage gain is found:

$$\frac{v_o}{v_1} = \frac{-R_E\mu\ (1 + h_{fe})}{R_E(1 + h_{fe}) + h_{ie} + r_d} = \frac{\mu R_E}{R_E + (h_{ie} + r_d)/(1 + h_{fe})} = K_v \tag{2.103}$$

Again, R_{in} is very high because of the MOSFET, and R_{out} can be found from $R_{out} = OCV/SCC$. It can be shown that R_{out} is R_E in parallel with $(h_{ie} + r_d)/(1 + h_{fe})$ ohms.

The MFSSM of the FET/FET SF-GG amplifier of Figure 2.35c is shown in Figure 2.37. Proceeding as before, we write the node equations for v_s and v_o, then use Cramer's rule to find the amplifier's MFSS gain: Note that $v_{gs1} = v_1 - v_s$ and $v_{gs2} = -v_s$:

$$v_s[2(g_d + g_m) + G_S] - v_o[g_d] = g_m v_1 \tag{2.104a}$$

$$-v_s[g_d + g_m] + v_o[G_D + g_d] = 0 \tag{2.104b}$$

$$\Delta = 2G_D(g_d + g_m) + g_d(g_m + G_S) + G_S G_D \tag{2.105}$$

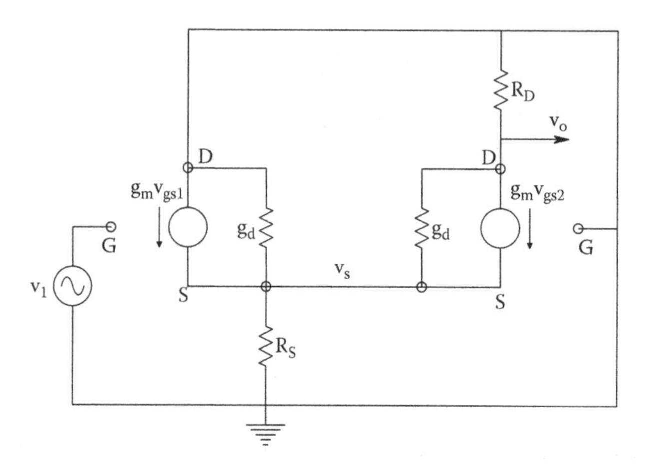

FIGURE 2.37 MFSSM for the two-MOSFET SF/GG amplifier. See Text for analysis.

$$\Delta v_o = v_1 g_m (g_d + g_m) \tag{2.106}$$

The voltage gain is found from Equations 2.105 and 2.106 using Cramer's rule:

$$\frac{v_o}{v_1} = \frac{+R_D \mu}{R_D + 2r_d + r_d(r_d + R_D)/[R_S(1+\mu)]} = K_v \tag{2.107}$$

Note that the gain is noninverting. R_{in} is on the order of 10^{13} Ω, and R_{out} is slightly lower than R_D.

The final 2-FET amplifier considered is the cascode amplifier using two JFETs, shown in Figure 2.35d. The MFSSM of the cascode is shown in Figure 2.38. Note that $v_{gs1} = v_1$, $v_{gs2} = -v_s$, the JFETs are matched, and $\mu \equiv g_m r_d$. The node equations are

$$v_s[2g_d + g_m] - v_o g_d = -g_m v_1 \tag{2.108a}$$

$$-v_s[g_d + g_m] + v_o[G_D + g_d] = 0 \tag{2.108b}$$

$$\Delta = 2g_d G_D + 2g_d^2 + g_m G_D + g_m g_d - g_d^2 - g_m g_d = G_D(2g_d + g_m) + g_d^2 \tag{2.109}$$

$$\Delta v_o = -v_1 g_m [g_d + g_m] \tag{2.110}$$

The cascode amplifier's midfrequency voltage gain is thus found to be

$$\frac{v_o}{v_1} = \frac{-R_D \mu(1+\mu)}{R_D + r_d(1+\mu)} = K_v \tag{2.111}$$

The JFET cascode amplifier's Rin is on the order of gigaohms; its R_{out} is slightly lower than R_D.

Two-transistor amplifiers using FETs generally have very high input resistances, gains that are not as high as equivalent 2-BJT amplifiers and more distortion in the output signal because of the nonlinear $I_D(V_{GS})$ characteristics of all FETs.

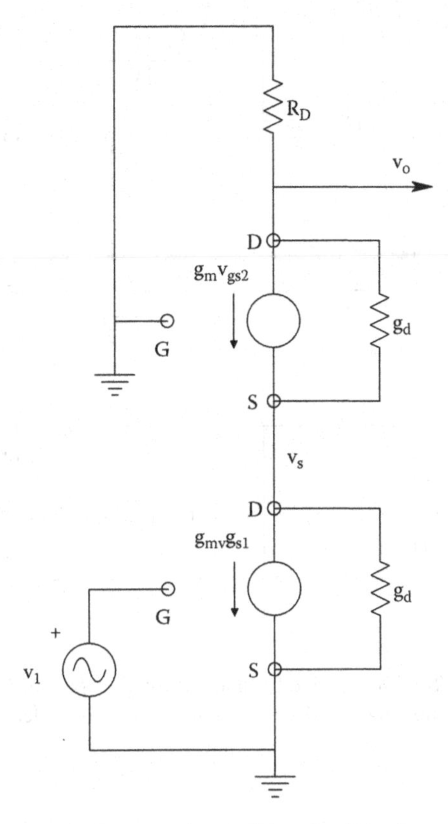

FIGURE 2.38 MFSSM for the two-JFET cascode amplifier. See Text for analysis.

2.5 HIGH-FREQUENCY MODELS FOR TRANSISTORS AND SIMPLE TRANSISTOR AMPLIFIERS

2.5.1 INTRODUCTION

The limitation of the high-frequency bandwidth of all transistor amplifiers can be modeled by small capacitances that shunt the transistor's small-signal model elements either to ground or that connect input to output. High bandwidth is certainly not required for conditioning recorded physiological signals such as the ECG, EMG, EEG, EOG, etc. Such signals require only a low audio bandwidth for faithful reproduction. High bandwidth (into the 10s of MHz) is required for ultrasound signals, both pulsed and CW. Pulse signals from sensors in imaging systems where radioactive emissions are measured (e.g., SPECT, PET, scintimammography) also require amplifiers with bandwidths in the 100s of MHz or higher. Emitted ionizing radiation is detected using scintillation crystal/photomultiplier tube systems or direct semiconductor radiation sensors (Northrop 2002).

A major goal of electronic amplifier design is to develop amplifier designs that overcome certain basic limitations on high-frequency bandwidth. A major limitation on high-frequency response is caused by the *Miller effect*. In the Miller effect, a small-signal parasitic capacitor couples the inverting output of an ideal VCVS amplifier to its input. The circuit is shown in Figure 2.39a. Clearly, $V_o = -\mu_{Vg}$, (the amplifier is inverting). Feedback to the input node is through the parasitic capacitance, C_{io}, (normally ca. 1–3 pF in small-signal transistors). A node equation is written on the V_g node:

$$V_g[G_s + j\omega\, C_{io}] - V_o j\omega\, C_{io} = G_s V_s \tag{2.112}$$

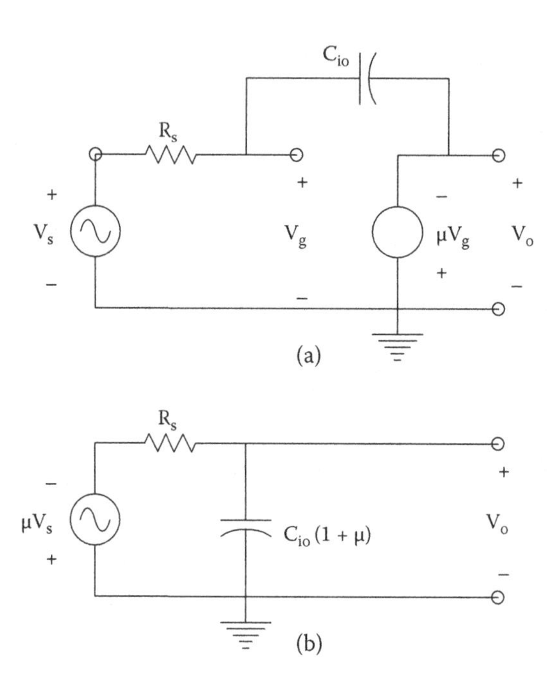

FIGURE 2.39 (a) Simple VCVS with negative feedback through capacitor C_{io} illustrating the cause of the Miller effect. (b) Simple circuit showing the Miller capacitor of the equivalent input low-pass filter. See Text for analysis.

from which one finds the frequency response function

$$\frac{V_o}{V_s}(j\omega) = \frac{-\mu}{1 + j\ C_{io}(1+\mu)R_s} \tag{2.113}$$

Equation 2.113 is the frequency response function of an equivalent, simple, R-C, low-pass filter shown in Figure 2.39b. Note that the equivalent capacitor shunting the V_g node to ground is (1 *minus* the voltage gain) times the parasitic feedback capacitor, C_{io}. This high-frequency attenuation of the input signal due to C_{io} is the *Miller effect.*

When the ideal, inverting VCVS is replaced by a Thevenin equivalent, as shown in Figure 2.40, the effect of C_{io} is more complex. Now two node equations must be written as

$$V_g[G_s + j\omega C_{io}] - V_o j\omega C_{io} = V_s G_s \tag{2.114a}$$

$$-V_g[j\omega C_{io} - \mu G_o] + V_o[G_o + j\omega C_{io}] = 0 \tag{2.114b}$$

Cramer's rule is used to solve for V_g and V_o:

$$\Delta = \begin{vmatrix} [G_s + j\omega C_{io} & -j\omega C_{io} \\ -[j\omega C_{io} - \mu G_o] & [G_o + j\omega C_{io} \end{vmatrix} = G_s G_o + j\omega C_{io}[G_s + G_o(1+\mu)] \tag{2.115}$$

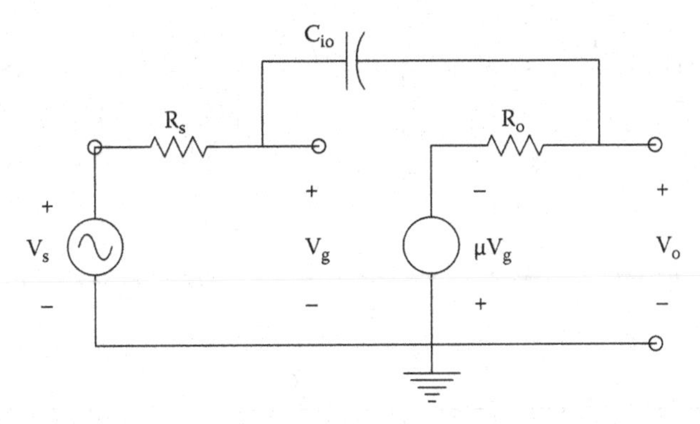

FIGURE 2.40 Another circuit illustrating the Miller effect; the effect of an output resistance is included.

$$\Delta V_o = V_s G_s [j\omega C_{io} - \mu G_o] \tag{2.116}$$

$$\Delta V_g = V_s G_s [j\omega C_{io} + G_o] \tag{2.117}$$

Thus,

$$\frac{V_o}{V_s}(j\omega) = \frac{-\mu[1 - j\omega C_{io} R_o / \mu]}{1 + j\omega C_{io}[(1+\mu)R_s + R_o]} \tag{2.118}$$

and

$$\frac{V_g}{V_s}(j\omega) = \frac{1 + j\omega C_{io} R_o}{1 + j\omega C_{io}[(1+\mu)R_s + R_o]} \tag{2.119}$$

From Equation 2.118 above, it can be seen that the break frequency of the pole still depends inversely on the Miller capacitance in the input circuit, $C_M \equiv C_{io}(1 + \mu)$. The Thevenin output resistance also contributes to the amplifier's time-constant. Note that the larger the gain magnitude, μ, the lower the break frequency. This property suggests a trade-off between gain and amplifier high-frequency bandwidth, called the *gain-bandwidth product* (GBWP). More will be said concerning the GBWP in the sections below.

Both BJTs and the various types of FETs have parasitic capacitances between the input and output nodes and ground, and between the input and output nodes (the latter able to form the evil Miller capacitance). In the following sections, the high-frequency SSMs for BJTs and FETs, and also the behavior of the three major, single-BJT amplifiers (the grounded-emitter, the grounded base, and the emitter-follower), and also the three major, single FET amplifiers (the grounded-source, the grounded-gate and the source-follower) will be examined.

2.5.2 High-Frequency SSMs for BJTs and FETs

The simplified, *hybrid-pi* (hy-pi) high-frequency, small-signal model (HFSSM) is widely used to model and predict the high-frequency behavior of both *npn* and *pnp* BJTs. The hy-pi model is illustrated in Figure 2.41a. The capacitance, C_μ, is largely due to the depletion capacitance of the normally reverse-biased, collector-base junction, and thus is voltage-dependent. The capacitance,

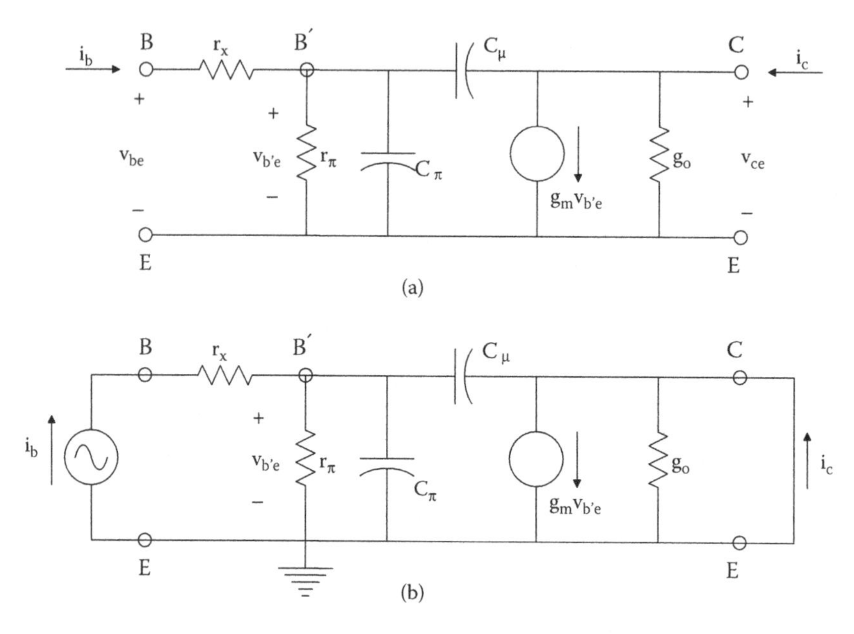

FIGURE 2.41 (a) The hybrid-pi, high-frequency SSM for a BJT. A common-emitter configuration is assumed. (b) A hy-pi HFSSM circuit used to calculate a BJT's complex short-circuit output current gain, $h_{fe}(j\omega)$, and f_T where $|h_{fe}(j2\pi f_T)| = 1$.

C_π, is the capacitance of the forward-biased, base-emitter junction, and its value can be considered to be dependent on the total emitter current. Note that the hy-pi SSM uses a Norton model for the BJT's collector–emitter port. The output conductance, g_o, can be related to the BJT's midfrequency, *h*-parameter, SSM by $g_o \cong (h_{oe} - g_m h_{re})$ (Northrop 1990). The VCCS has a small-signal transconductance, gm, given by

$$g_m = \left.\frac{\partial i_c}{\partial v_{b'c}}\right|_{v_{ce}=0} \cong \frac{h_{fe}}{r_x} = \frac{|I_{CQ}|}{V_T} \tag{2.120}$$

The g_m of BJTs is large compared with FETs, and depends on the DC operating point of the device; for example, if $I_{CQ} = 1$ mA, $g_m \cong 0.04$ S. g_m is measured under small-signal, short-circuit, collector–emitter conditions.

An important BJT parameter is its f_T, the frequency at which $|h_{fe}| = 1$. Recall that

$$h_{fe} = \left.\frac{\partial i_c}{\partial i_b}\right|_{v_{ce}=0} \tag{2.121}$$

When i_b and i_c are sine waves, h_{fe} can be written as a complex (vector) function of frequency

$$h_{fe}(j\omega) = \left.\frac{I_c}{I_b}(j\omega)\right|_{V_{ce}=0} \tag{2.122}$$

Thus, by definition of f_T, one has

$$|h_{fe}(j2\pi f_T)| \equiv 1 \tag{2.123}$$

To develop an expression for f_T in terms of the hy-pi SSM parameters, consider the model shown in Figure 2.41b. Because of the small-signal short-circuit conditions on the model, the collector current is

$$I_c(j\omega) = g_m V_{b'e} - j\omega C_\mu V_{b'e} \tag{2.124}$$

$V_{b'e}$ is found by writing a node equation on the B′ node. It is

$$V_{b'e} = \frac{I_b}{g_\pi + j\omega(C_\pi + C_\mu)} \tag{2.125}$$

Substituting Equation 2.125 into Equation 2.124, we obtain the final result for $h_{fe}(j\omega)$:

$$h_{fe}(j\omega) = \left.\frac{I_c}{I_b}(j\omega)\right|_{V_{ce}=0} = \frac{h_{fe}(0)}{1 + j\omega r_x(C_\pi + C_\mu)} \tag{2.126}$$

$h_{fe}(0)$ is the low- and midfrequency, common-emitter, h-parameter current gain, also known as the BJT's beta. Set the magnitude of the expression of Equation 2.126 equal to unity and solve for f_T:

$$f_T = \frac{g_m}{2\pi(C_\pi + C_\mu)} = \frac{h_{fe}(0)}{2\pi(C_\pi + C_\mu)r_\pi} = \frac{|I_{CQ}|}{2\pi(C_\pi + C_\mu)V_T}\ \text{Hz} \tag{2.127}$$

Thus, the f_T frequency for unity current gain magnitude is seen to be a function of both C_π and C_μ, as well as the BJT's Q-point. A Bode magnitude plot of $h_{fe}(j\omega)$ vs. ω is shown in Figure 2.42. Note that $h_{fe}(j\omega)$ has a (current) gain-bandwidth product. This is easily written from Equation 2.126:

$$\text{GBWP} = \frac{h_{fe}(0)}{2\pi r_\pi(C_\pi + C_\mu)}\ \text{Hz} \tag{2.128}$$

Note that the h_{fe} GBWP = f_T.

It is important to note that the hy-pi HFSSM is generally valid for frequencies below f_T /3. To examine high-frequency BJT circuit behavior above f_T/3, one must use *SPICE* or MicroCap™ computer simulations which use more detailed, nonlinear BJT models that include effects such as carrier transit times, charge storage, and how C_π changes with V_{CB}, etc.

A simple, linear, fixed-parameter model for FET high-frequency behavior is shown in Figure 2.43. For simple modeling of FET amplifier high-frequency response, the three voltage-dependent capacitances, C_{gs}, C_{gd}, and C_{ds}, are assigned values determined from the FET's quiescent operating point. Manufacturers of discrete FETs generally do not give specific values for C_{gs}, C_{gd}, and C_{ds}; instead they specify C_{iss}, the common-source, short-circuit input capacitance measured with $v_{ds} = 0$

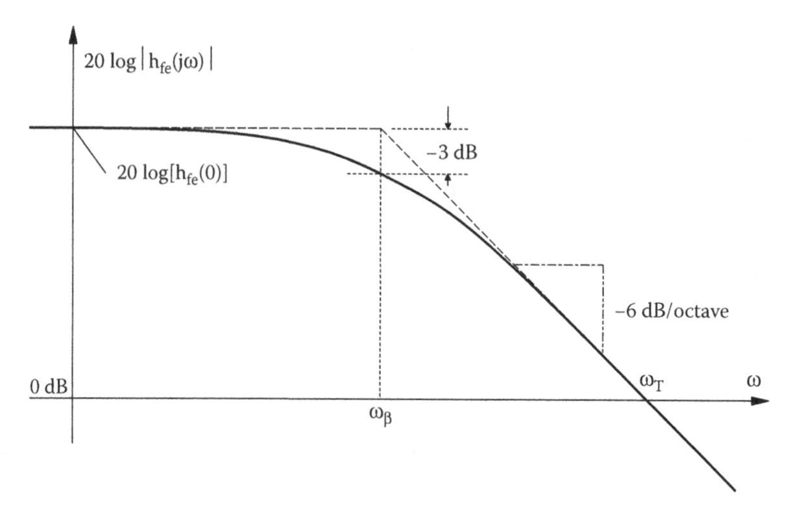

FIGURE 2.42 Bode frequency response magnitude of $|h_{fe}(j\omega)|$.

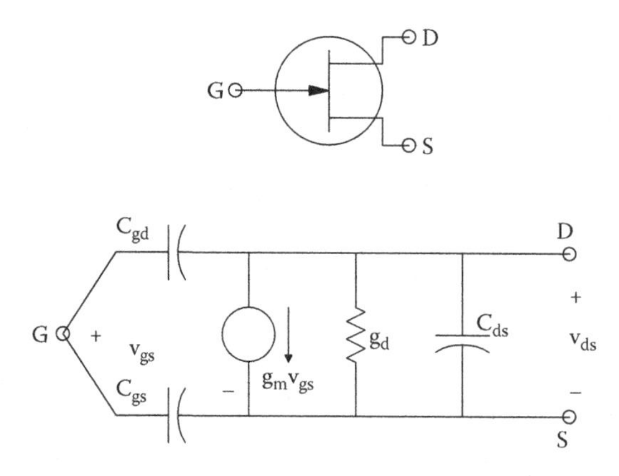

FIGURE 2.43 A simple, fixed parameter, HFSSM for *all* FETs. In JFETs in particular, C_{gd} and C_{gs} are voltage-dependent. Their values at the Q-point must be used.

(small-signal drain-source voltage = 0). From inspection of the FET HFSSM, it is obvious that $C_{iss} = C_{gd} + C_{gs}$, at some specific Q-point. Also given by manufacturers is C_{rss}, the reverse transfer capacitance measured with $v_{gs} = 0$. From the HFSSM, it is also obvious that $C_{rss} = C_{ds} + C_{gd}$. In general, $C_{gd} >> C_{ds}$, so $C_{rss} \cong C_{gd}$, and $C_{gs} \cong C_{iss} - C_{rss}$.

At VHF and UHF frequencies, the simple HFSSM of Figure 2.43 is no longer valid, and a two-port, *y*-parameter model is commonly used for computer modeling in which the four *y*-parameters are frequency-dependent. The y-parameter model is illustrated in Figure 2.44. Note that this a Norton 2-port. In general, $y_{fs}(j\omega) = g_{fs} + jx_{fs}$, and at mid- and low-frequencies, $y_{fs} = g_{fs} = g_m$, $y_{rs} \rightarrow 0$, $y_{is} \rightarrow 0$, and $y_{os} = g_d$ S.

FETs are characterized by a maximum operating frequency, f_{max}, at which the small-signal current magnitude into the gate node, $I_g(j\omega)$, equals the current magnitude, $|y_{fs} V_{gs}|$ with $v_{ds} = 0$. From the VHFSS y-model of Figure 2.44, it is clear that f_{max} satisfies

$$V_{gs}|y_{is}(j2\pi f_{max})| = V_{gs}|y_{fs}(j2\pi f_{max})| \tag{2.129}$$

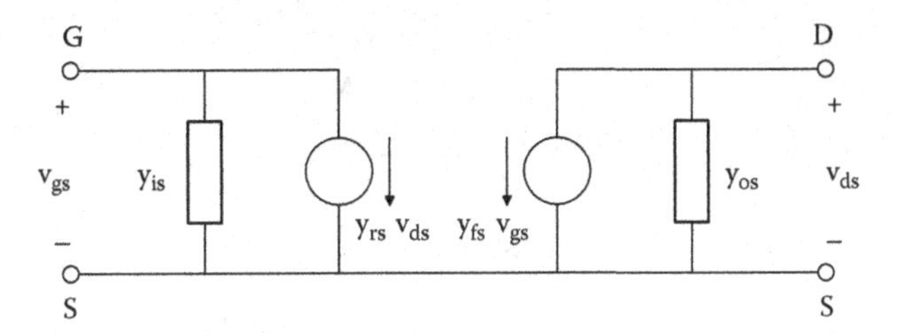

FIGURE 2.44 The more general, *y*-parameter HFSSM for FETs.

It is easily seen from the fixed-parameter, HFSSM of Figure 2.43, that

$$f_{max} \cong \frac{g_m}{2\pi C_{iss}} \tag{2.130}$$

Note that f_{max} is a *device* figure of merit, not a *circuit* figure of merit. The unity gain frequency for a grounded-source or grounded gate FET amplifier is apt to be lower than f_{max} because of the Miller effect and capacitive loading, etc.

2.5.3 Behavior of One-BJT and One-FET Amplifiers at High Frequencies

Figure 2.45a illustrates a simple, "grounded-emitter" (G-E) BJT amplifier. Note that the emitter is not actually grounded, but tied to ground through a parallel R_E,C_E. R_E provides temperature stabilization of the BJT's DC operating point; C_E bypasses the emitter to ground at signal frequencies, putting the emitter at small-signal ground. Figure 2.45b illustrates the HFSSM of the circuit. Note that some output capacitance is generally present; it has been omitted in the model for algebraic simplicity. The base spreading resistance, r_x, has also been eliminated so that there are two, rather than three node equations governing the amplifier's HF behavior. To analyze the circuit, begin by writing the phasor node equations for the V_b and V_o nodes:

$$V_b[G_s + g_\pi + j\omega(C_\pi + C_\mu)] + V_o[j\omega C_\mu] = V_s G_s \tag{2.131a}$$

$$-V_b[j\omega C_\mu - g_m] + V_o[j\omega C_\mu + G_c] = 0 \tag{2.131b}$$

Using Cramer's rule and a good deal of algebra, the mid- and high-frequency response function for the amplifier in time-constant form is found to be

$$\frac{\mathbf{V_o}}{\mathbf{V_s}}(j\omega) = \frac{-g_m R_C[r_\pi/(R_s + r_\pi)](1 - j\omega C_\mu/g_m)}{[1 - \omega^2 C_\mu C_\pi R_C(R_s r_\pi/(R_s + r_\pi))] + j\omega[C_\pi(R_s r_\pi/(R_s + r_\pi)) + C_\mu R_C + C_\mu(1 + g_m R_C)(R_s r_\pi/(R_s + r_\pi))]} \tag{2.132}$$

Note that this quadratic frequency response function has a zero at $\omega = g_m/C_\mu$ r/s, which is well above the BJT's ω_T, where the results predicted by the hy-pi model are no longer valid. It is therefore prudent to neglect the $(1 - j\omega C_\mu/g_m)$ term. Without the $(1 - j\omega C_\mu/g_m)$ term, the frequency response function is that of a second-order low-pass filter. The Miller capacitance is equal to $C_\mu(1 + g_m R_C)$; its presence provides a significant reduction of the amplifier's high-frequency – 3dB point.

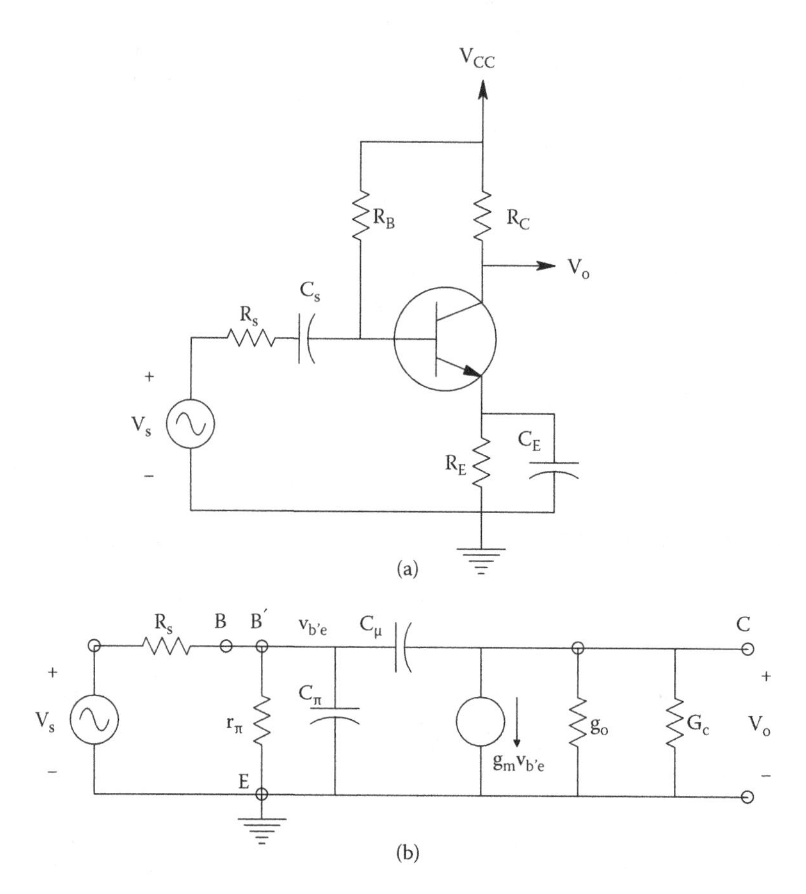

FIGURE 2.45 (a) A basic BJT grounded emitter amplifier; the emitter is assumed to be at small-signal ground at mid- and high-frequencies. (b) Hybrid-pi HFSSM for the amplifier. Note Cμ makes a Miller feedback path between the output node and the $v_{b'e}$ node.

A numerical evaluation of Equation 2.132 for the grounded-emitter BJT amplifier's frequency response is useful to appreciate its practical behavior. Let: $g_m = 0.01$ S, $r_\pi = 1.5$ kΩ, $R_C = 10^4$ Ω, $R_s = 1$ kΩ, $C_\pi = 20$ pF, $C_\mu = 2$ pF, $g_o = 0$ S, and $r_x = 0$. The zero is found to be at $\omega_o = g_m / C_\mu = 5 \times 10^9$ r/s, well over the amplifier's ω_T, which is found to be 4.55×10^8 r/s. Thus, the zero is ignored. The denominator is factored with MATLAB™ and is found to have two real poles: one at $\omega_1 = 6.60 \times 10^6$ r/s, the other at $\omega_2 = 6.32 \times 10^8$ r/s. ω_2 is also well-over $\omega_T/3$, and can be neglected. The midfrequency gain is $A_{vo} = -60$, and the Miller capacitance is $C_M = C_\mu\,(1 + g_m R_C) = 202$ pF. Finally, the G-E amplifier's high-frequency response function can be approximated by a one-pole, LPF frequency response:

$$\frac{V_o}{V_s}(j\omega) \cong \frac{-60.0}{(1 + j\omega/6.60 \times 10^6)} \tag{2.133}$$

The Hz –3 dB break frequency is $f_x = 6.60 \times 10^6 / 2\pi = 1.05$ MHz, not really very high. Recall that the amplifier's GBWP tends to remain constant. Hence to estimate f_x, we can divide the BJT's f_T by its midfrequency gain: $f_x = 7.24 \times 10^7 / 60 = 1.21 \times 10^6$ Hz. (Slightly higher than f_x, but in the same range.)

The next single-BJT amplifier circuit to be considered is the grounded-base amplifier, shown in Figure 2.46a and b. In the preceding treatment of the BJT G-E amplifier, it was seen that feedback from the collector to the base coupled through the small-signal, collector-to-base capacitance,

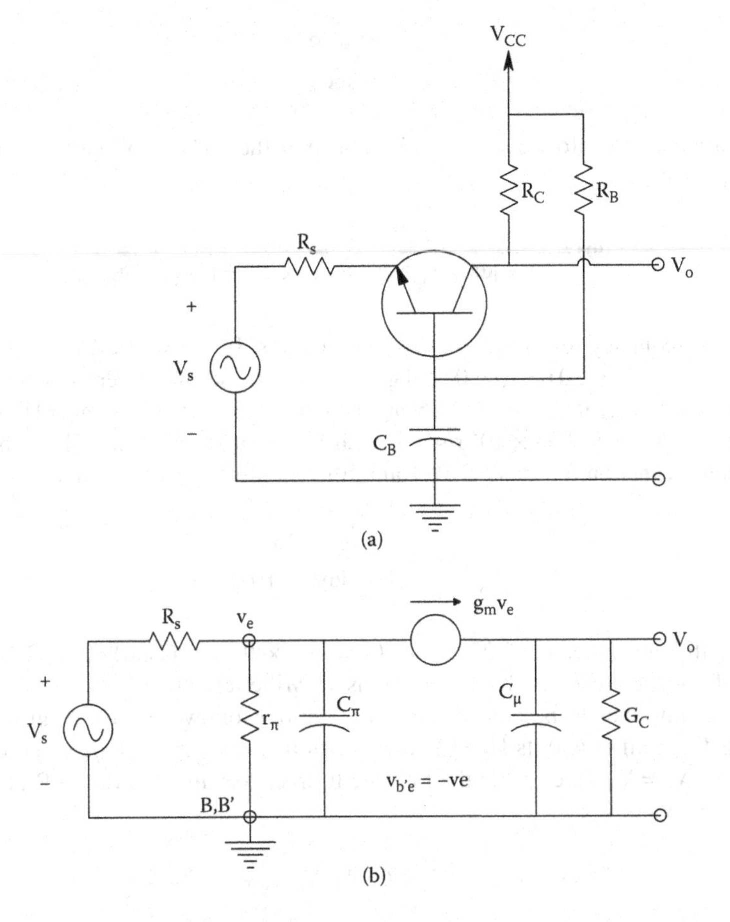

FIGURE 2.46 (a) A BJT grounded base amplifier. (b) The HFSSM for the amplifier. Note the model does not have a Miller feedback capacitor.

C_μ, gave rise to the Miller effect that caused a lowered high-frequency response. It will be shown that in the grounded-base (G-B) amplifier, no such feedback occurs, and there is no Miller effect. Consequently, a G-B amplifier's high-frequency response is generally better than that for a G-E amplifier, other conditions being equal.

To begin the analysis of the G-B amplifier, note that the transistor's base is bypassed to ground, causing the small-signal $v_b = 0$. Thus, $V_{b'e} = V_{be} = V_b - V_e = V_e$. Assume r_x and $g_o = 0$ for algebraic simplicity. Using the hybrid-pi HFSSM for the BJT, write node equations for the V_e and V_o nodes:

$$V_e[G_s + g_\pi + g_m + j\omega C_\pi] = V_s G_s \tag{2.134a}$$

$$V_o[G_C + j\omega C_\mu] - V_e g_m = 0 \tag{2.134b}$$

Note that the two node equations are independent. Thus, it is simple to write

$$V_e = \frac{V_s}{1 + R_s(g_\pi + g_m) + j\omega C_\pi R_s} \tag{2.135}$$

$$V_o = \frac{V_e g_m R_C}{1 + j\omega C_\mu R_C} \tag{2.136}$$

Substitute Equation 2.135 into Equation 2.136, and find the G-B amplifier's frequency response function:

$$\frac{V_o}{V_s}(j\omega) = \frac{g_m R_C/[1 + R_s(g_\pi + g_m)]}{(1 + j\omega C_\mu R_C)\{1 + j\omega C_\pi R_s/[1 + R_s(g_\pi + g_m)]\}} \tag{2.137}$$

Now evaluate the frequency response function's parameters: Let $R_s = 200\ \Omega$, $r_\pi = 2\ k\Omega$, $g_m = 0.01$, $R_C = 10^4\ \Omega$, $C_\mu = 2$ pF, $C_\pi = 20$ pF, $r_x = 0$, and $g_o = 0$. From these parameters, one finds that the non-inverting, midfrequency gain, $A_{vo} = +\ 32.26$, $\omega_1 = 1/(R_C C\mu) = 5 \times 10^7$ r/s, $\omega_2 = [1 + R_s(g\pi + g_m)]/R_s C\pi] = 7.75 \times 10^8$ r/s, $\omega_T = 4.55 \times 10^8$ r/s. Disregard ω_2 as it is above ω_T. Thus, the approximate frequency response function for the G-B BJT amplifier can finally be written as

$$\frac{V_o}{V_s}(j\omega) \cong \frac{+32.26}{(1 + j\omega/5 \times 10^7)} \tag{2.138}$$

The GBWP for this amplifier is $32.27 \times 5 \times 10^7 = 1.61 \times 10^9$ r/s. Clearly, the G-B amplifier has improved high-frequency response because there is no Miller effect.

The final BJT amplifier to be considered is the emitter-follower (E-F), or grounded-collector amplifier. An E-F amplifier and its HFSSM are shown in Figure 2.47. Node equations are written for the V_b and the $V_o = V_e$ nodes using the Laplace format. Assume that $R_b >> R_s$, and $r_x = g_o = 0$. Also, $V_{b'e} = V_{be} = (V_b - V_o)$:

$$V_b[(G_s + g_\pi) + s(C_\mu + C_\pi)] - V_o[g_\pi + sC_\pi] = V_s G_s \tag{2.139a}$$

$$-V_b[(g_\pi + g_m) + sC_\pi] + V_o[(G_E + g_\pi + g_m) + sC_\pi] = 0 \tag{2.139b}$$

From Cramer's rule,

$$\Delta V_o = V_s G_s[(g_\pi + g_m) + sC_\pi] \tag{2.140}$$

$$\Delta = s^2 C_\pi C_\mu + s[C_\pi(G_s + G_E) + C_\mu(G_E + g_m + g_\pi)] + G_s(G_E + g_m + g_\pi) + g_\pi G_E \tag{2.141}$$

The emitter-follower's frequency response function can then be written, letting $s \to j\omega$:

$$\frac{V_o}{V_s}(s) = \frac{R_E(g_m + g_\pi)[1 + sC_\pi/(g_m + g_\pi)]}{s^2 C_\pi C_\mu R_E R_s + s\{C_\pi(R_E + R_s) + C_\mu R_s[1 + R_E(g_m + g_\pi)]\} + \{[1 + R_E(g_m + g_\pi)] + g_\pi R_s\}} \tag{2.142}$$

Note that the transfer function above is *not* in time constant format; to put in standard time constant (TC) format, one must divide all terms by $\{[1 + R_E(g_m + g\pi)] + g\pi R_s\}$. The midfrequency gain of the E-F amplifier is simply

$$A_{vo} = \frac{R_E(1 + g_m r_\pi)}{R_E(1 + g_m r_\pi) + R_s + r_\pi} < 1 \tag{2.143}$$

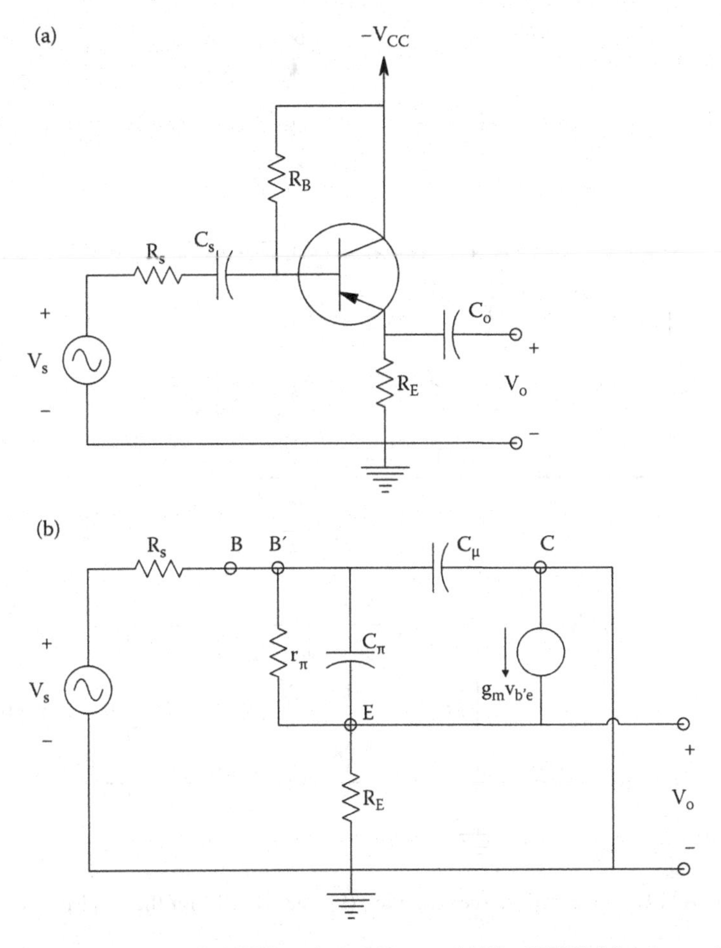

FIGURE 2.47 (a) A reactively coupled, BJT emitter-follower. (b) The HFSSM for the amplifier.

Note that there is *no Miller effect in an E-F amplifier;* there is no feedback from output to input, and the gain is positive and <1. Let: $C_\mu = 2$ pF, $C_\pi = 20$ pF, $g_m = 0.01$ S, $g_\pi = 5 \times 10^{-4}$ S, $R_s = 200\ \Omega$, and $R_E = 10^4\ \Omega$. The frequency of the zero is 5.25×10^8 r/s, and it can be neglected. The E-F's poles (break frequencies) are found to be at: 2.058×10^9 r/s, and 4.102×10^9 r/s. $\omega_T = 4.55 \times 10^8$ r/s. Because the break frequencies are $10 \times$ the transistor's ω_T, the results are not particularly valid. What they do illustrate, however, is that the E-F has amazing bandwidth. An external capacitance shunting G_C (an output capacitance) will lower the E-F's high-frequency response.

It is now appropriate to consider the high-frequency behavior of the three FET amplifiers analogous to the BJT amplifiers described earlier. These are the FET grounded-source (G-S) amplifier, the grounded gate (G-G) amplifier, and the source follower (S-F). Figure 2.48 illustrates a typical G-S amplifier and its HFSSM. It is clear that there will be a Miller effect for this amplifier because it has an inverting gain with magnitude >1, and a small capacitance Cgd coupling the output node to the input. The node equations for the G-S amplifier's HFSSM are

$$V_g[G_1 + s(C_{gs} + C_{gd})] - V_o[sC_{gd}] = V_1 G_1 \tag{2.144a}$$

$$-V_g[-g_m + sC_{gd}] + V_o[G_D' + s(C_{ds} + C_{gd})] = 0 \tag{2.144b}$$

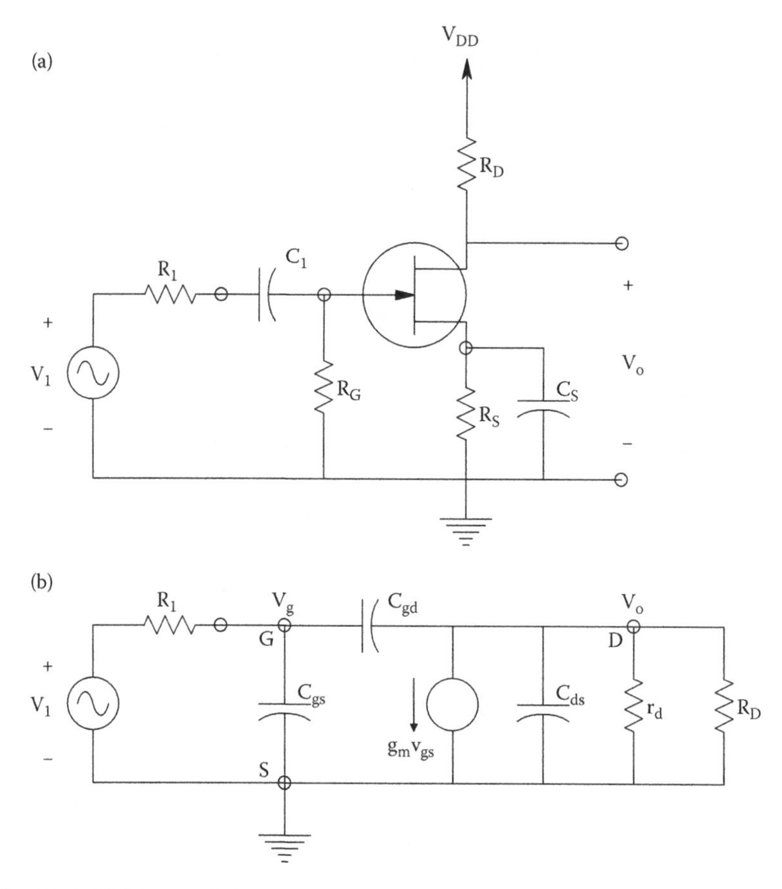

FIGURE 2.48 (a) A JFET grounded source amplifier. (b) The HFSSM for the amplifier.

where $G_D' = G_D + g_d$. These equations are solved with Cramer's rule:

$$\Delta = G_1 G_D' + s(C_{ds} + C_{gd})G_1 + s(C_{gs} + C_{gd})G_D' + s^2[(C_{gs} + C_{gd})C_{ds} + C_{gd}C_{gs}] \tag{2.145}$$

$$\Delta V_o = V_1 G_1[-g_m + sC_{gd}] \tag{2.146}$$

Hence, the detailed transfer function for the FET G-S amplifier is

$$\frac{V_o}{V_1}(s) = \frac{-g_m R_D'[1 - sC_{gd}/g_m]}{s^2[(C_{gs} + C_{gd})C_{ds} + C_{gd}C_{gs}]R_1 R_D' + s[R_1 C_{gd}(1 + g_m R_D') + R_D'(C_{gd} + C_{ds}) + R_1 C_{gs}] + 1} \tag{2.147}$$

Some reasonable parameters for the JFET are as follows: $g_d = 2 \times 10^{-5}$ S, $I_{DSS} = 10$ mA, $I_{DQ} = 5$ mA, $g_{mo} = 7 \times 10^{-3}$ S, $C_{gs} = C_{gd} = 2.5$ pF, $C_{ds} = 0.5$ pF, $R_1 = 600\ \Omega$, and $R_D = 3$ kΩ. Hence, $G_D' = 3.533 \times 10^{-4}$ S, and $G_D' = 3.533 \times 10^{-4}$ S, & $g_m = g_{mo}\sqrt{(I_{DQ}/I_{DSS})} = 4.423 \times 10^{-3}$ S. Now the zero is at $g_m/C_{gd} = 1.70 \times 10^9$ r/s, this is unrealistically high, so we can neglect it. The midfrequency gain is simply: $A_{vo} = g_m R_D' = -12.0$. To find the G-S amplifier's two break frequencies (poles), the denominator of Equation 2.147 is factored: The two break frequencies are found to be: $\omega_1 = 3.451 \times 10^7$ r/s or 5.492×10^6 Hz, and $\omega_2 = 1.950 \times 10^9$ r/s. The first, lower-frequency pole is dominant, the second pole is neglected, giving the approximate frequency response for the G-S amplifier:

$$\frac{V_o}{V_1}(j\omega) \cong \frac{-12}{[1 + j\omega/(3.451 \times 10^7)]} \tag{2.148}$$

The FET analog to the BJT grounded-base circuit is the *FET grounded-gate amplifier*, shown in Figure 2.49a. Assume that the DC IDQ flows through R_s and V_1, self-biasing the Q-point of the JFET so that V_{GSQ} is appropriately negative. Figure 2.49b shows the HFSSM of the G-G amplifier. One writes the node equations on V_s and V_o:

$$V_s[G_s + g_d + g_m + s(C_{gs} + C_{ds})] - V_o[g_d + sC_{ds}] = V_1 G_s \tag{2.149a}$$

$$-V_s[g_m + g_d + sC_{ds}] + V_o[G_D + g_d + s(C_{dg} + C_{ds})] = 0 \tag{2.149b}$$

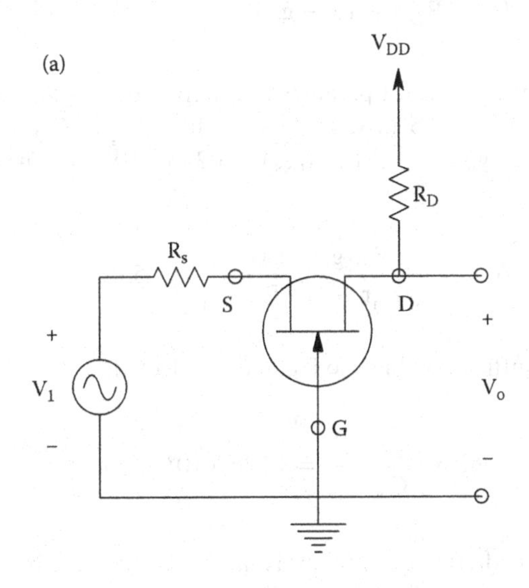

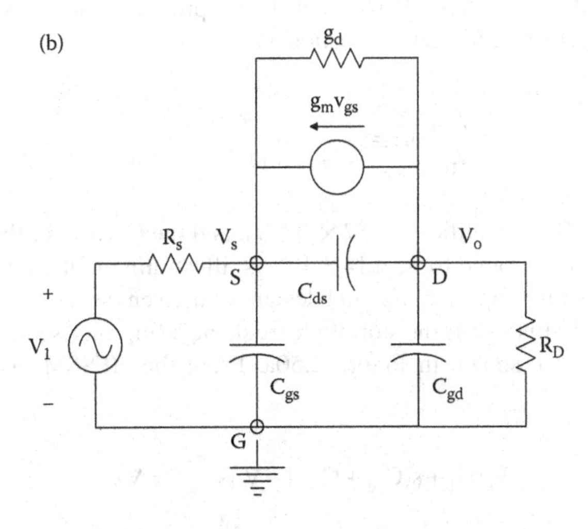

FIGURE 2.49 (a) A JFET grounded gate amplifier. (b) The HFSSM for the amplifier.

Using Cramer's rule,

$$\Delta = s^2[C_{ds}(C_{dg} + C_{gs}) + C_{gs}C_{dg}] + s[G_s(C_{dg} + C_{ds}) + g_d\ (C_{ds} + C_{gs})\ G_d(C_{ds} + C_{gs}) + g_m C_{dg}] + [G_s(G_D + g_d) + G_D(g_d + g_m)] \tag{2.150}$$

$$\Delta V_o = V_1 G_s[g_m + g_d + sC_{ds}] \tag{2.151}$$

The transfer function for the JFET G-G amplifier can finally be written after some algebra:

$$\frac{V_o}{V_1}(s) = \frac{+R_D(g_m + g_d)[1 + sC_{ds}r_d/(1 + g_m r_d)]}{s^2[C_{ds}(C_{dg} + C_{gs}) + C_{gs}\ C_{dg}]\ R_s R_D + s[G_s(C_{dg} + C_{ds}) + (G_D + g_d)(C_{ds} + C_{gs}) + g_m C_{dg}] + [1 + g_d R_D + R_s(g_d + g_m)]} \tag{2.152}$$

The numerical values of the FET HFSSM parameters are the same as for the G-S amplifier: Let: $g_d = 2 \times 10^{-5}$ S, $I_{DSS} = 10$ mA, $I_{DQ} = 5$ mA, $g_{mo} = 7 \times 10^{-3}$ S, $C_{gs} = C_{gd} = 2.5$ pF, $C_{ds} = 0.5$ pF, $R_s = 600\ \Omega$, and $R_D = 3\ \text{k}\Omega$ and $g_m = g_{mo}\sqrt{(I_{DQ}/I_{DSS})} = 4.243 \times 10^{-3}$ S. The G-G amplifier's mid-band gain is thus

$$A_{vo} = \frac{R_D(g_m r_d + 1)}{R_s(g_m r_d + 1) + R_D + r_d} = 3.535 \tag{2.153}$$

The frequency of the zero is sufficiently high so it can be neglected:

$$\omega_o = \frac{(g_m r_d + 1)}{C_{ds}\ r_d} = 8.526 \times 10^9\ \text{r/s} \tag{2.154}$$

Using numerical values, the quadratic denominator is factored to find the break frequencies. These are $\omega_1 = 1.29 \times 10^8$ and $\omega_2 = 1.78 \times 10^9$ r/s. Now the approximate low-pass frequency response function of the G-G JFET amplifier can be written as

$$\frac{V_o}{V_1}(j\omega) \cong \frac{3.535}{[1 + j\omega/(1.29 \times 10^8)]} \tag{2.155}$$

Note the GBWP for the G-G amplifier is 4.57×10^8 r/s, and the GBWP for the JFET G-S amplifier with the same parameters is found to be 4.14×10^8 r/s, illustrating that gain-bandwidth product is substantially independent of amplifier gain and design for a given device.

As a final example in this one-transistor, high-frequency amplifier section, let us consider the FET source-follower (S-F), shown in Figure 2.50a. From the HFSSM, we can write the node equations:

$$V_g[G_1 + s(C_{gd} + C_{gs})] - V_o[sC_{gs}] = V_1 G_1 \tag{2.156a}$$

$$-V_g[g_m + sC_{gs}] + V_o[g_m + G_s + g_d + s(C_{gs} + C_{ds})] = 0 \tag{2.156b}$$

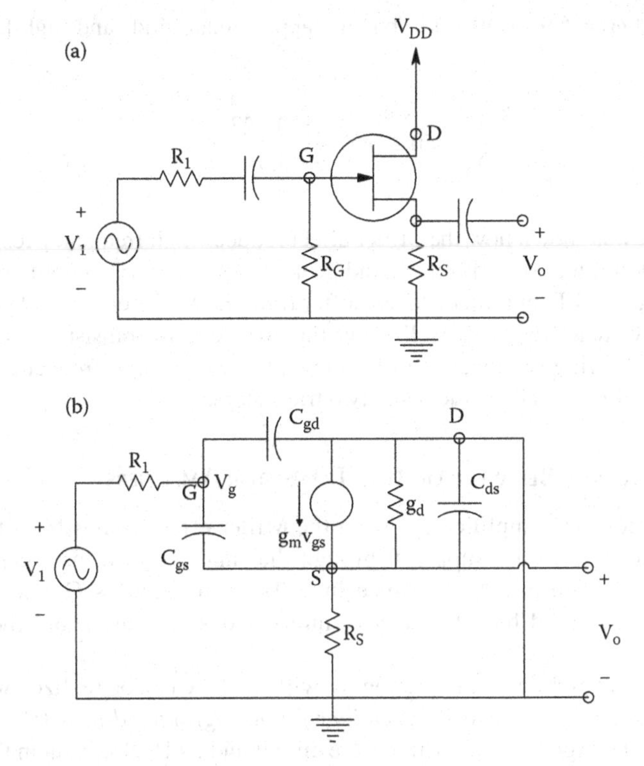

FIGURE 2.50 (a) A JFET source follower amplifier. (b) The HFSSM for the amplifier.

Using Cramer's rule, we get,

$$\Delta = s^2[C_{gd}(C_{gs}+C_{ds})+C_{gs}C_{ds}]+s[(C_{gs}+C_{ds})G_1+C_{gd}(g_m+g_d+G_s)+C_{gs}(G_s+g_d)] + [G_1(g_m+g_d+G_s)] \tag{2.157}$$

$$\Delta V_o = V_1 G_1[g_m + sC_{gs}] \tag{2.158}$$

After some algebra, the transfer function can be written as

$$\frac{V_o}{V_1}(s) = \frac{Rs\ g_m[1+sC_{gs}/g_m]}{s^2[C_{gd}(C_{gs}+C_{ds})+C_{gs}C_{ds}]R_1R_s + s\{R_s(C_{gs}+C_{ds})+R_1C_{gd}[1+R_s(g_m+g_d)]+R_1C_{gs}[1+g_dR_s]\}+[R_s(g_m+g_d+G_s)]} \tag{2.159}$$

From Equation 2.159, the midfrequency gain is found to be

$$A_{vo} = \frac{R_s(g_m r_d)}{R_s(g_m r_d+1)+r_d} = 0.923 \tag{2.160}$$

Using the parameters of the preceding FET amplifiers. The zero is at $\omega_o = g_m/C_{gs} = 1.70 \times 10^9$ r/s. The two poles are found by factoring the quadratic denominator in numerical form. They are

$\omega_1 = 1.26 \times 10^9$ and $\omega_2 = 5.96 \times 10^8$ r/s. Thus the approximate mid- and high-frequency response of the JFET S-F is thus

$$\frac{V_o}{V_1}(j\omega) \cong \frac{+\ 0.923}{[1 + j\omega/(5.96 \times 10^8)]} \tag{2.161}$$

In this section, it was shown how the Miller effect reduces high frequency response in both conventional grounded-emitter BJT amplifiers and grounded-source FET amplifiers. It was also seen that G-B, G-G, E-F, and S-F amplifiers do not suffer from the Miller effect, and generally have their first, high-frequency break frequency well-above that for the same transistors used in G-E and G-S amplifiers. In the following section, it will be shown that good, high-frequency amplifiers essentially free of Miller effect can be made using two transistors.

2.5.4 High-Frequency Behavior of Two-Transistor Amplifiers

The loss of high-frequency amplification from the Miller effect comes from the negative feedback from output to input nodes supplied through the small drain-to-gate capacitance in FETs or through the collector-to-base capacitance in BJTs, configured as G-S and G-E amplifiers, respectively. Clearly, a good high-frequency amplifier design must avoid the Miller effect at all costs.

The first broadband amplifier configuration we will examine can be realized with two BJTs, two FETs, or an FET and a BJT. It is called the *emitter-follower/grounded-base* (EF-GB) configuration when made from BJTs. Figure 2.51 illustrates the circuit and its HFSSM. As in the previous examples of single-transistor, high-frequency amplifier analysis, three node equations for the HFSSM of the amplifier are written in Laplace format:

$$V_o[G_C + sC_{\mu 2}] - V_e g_{m2} = 0 \tag{2.162a}$$

$$V_b[G_s + g_{\pi 1} + s(C_{\mu 1} + C_{\pi 1})] - V_e[g_{\pi 1} + sC_\pi] = V_s G_s \tag{2.162b}$$

$$-V_b[g_{m1} + g_{\pi 1} + sC_{\pi 1}] + V_e[(g_{\pi 1} + g_{\pi 2} + g_{m1} + g_{m2}) + G_E + S(C_{\pi 1} + C_{\pi 2})] = 0 \tag{2.162c}$$

Note that the V_o node equation is depends only on V_e. Hence,

$$\frac{V_o}{V_e}(s) = \frac{g_{m2} R_C}{1 + s\,C_{\mu 2} R_C} \tag{2.163}$$

To simplify the algebra, assume the transistors are identical, and have the same $I_{CQ.}$ Thus,

$$C_{\pi 1} = C_{\pi 2} = C_\pi,\ g_{m1} = g_{m2} = g_m,\ r_{\pi 1} = r_{\pi 2} = r_\pi,\ C_{\mu 1} = C_{\mu 2} = C_\mu,\ r_{x1} = r_{x2} = 0,\ \&\ g_{o1} = g_{o2} = 0. \tag{2.164}$$

Using Cramer's rule and a plethora of algebra, find the transfer function for V_e (let $s = j\omega$):

$$\frac{V_e}{V_s}(s) = \frac{(1 + g_m r_\pi)[1 + sC_\pi r_\pi/(1 + g_m r_\pi)]}{s^2[2C_\pi C_\mu + C_\pi^2]R_s r_\pi + s\{C_\pi[2r_\pi + R_s(g_m r_\pi + 2 + G_E r_\pi)] + C_\mu R_s[2(1 + g_m r_\pi) + G_E r_\pi]\} + [2(1 + g_m r_\pi) + G_E r_\pi + R_s(g_m + G_E)]} \tag{2.165}$$

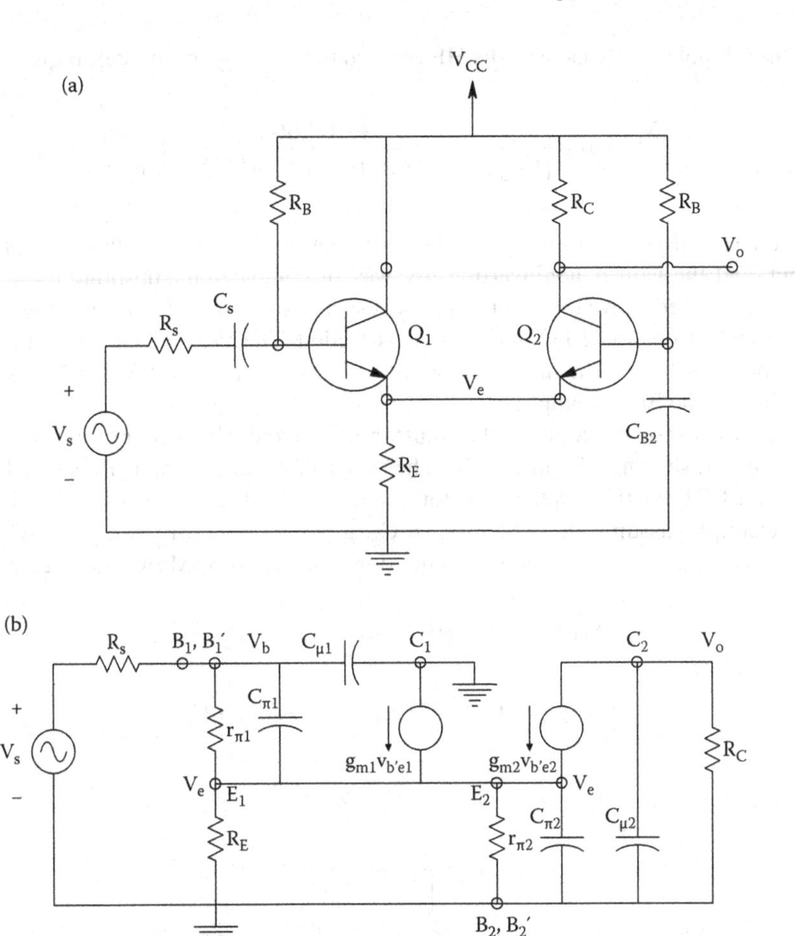

FIGURE 2.51 (a) A BJT emitter follower/grounded base amplifier. (b) The HFSSM for the amplifier.

The midfrequency gain of the amplifier is found by substituting Equation 2.165 into Equation 2.163, and letting $s = j\omega = 0$:

$$A_{vo} = \frac{V_o}{V_s} = \frac{g_m R_C}{\{2 + [r_\pi + R_s(1 + g_m R_E)]/[R_E(1 + g_m r_\pi)]\}} \tag{2.166}$$

Note that the small-signal term, $g_m r_\pi$, is equal to the BJT's beta or h_{fe}. Let us define reasonable numerical values for the EF/GB circuit's parameters: $I_{CQ} = 1$ mA, $g_m = 0.0384615$ S, $r_\pi = 2.6 \times 10^3\ \Omega$, $R_s = 300\ \Omega$, $R_C = 6$ kΩ, $R_E = 3$ kΩ, $C_\mu = 2$ pF, $C_\pi = 200$ pF. Substituting these parameters in the expressions above, one finds that $A_{vo} = +\ 108.66$. The frequency of the zero is $\omega_o = (1 + g_m r_\pi)/C_\pi r_\pi = 1.942 \times 10^8$ r/s. The collector break frequency is at: $\omega_3 = 1/C_\mu R_C = 8.333 \times 10^7$ r/s. The other two break frequencies are found from finding the roots of the denominator of Equation 2.165; they are $\omega_1 = 1.961 \times 10^8$ and $\omega_2 = 3.438 \times 10^7$ r/s. Thus, the overall frequency response function for the EF/GB amplifier is

$$\frac{V_o}{V_s}(j\omega) = \frac{108.66\ [1 + j\omega/(1.942 \times 10^8)]}{[1 + j\omega/(3.438 \times 10^7)][1 + j\omega/8.333 \times 10^7)][1 + j\omega/(1.961 \times 10^8)]} \tag{2.167}$$

Note that the HF pole nearly cancels the HF zero, so the final (approximate) frequency response is

$$\frac{V_o}{V_s}(j\omega) \cong \frac{+\ 108.66}{[1 + j\omega/(3.438 \times 10^7)][1 + j\omega/(8.333 \times 10^7)]} \tag{2.168}$$

Note from the HFSSM of the EF/GB amplifier that it has no Miller capacitance coupling the output to the input, and the gain is noninverting. By way of comparison, substitute the hy-pi transistor model parameters used above into the frequency response expression for a conventional, single, G-E amplifier, given by Equation 2.132 in the previous section. The midfrequency gain for this amplifier is found to be −230.8, and the dominant break frequency is at $\omega_1 = 5.348 \times 10^6$ r/s, considerably lower that that for the EF/GB amplifier.

A second two-transistor amplifier that substantially avoids the Miller effect is the well-known *cascode amplifier*, shown in Figure 2.52a. The two-BJT cascode amp is illustrated, but it is possible to use an FET for the lower transistor and a BJT for the top, or use two FETs. As in the preceding example, assume that $C_{\pi 1} = C_{\pi 2} = C_\pi$, $g_{m1} = g_{m2} = g_m$, $r_{\pi 1} = r_{\pi 2} = r_\pi$, $C_{\mu 1} = C_{\mu 2} = C_\mu$, $r_{x1} = r_{x2} = 0$, and $g_{o1} = g_{o2} = 0$. The node equations for the HFSSM of Figure 2.52b are

$$V_b[(G_s + g_\pi) + s(C_\pi + C_\mu)] - V_e[sC_\mu] = V_s G_s \tag{2.169a}$$

$$-V_b[-g_m + sC_\mu] + V_e[(g_\pi + g_m) + s(C_\pi + C_\mu)] = 0 \tag{2.169b}$$

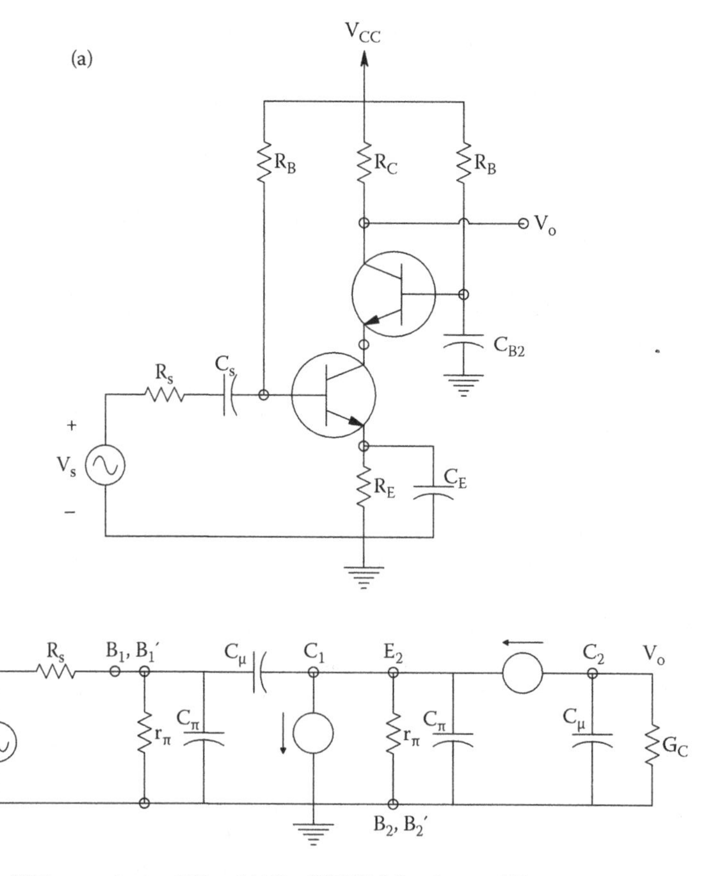

FIGURE 2.52 (a) A BJT cascode amplifier. (b) The HFSSM for the amplifier.

$$V_o[G_C + sC_\mu] - V_e g_m = 0 \tag{2.169c}$$

From Equations 2.169, one can easily write

$$\frac{V_o}{V_e}(s) = \frac{g_m R_c}{1 + s\, R_C C_\mu} \tag{2.170}$$

Using Cramer's rule on Equations 2.169A and B, one finds

$$\Delta = s^2[2C_\mu C_\pi + C_\pi{}^2] + s[g_\pi(C_\pi + C_\mu) + g_m(C_\pi + 2C_\pi)] + [G_s(g_\pi + g_m) + g_\pi(g_\pi + g_m)] \tag{2.171}$$

$$\Delta V_e = -V_s G_s g_m[1 - sC_\mu/g_m] \tag{2.172}$$

The transfer function for V_e can be written from the two equations, Equations 2.171 and 2.172:

$$\frac{V_e}{V_s}(s) = \frac{-g_m r_\pi[1 - s\, C_\mu/g_m]}{s^2[2C_\mu C_\pi + C_\pi{}^2] + s\, R_s[C_\pi(1 + g_m r_\pi) + C_\mu(1 + 2g_m r_\pi)] \;+\; [(1 + g_m r_\pi) + R_s(g_\pi + g_m)]} \tag{2.173}$$

From Equation 2.173 and Equation 2.169C, one can find the cascode amplifier's midfrequency gain, A_{vo}:

$$A_{vo} = \frac{V_o}{V_s} = \frac{-g_m R_C[g_m r_\pi/(1 + g_m r_\pi)]}{(1 \;+\; R_s/r_\pi)} \tag{2.174}$$

Now using the hy-pi HFSSM parameters that were used in the EF/GB HF amplifier, one evaluates the zero, poles, and gain, A_{vo}, for the cascode amplifier. They are $A_{vo} = -204.9$. The zero is at $\omega_o = 1.923 \times 10^{10}$ r/s (the zero is negligible). The collector pole for the upper BJT is $\omega_3 = 1/(R_C C_\mu) = 8.333 \times 10^7$ r/s. The two poles for the V_e frequency response function, Equation 2.173, are found to be: $\omega_1 = 1.739 \times 10^8$, and $\omega_2 = 2.036 \times 10^7$ r/s. Note that ω_2 is the dominant, lowest break-frequency. The simplified frequency response function is thus

$$\frac{V_o}{V_s}(j\omega) \cong \frac{-204.9}{[1 + j\omega/(2.036 \times 10^7)]} \tag{2.175}$$

The high break frequency for the BJT cascode amplifier compares favorably with that for the EF/GB amplifier analyzed above. There is no Miller effect for the upper (G-B) BJT, and the Miller effect for the lower (G-E) BJT is very small because the V_e/V_s voltage gain magnitude is <1. Namely,

$$\frac{V_e}{V_s}(0) = \frac{-g_m r_\pi/(1 + g_m r_\pi)}{1 + R_s/r_\pi} = -0.8877 \tag{2.176}$$

In summary, it is seen that certain one- and two-transistor amplifier designs are inherently broadband because they avoid the Miller effect. These designs include the emitter-follower, the grounded-base, the source-follower, the grounded gate, the EF/GB pair, and the cascode amplifier. In the following section, some other schemes for increasing high frequency response, also known as broadbanding will be examined. One way is to trade-off midband gain for high-frequency bandwidth by using negative feedback. Another is to use a high-pass zero to cancel a low-pass pole, effectively extending high-frequency bandwidth. Still another is to ensure that the Thevenin source resistance of the first stage's output is very low compared to the input resistance of the second stage; an emitter-follower is often used to realize low R_{s1}.

2.5.5 Broadbanding Strategies

In this section, we examine in detail two techniques used to extend amplifier bandwidths (other than choosing high-frequency transistors).

In op amps, instrumentation amplifiers, and other IC amplifiers, multiple transistor stages are used to achieve the requisite gain. The gain stages are generally direct-coupled (d-c), i.e., there is a DC pathway from the output of one stage to the input of the next gain stage. Thus, d-c amplifiers can amplify DC signals. To match appropriate DC bias voltages between the output of one stage and the input of the following stage, often a resistive voltage divider is used. Another strategy to match DC levels is to alternate *pnp* and *npn* BJTs in the stages (or *p*- and *n*-channel FETs). An advantage of the voltage divider is that it allows one to use *shunt capacitance frequency compensation.*

Figure 2.53 illustrates two stages of a d-c amplifier in general format; the first stage is represented by a frequency-independent, Thevenin model, coupled to the input of the second stage through a voltage divider, (R_1, R_2). The input resistance and capacitance of the second stage are R_i, C_i, respectively. V_2 drives the second stage. The shunt capacitor, C_1, can be used to cancel the low-pass effect of the input capacitance. To illustrate this effect, one finds the transfer function, V_2/V_1 using the simple voltage-divider relation:

$$\frac{V_2}{V_1}(s) = \frac{\dfrac{1}{G_{in} + sC_i}}{\dfrac{1}{G_{in} + sC_i} + R_{s1} + \dfrac{1}{G_1 + sC_1}} \tag{2.177}$$

$$\text{Where: } R_{in} = \frac{1}{G_2 + G_i} = 1/G_{in}. \tag{2.178}$$

Adjust C_1 so $C_1R_1 = C_iR_{in}$, and do algebra to find

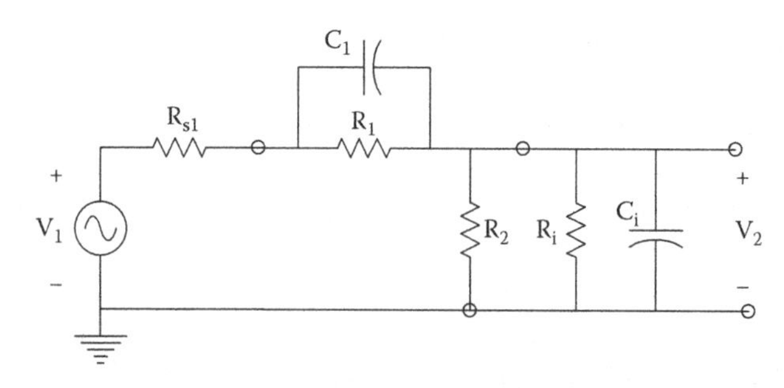

FIGURE 2.53 An R-C voltage divider model for direct coupling between amplifier stages. It is shown that a nearly flat frequency response occurs when we make $R_1C_1 = C_i(R_i||R_2)$.

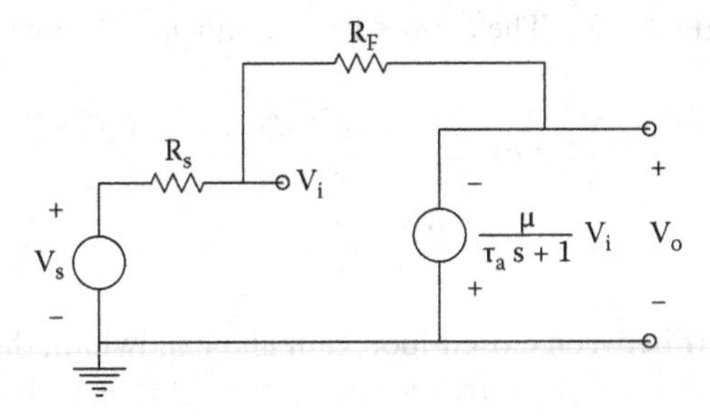

FIGURE 2.54 Circuit illustrating the trade-off of gain for bandwidth using negative feedback. See Text for analysis.

$$\frac{V_2}{V_1}(s) = \frac{\dfrac{R_{in}}{R_{in} + R_1 + R_{s1}}}{1 + \dfrac{s\, C_i R_{s1} R_{in}}{R_{in} + R_1 + R_{s1}}} \tag{2.179}$$

Note that if $R_{s1} \to 0$, $V_2/V_1 \to R_{in}/(R_{in} + R_1)$ (V_2/V_1 is independent of frequency), otherwise the break frequency is quite high.

Another general principle of extending the high-frequency bandwidth of a multistage, inverting-gain amplifier is to trade-off midband gain for bandwidth through the use of negative feedback. The classic illustration of the gain-bandwidth constancy is done with op amps in Section 6.3 of this text. A similar example will be examined here; see Figure 2.54 for the circuit. Without feedback ($R_F = \infty$), it can be seen by inspection that the amplifier's frequency response is

$$\frac{V_o}{V_s}(j\omega) = \frac{-\mu}{1 + j\omega\tau_a} \tag{2.180}$$

The gain-bandwidth product of this amplifier without feedback is

$$GBWP_o = \mu/\tau_a \ \text{r/s} \tag{2.181}$$

With feedback, V_i is given by the node equation

$$V_i[G_s + G_F] - V_o G_F = V_s G_s \tag{2.182a}$$

$$\downarrow$$

$$\frac{-(S\tau_a + 1)V_o}{\mu}[G_s + G_F] - V_o G_F = V_s G_s \tag{2.182b}$$

$$\downarrow$$

$$\frac{V_o}{V_s}(s) = \frac{-R_F\ \mu/[R_F + R_s(1+\mu)]}{\dfrac{s\tau_a(R_F + R_s)}{[R_F + R_s(1+\mu)]} + 1} \tag{2.182c}$$

The gain-bandwidth product with feedback is

$$GBWP_f = \mu/[\tau_a(1 + R_s/R_F)] \tag{2.183}$$

Now assume $\mu >> 1$, and $\mu R_s >> R_F$. The approximate frequency response function is

$$\frac{V_o}{V_s}(j\omega) \cong \frac{-R_F/R_s}{\dfrac{j\omega\tau_a}{\mu R_s/(R_s + R_F)} + 1} \qquad (2.184)$$

Note that there is a trade-off between closed-loop gain and bandwidth; the lower the midband gain magnitude, $-R_F/R_s$, the higher the break frequency, $\omega_b = \mu R_s/(R_s + R_F)/\tau_a$ r/s.

The choice of transistor for a high-frequency amplifier design is paramount. BJTs must be chosen to have high f_Ts, and FETs to have high f_{max}. While you may never be in the position of having to design either a discrete or IC multistage amplifier, you should appreciate the factors described above that go into the design of broadband amplifiers.

2.6 PHOTONS, PHOTODIODES, PHOTOCONDUCTORS, LEDS, AND LASER DIODES

2.6.1 Introduction

In this section, the properties of semiconductor devices that sense photon energy and others that emit photon energy will be examined. *Photons* are an alternate way to describe electromagnetic radiation (EMR) generally having wavelengths from 1×10^{-4} m to less than 3×10^{-12} m. These wavelengths include *infrared* (IR), *visible light, ultraviolet* (UV), *X-rays*, and *gamma rays.* The photon is a quantum EM "particle," used to describe physical interactions of low-power EMR with molecules, atoms, and subatomic particles, such as atomic shell electrons. The electromagnetic wave characterization of EM energy is used throughout the EM spectrum and finds application in describing the operation of antennas, transmission lines, fiber optic cables, and optical elements such as lenses, prisms, and mirrors used in the terahertz, IR, visible, and UV wavelengths. Maxwell's equations for EM wave propagation are also useful in describing such phenomena as diffraction, refraction and polarization of light (Balanis 1989, Hecht 1987). A photon has essentially zero mass, it moves at the speed of light in a medium and has an *individual energy* of $\varepsilon = hc/\lambda = h\nu$ J, where h is Planck's constant (6.6253×10^{-34} J-s), *c* is the speed of light in the supporting medium (c = 2.998 × 108 m/s in vacuo), λ is the wavelength of the EM radiation in meters, and ν is the Hz frequency of the EMR (ν of *visible* light is ca. 10^{14} Hz). Photon energy is also given in electron-volts (eV). To obtain the energy of a photon in eV, *divide* its energy in Joules by 1.602×10^{-19}. (1.602×10^{-19} is the magnitude of the charge on an electron.) For example, a photon of blue light having a wavelength of $\lambda = 450$ nm has an energy of: $e = (6.626 \times 10^{-34}$ J s$)(3 \times 10^{8}$ m/s$)/(450 \times 10^{-9}$ m$) = 4.41 \times 10^{-19}$ J, or 2.76 eV. Similarly, a photon of $\lambda = 700$ nm (red light) has an energy of 2.84×10^{-19} J or 1.77 eV. Figure 2.55 illustrates the EM spectrum.

There are many sensors that are used to measure photon EM energy in biomedical applications. These include, but are not limited to *photodiodes, phototransistors, photoconductors, pyroelectric IR sensors, photomultiplier tubes* (PMTs), *scintillation crystals plus PMTs*, etc. (Northrop 2002).

Below, *pn* junction photon sensors, photoconductors, and certain solid-state photon sources will be considered. It will be seen that the interaction of photons in a certain energy range with a semiconductor *pn* junction can cause the generation of a photovoltaic EMF; this EMF is the basis for photodiode behavior, and also the solar cell, which acts as an energy transducer (photons to electrical current flow), capable of doing work. Photodiodes and solar cells can be used to measure incident EM radiation intensity. Also treated in the sections below is the *generation* of photon energy by special semiconductor diode structures: the *light-emitting diode* (LED) and the *laser diode.* Both types of photon-emissive devices have found wide application in biomedical instrumentation (Northrop 2002).

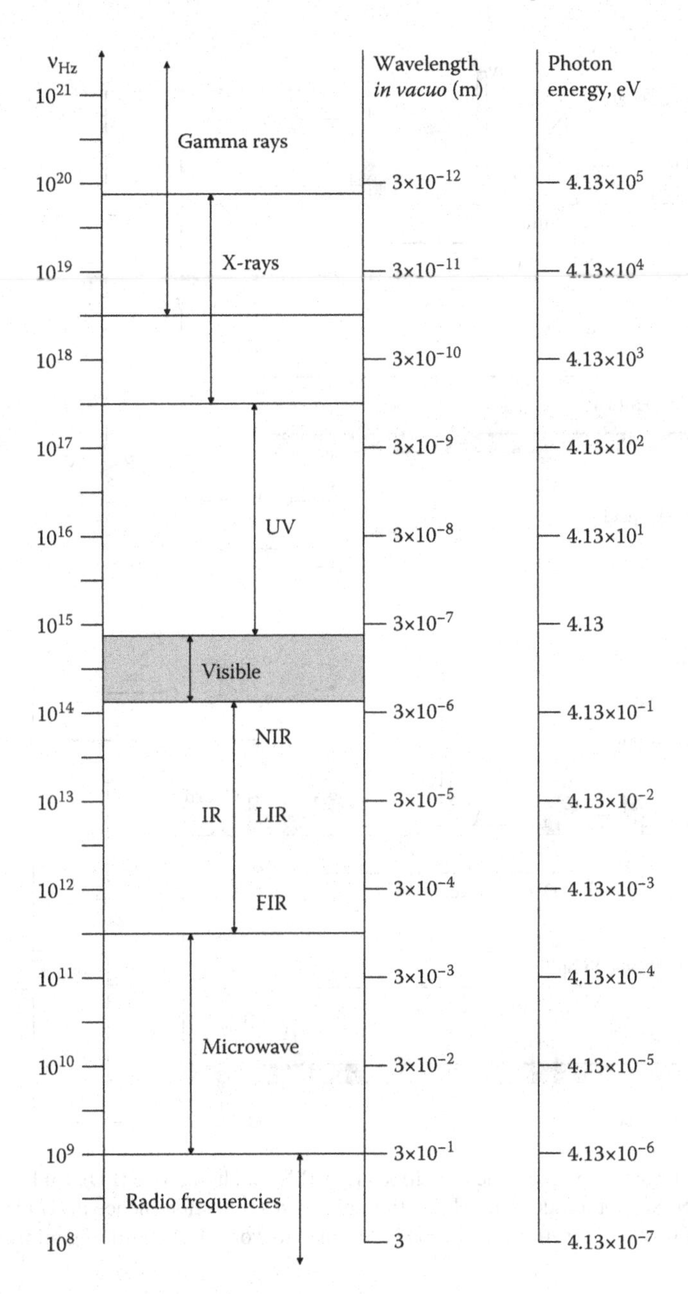

FIGURE 2.55 The upper electromagnetic spectrum.

2.6.2 PIN Photodiodes

Photodiodes are used as sensors for EMR ranging from near infrared (NIR) to near ultraviolet (UVA). Even a standard small-signal, silicon, *pn* junction diode with a transparent glass envelope will respond to incident EMR of appropriate wavelength, as will a reverse-biased LED. However, photodiodes used for photonic measurements have specialized junction structures that maximize the area over which incident photons are absorbed. Photodiodes are used in a broad range of biomedical instruments, including but not limited to *blood pulse oximeters; finger-tip heart-rate sensors; single-drop blood glucose meters; fiberoptic-based spectrophotometers* used to sense analytes in blood, urine, etc.; *spectrophotometric detection of tumors using endoscopes*, etc.

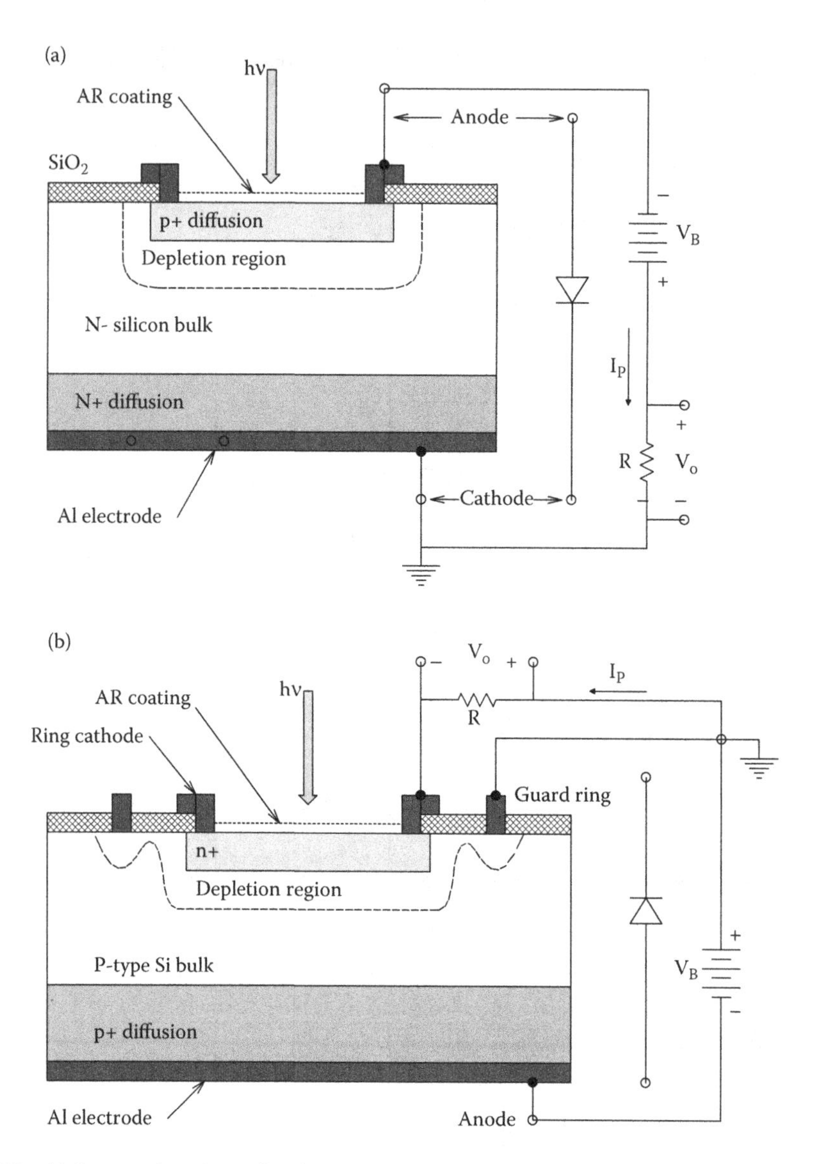

FIGURE 2.56 (a) Layer cake schematic of a three layer, PIN, Si photodiode (PD). (b) Layer cake schematic of a three layer, PIN, Si photodiode. The AR coating minimizes reflection (hence maximizes photon absorption) in the range of wavelengths in which the PD is designed to work. The guard ring minimizes dark current.

Photodiodes fall into two broad categories: 3-layer, PIN diodes (P stands for p-doped, I stands for intrinsic, and N stands for n-doped semiconductor), and *avalanche photodiodes* (APDs)—basically a 4-layer structure (P + IPN). Figure 2.56 illustrates schematic cross sections through two types of PIN devices. Note that to improve the efficiency of photon capture, a thin, $\lambda/4$ layer of antireflective (AR) coating is used on the surface of the PD, similar to the AR coatings commonly used on binocular and camera lenses. When an incident photon having the appropriate energy passes through the AR coating, it enters the p^+ diffusion layer, and interacts (collides) with a valence-band electron. If the electron gains energy greater than the band-gap energy, E_g, it is pulled up into the conduction band, leaving a mobile hole in the valence band. These electron-hole pairs are formed throughout the p^+ layer, the depletion layer, and the *n*-layer materials. In the depletion layer, the *E*-field accelerates these photoelectrons toward the *n*-layer, and the holes toward the *p*-layer. Electrons from the electron-hole pairs generated by photons in the *n*-layer, along with electrons that have arrived from the *p*-layer, are left in the n-layer conduction band. Meanwhile the holes diffuse through the *n*-layer up to the depletion layer while being accelerated and are collected in the *p*-layer valence band. By these mechanisms, electron-hole pairs which are generated in proportion to the amount of incident light are collected in the *n*- and *p*-layers of the PD. This results in a positive charge in the *p*-layer and a negative charge in the *n*-layer. When an external circuit is connected between the *p*- and *n*-layers, photocurrent electrons will flow away from the n-layer, and holes will flow away from the *p*-layer, toward the opposite electrode. The PIN PD and an external circuit is shown in Figure 2.56a. Note that in normal operation of the PD, it is reverse-biased, so *the photocurrent is a reverse current*, flowing in the same direction as the thermally generated leakage current which flows in a reverse-biased *pn* diode.

Figure 2.57 illustrates typical PIN PD volt–ampere curves. The load-line represents a graphical solution of the PD's (nonlinear) volt–ampere curves with the (linear) Thevenin circuit "seen" by the PD. The zero-current intercept of the load-line on the V_D axis is at the Thevenin open-circuit voltage; the zero-voltage intercept is the Thevenin short-circuit current. The load-line permits a graphical solution of

$$i_D(V_D) = \frac{V_B - V_D}{R} \tag{2.185a}$$

or

$$V_D = V_B - i_D R, \ (V_B < 0 \text{ in reverse-biased diode.}) \tag{2.185b}$$

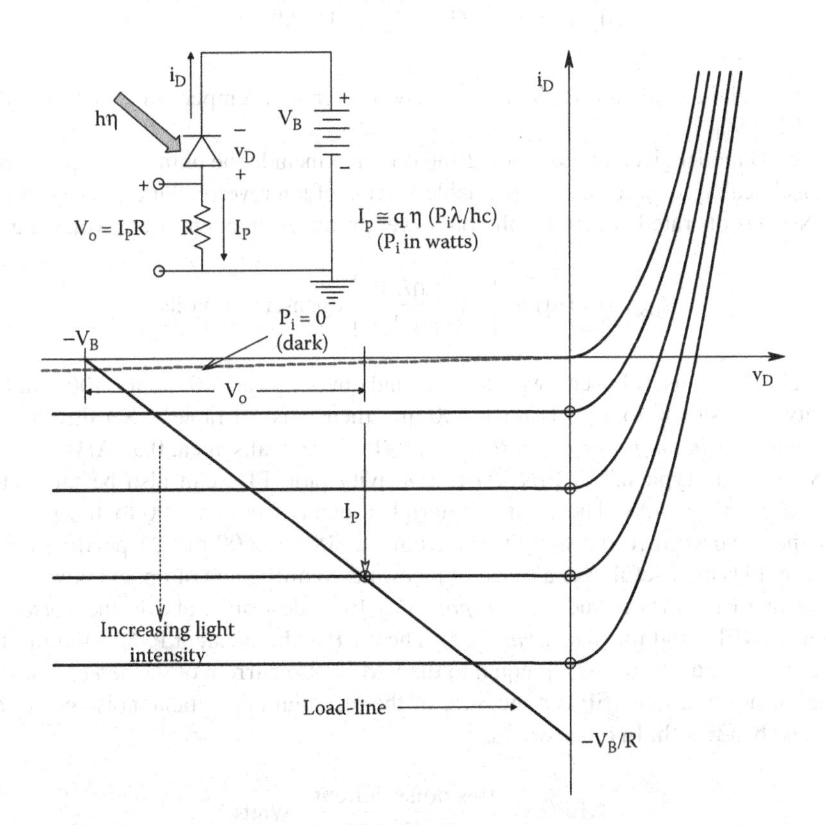

FIGURE 2.57 *Top:* Simple series circuit for PIN PD. *Bottom:* i_D vs. v_D curves as a function of absorbed photon power, P_i. The load-line is determined by the Thevenin equivalent circuit the PD "sees." Note that the PD's photocurrent, I_P, flows in the reverse direction. V_o across the load resistor can be determined graphically by the intersection of the $i_D = f(P_i)$ line with the load line.

The slope of the load-line is easily seen to be $-1/R$ and depends only on the Thevenin model parameters. Most PDs are operated in the third quadrant, either with a reverse-bias OCV, or under short-circuit conditions ($v_D = 0$). PD signal-conditioning circuits will be described below.

The total PD current can be modeled by

$$i_D = I_{rs}[\exp(v_D/V_T) - 1] - I_P \tag{2.186}$$

The photocurrent, I_P, flows in the reverse direction, and is given by

$$I_P = \frac{\eta\, q\, P_i \lambda}{h\, c} \text{ amperes} \tag{2.187}$$

where P_i is the total photon power incident on the PD active surface in watts, $V_T = kT/q$, η is the capture efficiency (ca. 0.8), I_{rs} is the *reverse saturation current,* k is Boltzmann's constant (1.380×10^{-23} J/°K), and h = Planck's constant (6.624×10^{-34} J s).

I_{rs} is very temperature-dependent; it can be approximated by (Navon 1975, Millman 1979)

$$I_{rs}(T) = I_{rs}(T_o)\, 2^{(T - To)/10} \tag{2.188a}$$

or

$$\Delta I_{rs}/I_{rs} = 1/2[3/T + \varphi/(kT^2)] \cong 0.08\ /^{o}K \tag{2.188b}$$

where T is the Kelvin temperature, T_o is the Kelvin reference temperature, and ϕ is the silicon energy gap (1.15 eV).

The simple PD model given by Equation 2.186 does not include the ohmic leakage of the reverse-biased PD. Such leakage can form an appreciable portion of the reverse, dark i_D for large reverse v_D.

If the PIN PD is operated at zero i_D, photon power produces an open-circuit voltage given by

$$V_{Doc} = (kT/q)\, \mathit{In}\left[1 + \frac{q\, \eta\lambda\, P_i}{h\, c\, I_{rs}}\right] \text{ open-circuit volts} \tag{2.189}$$

Silicon PIN PDs are useful over a wavelength band covering ca. 200 nm to 1100 nm; their spectral sensitivity rises slowly to a peak at ca. 800 nm, then falls off rapidly. Sensitivity is given by the PD's *responsivity in amps per watt:* $R(\lambda) = i_D(0)/Pi$. $R(\lambda)$ peaks at ca. 0.55 A/W @ ca. 850 nm. Figure 2.58 shows a "typical," Si PIN PD responsivity plot. PDs can also be fabricated using-germanium (Ge) and InGaAs. The former material responds from ca. 300 to 1600 nm, the latter composition has a spectral responsivity range from ca. 800 to 2600 nm. Depending on operating conditions, PIN PDs are useful over a range of picowatts to milliwatts of optical power.

Figures of merit for PDs include the *responsivity* $R(\lambda)$, described above, the *noise-equivalent* (optical) *power* (NEP), and the *detectivity* (D*). The NEP is the incident P_i @ λ required to generate a short-circuit response current, I_P, equal to the RMS noise current of the *detector system* (unity output signal-to-noise ratio.) NEP is a measure of the minimum detectable noise power at a given wavelength and bandwidth. In other words,

$$\text{NEP}(\lambda) = \frac{\text{rms noise current}}{\text{responsivity } @\lambda} \text{ Watts} \tag{2.190}$$

The noise generated by a PD operating under reverse bias is due to *shot noise* generated in the dark leakage current and *Johnson (thermal) noise* generated in the equivalent shunt resistance

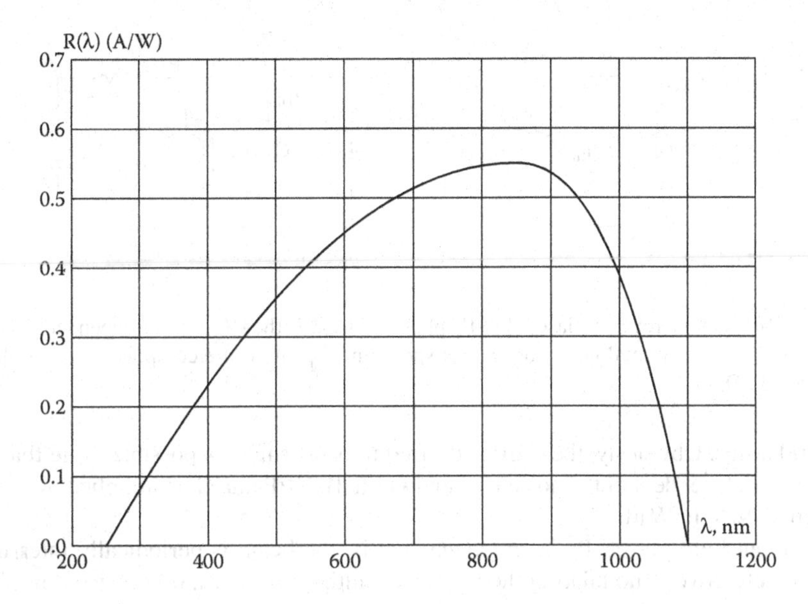

FIGURE 2.58 A typical responsivity plot for a Si PIN PD. See Text for discussion.

of the PD. Both the shot and thermal noise are broadband and are considered to have flat, *white, power density spectra* (see Chapter 9 in this text). The mean-squared shot noise can be shown to be given by

$$\overline{i_{sn}^2} = 2\ q\ I_{DL} B \text{ msA} \tag{2.191}$$

where q is the magnitude of the electron charge, I_{DL} is the dark leakage current in amperes (I_{DL} is zero for a zero-biased PD), and B is the equivalent Hz noise bandwidth over which the noise current is measured.

The mean-squared thermal noise can be shown to be given by

$$\overline{i_{tn}^2} = 4\ k\ T\ G \text{ msA/Hz} \tag{2.192}$$

where k = Boltzmann's constant (1.38×10^{-38} J/°K), T = Kelvin temperature of PD, B = equivalent Hz noise bandwidth, and G = net thermal noise producing conductance.

The total MS diode noise current is found by adding the two MS current noises:

$$\overline{i_n^2} = \overline{i_{sn}^2} + \overline{i_{tn}^2} \text{ msA/Hz} \tag{2.193}$$

Thus, the total RMS diode noise is

$$i_n = \sqrt{\overline{i_n^2}} = \sqrt{(2\ q\ I_{DL} + 4\ k\ T\ G)}\sqrt{B} \text{ rmsA} \tag{2.194}$$

Johnson noise dominates as the dark current → 0. Note that the NEP depends on λ, I_{DL} (hence the PD operating circuit), the noise bandwidth B, T, and the net (Norton) conductance, G, in parallel with the photocurrent and noise current sources. The NEP for Si PIN PDs ranges from ca. 10^{-14} W/$\sqrt{\text{Hz}}$ for small-area (A = 1 mm²), low-noise PDs, to over 2×10^{-13} W/$\sqrt{\text{Hz}}$ for very large area

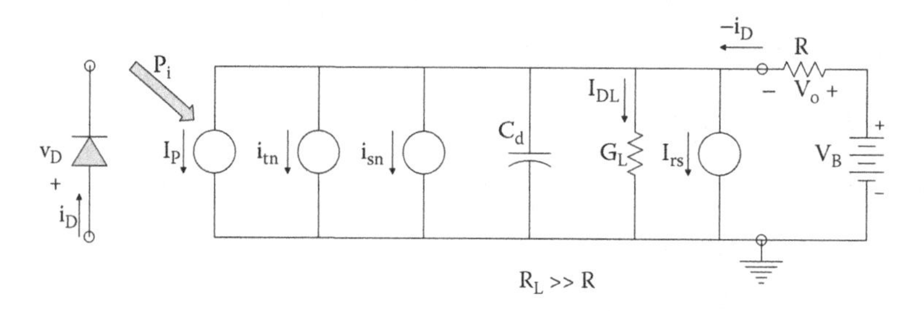

FIGURE 2.59 Model for a reverse-biased, Si PIN photodiode. i_{sn} is the DC current-dependent shot noise root power spectrum; i_{tn} is the thermal noise root power spectrum. V_B and R are components of the dc Thevenin circuit biasing the PD.

cells (A = 100 mm^2). Obviously, the NEP is desired to be as small as possible. Note that manufacturers give NEP independent of the noise Hz bandwidth, B. NEP must be multiplied by the $\sqrt{B}$ used to get the actual NEP in Watts.

Often the input light power, P_i, is *chopped.* That is, the beam is periodically interrupted by a chopper wheel, effectively modulating the beam by multiplying it by a 0,1 square wave. The chopping rate is generally at audio frequencies (e.g., 1 kHz), and the bandwidth of the associated band-pass filter used to condition the PD output determines B. Chopping is used to avoid the excess, 1/f diode noise present near DC and at very low frequencies.

Figure 2.59 illustrates the equivalent model for a reverse-biased, Si PIN PD, showing signal, noise and dark current sources, the diode small-signal capacitance, C_d, which is a depletion capacitance that depends on $-v_{DQ}$, and diode semiconductor doping and geometry. Note that the DC reverse leakage current has two components; a constant, small I_{rs}, and a voltage-dependent dark current, I_{DL}. $(I_{DL} + I_{rs})$ are used to calculate i_{sn}. Normally, $R_L >> R$, so the thermal noise current is found using the external load resistor, R (1/R = G). The junction depletion capacitance, C_d, *decreases* as v_{DQ} goes more negative. Large C_d is deleterious to PD high-frequency response because it shunts $I_P(j\omega)$ to ground. Note that C_d *increases with illumination*, being smallest in the dark (using the circuit of Figure 2.57). C_d is on the order of pF. For example, one Si PIN PD with 1 mm^2 active area and a $v_{DQ} = -10$ V, has a $C_d \cong 4$ pF.

The detectivity, D* is 1/NEP for the detector element only, normalized to a 1 cm^2 active area. D* is used only for comparisons between PDs of different active areas. D* units are cm$\sqrt{\text{Hz}}$/W. (A "better" PD has a higher D*).

2.6.3 Avalanche Photodiodes

A cross-sectional schematic of an *avalanche PD* (APD) is shown in Figure 2.60. In an APD, a large, reverse biasing voltage is used, about 100 V or more, depending on diode design. The internal E-field completely depletes the π-region of mobile carriers. The *E*-field in the π-region causes any injected or thermally generated carriers to attain a saturation velocity, giving them enough kinetic energy so that their impact with valence-band electrons causes ionization—the creation of other electron-hole pairs, which in turn are accelerated by the E-field, causing still more impact ionizations, etc.

Photon-generated electron-hole pairs are separated by the E-field in the p- and π-regions; electrons move into the n+ layer, holes drift into the p+ layer, which are boundaries of the APD's space-charge region. These photon-generated carriers are *multiplied* as they pass through the avalanche region by the impact ionization process. At a given reverse operating voltage, $-v_{DQ} = V_R$, one electron generated by photon collision produces M electrons at the APD's anode. The contribution of electrons to I_P is much greater than that from holes because electrons generated in the *p*- and π-regions are pulled into the avalanche region, whereas holes are swept back into the p+ region (including the holes generated in the avalanche process).

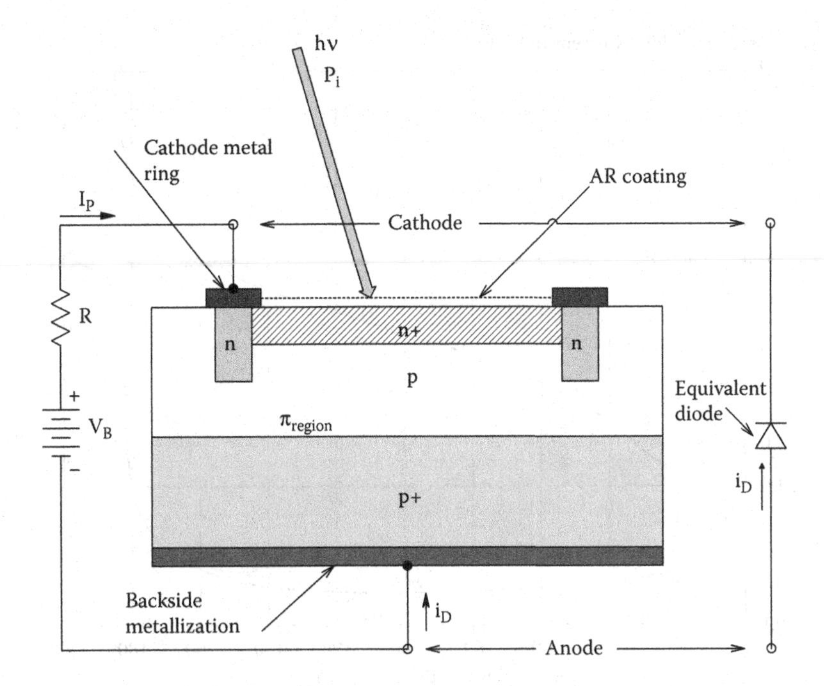

FIGURE 2.60 Cross-sectional, layer cake model of an avalanche photodiode.

APD noise is mostly due to *shot noise.* As in the case of the PIN PD, the shot noise is a broadband (white) Gaussian noise whose mean-squared value is proportional to the net DC component of the APD's anode current, I_{Dtot}. The DC anode current has two components; dark leakage current, I_L, and DC photo-current, I_P. The mean-squared shot noise current is given by

$$\overline{i_n^{\,2}} = 2\,q\,I_{Dtot}B \text{ msV} \tag{2.195}$$

It is clear that the lowest APD shot noise occurs when the APD is operated at very low (average) light levels. Figure 2.61 illustrates the peak gain and RMS shot noise current as a function of the DC reverse bias voltage on a "typical" Si APD.

The total leakage current, I_L, can be written as

$$I_L = I_{LS} + MI_{LB} \tag{2.196}$$

where I_{LS} is the dark surface leakage current (not amplified), and I_{LB} is the bulk leakage current (which gets amplified by the avalanche process).

The theoretical MS shot noise current may also be written as

$$\overline{i_n^{\,2}} = 2qB\{I_{LS} + [I_{LB}M^2 + P_i\ R_1(\lambda)M]\ F\} \text{ msA} \tag{2.197}$$

where q is the electron charge magnitude, I_{LS} is the *dark surface leakage current,* I_{LB} is the *dark bulk leakage current.* $I_P = P_i\,R_1(\lambda)\,M$ is the amplified dc photocurrent. F is the *excess noise factor.* In general, $F = \rho M + (1 - \rho)(2 - 1/M)$. Since $M \approx 100$, $F \cong 2 + \rho M$. The parameter ρ is the ratio of hole-to-electron ionization probabilities and is <1. M is the *voltage-dependent, APD internal*

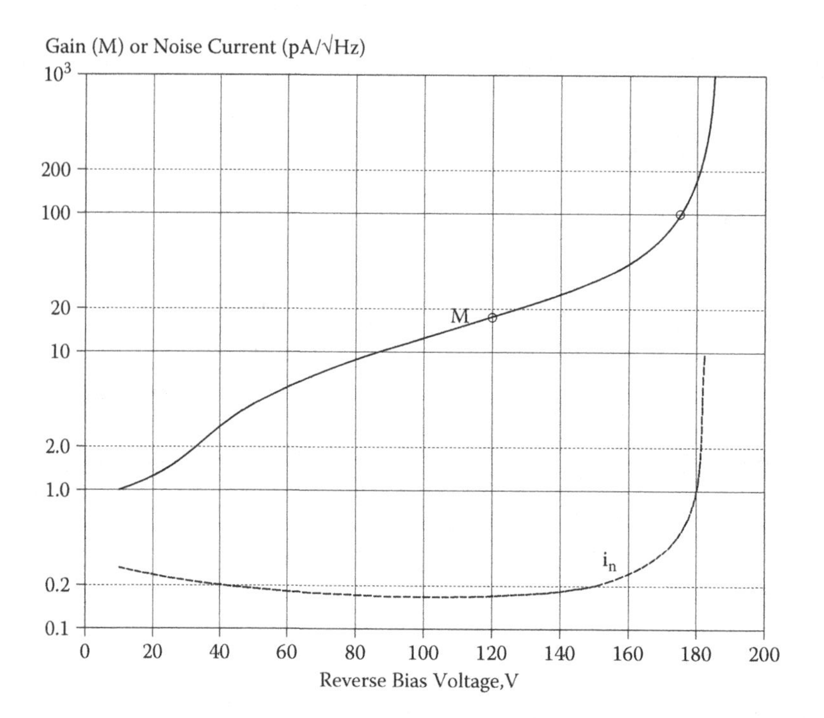

FIGURE 2.61 Plot of peak photonic gain, M, and shot noise root power spectrum, i_n, for a typical avalanche PD.

gain. It is defined as the ratio of the output current at a given P_i, λ, and dc reverse-bias voltage, V_R, to the output current for the same input (P_i and λ), but at a low DC reverse-bias voltage, say 10 V. P_i is the *incident optical power* at wavelength λ, $R(\lambda,V_D)$ is the *spectral responsivity* in A/W, and B is the *Hz noise bandwidth*.

The Perkin-Elmer PE C30902S APD has the following parameters at a reverse voltage of ca. 225 V: F = 0.02M + 0.98(2 − 1/M). M = 250 at 830 nm. Thus, F = 6.956. The responsivity at 830 nm is R(λ) = 128 A/W. (Divide the responsivity at 830 nm by M and we have $R_1(830) = 0.512$ A/W.) Total dark current is $I_D = 1 \times 10^{-8}$ A. The *noise current root spectrum*, $i_n = 1.1 \times 10^{-13}$ rmsA/$\sqrt{\text{Hz}}$. The *shunt capacitance* is $C_d = 1.6$ pF. The *rise time* and *fall time* to an 830 nm light pulse with a 50 Ω R_L (10—90%), $t_r = t_f = 0.5$ ns.

The wavelength range of the APD responsivity curve, R(λ), depends on the APD material: Si APDs are useful between 300 to 1100 nm, Ge APDs between 800 and 1600 nm, and InGaAs devices respond between 900 to 1700 nm. The peak responsivity depends on the average reverse bias voltage on the APD. $R_1(\lambda)$ is defined as the APD's responsivity at a low V_R such that M = 1. Thus, the APD's (amplified) photocurrent at a given λ and V_R, can be written as

$$I_P = P_i R_1(\lambda)\, M = P_i R(\lambda) \text{ amps} \tag{2.198}$$

As pointed out above, the total shot noise from an APD depends not only on DC leakage current, but also on DC photocurrent. There is also a noise current from any Thevenin conductance shunting the APD. Thus, the total diode noise in MS amps is given by

$$\overline{i_n^2} = 2qB\{I_{LS} + [I_{LB}M^2 + P_i\; R_1(\lambda)\; M]\; F\} + 4kTG_L B \; msA \tag{2.199}$$

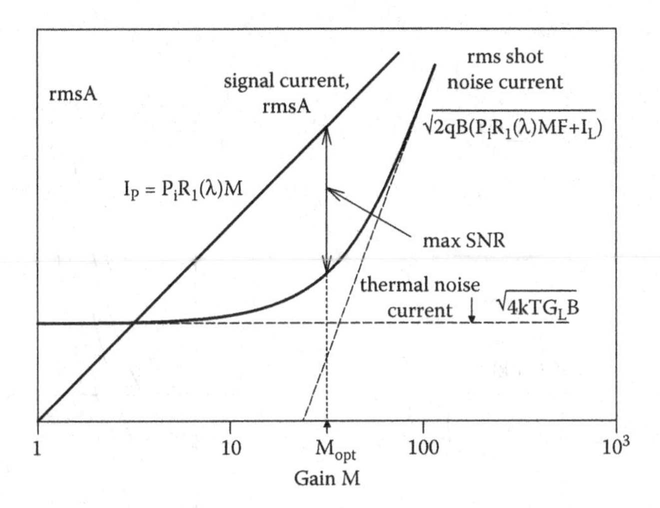

FIGURE 2.62 Plot of signal current and rms shot noise current for a typical APD vs. gain M, showing the optimum M where the diode's RMS SNR is maximum.

The APD's msSNR can be written, noting that $F \cong 2 + \rho M$:

$$SNR = \frac{P_i^2 R_1^2(\lambda)\, M^2}{2qB\{I_{LB}M + P_i R_1(\lambda)]\, MF\} + 4kTG_L B}$$

$$= \frac{P_i^2 R_1^2(\lambda)/B}{2q\{I_{LS}/M^2 + [I_{LB} + P_i R_1(\lambda)/M](2 + \rho M)\} + 4kTG_L/M^2} \tag{2.200}$$

Inspection of the *denominator* of the right-hand *SNR* expression shows that it has a minimum at some $M = M_o$, which results in a *maximum SNR*, other factors remaining constant. This optimum M_o is illustrated in Figure 2.62. Recall that M is set by the DC reverse bias on the APD, V_R, so finding the optimum V_R and M to optimize the APD SNR can be challenging.

2.6.4 Signal Conditioning Circuits for Photodiodes

The most basic signal conditioning circuit for a PD is the simple DC Thevenin circuit shown in Figure 2.57. As discussed in the text, the output voltage from the photocurrent can be found graphically using the load-line determined by V_B and R. Neglecting dark current, it is simply

$$V_o = q\eta(P_i\lambda/hc)\, R \text{ Volts} \tag{2.201}$$

A commonly used active circuit used to condition PD output is shown in Figure 2.63. Because the summing junction of the op amp is at virtual ground, the PD is held at a constant reverse-bias, V_B. Since I_P flows through R_F, Ohm's law tells that $V_o = q\eta(P_i\,\lambda\,/hc)\,R_F$, neglecting leakage (dark) current. By operating a PIN PD at reverse bias, the junction depletion capacitance, C_d, is made smaller and the diode's bandwidth is increased. Unfortunately, reverse-bias also increases the leakage current, hence the device's shot noise. If V_B is made zero, then C_d is maximum and the PD's bandwidth is lowest. At zero bias, the leakage current → 0, and the diode's shot noise is minimal, depending only on the photocurrent. As will be seen in Chapter 9, R_F and the op amp itself contribute noise to V_o; this noise will not be discussed here, however. Sometimes a resistor is added in series with V_B to limit the current through the PD. This circuit is shown in Figure 2.64. Note that the maximum

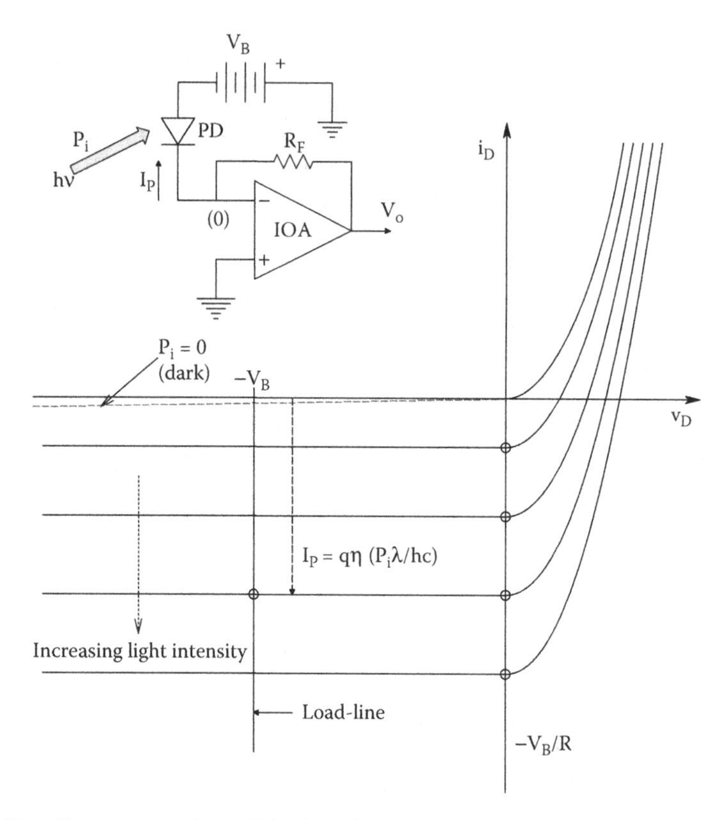

FIGURE 2.63 *Top:* Op amp signal conditioning circuit for a PIN PD operated at constant bias voltage. *Bottom:* Plot of PD i_D vs. v_D curves showing the constant voltage load-line.

PD current is determined by the load-line and is $i_D = -V_B/R$. APDs are run with the same circuit, except V_B is on the order of 100s of volts, and the series R (typically ≥1 MΩ) serves to protect the APD from excess reverse current which for most APDs is on the order of 100s of μA. While the series resistor protects the APD from excess reverse current, it also produces thermal (Johnson) noise over and above the APD's shot noise, and the noise which is produced in the op amp circuit.

An op amp circuit can be used to condition the output of a PIN PD to yield a *logarithmic output* proportional to P_i is shown in Figure 2.65. The PD is operated in the zero current mode. We solve for v_{Doc}

$$i_D = 0 = I_{rs}[\exp(V_{DOc}/V_T) - 1] - q\eta(P_i\lambda/hc) \tag{2.202a}$$

$$\downarrow$$

$$V_{Doc} = V_T \ln\left[1 + \frac{q\eta(P_i\lambda/hc)}{I_{rs}}\right] \tag{2.202b}$$

And because of the R_1, R_F voltage divider, one finally obtains

$$V_o = (1 + R_F/R_1)V_T \ln\left[1 + \frac{q\eta(P_i\lambda/hc)}{I_{rs}}\right] \tag{2.203}$$

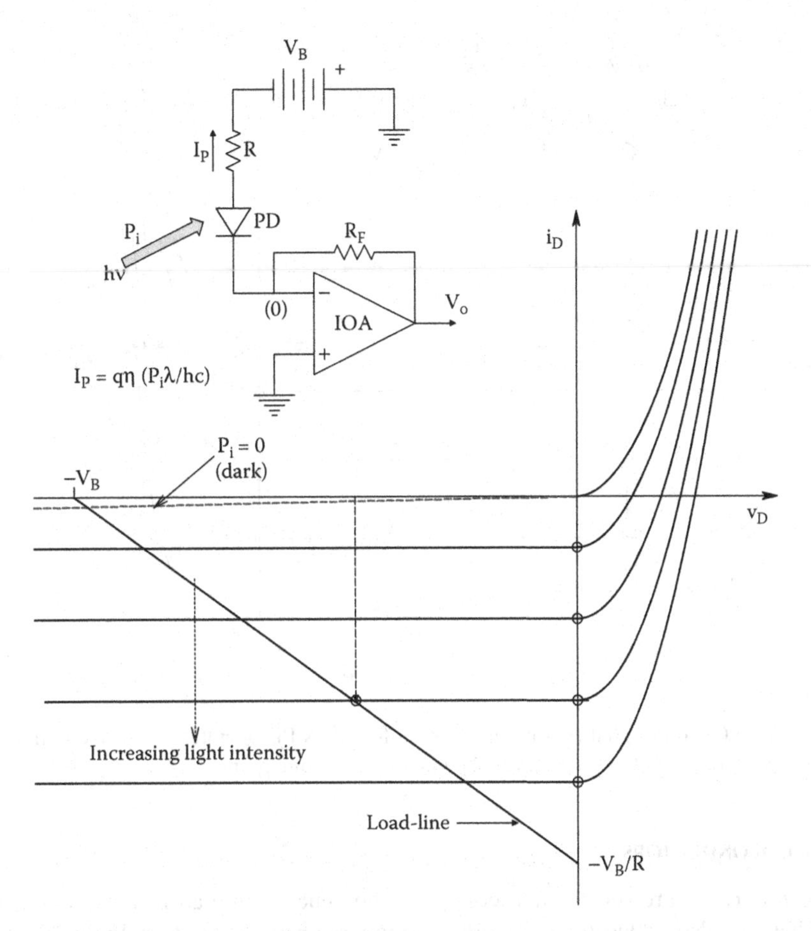

FIGURE 2.64 *Top:* Op amp signal conditioning circuit for a PIN PD biased from a Thevenin dc source. *Bottom:* Plot of PD i_D vs. v_D curves showing the load-line.

At very low light powers, using the relation $\ln(1 + \varepsilon) \cong \varepsilon$, V_o can be approximated by

$$V_o \cong (1 + R_F/R_1)V_T\left(\frac{q\eta(P_i\lambda/hc)}{I_{rs}}\right) \tag{2.204}$$

Typical parameter values are as follows: $(1 + R_F/R_1) = 10^3$, $V_T = kT/q = 0.0258$, $q = 1.602 \times 10^{-19}$ Cb, $\eta \cong 0.8$, $\lambda = 512$ nm, $h = 6.625 \times 10^{-34}$ J.sec., $c = 3 \times 10^8$ m/s, $I_{rs} \cong 1$ nA, NEP $\cong 5 \times 10^{-14}$ W. Neglecting leakage (dark) current, one can calculate V_o for $P_i = 1$ pW @ $\lambda = 512$ nm: Thus, $V_o = 8.51$ mV.

Several manufacturers make ICs containing a PIN photodiode with an on-chip amplifier. For example, Burr-Brown (acquired by Texas Instruments in 2000) makes the OPT202 photosensor, which has a 2.29 × 2.29 mm PD coupled to an op amp having an internal 1 MΩ feedback resistor, as shown in Figure 2.66. This IC works over a wide supply voltage range (±2.25 to ±18 V) and has a voltage output responsivity of 0.45 V/μW at $\lambda = 650$ nm with its internal $R_F = 1$ MΩ. It has a −3 dB bandwidth of 50 kHz, and a 10 to 90% rise time of 10 μs. To alter system responsivity, the R_F can be either be made larger or smaller than the internal 1 MΩ R_F. The IC's NEP is 10^{-11} W for B = 1 kHz and $\lambda = 650$ nm with $R_F = 1$ MΩ.

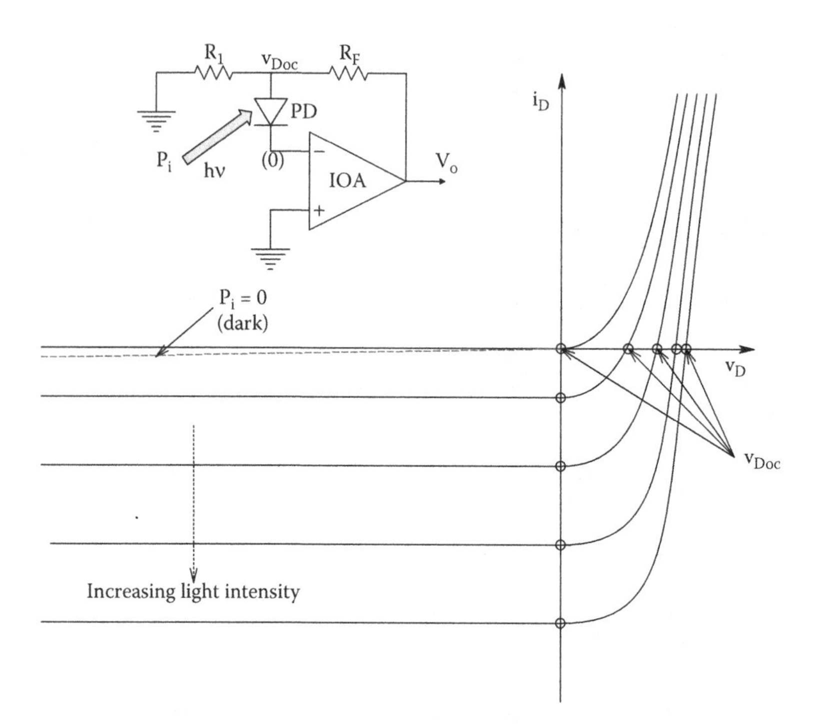

FIGURE 2.65 *Top:* Op amp signal conditioning circuit for a PIN PD operated in the open-circuit photovoltage mode. *Bottom:* Plot of PD i_D vs. v_D curves showing the operating points.

2.6.5 Photoconductors

Photoconductors (PCs) are sensors that convert photon energy into an increase in electrical conductance. They are also called *light-dependent resistors or photoresistors.* Figure 2.67 illustrates the cross-sectional schematic of a typical PC device. PCs can be made from a number of intrinsic and doped semiconductor materials. Each semiconductor has a distinct spectral response to light, ranging from UV to FIR. Table 2.1 lists some of the materials used in PCs, their bandgap energies in eV, and the wavelength of their peak spectral response.

In general, the total current in a PC can be written using Ohm's law:

$$I_{PC} = V_s[G_D + G_P] \tag{2.205}$$

where V_s is the bias voltage, G_D is the equivalent dark conductance, and G_P is the photoconductance. G_P can be shown to be given by (Yang 1988):

$$G_P = \frac{I_P}{V_s} = \frac{q\,\eta\,\tau_p(\mu_p + \mu_n)}{l^2}\left[\frac{P_i\lambda}{hc}\right] \text{ Siemens} \tag{2.206}$$

where τ_p is the *mean lifetime of holes*, $\mu_p = |\mathbf{v_p}/E|$ = *hole mobility* in cm²/V s, $\mu_n = |\mathbf{v_n}/E|$ = electron mobility in cm²/V s, v_p and v_n are the mean drift velocities of holes and electrons, respectively, in cm/s, E is the uniform **E**-field in the semiconductor, and q, η, P_i, λ, h, and c have been defined earlier. Note that in general, $\mu_n > \mu_p$. The expression for G_P is an approximation, valid up to the cut-off wavelength, λ_c. $[P_i\lambda/hc] = \Phi_i$, the incoming number of photons/second on area wl cm².

The dark conductance of a Si PC can be found simply from the room temperature resistivity of Si, ρ, and the geometry of the PC. For example,

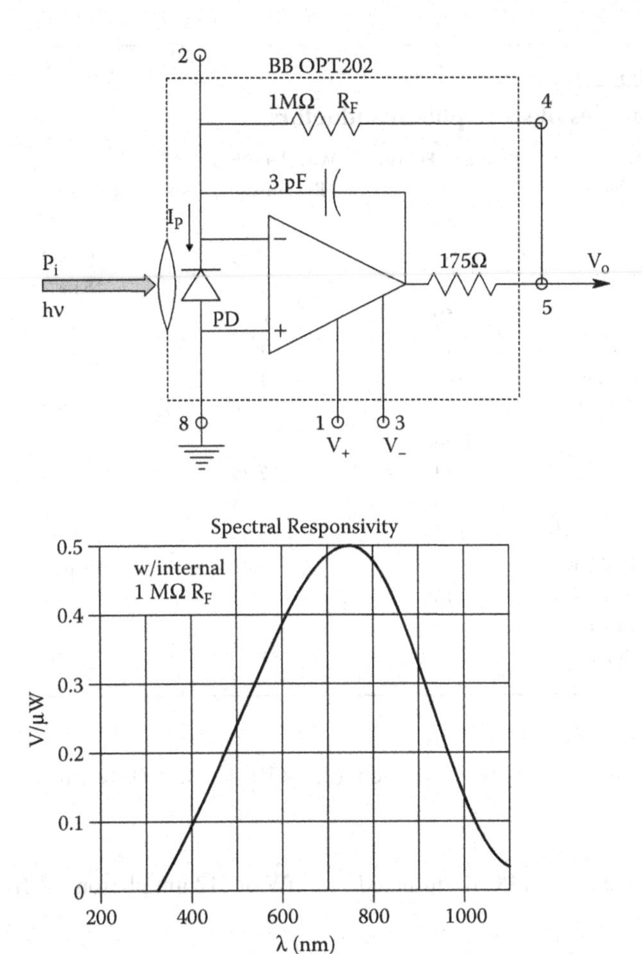

FIGURE 2.66 *Top:* Schematic of the Burr-Brown OPT202 IC photosensor. *Bottom:* Spectral sensitivity of the OPT202 sensor. See Text for details.

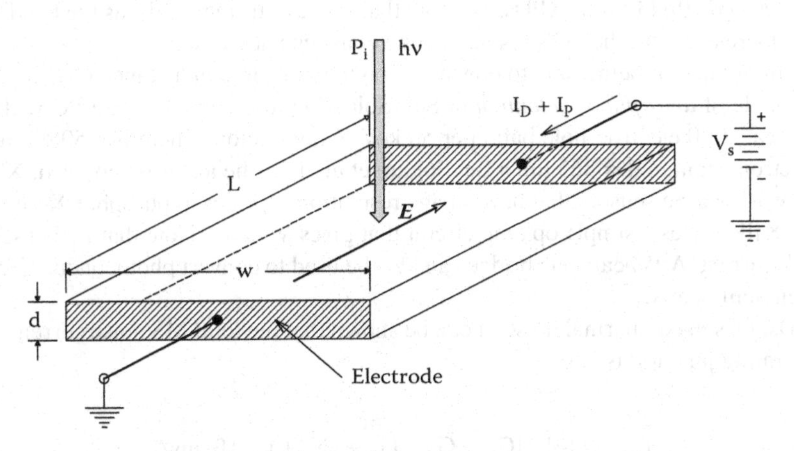

FIGURE 2.67 Geometry of a photoconductor slab.

TABLE 2.1
Properties of some photoconductors

PC Material	Bandgap Energy, eV	Wavelength of Peak Response, λ_c, μm	Rise time/Fall time
ZnS	3.60	0.345	
CdS	2.40	0.52	30 ms/10 ms
CdSe	1.80	0.69	15 ms/15 ms
CdTe	1.50	0.83	
Si (intrinsic)	1.12	1.10	1 μs/1 μs
Ge (intrinsic)	0.67	1.85	0.1 μs/0.1 μs
PbS	0.37	3.35	
InAs	0.35	3.54	≈ 1 ns
Te	0.33	7.75	
PbTe	0.30	4.13	
PbSe	0.27	4.58	2 μs
HgCdTe (77 K)		5.0	*/5 μs
InSb (77 K)	0.18	6.90	
GeCu (4 K)		25	
GeBe (3 K)		55	

$$G_D = A/\rho l = w\,d/\rho l = 0.2\text{ cm} \times 0.001\text{ cm}/(2.3 \times 10^3\ \Omega\text{ cm} \times 0.02\text{ cm}) = 4.348 \times 10^{-6}\text{ S.} \tag{2.207}$$

The photoconductance for a Si PC illuminated by 1 μW of 512 nm photons is, from Equation 2.206,

$$G_P = \frac{\overset{\text{Cb}}{1.6 \times 10^{-19}} \times \overset{\eta}{0.8} \times \overset{\tau_p}{10^{-4}}\ \overset{\text{cm}^2/\text{V.sec.}}{(1350 + 450)}}{\underset{\text{cm}^2}{10^{-4}}} \left[\frac{\overset{\text{W}}{10^{-6}} \times \overset{\text{m}}{512 \times 10^{-9}}}{\underset{\text{joule.sec}}{6.625 \times 10^{-34}} \times \underset{\text{m/sec.}}{3 \times 10^{8}}} \right] = 5.935 \times 10^{-4}\ \text{Siemens} \tag{2.208}$$

A great advantage of PCs is their unique ability to respond to MIR and FIR photons at wavelengths not sensed by PIN PDs or APDs. We note that for various materials, as the band-gap energy decreases, λ_c increases, and the PC's response time constants decrease.

PCs also are unique in being able to convert X-ray photons to conductance change. X-ray sensing PCs are made of *amorphous selenium* (a-Se) (Soltani et al. 1999). An a-Se PC with $E = 10$ V/μm produces ca. 1000 electron-hole pairs per 50 keV X-ray photon. There is a 50% attenuation of a 50 keV electron beam in d = 365 μm a-Se. Soltani et al. describe a charge-coupled, X-ray photon sensing *array* using a-Se sensors that have image resolution superior to phosphor X-ray sensors.

Figure 2.68 illustrates a simple op amp circuit that gives Vo ∝ Pi. Note that R_C is used to cancel the PC's dark current. A Wheatstone bridge can also be used to convert photoconductance to output voltage, albeit nonlinearly.

Unlike PDs, PCs make thermal noise. It can be shown that the total MS noise current input to the op amp's summing junction is

$$\overline{i^2_{ntot}} = \{4kT[G_D + G_P + G_C + G_F] + i_{na}^2\}B \text{ msA} \tag{2.209}$$

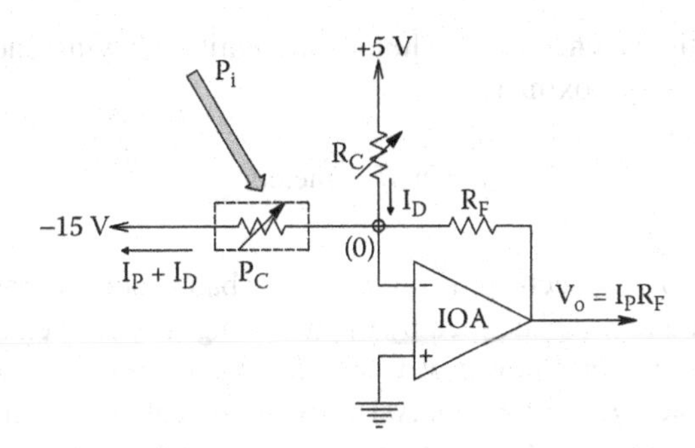

FIGURE 2.68 Op amp circuit for conditioning a photoconductive sensor's output. The current through R_C compensates for the PC's dark current.

Note that the MS noise increases with input light power because G_P increases with P_i. In addition to the noise current, the op amp also has an equivalent, short-circuit input noise voltage, e_{na}^2 B ms V. However, such noise will be considered in Chapter 9 of this text.

2.6.6 LEDs

LEDs are widely used in all electronic applications as pilot lights, status indicators, and warning signals. They are also used in biomedical applications as (approximately) monochromatic light sources for chemical analysis by nondispersive spectrophotometry. LEDs can be purchased that not only emit near IR, but also visible red, orange, yellow, green, blue, near UV, and white light. An important application for LEDs in Biomedicine is in the *pulse oximeter*, which is basically a two-wavelength, nondispersive spectrophotometer used to measure blood oxygen saturation (Northrop 2002). One NIR LED emits at 805 nm, the isobestic wavelength for *deoxyhemoglobin* (Hb) and *oxyhemoglobin* (HbO_2) absorbance (the wavelength where both Hb and HbO_2 absorbances are equal). The other wavelength is at ca. 650 nm (red), where there is a large difference between the absorbances of Hb and HbO_2. LEDs are also used as the light sources in some designs of the paper strip, blood glucose sensors. Again, a two-λ spectrophotometer is used. Even though LEDs are relatively broad-band emitters, their spectral purity is good enough for simple spectrophotometric measurements.

An LED is a solid-state, *pn* junction device that emits photons upon the application of a forward-biasing current. It converts electric energy directly into photon energy without the intermediate step of thermal conversion. LED *p*-material is typically doped gallium aluminum arsenide (dGaAlAs), while the *n*-material is doped gallium arsenide (dGaAs). Between the *p*- and *n*- layers is an *active layer.* When a forward voltage (and current) are applied to the LED, holes from the *p*-region (GaAlAs) meet electrons from the *n*-doped GaAs layer in the active layer and recombine, producing photons. Photon wavelength is dependent on the chemical composition and relative energy levels of the two doped semicon layers. It also depends to a small degree on the junction temperature and I_D. Visible-light LEDs typically have plastic dome lenses that serve to expand and diffuse the light from the LED's active layer. The plastic is colored to indicate the color of the emitted light. Clear plastic lenses are used for NIR LEDs.

The wavelength of the emitted light can be altered by varying the composition of the doped semicon materials used in the LED. Typical materials used in LED construction include Al, As, Ga, In, P, and N (as nitrides). White light can be made by several mechanisms, but one way is to make a blue LED and use the blue light to excite a mixture of phosphors in the reflector cup that emit at several longer wavelengths; the mixture of wavelengths appears white.

LED forward voltage is on the order of 1.5 V, and operating currents range from a few mA to 10s of mA. When a forward current is applied through a *pn* junction, carriers are injected across the junction to establish excess carriers above the thermal equilibrium values. The excess carriers recombine, and in so doing, some energy is released in the form of heat, and light (photons). The injected electrons in the *p* side make a downward energy transition from the conduction band to recombine with holes in the valence band. Photons are emitted having energy about Eg in Joules. The emission wavelength is approximately

$$\lambda = hc/E_g \text{ meters} \quad (2.210)$$

In practice, the emission power spectrum is not a narrow band such as produced by lasers, but is a curve with a smooth peak and a "Q" defined by the wavelength of the peak emission power density divided by the $\Delta\lambda$ between the half-power wavelengths on either side of the peak (Table 2.2). That is, $Q = \lambda_{pk}/\Delta\lambda$. For example, $Q \cong 16$ for a GaAsP LED with peak emission at 650 nm (Yang 1988). The Qs for Siemens LEDs LS5421, LO5411, LY5421, and LG5211 emitting power peaks at 635, 610, 586, and 565 nm with spectral bandwidths of 45, 40, 45, and 25 nm, respectively.

Figure 2.69a illustrates the I-V characteristics of a green, gallium phosphide (GaP) LED. Compare this curve with the I-V curve for a typical small-signal, Si *pn* junction diode, as shown on Figure 2.69b. Figure 2.69c illustrates the light intensity vs. I_D for a green LED. Figure 2.70 illustrates the relative spectral emission of a GaP green LED. The peak is at ca. 561 nm, and the half intensity width is measured at ca. 26 nm, giving an LED Q = 21.6.

Modern LEDs are now available in the *near UV*, which provides excellent application in biochemical fluorescence analysis as an inexpensive source of excitation for DNA microarrays (gene chips) and many other modes of fluorescent chemical analysis. Their UV can also be used to catalyze the polymerization of dental fillings, and for spot sterilization. For example, the Nichia NSHU550E UV LED (gallium indium nitride) has an UV spectral emission peak centered at 370 nm, quite invisible to the human eye. Nichia also makes gallium nitride (GaN) single quantum well LEDs that emit blue with a peak at ca. 470 nm that are intended for excitation in fluorescence applications including protein and DNA analysis using SYBR® green and SYPRO® orange molecular tags.

It will be seen in the following section that laser diodes (LADs) have much narrower spectral emission lines, but also can have, under certain operating conditions, many closely spaced emission lines.

2.6.7 Laser Diodes

The basic difference between an LED and a laser diode (LAD) is that the latter has an optical resonance cavity which promotes lasing. The optical cavity has two *end facet partial mirrors* that reflect

TABLE 2.2
Semiconductor LED Materials And Approximate Emission Peaks Wavelengths

Material	Peak Wavelength (μm)	Photon Energy (eV)
GaP (Zn, diffused green)	0.553	2.24
$Ga_{1-x}Al_xAs$ (red)	0.688	1.78
GaP (Zn, 0-doped red)	0.698	1.76
GaAs (NIR)	0.84	1.47
InP	0.9	1.37
Ga (As_xP_{1-x})	1.41–1.95	
GaSb	1.5	0.82
PbS (MIR)	4.26	0.29
InSb	5.2	0.23
PbTe	6.5	0.19
PbSe	8.5	0.145

Peak emission λ depends on temperature and diode current.

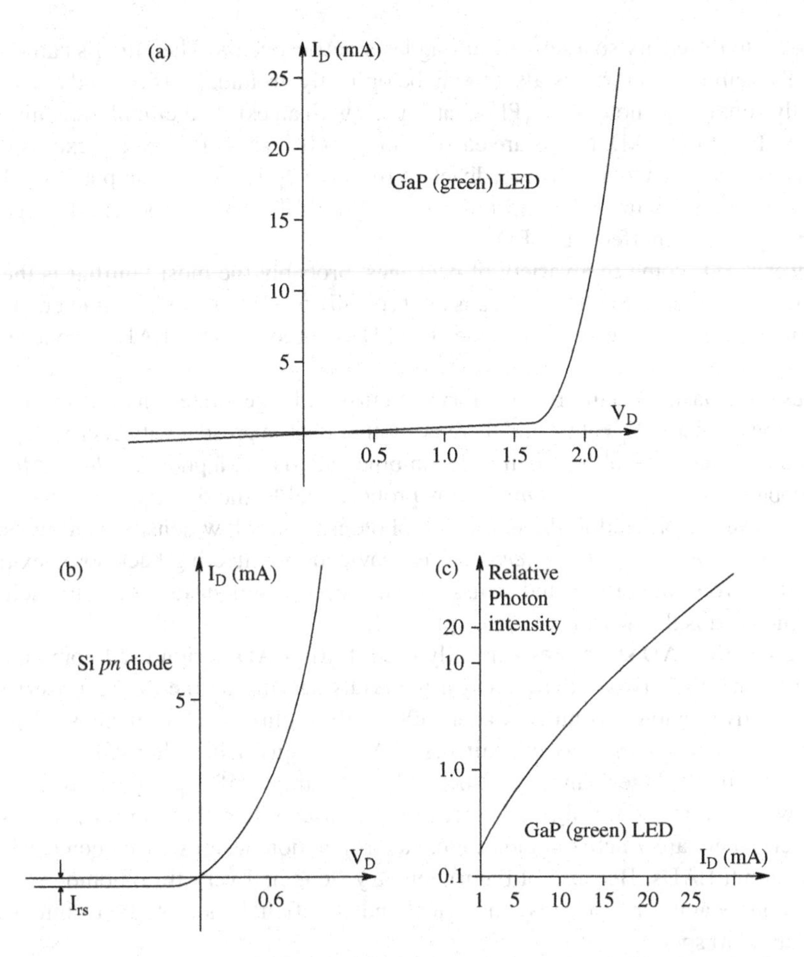

FIGURE 2.69 (a) i_D vs. v_D curve for a GaP (green) LED. Note the high threshold voltage for forward conduction. (b) For comparison, the i_D vs. v_D curve for a typical Si, small-signal *pn* diode. (c) Relative light intensity vs. forward current.

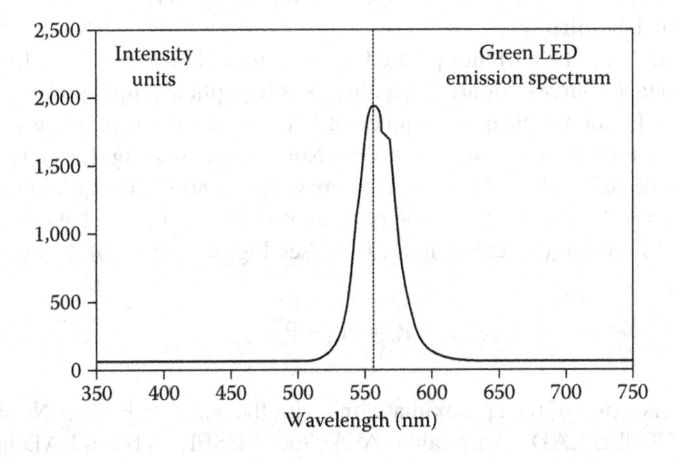

FIGURE 2.70 Spectral emission characteristic of a GaP green LED.

photons back into the cavity so a self-sustaining laser action occurs. The mirrors can be the cleaved surfaces of the semiconductor crystals, or may be optically ground, polished and coated. The LAD unit generally contains a photodiode (PD) that is used with an external circuit to monitor the optical power output, P_o, of the LAD. LADs are easily damaged by excess ID causing excess P_o. Often the PD output is used to provide negative feedback to limit the optical power output of the LAD so that the end mirrors are not damaged by heat or excess light. If the end mirrors are damaged, the LAD becomes an expensive, ineffective, LED.

Low power LADs come in a variety of packages, probably the most familiar is the cylindrical can with top (end) window. Such "TO-" cans are typically 5.6 or 9.0 mm in diameter, and have three leads; common, LAD cathode and PD anode. The PD's cathode and the LAD's anode are connected to the common lead.

How does diode lasing occur? If some forward current, I_D, generates an electron-hole pair ready to emit a photon of energy $E_g = h\nu_o$, and there is another photon present with energy $h\nu_o$, the existing photon stimulates the electron-hole pair to recombine and to emit a photon *coherent to* the existing one. The probability of *stimulated emission* is proportional to the density of excess electrons and holes in the active region, and to the density of photons. Under low density conditions, it is negligible. However, if *coherent positive feedback* is provided by reflecting back some exiting photons with the end mirrors, the stimulated emission can become self-sustaining. This self-sustaining, stimulated emission is the heart of the laser principle.

There are several LAD structures currently used. Early LAD design used homojunction architecture; the boundary between the *p*- and *n*-materials serving as the *active* (laser) *region*. The length of the active region was much longer (300 to 1000 μm) than its thickness (1 μm) or width (3 μm). The end facets served as the mirrors. LAD designs using alternating layers of *p*- and *n*-materials is called a heterojunction structure. For example, if 3 *p*-layers are alternated with 3 *n*-layers, we see that there are 5 active regions to lase. When there are 4 *p*-layers alternated with 4 *n*-layers, there are 7 active regions, etc. Heterojunction designs have been used to fabricate high-power output LADs. Because of their geometry (long and very thin) homo- and heterojunction LAD output beams tend to be asymmetrical and are often difficult to focus into a small, symmetrical (Gaussian) spot.

The newer, *vertical cavity, surface-emitting laser* (VCSEL) diodes consist of a (top) light exit window (it can be round, 5 to 25 μm diameter), a top distributed Bragg reflector, a gap to set the emission wave-length, two λ-spacers surrounding a GaAs active region, then a bottom distributed Bragg reflector sitting on the bottom substrate. VCSEL lasers operate in a single longitudinal mode. They can be designed to have an anastigmatic Gaussian beams, which are easy to focus with simple lenses. Because the mirror area is larger, VCSEL lasers are not as prone to overpower damage, and there is no need for optical feedback as in edge-emitting LADs. They also lase at much lower IDs because of their efficient mirrors.

LADs are considered to be current-operated devices; they should be driven from regulated current sources, not voltage sources. Figure 2.71a illustrates the optical output power P_o from a LAD vs. the forward current, I_D, for a typical heterojunction LAD I_{Dt} is the *threshold current* where enough electron-hole pairs are produced to sustain lasing. Note that increasing device temperature moves the $P_o(I_D)$ curve to the right. The steep part of the curve is essentially linear and is characterized by its slope: $\Delta P_o / \Delta I_D = \rho$ W/amp. In the region of I_D between 0 and I_{Dt}, the LAD is basically a LED. An algebraic model for the $P_o(I_D)$ curve above I_{Dt} is (see Figure 2.75 (top)):

$$P_o = \rho I_D - P_x \qquad (2.211)$$

where P_x is the intersection of the approximate line with the negative P_o axis. Needless to say, I_{Dt} is much lower for a VCSEL LAD. (An Avalon, AVAP760, VCSEL, 760 nm LAD has $I_{Dt} = 2.0$ mA, and $I_{DQ} = 3.0$ mA. I_{DQ} is the operating current for this LAD.)

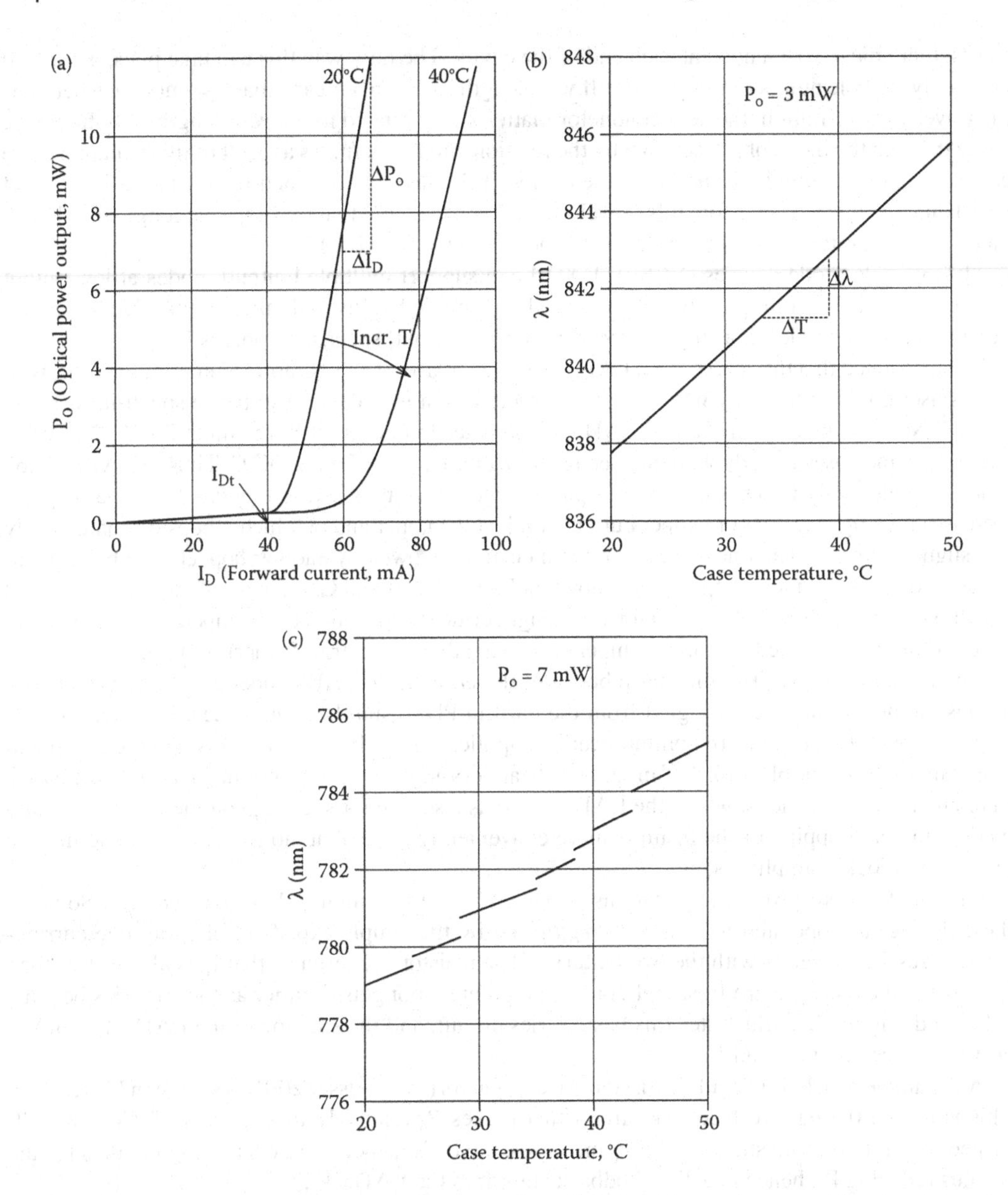

FIGURE 2.71 (a) Optical power output from a laser diode (LAD) vs. forward current. Note that increasing the heterojunction temperature decreases the output power at constant I_D. (b) Increase in output wavelength of a LAD at constant P_o with increasing case temperature. (c) Mode-hopping behavior of LAD output wavelength with increasing case temperature.

While VCSEL LADs have a *single mode output* (the 760 nm VCSEL above has a line Q of 3.95×10^{14} Hz/100 $\times$ 10^6 Hz = 3.95×10^6), homo- and heterojunction LADs generally emit a multimode, "comb" spectral output. The number of spectral lines that appear at the output of a gain-guided LAD depends on the properties of the cavity and mirrors, the operating current, and the temperature. Quoting the *Newport Laser Diode Tutorial* 2011:

"The result is that multimode laser diodes exhibit spectral outputs having many peaks around their central wavelength. The optical wave propagating through the laser cavity forms a standing wave between the two mirror facets of the laser. The period of oscillation of this curve is determined by the distance L between the two mirrors. This standing optical wave resonates only when the cavity length L is an integer number m of half wavelengths existing between the two mirrors. In other words, there must exist a node at each end of the cavity. The only way this can take place is for L to be exactly a whole number multiple of half wavelengths $\lambda/2$. This means that $L = m(\lambda/2)$, where λ is the wavelength of light in the semiconductor matter and is related to the wavelength of light in free space through the index of refraction n by the relationship $\lambda = \lambda_o/n$. As a result of this situation there can exist many longitudinal modes in the cavity of the laser diode, each resonating at its distinct wavelength of $\lambda_m = 2L/m$. From this [development] you can note that two adjacent longitudinal laser modes are separated by a wavelength [difference] of $\Delta\lambda = \lambda_o^2/(2nL)$."

"Even single-mode devices [VCSEL LADs] can support multiple [output] modes at low output power .... As the operating current is increased, one mode begins to dominate until, beyond a certain operating power level, a single narrow linewidth [output] spectrum appears."

It is also noted that the center λ of a LAD's output increases with operating temperature. This property is useful in spectroscopy where the fine structure of a molecular absorbance spectrum is being studied. Newport givers data for one LAD with a center frequency of 837.6 nm at 20°C. The center wavelength increases linearly with increasing temperature to 845.5 nm at 50°C. Thus, $\Delta\lambda/\Delta T = 0.263$ nm/°C. Single-mode LADs can exhibit a phenomenon known as *mode-hopping*. Here the output λ increases linearly over a short temperature interval, at the upper end of which it hops discontinuously to a slightly larger λ. The linear behavior again occurs, followed by another hop, etc. Both the linear behavior of $\lambda(T)$ and mode-hopping are shown in Figure 2.71B and C. Because of mode-hopping and λ drift with temperature, LADs used for wavelength critical applications are temperature stabilized to ca. 0.1°C around a desired operating temperature using thermoelectric (Peltier) cooling.

There are many circuits which have been developed to drive LADs under constant-current conditions. Some circuits use the signal from the built-in PD to stabilize the diode's P_o when CW AC or pulsed output is desired. In communications applications, where the LAD is driving an optical fiber cable, it is desirable to on/off modulate Po at very high rates, up into the GHz in some cases. In biomedical applications, where the LAD is used as a source for spectrophotometry, the intensity modulation or chopping of the beam is more conveniently done at audio frequencies to permit the operation of lockin amplifiers, etc.

One of the more prosaic applications of LADs is the common (CW) *laser pointer.* Some of these devices are operated *without any regulation* by the simple expedient of using one current-limiting resistor in series with the two batteries. The resistor is chosen so that I_D is always less than I_{Dmax} when the batteries are fresh. Of course the pointer spot gets dimmer as the batteries become exhausted. Figure 2.72 illustrates this basic series circuit, and the solution of the LAD's $I_D = f(V_D)$ curve with the circuit's load-line.

An example of a 2-BJT regulator used in laser pointers (Goldwasser 2001) is shown in Figure 2.73. This is a type 0, negative feedback circuit that makes P_o relatively independent of ΔV_B and ΔT. Inspection of this circuit shows that if P_o increases, the PD's I_P increases, decreasing I_{B2}, thus I_{B1} and I_D, thus reducing P_o; hence negative feedback stabilizes the LAD's P_o.

When it is desired to modulate a LAD at hundreds of MHz to GHz for communications applications, very special circuits indeed are used. LADs can be modulated around some 50% P_o point much faster than from fully off to fully on. Several semiconductor circuit manufacturers offer high frequency single-chip LAD regulator/drivers. For example, the Analog Devices AD9661A driver chip allows LAD on/off switching up to 100 MHz, and has <2 ns rise/fall times. The Maxim MAX3263 is a 155 Mbps LAD driver with < 1 ns rise/fall times. Needless to say, getting a LAD to switch at such rates can involve the artful use of ferrite beads, and consideration of parasitic distributed parameters such as LAD lead inductance and stray capacitances. The MAX3263 IC also has a "slow start" feature to protect the LAD at turn-on. The design of GHz modulation circuits are beyond the scope of this text and will not be treated here.

Figure 2.74 illustrates the architecture of an op amp feedback/modulation circuit designed by the author for spectrophotometric LAD applications. It uses a VCCS to drive the LAD, and a feedback loop containing signal conditioning for the on-board PD, a difference amplifier (DA), an integrator, and another DA. The input that sets the LAD's output power is V_{oQ}, which can be an audio-frequency

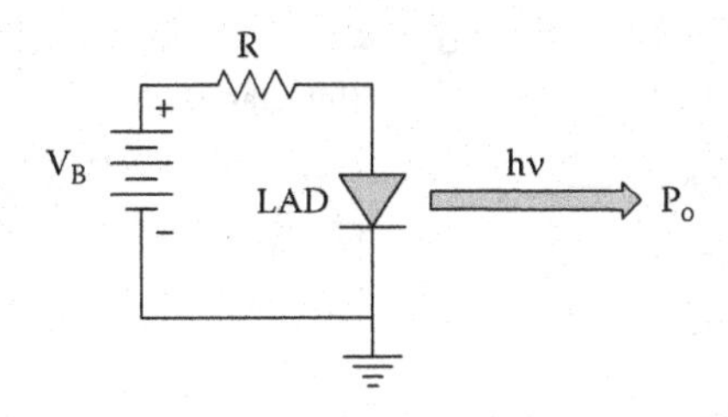

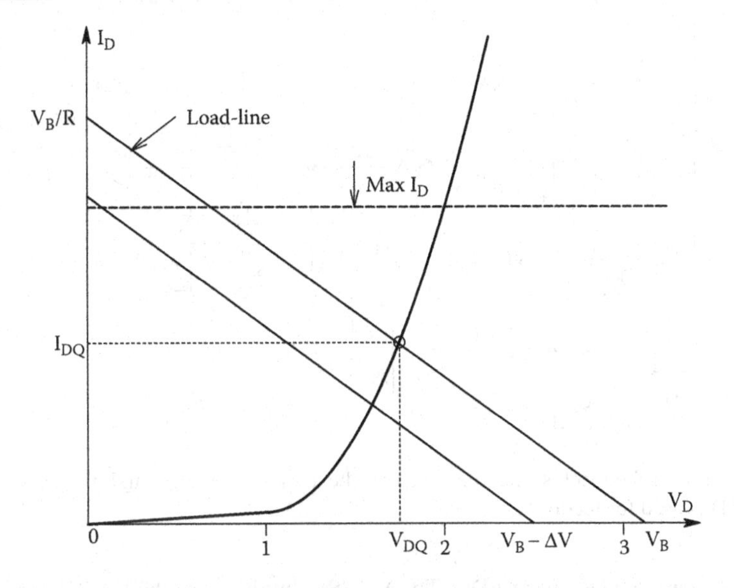

FIGURE 2.72 *Top:* LAD powered from a simple DC Thevenin circuit. *Bottom:* A LAD's i_D vs. v_D curve showing max i_D, load-lines and operating point.

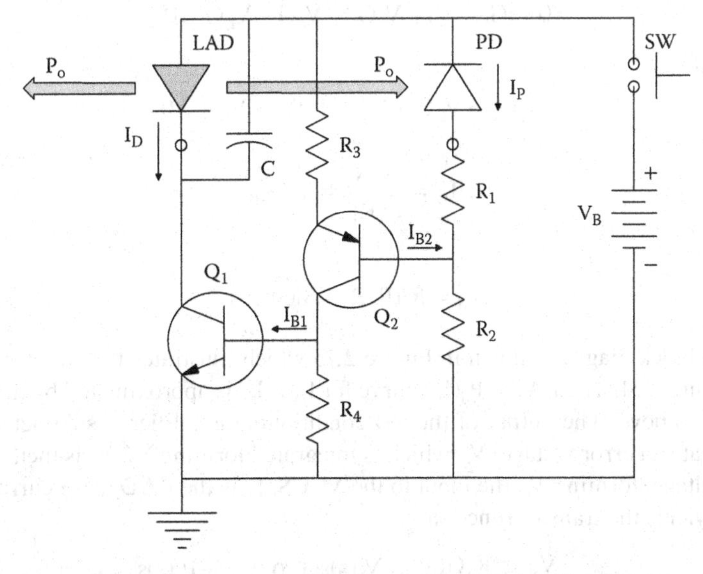

FIGURE 2.73 A simple LAD P_o (hence i_D) regulator circuit. The LAD's built-in PD is used to make a type-0 feedback, intensity regulator.

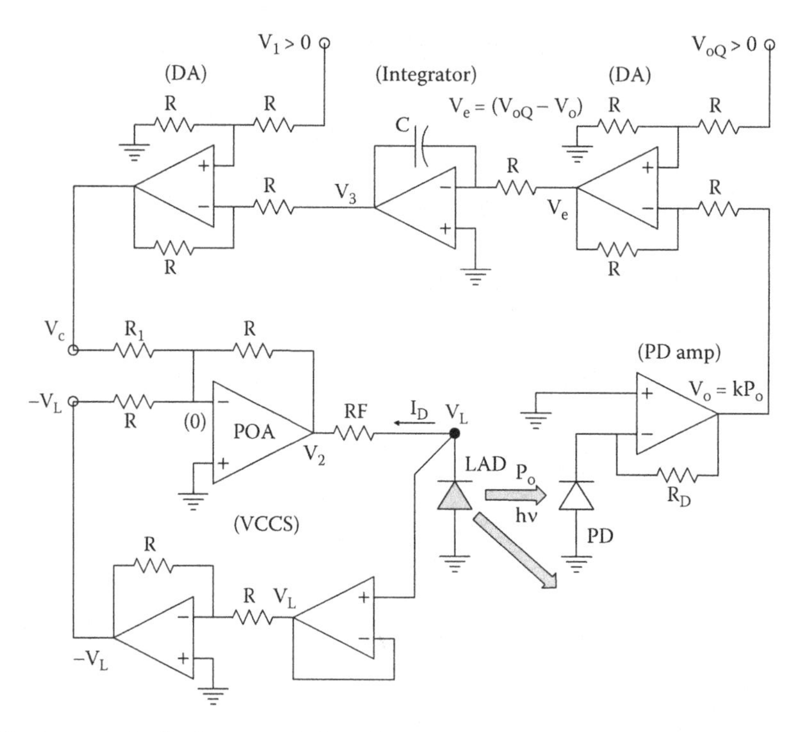

FIGURE 2.74 A type-1 feedback system designed by the author to regulate and modulate a LAD's P_o. The LAD's built-in PD is used for feedback.

square-wave, a sinewave +DC, or just DC. The VCCS subunit drives the LAD. Its transconductance can be found by KVL, noting:

$$V_2 = -(I_D\ R_F + V_L) \tag{2.212}$$

The node equation for the power op amp's summing junction can be written as

$$(0)[2G + G_1] - V_c G_1 - V_2 G - V_L G = 0 \tag{2.213}$$

Substituting for V_2,

$$-V_c G_1 - V_L G - G[-(I_D R_F + V_L)] = 0 \tag{2.214a}$$

$$\downarrow$$

$$I_D = \frac{V_c R}{R_1 R_F} = V_c G_M \tag{2.214b}$$

$$\downarrow$$

$$G_M = R/(R_1 R_F)\ \text{Siemens} \tag{2.214c}$$

Now refer to the block diagram shown in Figure 2.75 which illustrates the simplified dynamics of the circuit of Figure 2.74. The LAD's $P_o(I_D)$ curve for $I_D > I_{Dt}$ is approximated by the linear relation of Equation 2.211 above. The output of the PD conditioning amplifier is subtracted from the set-point, V_{oQ}, to create an error voltage, V_e, which is integrated forming V_3. V_3 is then subtracted from $V_1 > 0$, a bias voltage, forming V_c, the input to the VCCS. I_D is the LAD drive current. Application of Mason's rule yields the transfer function:

$$P_o = \frac{V_{oQ}(s) K_i G_M \rho}{s + K_i G_M \rho k} + \frac{V_1(s) s G_M \rho}{s + K_i G_M \rho k} + \frac{-P_x(s) s}{s + K_i G_M \rho k} \tag{2.215}$$

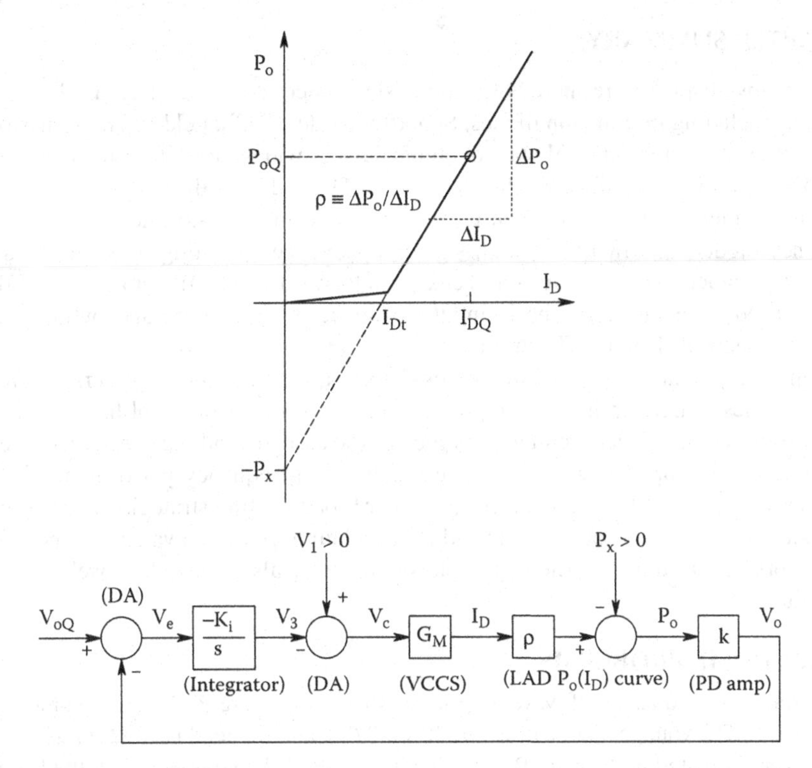

FIGURE 2.75 *Top:* Typical LAD i_D vs. v_D curve, showing desired P_{oQ}. *Bottom:* Simplified block diagram of the regulator/modulator of Figure 2.74. See Text for analysis.

Note that V_1 and P_x are DC levels. At turn-on, they can be considered to be steps. Using the *Laplace initial value theorem,* one finds

$$\underset{\lim s\to\infty}{P_o(0+)} = s\frac{V_{oQ}}{s}\frac{K_i G_M \rho}{s + K_i G_M \rho k} + s\frac{V_1}{s}\frac{s\, G_M \rho}{s + K_i G_M \rho k} - s\frac{P_x}{s}\frac{s}{s + K_i G_M \rho k} \tag{2.216a}$$

$$\downarrow$$

$$P_o(0+) = 0 + (V_1 G_M \rho - P_x) \tag{2.216b}$$

In other words, the *initial* P_o is set by V_1.

Next, we use the Laplace final *value theorem* to find P_{oSS}:

$$\underset{\lim s\to 0}{P_o SS} = s\frac{V_{oQ}}{s}\frac{K_i G_M \rho}{s + K_i G_M \rho k} + s\frac{V}{s}\frac{s\, G_M \rho}{s + K_i G_M \rho k} - s\frac{P_x}{s}\frac{s}{s + K_i G_M \rho k} \tag{2.217a}$$

$$\downarrow$$

$$P_o SS = \frac{V_{oQ} K_i G_M \rho}{K_i G_M \rho k} + 0 + 0 = V_{oQ}/k \tag{2.217b}$$

Note that the final value of P_o is independent of V_1 and P_x, and is set by V_{oQ}.

It has been shown that driving laser diodes safely is a complicated matter; it requires a VCCS and feedback to stabilize P_o against changes in temperature and supply voltage. It also requires a mechanism to protect the LAD against over-current surges at turn-on, and when switching I_D. Fortunately, several manufacturers now offer special ICs that both stabilize P_o and permit high-frequency modulation of the laser output intensity.

2.7 CHAPTER SUMMARY

Introduced in this chapter were models for the basic semiconductor devices used in analog electronic circuits, including *pn* junction diodes, Schottky diodes, BJTs, field-effect transistors (JFETs, MOSFETs), and some common solid-state photonic devices widely used in biomedical instrumentation, e.g., PIN photodiodes, avalanche photodiodes, LEDs, and laser diodes.

The circuit element models were seen to be subdivided into DC-to-midfrequency models and high-frequency models that included small-signal capacitances resulting from charge depletion at reverse-biased *pn* junctions, and from stored charge in forward-conducting junctions. Midfrequency models were used to examine the basic input resistance, voltage gain, and output resistance of simple, one-transistor BJT and FET amplifiers.

Also examined as analog IC "building blocks" were two-transistor amplifiers. High-frequency behavior of diodes, single transistor amplifiers, and two-transistor amplifiers were examined. Certain two-transistor amplifier architectures such as the cascode and the emitter (source) follower/grounded base (gate) amplifier were to give excellent high-frequency performance because they minimized or avoided the Miller effect. Certain other broadbanding strategies were described.

Semiconductor photon sensors were introduced including *pin* and avalanche photodiodes, and photoconductors. LEDs and laser diode photon sources were also covered, as well as circuits used in their operation.

CHAPTER 2 HOME PROBLEMS

2.1 A diode is used as a half-wave rectifier as shown in Figure P2.1a. (a) Assume the diode is ideal. The voltage source is $v_s(t) = 10\sin(377t)$, and the load is 10 Ω. *Find* the average power dissipated in the load, R_L. (b) Now let the diode be represented by the I-V curve in Figure P2.1b. *Find* the average power dissipated in the load, and also in the diode.

2.2 A diode bridge rectifier is shown in Figure P2.2. Each diode has the I-V curve of Figure P2.1b. *Find* the average power in the load, R_L, and also in each diode.

2.3 A zener diode power supply is shown in Figure P2.3. Its purpose is to deliver 5.1 VDC to an 85 Ω load, where a 9 V battery is the primary DC source. A 1N751 zener diode is used; its rated voltage is 5.1 V when a 20 mA reverse (zener) current, I_Z, is flowing. *Find:* The required value for R_s. Also *find* the power dissipation in the diode, R_s and R_L, and the power supplied by the battery.

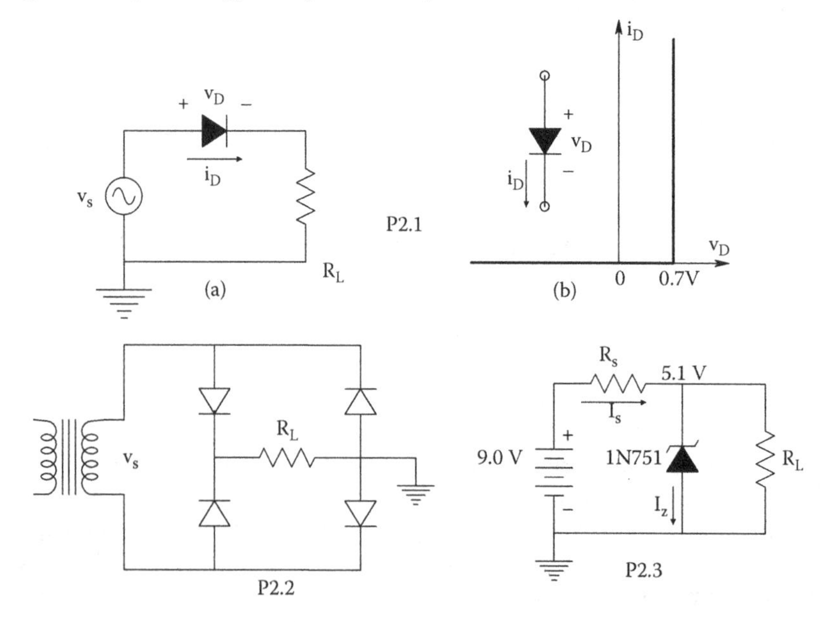

2.4 Refer to the emitter-follower in Figure P2.4. Given: $h_{FE} = 99$, $V_{BEQ} = 0.65$ V. (a) Find I_{BQ} and R_B required to make $V_{EQ} = 0$ V. (b) Calculate the quiescent power dissipation in the BJT and in R_E. (c) Calculate the small-signal h_{ie} for the BJT at its Q-point.

2.5 A *pnp* BJT grounded base amplifier is shown in Figure P2.5. Given: $h_{FE} = 149$, $V_{BEQ} = 0.65$ V. *Find* R_B and R_C so the amplifier's Q-point is at $I_{CQ} = -1.0$ mA, $V_{CEQ} = -5.0$ V. *Find* V_{EQ}.

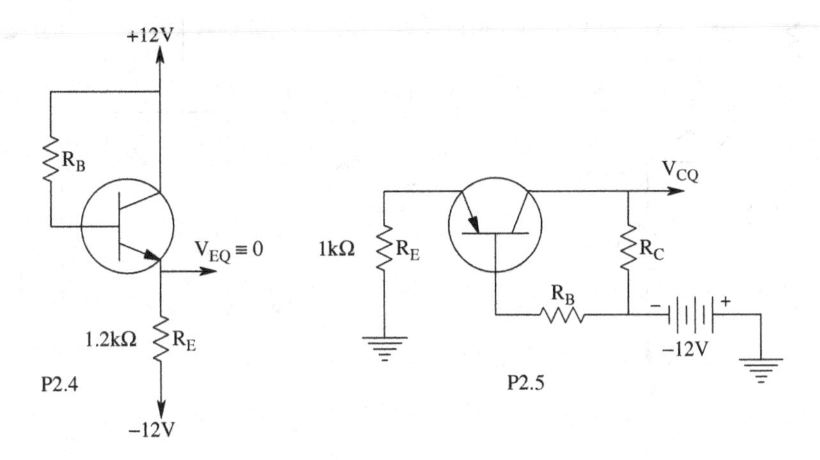

2.6 The circuit shown in Figure P2.6 is a *current mirror.* Given: $h_{FE} = 100$ (all 3 BJTs), $V_{CC} = +6.0$ V, $R = 12$ kΩ, $V_{BE1} = 0.65 = V_{BE2}$, $V_{BE3} = 0.60$ V, $V_{CE2} >> V_{CE2sat}$. (a) Find V_{CE1}. (b) Find I_R. (c) Find I_{E3}. (d) Find I_{B3}. (e) Find I_{C1} and I_{C2}.

2.7 An *npn* BJT grounded base amplifier is shown in Figure P2.7. Given: $V_{BEQ} = 0.65$ V, $h_{FE} = 119$. *Find* R_B and R_C so the Q-point is at $I_{CQ} = 2.5$ mA, $V_{CEQ} = 7$ V.

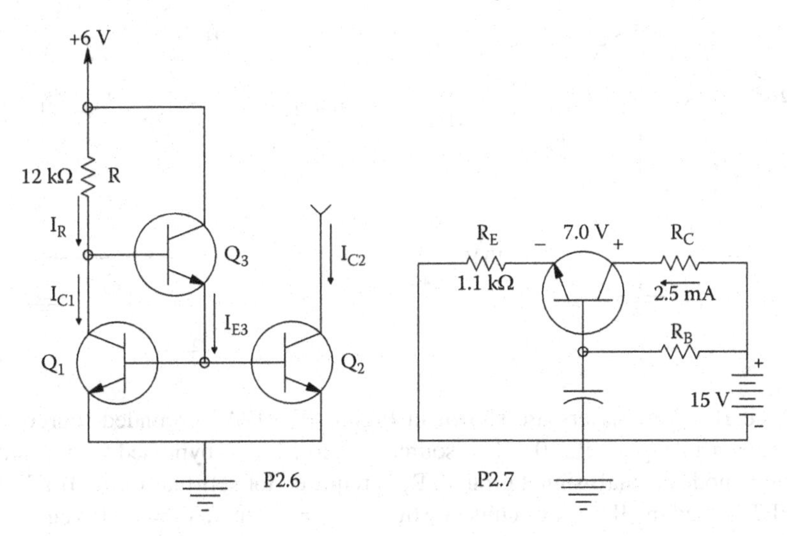

2.8 A *pnp* BJT emitter-follower is shown in Figure P2.8. *Given:* $h_{FE} = 99$, $V_{BEQ} = -0.65$ V.
(A) *Find:* R_B and I_{BQ} required to make $V_{CEQ} = -10$ V.
(B) Find the quiescent power dissipated in the BJT and in R_E.

2.9 Consider the three basic BJT amplifiers shown in Figure P2.9. In each amplifier, find the R_B required to make $I_{CQ} = 1$ mA. Also find V_{CEQ} in each circuit. Given: $h_{FE} = 100$ and $V_{BEQ} = 0.65$ V.

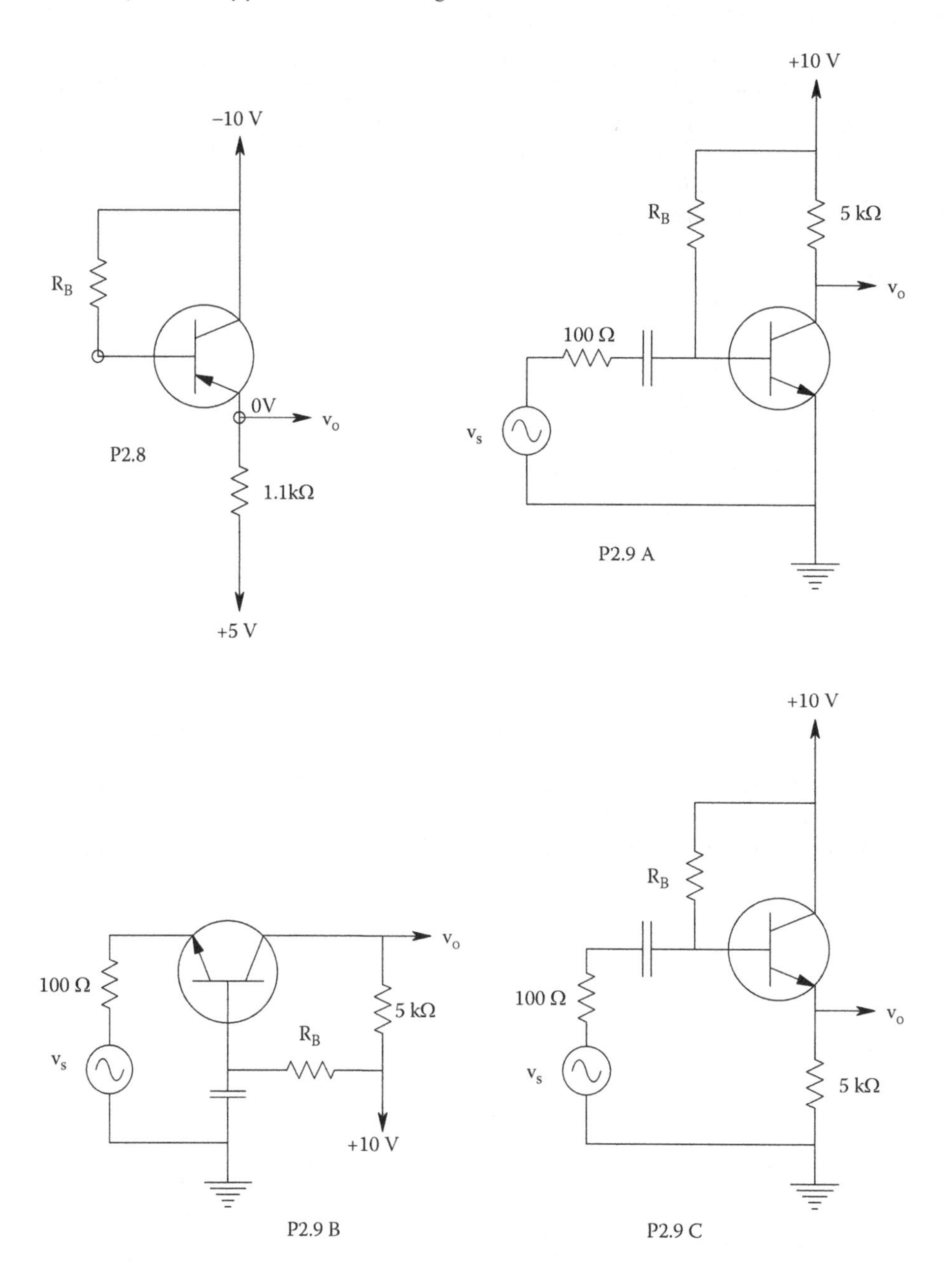

2.10 Three JFET amplifiers are shown in Figure P2.10. A "grounded-source" amplifier is shown in Figure P2.10a. The source resistor, R_S, is bypassed by C_S, making the source node at small-signal ground. R_S is required for self-bias of the JFET. The same JFET is used in all three circuits in which: $I_{DSS} = 6.0$ mA, $V_P = -3.0$ V, $g_{mo} = 4 \times 10^{-3}$ Siemens. In circuits A and B, *find* g_{mQ}, R_S and R_D so $I_{DQ} = 3.0$ mA, and $V_{DQ} = 8.0$ V. Give V_{DSQ}. Circuit C is a source-follower. *Find* R_1, and R_S required to make $I_{DQ} =$ 3.0 mA, and $V_{SQ} = 8.0$ V. Neglect gate leakage current.

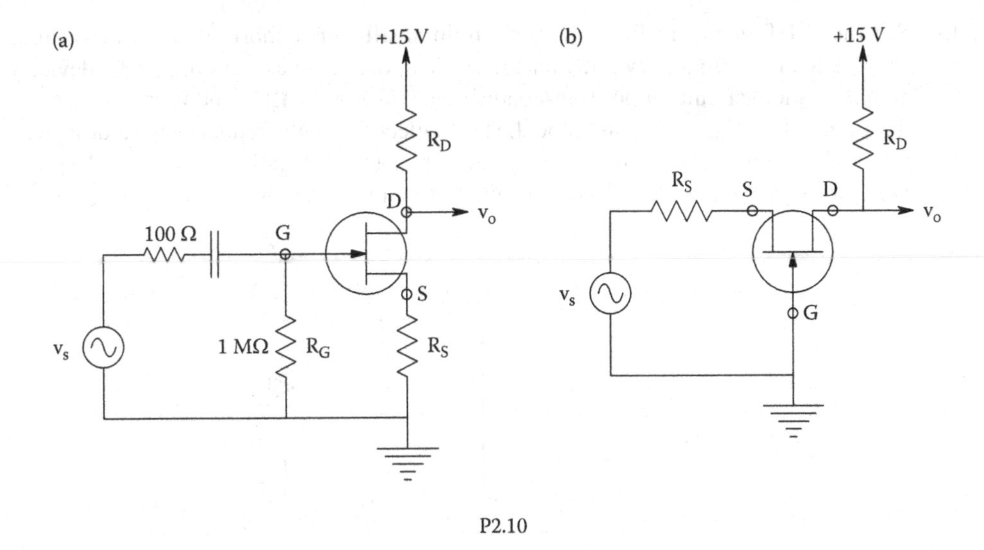

P2.10

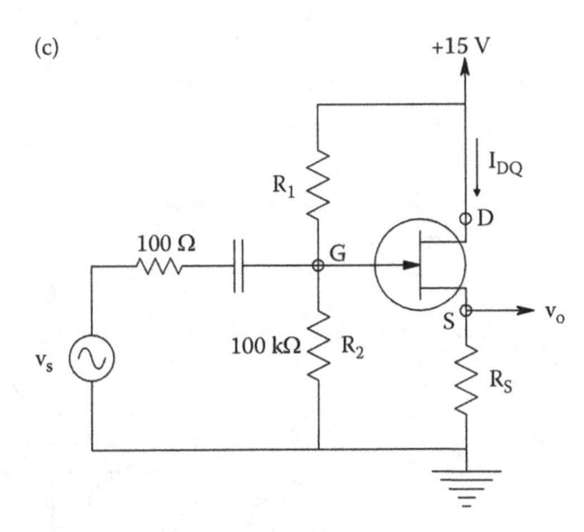

2.11 The circuit of Figure P2.11 is an emitter-follower/grounded base amp. pair, normally used to amplify video frequency signals because it has no Miller effect. We will examine its gain at midfrequencies.

(A) Draw the midfrequency SSM for the amplifier. Let $h_{oe} = h_{re} = 0$ for both BJTs.

(B) Find an expression for $A_{vo} = v_o/v_1$. Show what happens to A_{vo} when $R_E \to \infty$ and $\beta_1 = \beta_2 = \beta$.

2.12 A simplified MOSFET feedback pair amplifier is shown in Figure P2.12. (A) Draw the MFSSM for the amplifier. Assume the MOSFETs have different g_ms (g_{m1}, g_{m2}), and $g_{d1} = g_{d2} = 0$ for simplicity. (B) Find an algebraic expression for the amplifier's midfrequency voltage gain, $A_{vo} = v_o/v_1$. (C) Find an algebraic expression for the amplifier's small-signal, Thevenin output resistance. Use the OCV/SCC method. Note that the OCV is $v_1 A_{vo}$, and to find the SCC, replace R_L with a short-circuit to small-signal ground and find the current in it.

2.13 See the JFET in Figure P2.13 with its drain small-signal short-circuited to ground. (A) Use the high-frequency SSM for the JFET to derive an expression for the device's complex, short-circuit output transconductance, $\mathbf{G_M}(j\omega) = \mathbf{I_d}/\mathbf{V_1}$, at $\mathbf{V_{ds}} \equiv 0$. Assume: g_m, g_d, C_{gs}, C_{gd}, C_{ds}, > 0 in the model. (B) Neglect the high-frequency zero at g_m/C_{gd} r/s. Find an expression for the Hz frequency, f_T, such that $r_d|\mathbf{G_M}(j2\pi f_T)| = 1$. Express f_T in terms of the quiescent drain current, I_{DQ}. Plot f_T vs. I_{DQ} for $0 \le I_{DQ} \le I_{DSS}$.

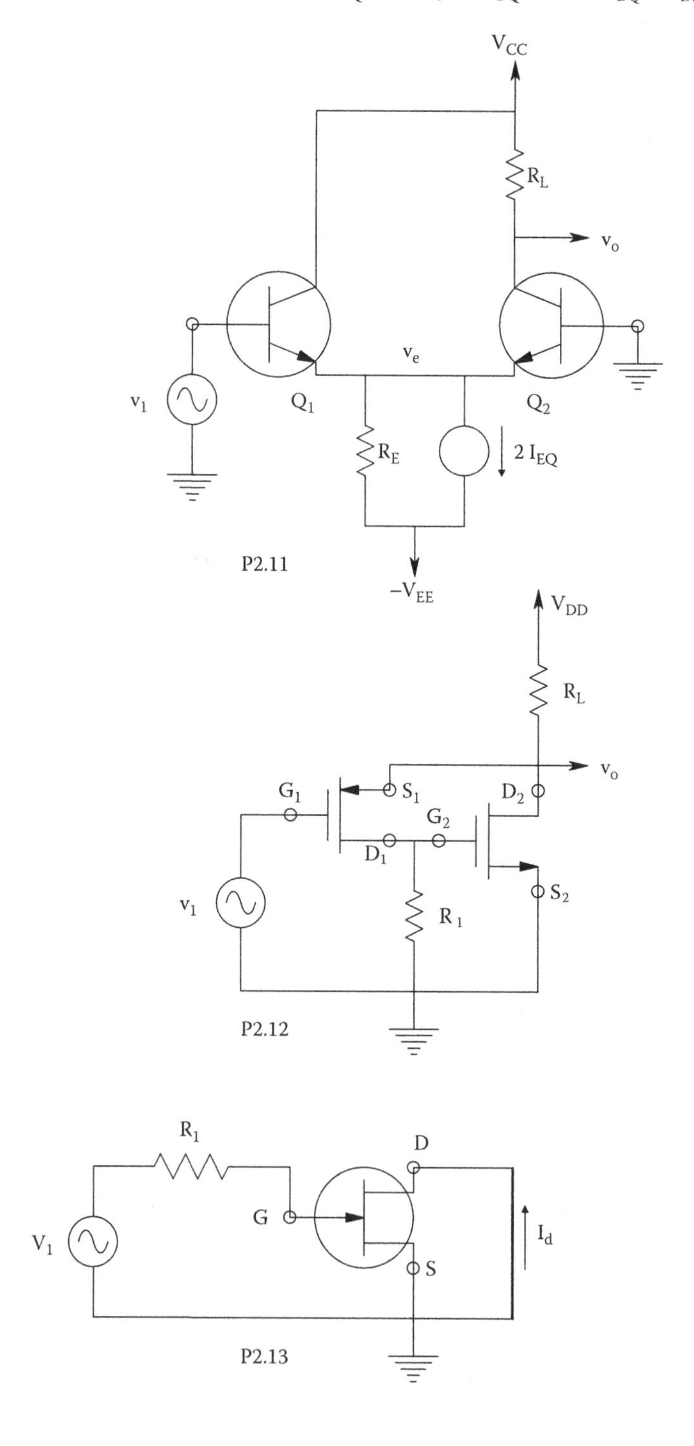

2.14 An emitter-coupled cascode amplifier uses three 2N2369 BJTs as shown in Figure P2.14.

(A) Use an ECAP to do a DC biasing analysis. Plot the DC V_o vs. V_1. Use a 0–15 V scale for V_o, and a ± 0.25 V scale for the dc input, V_1. Find the amplifier's maximum dc gain.

(B) Make a Bode plot of the amplifier's frequency response, $20 \log|\mathbf{V}_o/\mathbf{V}_1|$ vs. f for $10^5 \le f \le 10^9$ Hz. Give the midfrequency gain, the –3 dB frequency, and f_T for the amplifier.

(C) Now put a 300 Ω resistor in series with V_1. Repeat B).

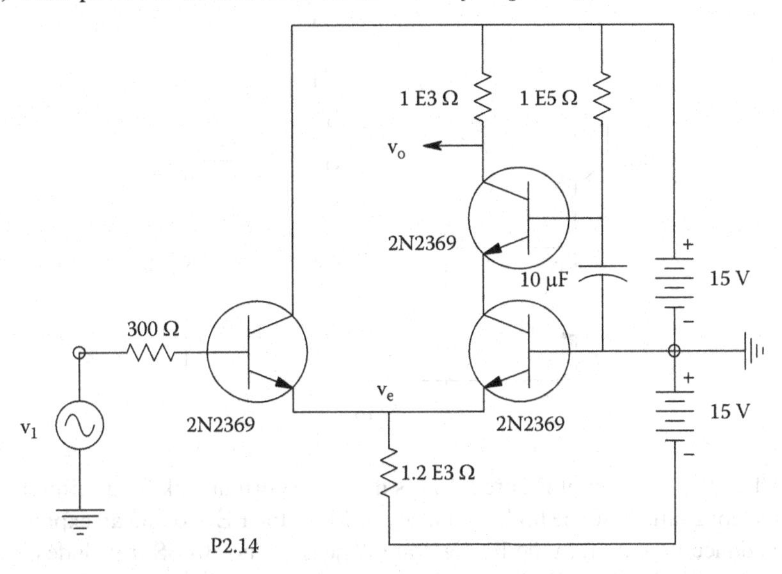

P2.14

2.15 An EF/GB amplifier, shown in Figure P2.15, uses capacitance "neutralization" to effectively cancel its input capacitance and extend its high frequency –3 dB bandwidth. Use an ECAP to investigate how C_N affects the amplifier's high frequency response. First try $C_N = 0$, then see what happens with C_N values in the tenths of a pF. Find C_N that will give the maximum –3 dB frequency with no more than a +3 dB peak to the frequency response Bode plot.

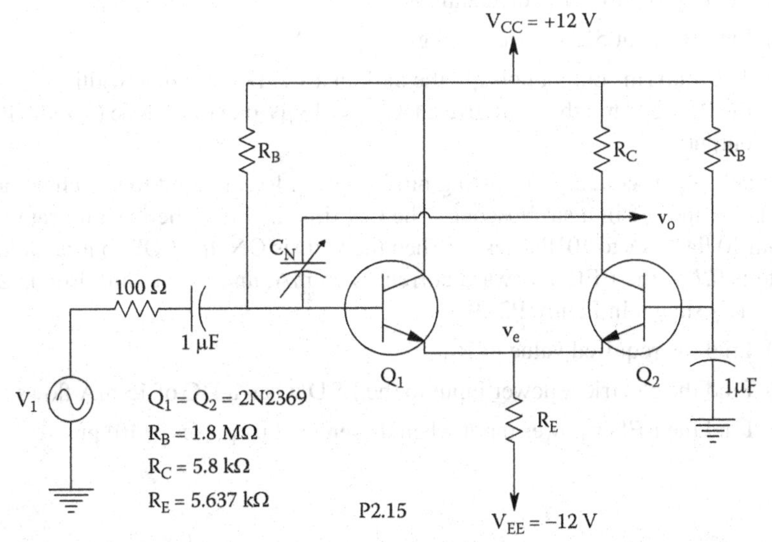

P2.15

2.16 The MOSFET source-follower in Figure P2.16 uses a current mirror to obtain a high equivalent R_S looking into the drain of Q_2. The three MOSFETs have identical MFSSMs (identical g_{mo}, I_{DSS} and V_P).

(A) Draw the MFSSM for the circuit.

(B) Find and expression for the midfrequency gain, $A_{vo} = v_o/v_1$.

(C) Find an expression for the Thevenin output resistance presented at the v_o node.

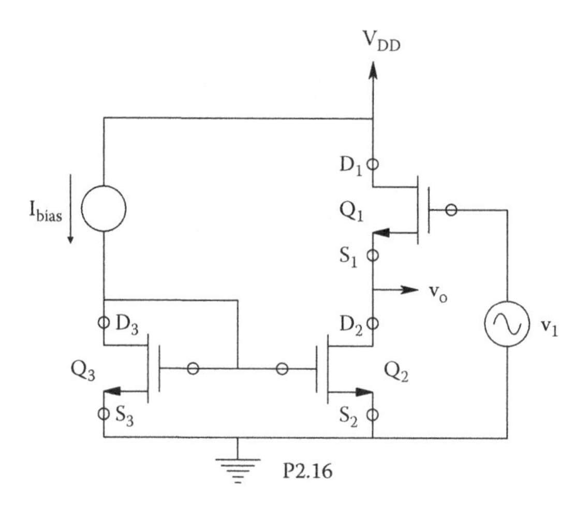

P2.16

2.17 (A) The JFET circuit of Figure P2.17 is used as a current sink for a differential amplifier's "long tail." Use the high-frequency SSM for the FET to find an expression for the impedance looking into the FET's drain, $\mathbf{Z}_{id}(j\omega)$. (The HiFSSM includes: g_m, g_d, C_{ds}, C_{gd}, C_{gs}.). (B) Find the FET's short-circuit, DC drain current, I_{Dsc}. Assume the FET's drain current is given by $I_D = I_{DSS}(1 - V_{GS}/V_P)^2$. Assume saturated drain operation. I_{DSS} and V_P are known.

2.18 A Si avalanche photodiode (APD) is connected as shown in Figure P2.18. The total dark current of the APD is $I_D = 10$ nA, Its spectral responsivity at $\lambda = 512$ nm is $R(\lambda) = 12$ A/W at a reverse $v_D = -150$ V. R_F of the ideal op amp is 1 MΩ.

(A) Find V_o due to dark current alone.

(B) Find the P_i at 512 nm that will give $V_o = 1$ V.

(C) The total rms output noise in the dark in a 1 kHz noise bandwidth is 4.33 μV. Find the P_i @ 512 nm that will give a DC $V_o = 13$ μV due to I_P alone (3 × the RMS noise output).

2.19 A single, open-collector, inverting buffer gate (7406) is used to switch a GaP (green) LED on and off in a stroboscope. The ON time is 2 μs. The flashing rate is variable from 10 flashes/s to 10^4 flashes/s. When the LED is ON, the LOW output voltage of the gate is 0.7 V, the LED's forward current is 15 mA, and its forward drop is 2.0 V. The circuit is shown in Figure P2.19.

(A) Find the required value of R_D.

(B) Find the electrical power input to the LED when a DC of 15 mA flows.

(C) Find the LED's power input when driven by 2 μs pulses at 10^4 pps.

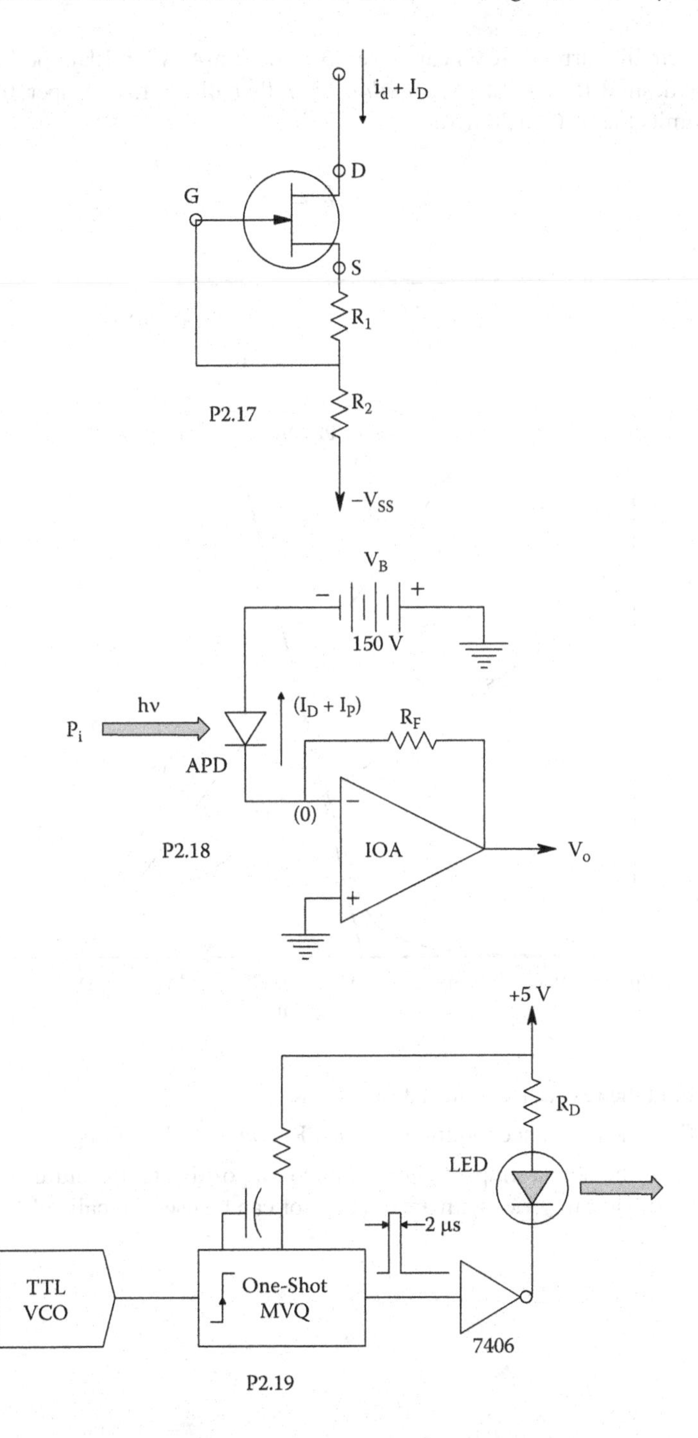

2.20 A laser pointer is to be run CW from a 3.1 V (max) alkaline battery. The simple series circuit is shown in Figure P2.20A is to be used to save money. Figure P2.20B shows the LAD's $i_D = f(v_D)$ curve and its linear approximation. The maximum (burnout) $i_D = 20$ mA. The desired operating current with the 3.1 battery is 15 mA. Three load lines are shown: LL_1 gives the desired operating point; LL_2 is always safe because the short-circuit current (SCC) can never exceed 20 mA. With LL_2, the LAD cannot run at the desired 15 mA. LL_3 is a *nonlinear LL* that allows 15 mA operation of the LAD, but limits the SCC to 20 mA.

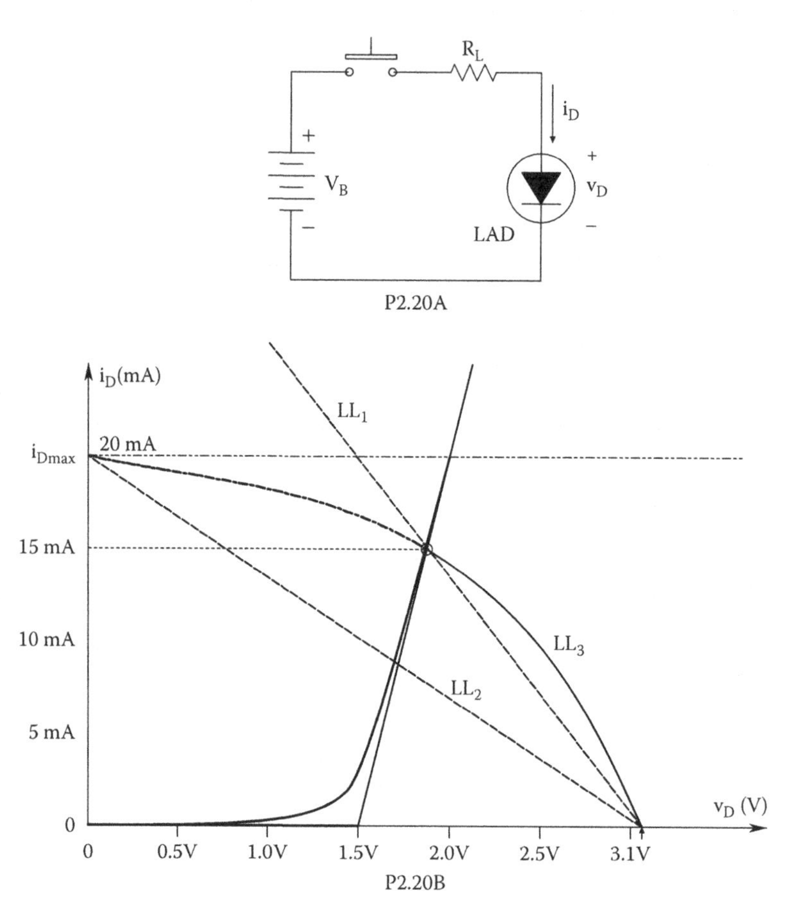

(A) Find the resistance required for LL_1, R_{L1}.
(B) Find the resistance required for LL_2, R_{L2}, and the LAD's operating point at Q_2.
(C) Describe how a simple tungsten lamp or a positive temperature coefficient (PTC) thermistor in series with a fixed resistor can be used to realize LL_3.

3 Differential Amplifier

3.1 INTRODUCTION

The *differential* or *difference amplifier* (DA) is a cornerstone element in the design of most analog signal conditioning systems used in biomedical engineering applications, as well as in general instrumentation applications. Nearly all instrumentation and medical isolation amplifiers are DAs; also, nearly all operational amplifiers are DAs. Why are DAs so ubiquitous? The answer lies in their inherent ability to reject unwanted DC levels, interference, and noise voltages common to both inputs. An *ideal* DA responds only to the so-called difference-mode signal at its two inputs. Most DAs have a single-ended, complex output voltage, $\mathbf{V}_o$, given by the phasor relation:

$$V_o = A_1V_1 - A_1' V_1' \tag{3.1}$$

where $\mathbf{V}_1$ is the complex (phasor) AC voltage at the DA's noninverting input terminal, and $\mathbf{V}_1'$ is the complex AC voltage at the DA's inverting input terminal.

Ideally, it is desired that the complex gains $\mathbf{A}_1$ and $\mathbf{A}_1'$ be exactly equal over as wide a frequency range as possible. In reality, this does not happen, and $\mathbf{V}_o$ is more generally given by the relation

$$V_o = A_D V_{ld} + AcV_{lc} \tag{3.2}$$

where

$$V_{id} \equiv (V_1 - V_1')/2 \quad \text{(Difference-mode input voltage)} \tag{3.3a}$$

$$V_{lc} \equiv (V_1 + V_1')/2 \quad \text{(Common-mode input voltage)} \tag{3.3b}$$

and $\mathbf{A}_D$ is the *complex difference mode gain*, and $\mathbf{A}_C$ is the *complex common-mode gain.*

From Equation 3.1, it can easily be shown by vector summation that

$$A_D = A_1 + A_1' \tag{3.4a}$$

$$A_C = A_1 - A_1' \tag{3.4b}$$

Clearly, if $\mathbf{A}_1 = \mathbf{A}_1'$, then $\mathbf{A}_C \to 0$.

3.2 DA CIRCUIT ARCHITECTURE

Figure 3.1 illustrates a simplified circuit of the Burr-Brown, OPA606, JFET-input op amp (OA). (The circles with arrows in them represent BJT transistor DC current sources.) Note that a pair of *p*-channel JFETs connected as a DA is used as a *differential input headstage* in the OA. The single-ended signal output from the left-hand (inverting input) JFET drives the base (input) of a BJT emitter-follower which drives a second BJT connected as a grounded-base amplifier. Its output, in turn, drives the OA's output stage.

To appreciate how the differential headstage works, consider the simple JFET DA circuit of Figure 3.2. Note that in the op amp schematic, the resistors R_s, R_d, and R_d' are shown as active

DC current sources and thus can be assumed to have very high Norton resistances on the order of megohms. (See Northrop 1990, Section 5.2, and Section 2.3.5 in this text for a description on active current sources and sinks used in IC DA designs.) Figure 3.3a illustrates the *midfrequency, small-signal model* (MFSSM) of the JFET DA. To make the circuit bilaterally symmetric so that the *bisection theorem* (cf. this text, Glossary; Northrop 1990, Chapter 2) can be used in its analysis, we put two $2R_s$ resistors in parallel to replace the one R_s in the actual circuit. Note that *all DC voltage sources are represented by small-signal grounds in all SSMs.* We wish to evaluate the scalar A_D and A_C in Equation 3.2 above using the DC SSM. The simplest way to do this is to use the *bisection*

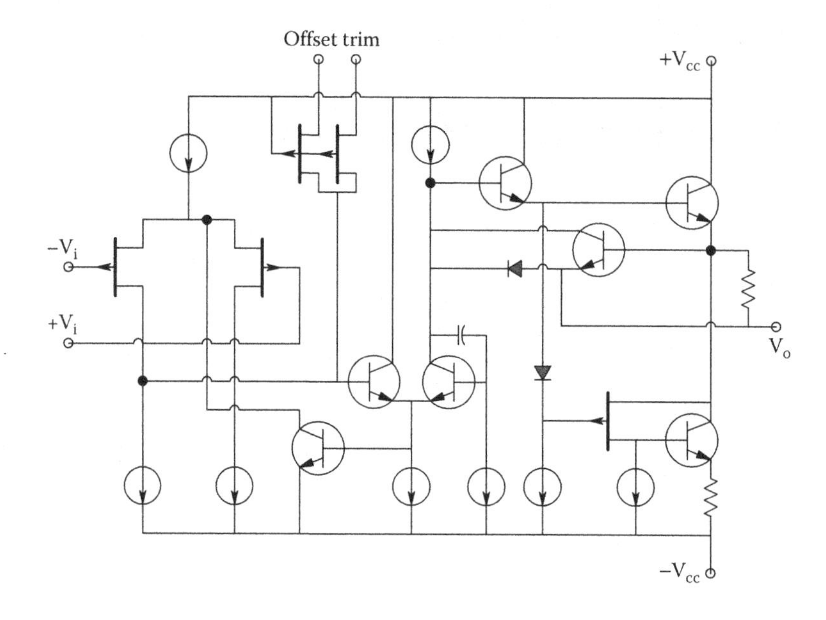

FIGURE 3.1 Simplified schematic of a Burr-Brown OPA606 JFET-input, differential amplifier (DA). The circles with arrows are current sources and sinks.

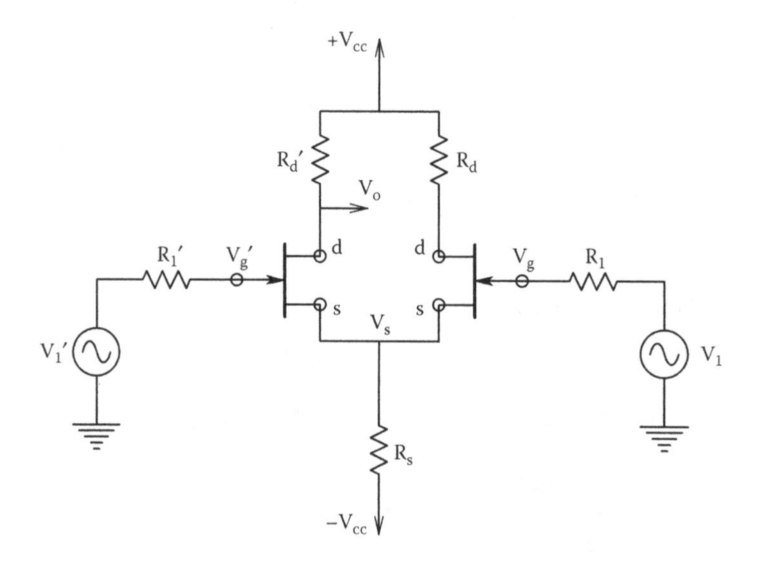

FIGURE 3.2 A JFET differential amplifier. The circuit must be symmetrical to have a high common-mode rejection ratio.

theorem on the DA's MFSSM. First, one applies pure DM excitation where $v_s' = -v_s$. Thus, $v_{sc} = 0$, and the revised MFSSM is shown in Figure 3.3b. One writes a node equation at the drain (v_{od}) node

$$v_{od}[G_d + g_d] = -g_m v_{sd} \tag{3.5}$$

Thus,

$$A_D = v_{od} / v_{sd} = \frac{-g_m}{G_d + g_d} = \frac{-g_m r_d R_d}{R_d + r_d} \tag{3.6}$$

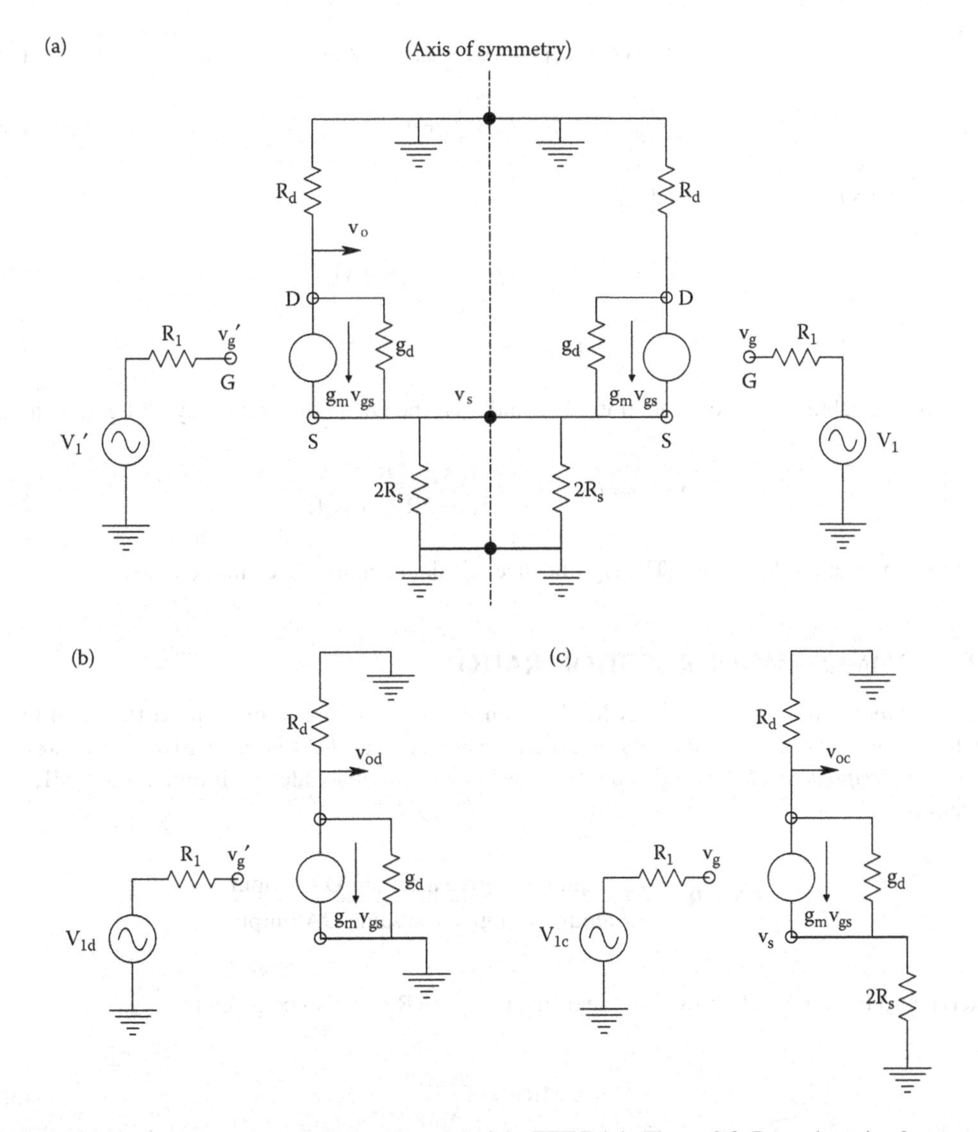

FIGURE 3.3 (a) Midfrequency small-signal model of the FET DA in Figure 3.2. R_s on the axis of symmetry is split into two, parallel $2R_s$ resistors. (b) Left-half-circuit of the DA following application of the bisection theorem for difference-mode excitation. Note that DM excitation makes $v_s = 0$, so The FET sources can be connected to small-signal ground. (c) Left-half-circuit of the DA following application of the bisection theorem for common-mode excitation. See Text for analysis.

Now consider pure CM input, where $v_s' = v_s$, and $v_{sd} = 0$. The *bisection theorem* gives us the MFSSM shown in Figure 3.3c. Now two node equations are required; for the v_{oc} node,

$$v_{oc}[G_d + g_d] - v_s g_d + g_m(v_{sc} - v_s) = 0 \tag{3.7}$$

For the v_s node,

$$v_s[G_s / 2 + g_d] - v_{oc} g_d - g_m(v_{sc} - v_s) = 0 \tag{3.8}$$

The two node equations are rewritten as simultaneous equations in v_{oc} and v_s:

$$v_{oc}[G_d + g_d] - v_s[g_m + g_d] = -v_{sc} g_m \tag{3.9a}$$

$$-v_{oc} g_d + v_s[G_s / 2 + g_d + g_m] = v_{sc} g_m \tag{3.9b}$$

Now *Cramer's rule* is used to find v_{oc}:

$$\Delta = G_d G_s / 2 + G_d g_d + g_d g_m + g_d G_s / 2 \tag{3.10}$$

$$\Delta v_{oc} = -v_{sc}\, g_m G_s / 2 \tag{3.11}$$

After some algebra is used on Equations 3.10 and 3.11, the DC to midfrequency CM gain is found:

$$A_c = v_{oc} / v_{sc} = \frac{-g_m r_d R_d}{r_d + R_d + 2R_s(1 + g_m R_d)} \tag{3.12}$$

Note that in general, $A_D >> A_C$. The significance of this inequality is examined next.

3.3 COMMON-MODE REJECTION RATIO

The *common-mode rejection ratio* (CMRR) is an important figure of merit for differential instrumentation and operational amplifiers. A general property of all DAs is that CMRR *decreases* with *increasing frequency*. CMRR is desired to be as large as possible; ideally, infinite. The CMRR can be defined as

$$\text{CMRR} \equiv \frac{v_{1c} \text{ required to give a certain DA output.}}{v_{1d} \text{ required to give the same DA output.}} \tag{3.13}$$

Referring to Equation 3.2 above, it is clear that the CMRR can also be given by

$$\text{CMRR} \equiv \frac{|A_D(f)|}{|A_C(f)|} \tag{3.14}$$

Note that the CMRR is a positive real number and is a function of frequency. Generally, the CMRR is given in dB; i.e., $\text{CMRR}_{dB} = 20 \log \text{CMRR}$. For the MFSSM of the JFET DA in the section above, the CMRR can be shown to be

$$\text{CMRR} = \frac{\dfrac{-g_m r_d R_d}{R_d + r_d}}{\dfrac{-g_m r_d R_d}{r_d + R_d + 2R_s(1 + g_m R_d)}} = 1 + \frac{2R_s(1 + g_m r_d)}{R_d + r_d} \quad (3.15)$$

By making R_s very large by using a *dynamic current source* in the "long tail," (Northrop 1990), the low-frequency CMRR of the simple JFET DA can be made about 10^4, or 80 dB.

The CMRR_{dB} of a typical, commercial, *differential instrumentation amplifier,* e.g., a Burr-Brown INA111, is given as 90 dB at a gain of 1, and 110 dB at a gain of 10, and 115 dB at gains from 10^2 to 10^3, all measured at 100 Hz. At a break frequency close to 200 Hz, the $\text{CMRR}_{\text{dB}}(f)$ of the INA111 begins to roll off at ca. 20 dB/decade. For example, at a gain of 10, the $\text{CMRR}_{\text{dB}}(f)$ is down to 80 dB at 6 kHz. Because most input common-mode interference picked up in biomedical applications of DAs is either at DC or power line frequency, it is important for such DAs to have a high CMRR that remains high (80–120 dB) from DC to over 120 Hz. Modern, IC, instrumentation amplifiers easily meet these criteria.

The major reason for the frequency dependence of the CMRR of DAs can be attributed to the frequency dependence of $\mathbf{A_D}(f)$ and $\mathbf{A_C}(f)$, as described in Section 3.5. Figure 3.4 illustrates Bode AR asymptote plots for these parameters for a typical DA. For example, $20 \log |\mathbf{A_D}(f)|$ starts out at +40 dB at DC (gain of 100) and its Bode AR has its first break frequency at f_3 Hz. $20 \log |\mathbf{A_C}(f)|$ starts at −60 dB at DC (gain of 0.001) and has a zero at approximately the open-loop amplifier's break frequency, f_1; its Bode AR increases at +20 dB/decade until it reaches a high frequency pole at f_2 where it flattens out. Since the numerical $\text{CMRR} = |\mathbf{A_D}(f)|/|\mathbf{A_C}(f)|$, the CMRR_{dB} is simply

$$\text{CMRR}_{\text{dB}} = 20 \log |A_D(f)| - 20 \log |A_C(f)| \quad (3.16)$$

Thus, $\text{CMRR}_{\text{dB}} = 100$ dB at DC, decreases at −20 dB/decade from f_1 to f_2, where it levels off at 30 dB. At f_3, the CMRR_{dB} again drops off at −20 dB/decade. Good DA design tries to make f_1 as

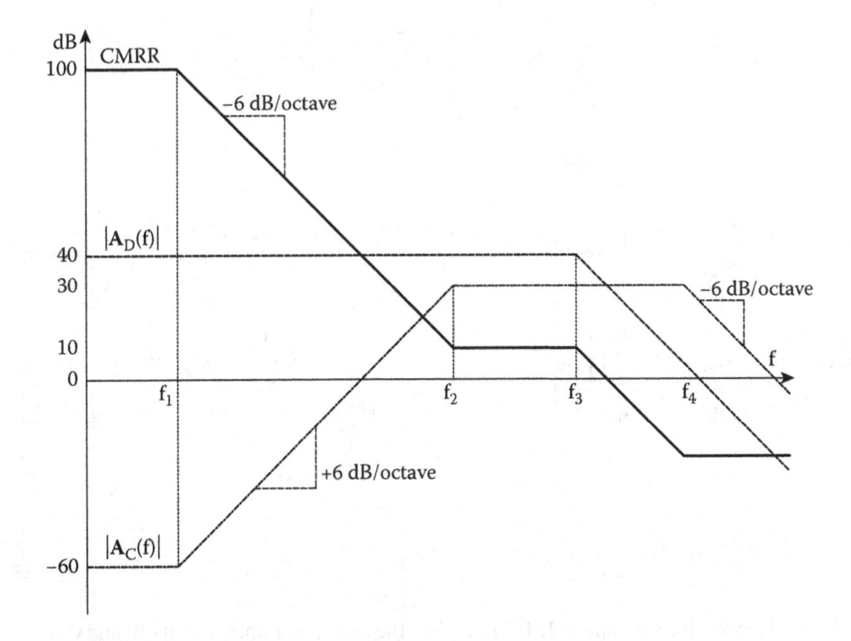

FIGURE 3.4 Typical Bode plot asymptotes for the common-mode gain frequency response, the difference-mode gain frequency response, and the common-mode rejection ratio frequency response.

large as possible to extend the high CMRR region well into the frequency range of common-mode interference and noise.

3.4 CM AND DM GAIN OF SIMPLE DA STAGES AT HIGH FREQUENCIES

3.4.1 INTRODUCTION

Figure 3.5a–c illustrate the small-signal, high-frequency models for a JFET DA. Note that the *small-signal, high-frequency model* (SSHFM) for *all* FETs includes three, small, internal capacitors: the drain-to-source capacitance, C_{ds}, the gate-to-drain capacitance, C_{gd}, and the gate-to-source capacitance, C_{gs}. It is these capacitors, in particular C_{gd}, that effectively limit the high-frequency performance of the JFET DA. The small-signal, drain-source conductance, g_d, is also quiescent operating point-dependent; it is determined by the upward slope of the FET's i_D vs v_D curves as a function of v_{GS} (cf. Northrop 1990, Section 1.6). The transconductance, g_m, of the small-signal, voltage-controlled current source is also Q-point dependent, as shown in Chapter 2.

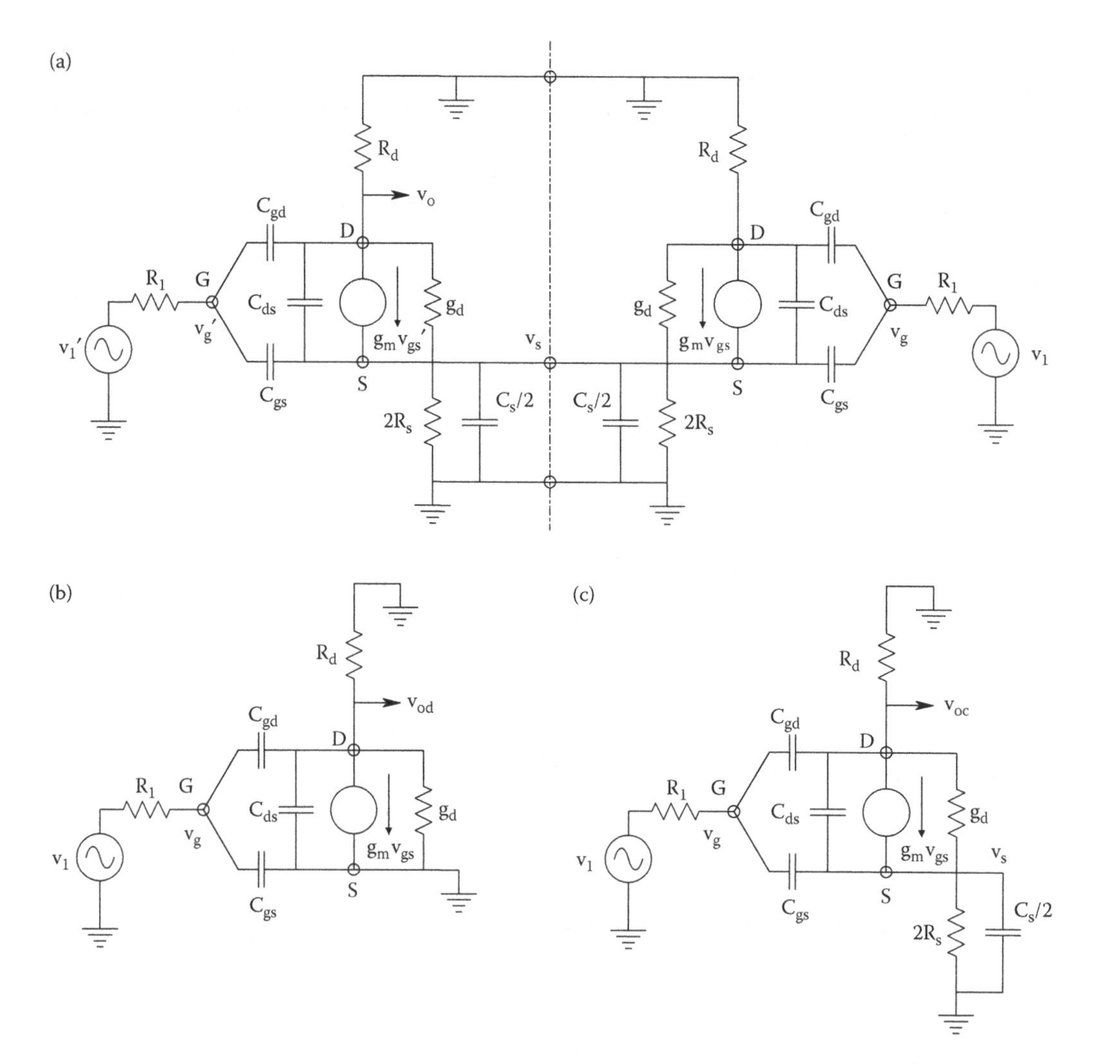

FIGURE 3.5 (a) HFSSM for a complete JFET DA. Note the axis of symmetry splits R_s and C_s symmetrically. C_s is the stray capacitance from the common source nodes to ground. (b) HFSSM for the left half of the DA given pure DM excitation. (c) HFSSM for the left half of the DA given pure CM excitation.

Figure 3.6 illustrates a simple BJT DA. The *hybrid-pi,* HFSSMs for CM and DM inputs are illustrated in Figure 3.7a and b after application of the bisection theorem. In both the CM and DM HFSSMs, we see two lumped-parameter, small capacitors: C_μ is the collector-to-base capacitance. It is on the order of single pF, and is largely due to the depletion capacitance of the reverse-biased *pn* junction between collector and base; its value is a function of the collector-to-base voltage. However, given a fixed quiescent operating point (Q-point) for the amplifier, and small-signal, linear operation, it is possible to approximate C_μ with a fixed value for pencil-and-paper calculations. C_π models the somewhat larger capacitance of the forward-biased, base-emitter *pn* junction. It, too, depends on v_{BE}, and is generally approximated by its value at V_{BEQ}. C_μ is generally on the order of 10 to 100 pF; it is larger in power transistors having larger base and emitter junction areas.

C_s and C_e shunting the common source or emitter resistance to ground, respectively, is on the order of single pF, but R_s and R_e are generally the product of very dynamic current sources (with Norton resistances on the order of 10s of megaohms), so these capacitances can be very important in determining the high-frequency behavior of the CM gain.

3.4.2 High-Frequency Behavior of A_C and A_D for the JFET DA

Let us first find an algebraic expression for the DM gain of the FET DA at high frequencies. This calculation requires the solution of two, simultaneous, linear algebraic node equations. Refer to Figure 3.5b; the node voltages are v_g and v_{od}. Sum all the currents *leaving* these nodes as positive. After rearranging terms, there results

$$v_g[s(C_{gd}+C_{gs})+G_1]-v_{od}\,s\,C_{gd}=v_{1d}G_1 \quad (3.17a)$$

$$-v_g[sC_{gd}-g_m]+v_{od}[(g_d+G_d)+s\,(C_{ds}+C_{gd})]=0 \quad (3.17b)$$

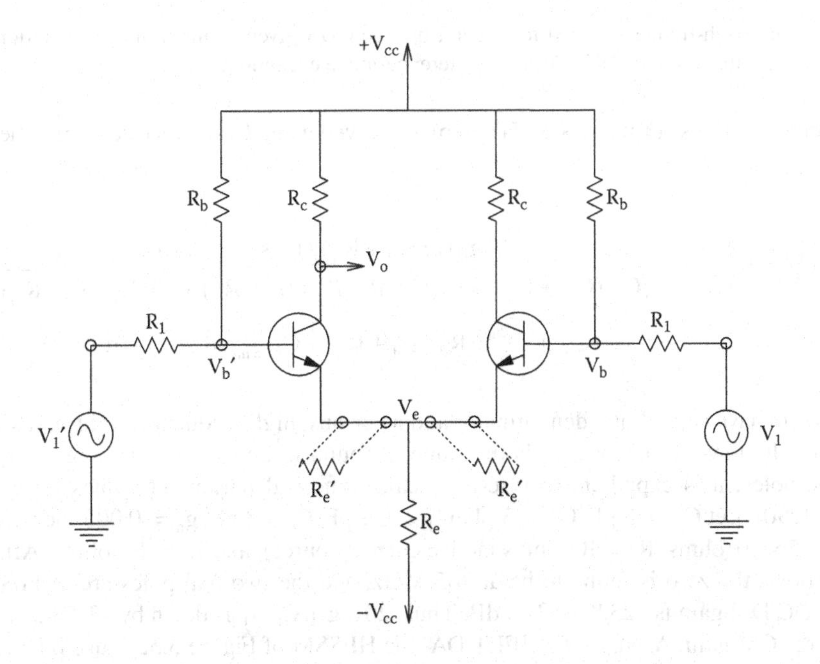

FIGURE 3.6 Schematic of a BJT DA. Note its bilateral symmetry. The resistors R_e' can be used to raise the DM input resistance.

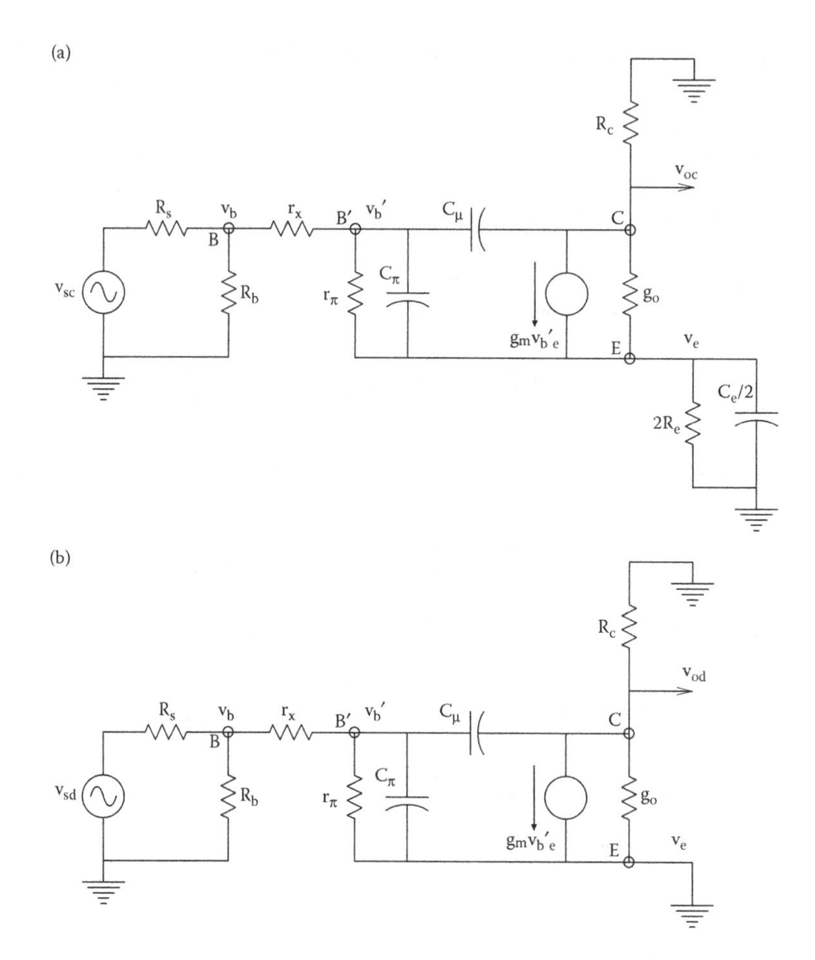

FIGURE 3.7 (a) High-frequency SSM for the left half BJT DA given common-mode excitation. (b) High-frequency SSM for the left half BJT DA given difference-mode excitation.

The two node equations (Equations 3.17a and b) are solved using Cramer's rule to find the DM gain, $A_D(s)$:

$$A_D(s) = \frac{v_{od}}{v_{1d}} = \frac{[-g_m r_d / (r_D + R_d)](1 - s\, C_{gd} / g_m)}{s^2[C_{gd}(C_{gs} + C_{ds}) + C_{ds}C_{gs}]R_1 r_d R_d / (r_d + R_d) + s[(C_{gd} + C_{gs})R_1 + (C_{ds} + C_{gd})r_d R_d / (r_d + R_d) + C_{gd} g_m r_d R_1 / (r_d + R_d)] + 1} \tag{3.18}$$

$A_D(s)$ is seen to have a quadratic denominator and a curious, high-frequency, right-half s-plane zero at g_m / C_{gd} r/s. Its low-frequency gain is the same as found in Section 3.2, i.e., $-g_m\, r_d\, R_d/(r_d + R_d)$. To find the poles, it is expedient to insert typical, numerical parameter values for a JFET DA (Northrop 1990). Let $C_{gd} = 3$ pF, $C_{gs} = 3$ pF, $C_{ds} = 0.2$ pF, $C_s = 3$ pF, $g_m = 0.005$ Siemens, $r_d = 10^5$ ohms, $R_d = 5 \times 10^3$ ohms, $R_s = 10^6$ ohms (active current source), and $R_1 = 10^3$ ohms. After numerical calculations, the zero is found to be at 265 MHz, and the two real poles are at 1.687 and 309 MHz. The DC DM gain is –23.8, or 27.5 dB. Thus, $20 \log |\mathbf{A_D}(f)|$ is down by –3 dB at 1.687 MHz.

To find the CM gain, $A_C(s)$, for the JFET DA, the HFSSM of Figure 3.5c is used. Unfortunately, the bisection theorem tells us that the voltage, v_s, on the axis of symmetry is nonzero, so there is a third (v_s) node equation to write when finding v_{oc}. The three node equations are

$$v_g[G_1 + s(C_{gd} + C_{gs})] - v_{oc}[s\,C_{gd}] - v_s[s\,C_{gs}] = v_{1c}G_1 \quad (3.18a)$$

$$-v_g[sC_{gd} - g_m] + v_{oc}[(g_d + G_d)] + s(C_{ds} + C_{gd})] - v_s[g_m + g_d + sC_{ds}] = 0 \quad (3.18b)$$

$$-v_g[g_m + sC_{gs}] - v_{oc}[g_d + sC_{ds}] + v_s[s(C_s/2 + C_{ds} + C_{gs}) + G_s/2 + g_d + g_m] = 0 \quad (3.18c)$$

Now no one in their right mind would attempt an *algebraic* solution on paper of a third-order system such as described by Equations 3.18A–C. Clearly, a computer (numerical) simulation is indicated; a circuit analysis program such as *pSPICE* or *MicroCap*™ should be used. Figures 3.8 and 3.9 show Bode plots of the DM and CM HFSSM frequency responses calculated using the venerable MicroCap™ III circuit analysis software. Note that the CM frequency response gain is ca. –46 dB at low frequencies. A zero at ca. 120 kHz causes the CM AR to rise at +20 dB/decade until a pole at ca. 10 MHz causes it to level off. A second pole at ca. 300 MHz causes the CM frequency response to again fall off. On the other hand, the DM frequency response is flat at +27.5 dB from DC out to the first real pole at ca. 1.7 MHz. The DM AR then rolls off at –20 dB/decade until the second pole, estimated to be at 310 MHz. However, the zero at 265 MHz pretty much cancels out the effect of the 310 MHz pole on the DM AR.

Note that the $CMRR_{dB}(f)$ for this amplifier is simply $20 \log|\mathbf{A}_D(f)| - 20 \log |\mathbf{A}_C(f)|$. At low frequencies, the CMRR is 27.5 – (–46) = 73.5 dB. It stays this high up to ca. 100 kHz, when it begins to drop off due to the rise in $|\mathbf{A}_C(f)|$. At 10 MHz, the $CMRR_{dB}(f)$ has fallen to 21 dB, etc.

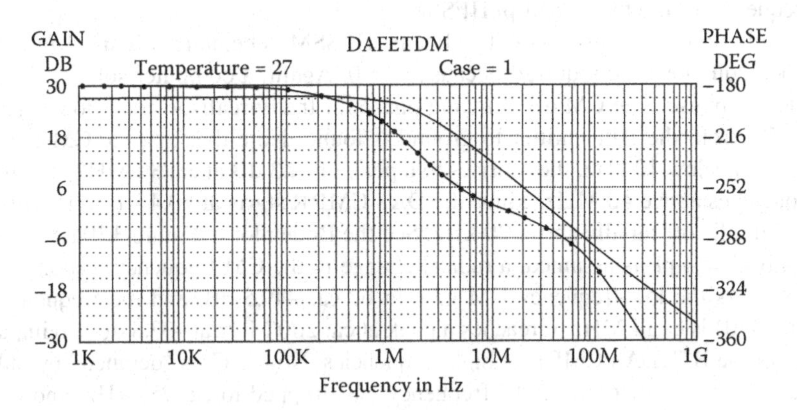

FIGURE 3.8 Difference-mode frequency response of the JFET DA of Figure 3.5a. The –3 dB frequency is ca. 1.9 MHz. Phase is bold trace with dots. See text for details.

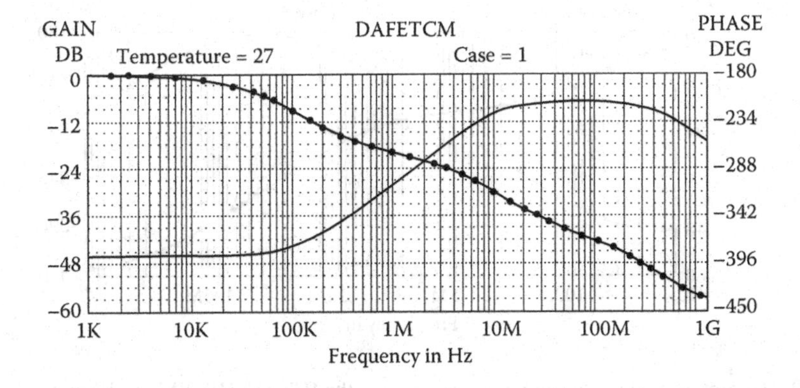

FIGURE 3.9 Common-mode frequency response of the JFET DA of Figure 3.5a. Note that the AR rises at +6 dB/octave from –46 dB at 110 kHz, to a maximum of –7 dB at ca. 20 MHz, then falls off again by –6 dB/octave at ca. 400 MHz.

3.4.3 High-Frequency Behavior of A_D and A_C for the BJT DA

Next, examine the high-frequency gain of the simple BJT DA shown in Figure 3.6 for DM and CM inputs. The hybrid-pi HFSSM for BJTs is used. After application of the bisection theorem, one obtains the reduced CM and DM HFSSMs shown in Figure 3.7a and b.

First, the HF DM gain will be found. The DM circuit of Figure 3.7b has three nodes: v_b, v_b', and v_{od}. The v_b node can be eliminated by noting that $R_b >> (r_x, R_s)$, so R_b can be set to ∞, and a new Thevenin resistance, $R_s' = R_s + r_x$ is defined. v_b' and v_{od} will be solved for. Note that $v_e = 0$. Writing the two node equations

$$v_b' [G_s' + g_\mu + s(C_\mu + C_\mu)] + v_{od}[sC_\mu] = v_{sd}G_s' \tag{3.20a}$$

$$v_b'[g_m - s\, C_\mu] + v_{od}[g_o + G_c + s\, C_\mu] = 0 \tag{3.20b}$$

Even though the admittance matrix, Δ, is second-order, its paper-and-pencil solution is tedious, so it is best to use MicroCap to find the linear, DM, BJT DA's HFSSM frequency response. In this example, the parameter values were taken to be: $R_c = 6.8$ kΩ, $r_o = \infty$, $g_m = 0.05$ S, $r_\pi = 3$ kΩ, $R_e = 10^6$ Ω, $C_e = 5$ pF, $C_\mu = 2$ pF, $C_\pi = 30$ pF, $r_x = 10$ Ω, and $R_s = 50$ Ω. Thus, $R_s' = 60$ Ω. From the Bode plot, it is seen that the DM frequency response has a low- and midfrequency gain of 50.4 dB, the –3 dB frequency is ca. 2.0 MHz, and the 0 dB frequency is ca. 410 MHz (this is a frequency well beyond the upper frequency where the hybrid-pi HFSSM is valid).

For CM excitation of the BJT DA, the linear, HFSSM schematic, Figure 3.7a is used. Note that three node equations are required because $v_e \neq 0$. Again, a computer solution is used for the CM frequency response. The CM dB gain and phase for the unrealistic condition of *zero* parasitic capacitance (C_e) from the BJT emitter to ground is found. Note that that the CM gain is ca. –49 dB at frequencies below 10 kHz, then it rises to a peak of –1.3 dB at ca. 30 MHz, and then falls off again at frequencies above 40 MHz. Thus, the DA's CMRR starts at 50.4 – (–49) = 99.4 dB at low frequencies and falls off rapidly above 20 kHz. See the Bode plot in Figure 3.10a.

Curiously, if $C_e = 4$ pF is assumed, a radical change in the CM frequency response is observed. Figure 3.10b shows the low-frequency CM gain to be ca. –49.5 dB, and the frequency where the CM gain is up 3 dB is ca.14 MHz, it reaches a peak at ca. 200 MHz at –33.8 dB, giving a significant improvement in the BJT DA's CMRR at high frequencies. Now if C_e is "detuned" by only ± 0.2 pF, Figure 3.10c and d show that the +3 dB frequency has dropped to ca. 750 kHz, and the peak CM gain has risen to –27.2 dB at ca. 320 MHz. What is amazing, and can also be shown when simulating

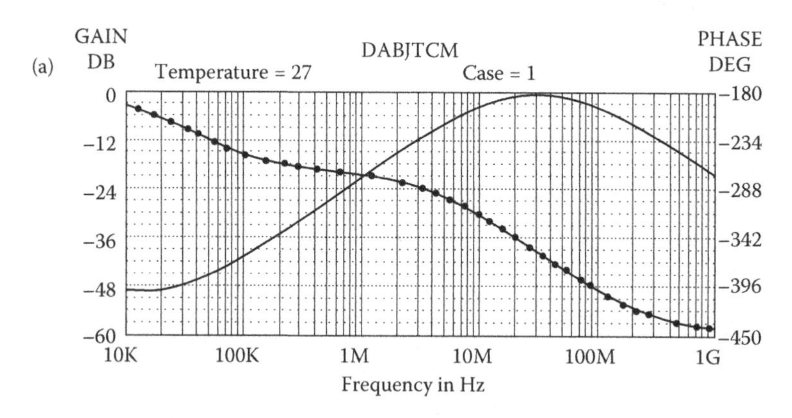

FIGURE 3.10 Common-mode gain frequency response of the BJT DA HFSSM of Figure 3.7 A with various values of parasitic emitter capacitance, C_e, showing how C_e can improve the DA's CMRR by giving a low CM gain at high frequencies. (a) CM gain frequency response (FR) with $C_e = 0$. (b) CM gain FR with an optimum $C_e = 4$ pF. (c) CM gain FR with $C_e = 4.2$ pF. (d) CM gain FR with $C_e = 3.8$ pF.

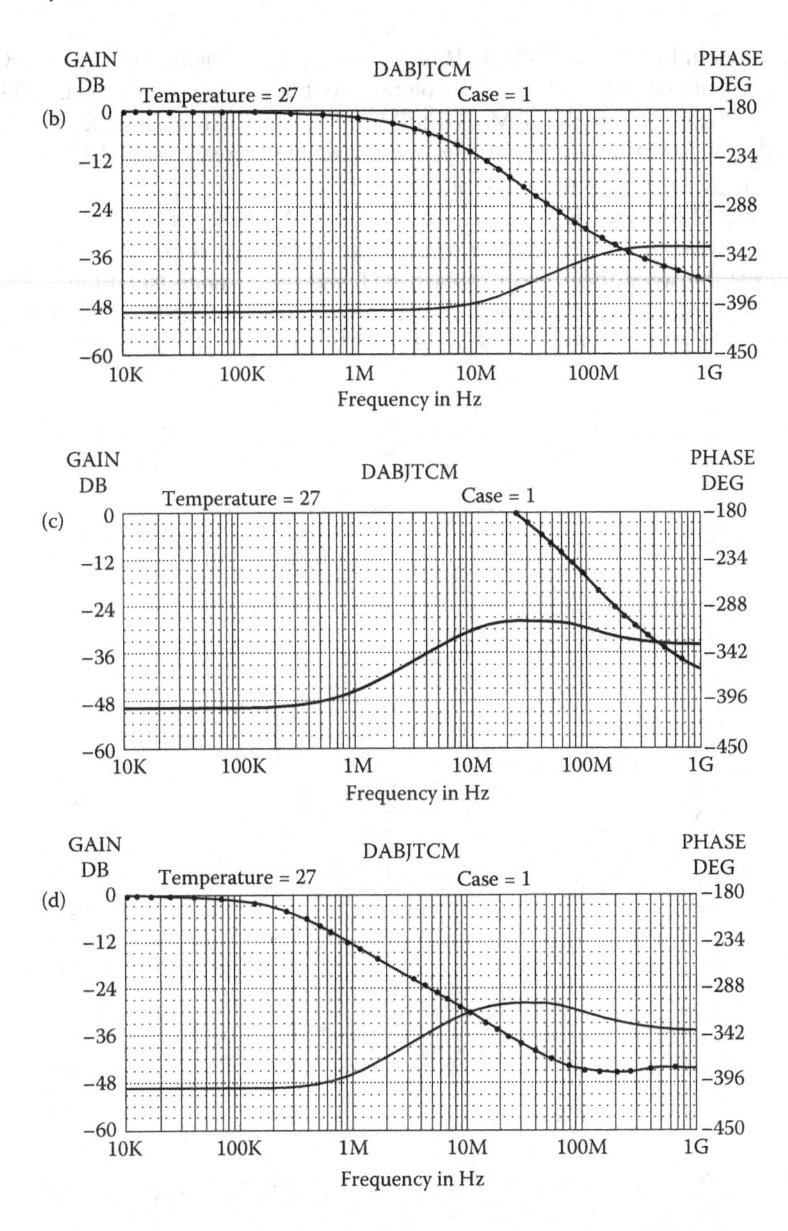

FIGURE 3.10 (CONTINUED) Common-mode gain frequency response of the BJT DA HFSSM of Figure 3.7a with various values of parasitic emitter capacitance, C_e, showing how C_e can improve the DA's CMRR by giving a low CM gain at high frequencies. (a) CM gain frequency response (FR) with $C_e = 0$. (b) CM gain FR with an optimum $C_e = 4$ pF. (c) CM gain FR with $C_e = 4.2$ pF. (d) CM gain FR with $C_e = 3.8$ pF.

transistor DAs with real transistor models instead of linear HFSSMs, is that the DM gain frequency response is extremely sensitive to C_e, a parasitic parameter which we have little control over. Note that subtle changes in C_e can radically improve or spoil the high-frequency CMRR of a transistor DA!

3.5 INPUT RESISTANCE OF SIMPLE TRANSISTOR DAS

In general, simple, two-transistor DAs have much lower $\mathbf{R_{in}}$ for DM signals than for CM inputs. This is true over the entire frequency range of the DA. This effect is more pronounced for BJT DA stages than for JFET or MOSFET DAs. By way of illustration, consider the CM HIFSSM of the BJT amplifier illustrated in Figure 3.7a. When $|\mathbf{R_{in}}(f)|_{DM} = |\mathbf{V_{sc}}/\mathbf{I_{sc}}|$ is plotted using MicroCap, we see that at low frequencies $|\mathbf{R_{in}}| \cong r_\pi + r_x = 3\,E3$ ohms, and it begins to roll off at ca. 100 kHz.

On the other hand, when the DM HIFSSM of Figure 3.7b is simulated, the low frequency $|\mathbf{R_{in}}(f)|_{CM} \cong 3.0\,E8\ \Omega$, or $2R_E\,(1 + g_m\,r_\pi)$, a sizeable increase over the DM $|\mathbf{R_{in}}(f)|$. The low-frequency $|\mathbf{R_{in}}(f)|_{CM}$ begins to roll off at only 200 Hz.

Ideally, one would like the $|\mathbf{R_{in}}(f)|$ for *both* CM and DM to be very large, to prevent loading of the source(s) driving the DA. There are several ways to achieve high $|\mathbf{R_{in}}(f)|_{DM.}$ One way is to insert a resistor R_e' between the emitter of each BJT and the V_e node (see Figure 3.6). It is easy to show from the midfrequency, common-emitter *h*-parameter, MFSSM of the BJT DA for DM inputs (see Figure 3.11b) that $R_{inDM} = V_{sd}/I_b = h_{ie} + R_e'\,(1 + \beta)$. The practical upper bound on

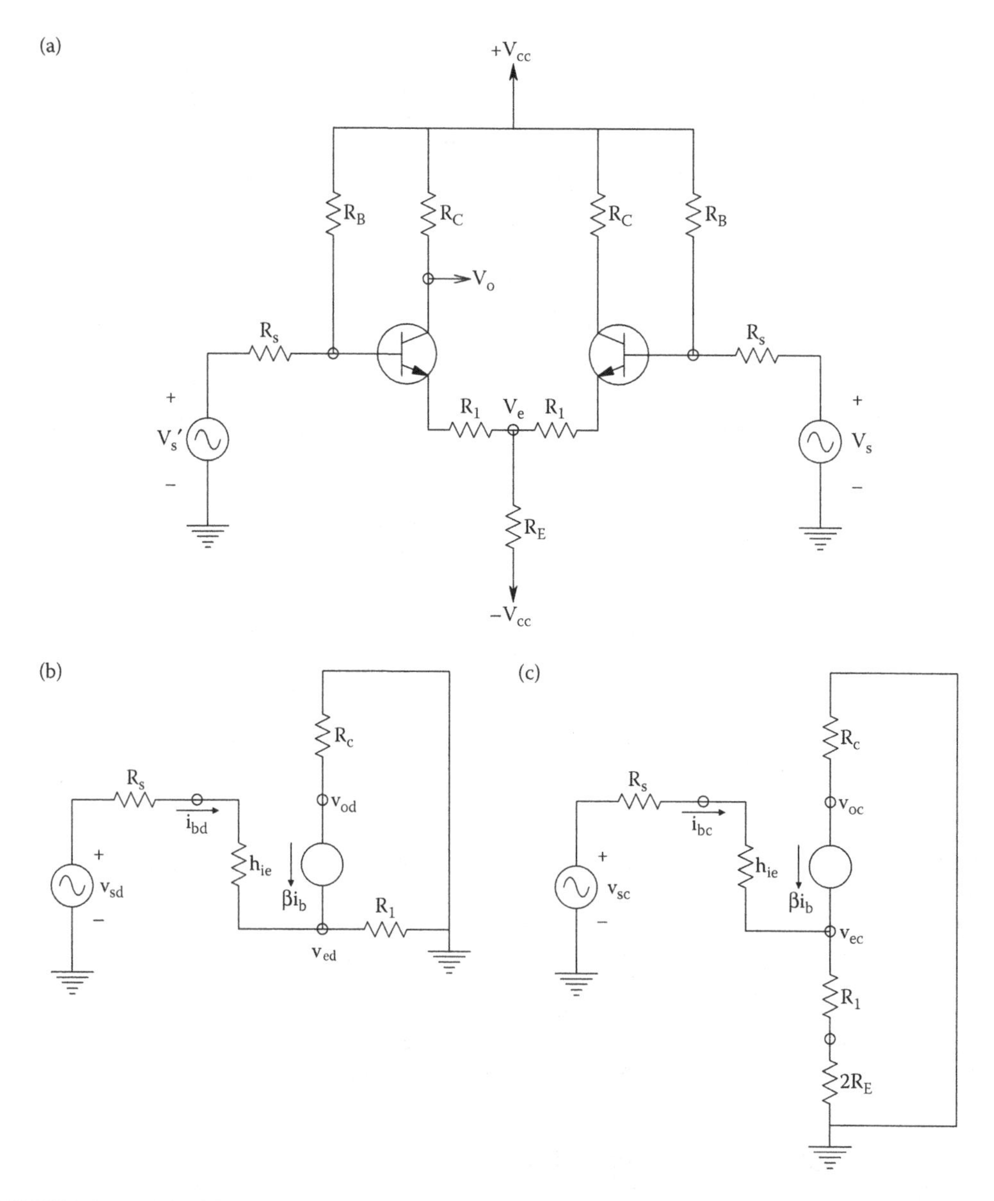

FIGURE 3.11 (a) A BJT DA with extra emitter resistances, R_1, which lower DM gain and increase DM input resistance. (b) Simplified MFSSM of the left side of the DA given DM inputs. (c) Simplified MFSSM of the left side of the DA given CM inputs.

R'_e is set by DC biasing considerations. The small-signal input resistance h_{ie} can be shown to be approximated by

$$h_{ie} \cong V_T h_{fe} / I_{CQ} \text{ Ohms} \tag{3.21}$$

where $V_T = kT/q$, h_{fe} is the transistor's current gain, and I_{CQ} is the collector current at the BJT's quiescent (Q) operating point. T is the Kelvin temperature. k is Boltzmann's constant = 1.38×10^{-23} J/°K.

Another approach is to use BJT Darlington amplifiers in the DA; A Darlington circuit and its simplified MFSSM is shown in Figure 3.12. Darlingtons can easily be shown to have a small-signal input resistance of

$$R_{in} = h_{ie1} + h_{ie2}(1 + h_{fe1}) \tag{3.22}$$

If an emitter resistor R_1 is used as in the first case, R_{in} can be shown to be

$$R_{in} = h_{ie1} + (1 + h_{fe1})[h_{ie2} + R_1(1 + h_{fe2})] \cong h_{fe1}\ h_{fe2}\ R_1 \tag{3.23}$$

So, if $h_{fe1} = h_{fe2} = 100$ and $R_1 = 200\ \Omega$, $R_{in} > 2\ \text{M}\Omega$.

Another obvious way to increase R_{in} for DM excitation (and CM, as well) is to design the DA headstage using JFETs or MOSFETs. Using these devices, the low- and midfrequency R_{in} is on the order of 10^9–$10^{12}\ \Omega$.

3.6 HOW SIGNAL SOURCE IMPEDANCE AFFECTS THE LOW-FREQUENCY CMRR

Figure 3.13 illustrates a generalized input circuit for an instrumentation DA. Note that the two Thevenin sources v_s and v'_s can be broken into DM and CM components. As we defined above

$$v_{sd} \equiv (v_s - v'_s)/2 \tag{3.24a}$$

$$Av_{sc} \equiv (v_s + v'_s)/2 \tag{3.24b}$$

Superposition is used to compute the effects of v_{sc} and v_{sd} on the output of the DA. When v_{sc} is considered, we replace both v_s and v'_s with v_{sc} in Figure 3.13. When v_{sd} is considered, we replace v_s with v_{sd} and v'_s with $-v_{sd}$.

Note that manufacturers usually specify a common-mode input impedance, $\mathbf{Z_{ic}}$, measured from one input lead to ground under pure CM excitation, and a difference-mode input impedance, $\mathbf{Z_{id}}$, measured under pure DM excitation from either input to ground. The input Zs are generally given by manufacturer's specs as a resistance in parallel with a small, shunting capacitance. For example, $\mathbf{Z_{ic}} = 10^{11}\ \Omega \,||\, 5$ pF. In the following development, it will be assumed that the signal frequency is sufficiently low so that the currents through the input capacitances are negligible compared to the parallel input resistance. Thus, only input resistances will be used.

By Ohm's Law, the DM current into the non-inverting input node is just

$$i_d = 2v_{sd}/R_1 + v_{sd}/R_{ic} \tag{3.25}$$

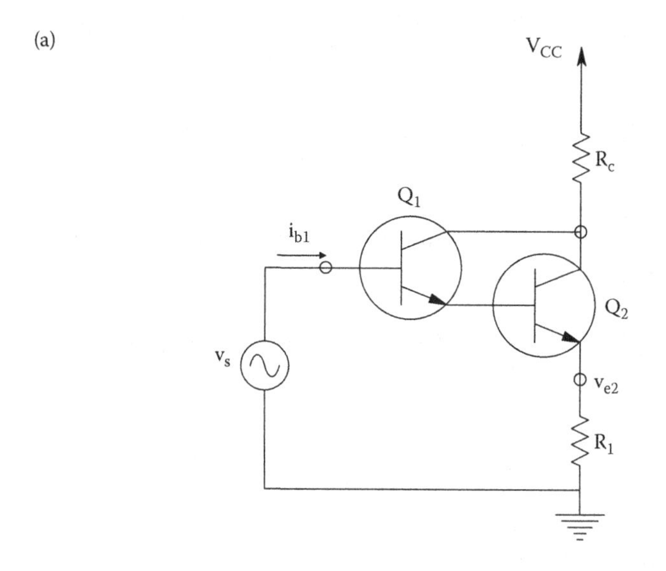

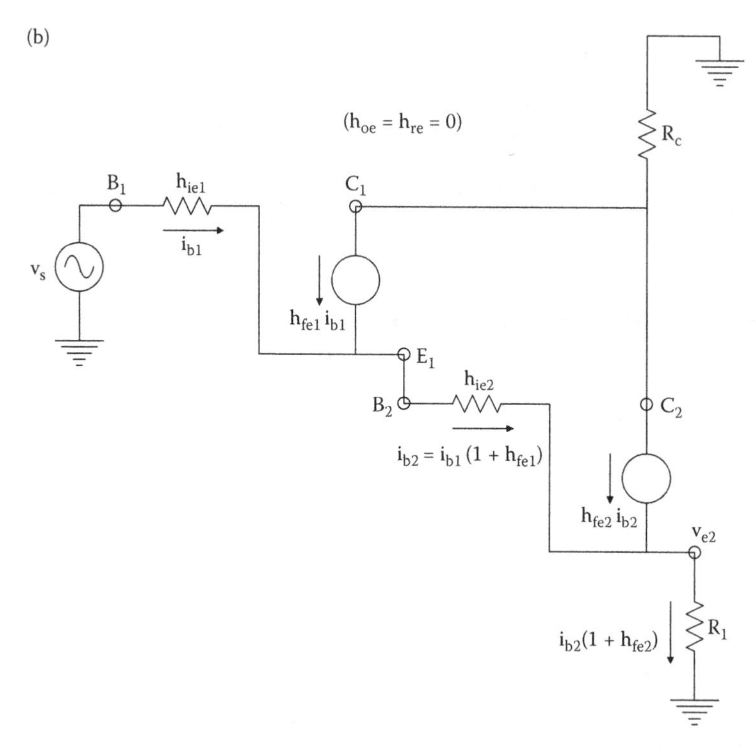

FIGURE 3.12 (a) A Darlington stage which can replace the left-hand BJT in the DA of Figure 3.11a. (b) MFSSM of the Darlington valid for DM excitation of the DA. The input resistance for the Darlington DA given DM excitation is derived in the Text.

From which one can write

$$i_d / v_{sd} = 1 / R_{sd} = 2 / R_1 + 1 / R_{ic} \tag{3.26}$$

Solving for the equivalent shunting resistance in Equation 3.26, one gets

$$R_1 = 2\ R_{id} R_{ic} / (R_{ic} - R_{id}) \tag{3.27}$$

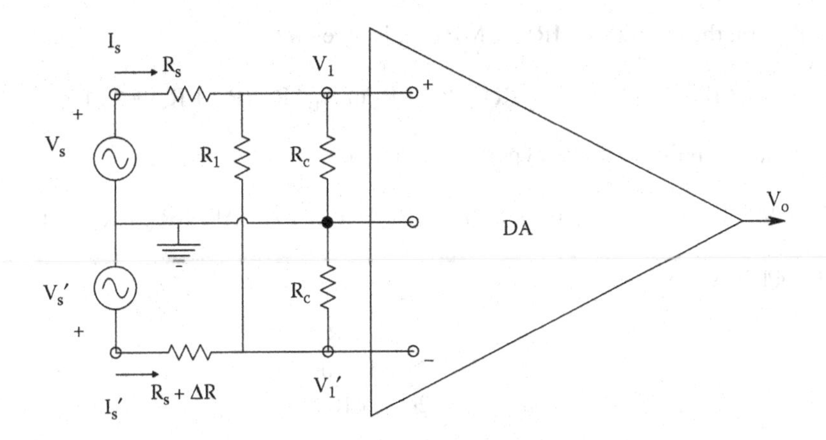

FIGURE 3.13 A generalized input equivalent circuit for an instrumentation DA.

In many differential amplifiers, $R_{ic} > R_{id}$. In others, $R_{ic} \cong R_{id}$, and from Equation 3.27, $R_1 = \infty$. Hence,

$$Z_{ic} = Z_{id} \cong R_{ic}. \tag{3.28}$$

Assume that $R_{ic} = R_{id}$. Thus, R_1 may be eliminated from Figure 3.13, which illustrates two Thevenin sources driving the DA through unequal source resistances, R_s and $R_s + \Delta R$. Using superposition and the definitions in Equations 3.24A and B, it is possible to show that a purely CM excitation, v_{sc}, produces an unwanted difference-mode component at the DA's input terminals:

$$v_{id} / v_{sc} = R_{ic}\Delta R / 2(R_{ic} + R_s)^2 \tag{3.29}$$

Also, v_{sc} produces a large CM component; the ΔR term is numerically negligible:

$$v_{ic} / v_{sc} = R_{ic} / (R_{ic} + R_s) \tag{3.30}$$

For purely DM excitation in v_s, it also can be shown that

$$v_{id} / v_{sd} = R_{ic} / (R_{ic} + R_s) \tag{3.31}$$

and

$$v_{ic} / v_{sd} = R_{ic}\Delta R/2(R_{ic} + R_s)^2 \tag{3.32}$$

In order to find the CMRR of the circuit of Figure 3.13, Equation 3.2 for v_o will be used, and the definition for CMRR, relation 3.13. Thus,

$$v_{oc} = A_D v_{sc} R_{ic}\Delta R/2(R_{ic} + R_s)^2 + A_C v_{sc} R_{ic} / (R_{ic} + R_s) \tag{3.33}$$

and

$$v_{od} = A_D v_{sd} R_{ic} / (R_{ic} + R_s) + A_C v_{sd} R_{ic}\Delta R/2(R_{ic} + R_s)^2 \tag{3.34}$$

After some algebra, the circuit's CMRR, $CMRR_{sys}$, is given by

$$CMRR_{sys} = [A_D + A_C \Delta R/2(R_{ic} + R_s)]/A_D \Delta R/2(R_{ic} + R_s) + A_C] \quad (3.35)$$

Equation 3.35 may be reduced to the hyperbolic relation:

$$CMRR_{sys} = [(A_D/A_C) + \Delta R/2(R_{ic} + R_s)]/[(A_D/A_C)\Delta R/2(R_{ic} + R_s) + 1] \quad (3.36)$$

which can be approximated by

$$CMRR_{sys} \cong \frac{CMRR_A}{\dfrac{CMRR_A \Delta R}{2(R_{ic} + R_s)} + 1} \quad (3.37)$$

in which the manufacturer-specified CMRR is $CMRR_A = A_D/A_C$, and $CMRR_A >> DR/2(R_{ic} + R)$.

A plot of $CMRR_{sys}$ vs $\Delta R/R_s$ is shown in Figure 3.14. Note that when the Thevenin source resistances are matched, $CMRR_{sys} = CMRR_A$. Also, when

$$\Delta R/R_s = -2(R_{ic}/R_s + 1)/CMRR_A, \quad (3.38)$$

the $CMRR_{sys} \to \infty$. This implies that a judicious addition of an external resistance ΔR in series with one input lead or the other may be used by trial and error to increase the effective CMRR of the system. For example, if $R_{ic} = 100\ M\Omega$, $R_s = 10\ k\Omega$, and $CMRR_A = 100$ dB, then $\Delta R/R_s = -0.2$ to give ∞ $CMRR_{sys}$. Since it is generally not possible to reduce R_s', it is easier to externally add a 2 kΩ ΔR in series with R_s.

Again, it is stressed that an amplifier's $CMRR_A$ is a decreasing function of frequency because of the frequency dependence of the gains, $\mathbf{A_D}$ and $\mathbf{A_C}$. Also, the AC equivalent input circuit of a DA contains capacitances in parallel with R_1, R_{ic}, and R_{ic}' and the source impedances often contain a reactive, frequency-dependent component. Thus, in practice, at low frequencies, $CMRR_{sys}$ can often be maximized by the ΔR method, but seldom can be drastically increased at high frequencies because of reactive unbalances in the input circuit.

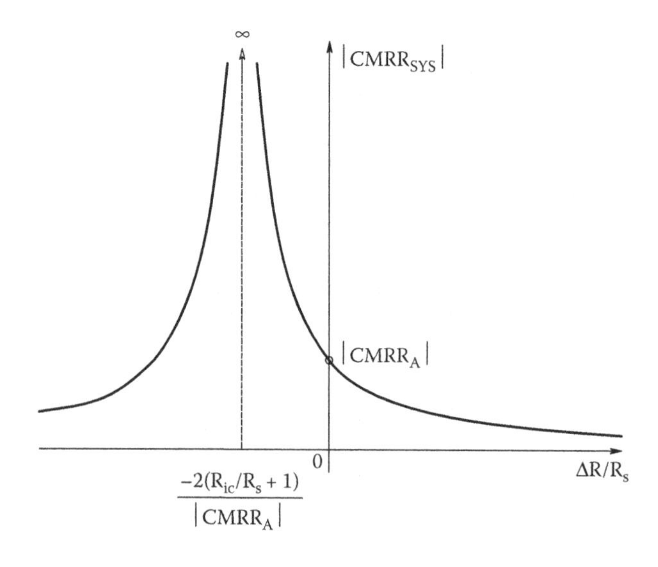

FIGURE 3.14 The CMRR of a balanced input DA as a function of the incremental change in one input (Thevenin) resistance. Note that a critical value of $\Delta R/R_s$ exists that theoretically gives infinite CMRR.

3.7 HOW OP AMPS CAN BE USED TO MAKE DAS FOR MEDICAL APPLICATIONS

3.7.1 Introduction

It is true that op amps themselves are differential amplifiers, but several practical factors make their *direct use* in instrumentation highly impractical. The first factor is their extremely high open-loop gain and relatively low signal bandwidth. As will be seen in Chapters 6 and 7, op amps are designed to be used with massive amounts of negative feedback which acts to reduce their gain, increase their bandwidth, reduce their output signal distortion, etc. When used without feedback, their extremely high, open-loop gain generally produces unacceptable signal levels at their outputs, as well as DC levels that drift because of temperature-sensitive input DC offset voltage and DC bias currents. Consequently, circuits have evolved which use two or three op amps with feedback to make DAs with gains typically ranging from 1 to 10^3, wide bandwidths, low noise, high input Z, high CMRR, etc.

Why would one want to build a DA from op amps, when instrumentation amplifiers (IAs) are readily available from manufacturers? One reason is that one can select ultra low-noise op amps for the circuit, and can tweak resistor values to maximize the DA's CMRR. If one is building only a few DAs, one should be able to achieve a higher performance-to-cost ratio by doing a custom design with op amps, rather than purchasing commercial IAs.

3.7.2 Op Amp DA Designs for Instrumentation

A *2-op amp DA* is shown in Figure 3.15. All resistors "R" are closely matched to <0.02% to maintain a high CMRR. Analysis is easy if we assume ideal op amps. Node equations are written for the V_2 and V_3 nodes, which by the ideal op amp assumption, are V_s' and V_s, respectively. The unknowns are V_o and V_4:

$$V_s'[2G+G_F] - V_sG_F - V_4G = 0 \tag{3.39a}$$

$$-V_s' G_F V_s[2G+G_F] - V_oG - V_4G = 0 \tag{3.39b}$$

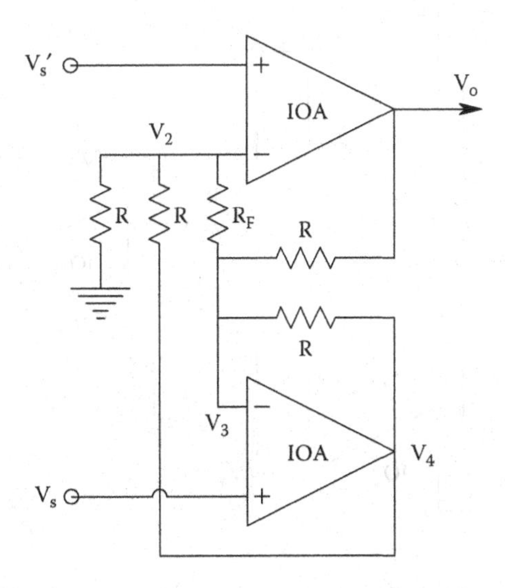

FIGURE 3.15 A two-operational amplifier DA. Resistors must be precisely matched to obtain maximum CMRR.

Clearly, from Equation 3.39a, $V_4 G = V_s'[2G + G_F] - V_s G_F$. This equation is substituted into Equation 3.39B, yielding

$$V_o = (V_s - V_s')2(1 + R/R_F) = \frac{(V_s - V_s')}{2} 4(1 + R/R_F) = V_{sd} 4(1 + R/R_F) \tag{3.40}$$

Thus, the two-op amp DA configuration can have DM gains, $A_D \geq 4$. (This analysis does not treat the CM gain.)

A 3-op amp DA circuit is shown in Figure 3.16. In this circuit, it is assumed that all $R_j = R_j'$, i.e., corresponding resistors are perfectly matched in order to make the CMRR $\to \infty$. Analysis of the 3-op amp DA can be done with superposition but is easier if one assumes pure CM and DM excitations and use the bisection theorem. For pure CM excitation, $V_s' = V_s = V_{sc}$. By symmetry and the IOA assumption, $V_2 = V_2' = V_{sc}$, hence there is no current in $R_1 + R_1'$, and $V_c = V_{sc}$. There is also no current in R_2 and R_2', so there is no voltage drop across these feedback resistors, and thus $V_3 = V_3' = V_{sc}$. When the right-hand IOA circuit has matched resistors, it is a DA with gain:

$$V_o = (V_3 - V_3')(R_4 / R_3) \tag{3.41}$$

Clearly, for CM signals,

$$A_C = \frac{V_o}{V_{sc}} = 0 \tag{3.42}$$

For pure DM excitation, $V_s' = -V_s$, $V_2 = V_s = V_{sd}$, and $V_2' = -V_s$. Thus, a potential of 2Vs exists across resistors $(R_1 + R_1')$, and by Kirchoff's voltage law, $V_c = 0$ on the *axis of symmetry*. Since current flows through R_1 and R_2, also R_1' and R_2', the input IOAs each have a gain of $(1 + R_2/R_1)$. Now $V_3' = -V_{sd}(1 + R_2/R_1)$, and $V_3 = V_{sd}(1 + R_2/R_1)$. Using superposition on the output IOA circuit, we have,

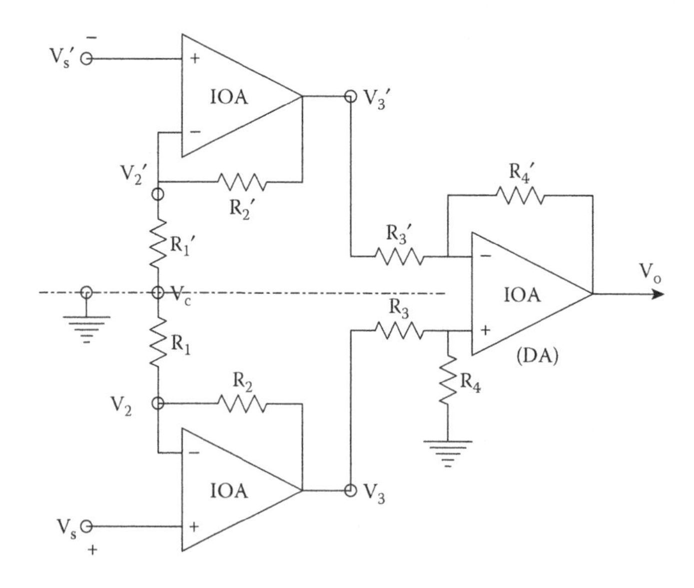

FIGURE 3.16 The symmetrical, 3-op amp DA. Again, for max CMRR, the primed resistors must precisely equal the corresponding nonprimed resistors.

$$\frac{V_o}{V_{sd}} = A_D = (R_4 / R_3)2(1 + R_2 / R_1) \tag{3.43}$$

IC versions of this DA circuit generally make $R_3 = R_4$, set the R_2s = 25 k, and replace $(R_1 + R_1')$ with a single external resistor to set A_D between 1 and 10^3. An example of such an IC DA is the Burr-Brown INA111.

In practice, the OAs are not ideal and have different, finite CMRRs, and also, the resistors are not perfectly matched. For example, the "off-the-shelf" CMRR is 106 dB at an $A_D = 100$ for the INA111.

3.8 CHAPTER SUMMARY

Because of their great importance in many aspects of biomedical measurements, differential amplifiers have been treated here in their own chapter. DAs are essential electronic subsystems for such ICs as op amps, instrumentation amplifiers, and analog voltage comparators. DAs are widely used in instrumentation systems to condition signals because of their ability to reject, by subtraction, interference, and noise that is exactly common to both inputs.

In describing DA circuit architecture, we introduced the important definitions of differential and common-mode input signals, differential and common-mode gains, and the common-mode rejection ratio (CMRR(f)) as a DA figure of merit. Internal and external factors affecting the DA's CMRR at low frequencies were described.

The mid- and high-frequency behavior of DA difference-mode and common-mode gains was explored by circuit simulation, and we discussed factors affecting the CMRR at high frequencies. Circuits using two and three op amps to make instrumentation DAs were described and analyzed.

CHAPTER 3 HOME PROBLEMS

3.1 A pair of matched JFETs and an ideal op amp are used to make a DA as shown in Figure P3.1. Both JFETs are described at midfrequencies by the simple Norton (g_m, g_d) MFSSM.

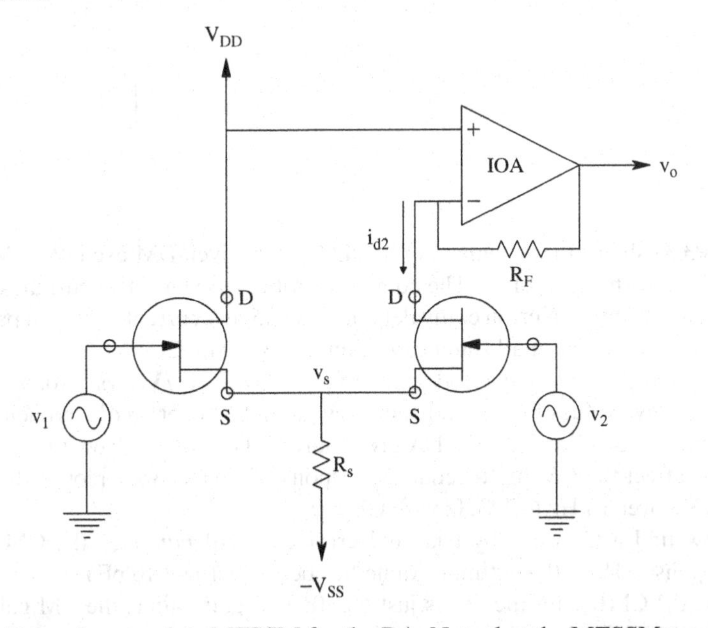

(A) Draw the complete MFSSM for the DA. Note that the MFSSM treats all ideal DC voltage sources as small signal grounds, and all ideal DC current sources as open circuits.

(B) Use superposition to derive an expression for $v_o = f(v_1, v_2)$. Show what happens to v_o when R_S is replaced with an ideal DC current source.

3.2 The schematic of a JFET/BJT cascode DA is shown in Figure P3.2. In this DA, $Q_1 = Q_2$ with $h_{oe} = h_{re} = 0$, $h_{fe} = 120$, $I_{CQ} = 1$ mA, $R_C = 7$ kΩ, $R_s = 25$ MΩ (dynamic load), and $R_B = 1.24$ MΩ. Also, $Q_3 = Q_4$ with $g_m = 5 \times 10^{-3}$ S, $g_d = 1 \times 10^{-4}$ S.

(A) Use the bisection theorem to draw the MFSSMs for both pure CM and pure DM excitation.

(B) Find an expression for the CM gain, v_o/v_{1c}.

(C) Find an expression for the DA's DM gain, v_o/v_{1d}.

(D) Find an expression for and evaluate numerically the DA's CMRR.

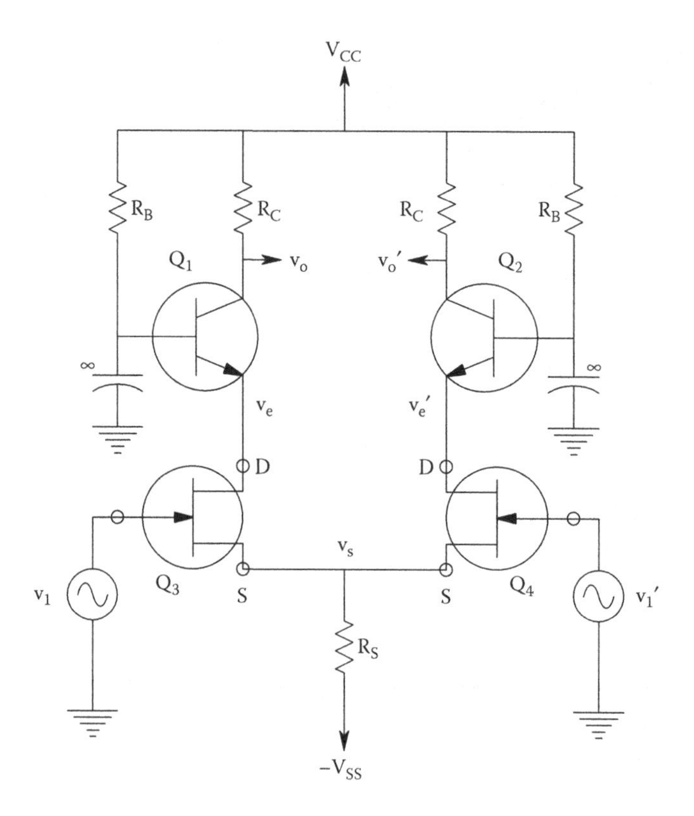

3.3 Figure P3.3a shows the schematic of a 2N2369 DA given DM excitation. VINV is an ideal VCVS with a gain of −1. The common emitters use an active current sink, which can be replaced by its Norton equivalent of a 2.0125 mA current source in parallel with a 2 MΩ resistor and a small shunt capacitance to ground, C_E.

(A) Use an ECAP to make a Bode plot of the *DM gain*, $\mathbf{V}_o/\mathbf{V}_{1d}$, vs f from 10 kHz to 10 GHz. Give values for the midfrequency gain, the upper −3 dB frequency, and f_T.

(B) Figure P3.3B illustrates the DA given pure CM excitation. Now the capacitor, C_E, will affect the CM high-frequency response. Make a Bode plot of the *CM gain*, $\mathbf{V}_o/\mathbf{V}_{1c}$ over 1 kHz to 1 GHz with CE ≡ 0.

(C) Now find a C_E value by trial and error that will *minimize* the CM frequency response. (Hint: the optimum value lies between 1 and 10 pF.)

(D) The dB CMRR for the DA is just the dB DM gain minus the CM gain. Plot the dB CMRR for the amplifier with $C_E = 0$, and C_E = the optimum value, for 10 kHz ≤ f ≤ 1 GHz.

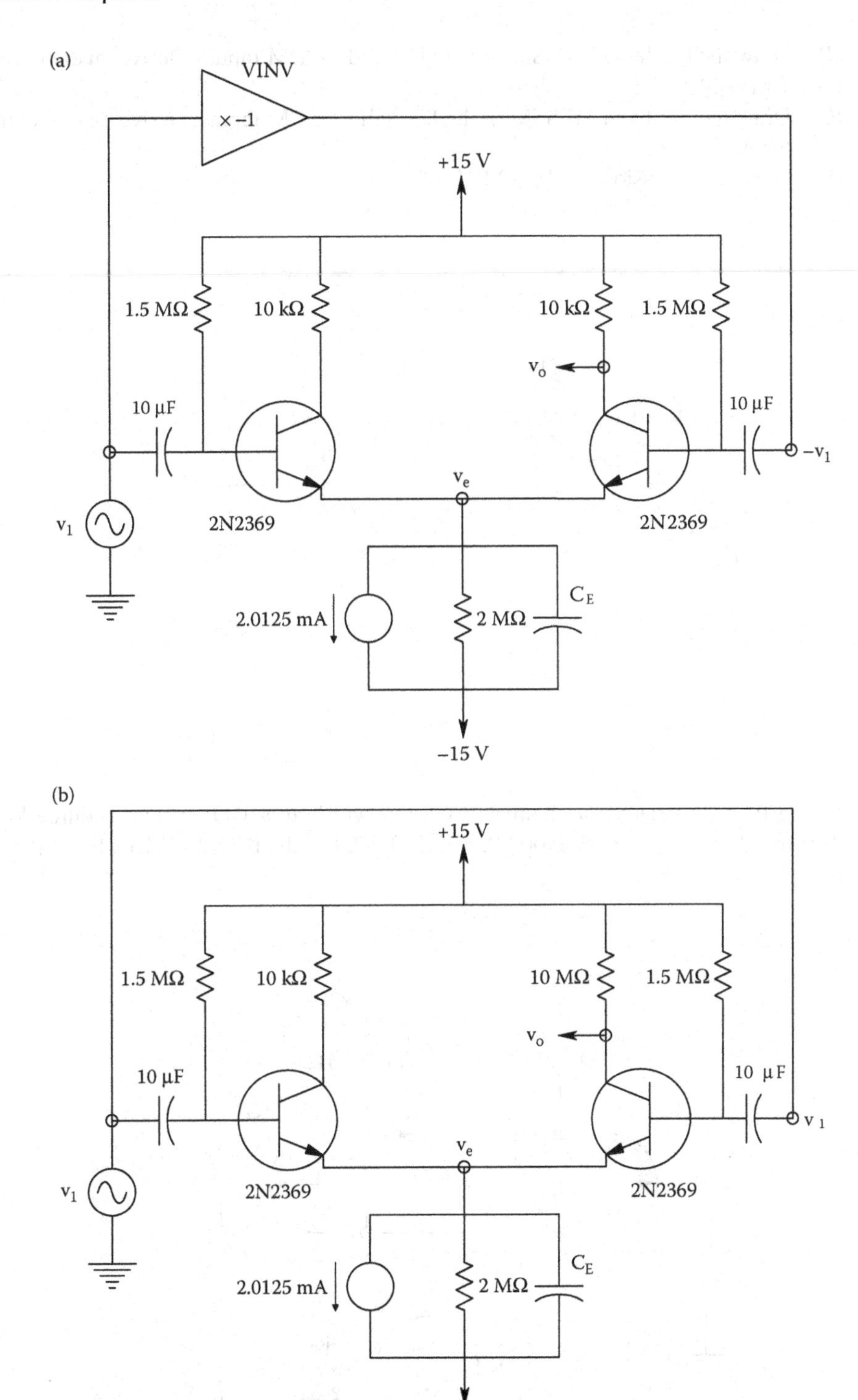

3.4 A MOSFET DA is shown in Figure P3.4.

(A) Draw the complete MFSSM for the DA. Use the Norton model (g_m, g_d) for the MOSFETs.

(B) Draw the left-hand MFSSM of the DA valid for DM inputs. Derive an expression for the MF $A_d = v_o / v_{1d}$.

(C) Draw the left-hand MFSSM of the DA valid for CM inputs. Derive an expression for $A_c = v_o / v_{1c}$.

(D) Give an expression for the CMRR of the DA.

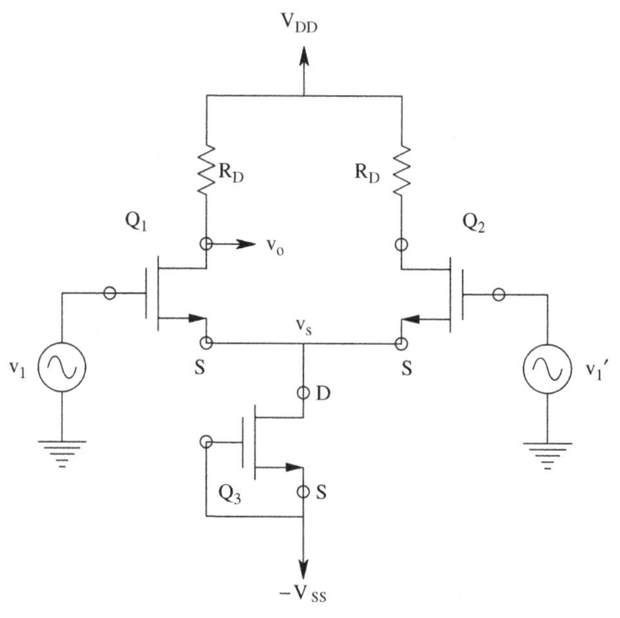

3.5 Figure P3.5 illustrates a ***p***-channel JFET DA with a ***pnp*** BJT dynamic source load. Assume $Q_1 = Q_2$ with $g_m = 0.002$ S, $r_d = 250$ kΩ. For the BJT: $h_{fe} = 150$, $h_{oe} = 10^{-6}$ S, $h_{ie} = 1.5$ kΩ, $h_{re} = 0$.

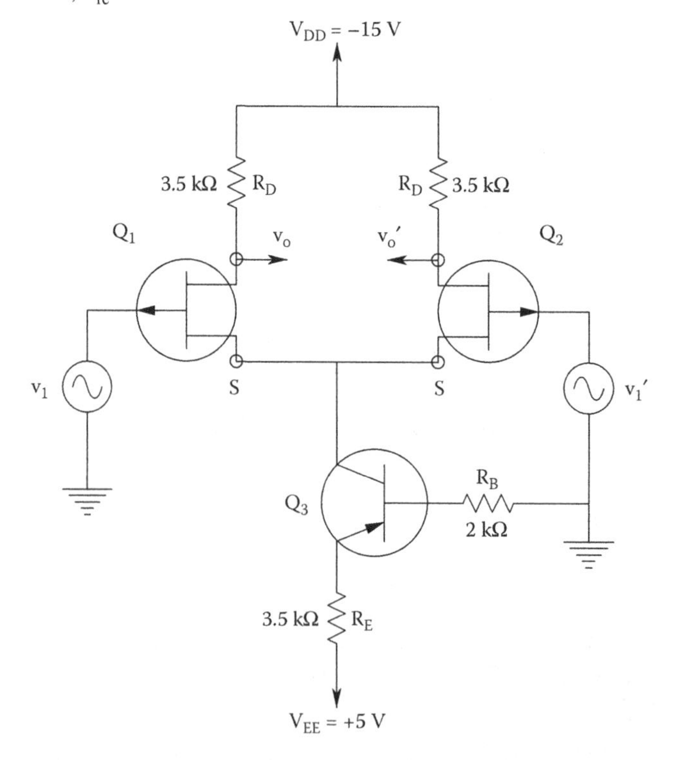

(A) Draw the MFSSM for the DA.
(B) Find an expression and the numerical value for the small-signal resistance, R_S, looking into the collector of the BJT.
(C) Find the expression and numerical value for $A_d = v_o/v_{1d}$, $A_c = v_o/v_{1c}$, and the DA's CMRR.

3.6 The DA shown in Figure P3.6 uses common-mode negative feedback between the output and the dynamic load BJT, Q_3. Assume $Q_1 = Q_2$ with $h_{fe} = 200$, $h_{ie} = 2.5\ k\Omega$, $h_{oe} = h_{re} = 0$, $R_1 = 70\ k\Omega$, $R_C = 4\ k\Omega$. For Q3: $h_{fe} = 200$, $h_{oe} = 10^{-5}$ S, $h_{ie} = 1.2\ k\Omega$, $h_{re} = 0$. The numbers in parentheses are quiescent DC bias voltages. The zener diode drops 14.3 V at 0.2 mA. Treat it as an ideal DC voltage source.

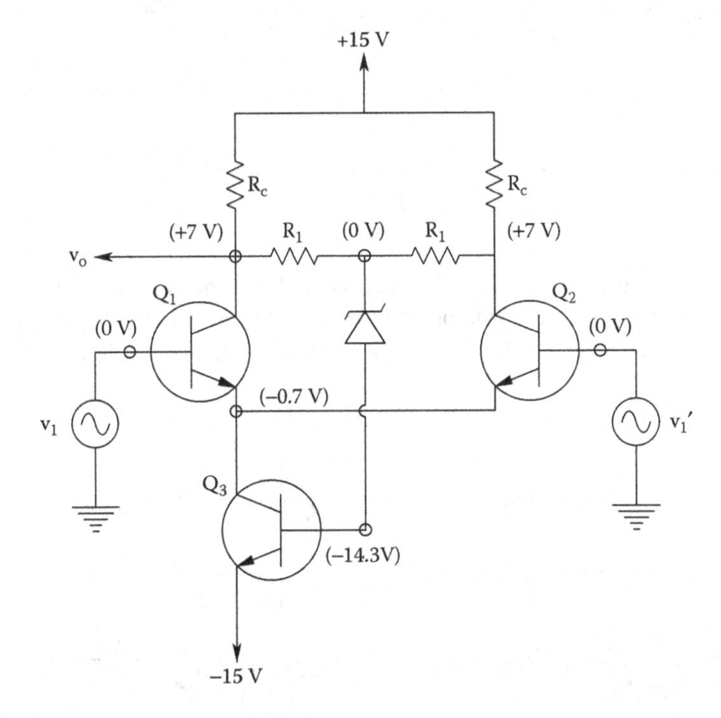

(A) Use the bisection theorem to draw the MFSSM for the DA given pure DM excitation.
(B) Use the bisection theorem to draw the MFSSM for the DA given pure CM excitation.
(C) Give algebraic expressions for $A_d = v_o/v_{1d}$ and $A_c = v_o/v_{1c}$. Evaluate numerically.
(D) Evaluate the DA's CMRR.
(E) By way of comparison, repeat parts A–D when the zener diode is removed and Q_3's base is tied to small-signal ground.

3.7 The DA shown in Figure P3.7 uses feedback pair amplifiers. For symmetry, $Q_1 = Q_3$ and $Q_2 = Q_4$, but $Q_1 \neq Q_2$, etc. Q_1 and Q_3 have h_{fe1}, $h_{ie1} > 0$ and $h_{re1} = h_{oe1} = 0$. Likewise, Q_2 & Q_4 have h_{fe2}, $h_{ie2} > 0$ and $h_{re2} = h_{oe2} = 0$.
(A) Draw the complete MFSSM for the DA given pure DM excitation.
(B) Draw the complete MFSSM for the DA given pure CM excitation.
(C) Find an expression for Ad = vo /v1d.
(D) Find an expression for Ac = vo /v1c.
(E) Find an expression for the DA's CMRR.
(F) Find an expression for the DA's small-signal input resistance when it is given DM input. Let $R_{ind} = v_{1d}/i_{1}$.
(G) Find an expression for the DA's small-signal input resistance when it is given CM input. Let $R_{inc} = v_{1c}/i_1$.

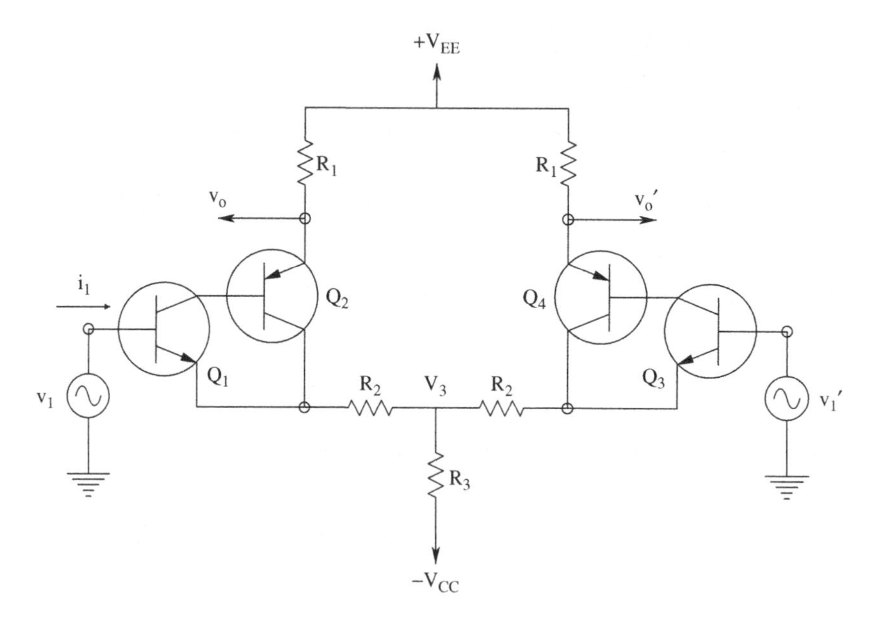

3.8 Figure P3.8 illustrates a DA using Darlington modules, the purpose of which is to raise the DM input resistance. For symmetry, $Q_1 = Q_3$ and $Q_2 = Q_4$. Q_1 & Q_3 have h_{fe1}, $h_{ie1} > 0$, $h_{re1} = h_{oe1} = 0$. Q_2 & Q_4 have h_{fe2}, $h_{ie2} > 0$, $h_{re2} = h_{oe2} = 0$. Q_5 has h_{fe5}, h_{ie5}, $h_{oe5} > 0$, $h_{re5} = 0$.

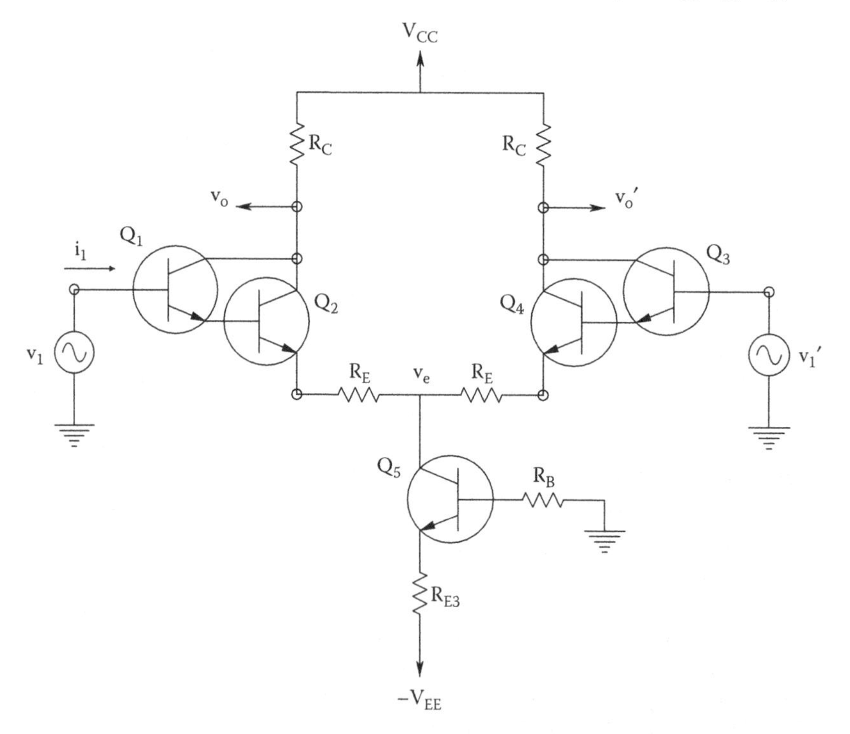

(A) Draw the MFSSMs for the DA for pure CM and DM excitations.
(B) Find an expression for $A_d = v_o/v_{1d}$.
(C) Find an expression for $A_c = v_o/v_{1c}$.
(D) Find an expression for the DA's CMRR.
(E) Find an expression for the DA's small-signal input resistance when it is given DM input. Let $R_{ind} = v_{1d}/i_1$.

(F) Find an expression for the DA's small-signal input resistance when it is given CM input. Let $R_{inc} = v_{1c}/i_1$.

(G) Now let $h_{fe1} = 100$, $h_{ie1} = 6$ kΩ, $h_{fe2} = 50$, $h_{ie2} = 1$ kΩ, $h_{fe5} = 100$, $h_{oe5} = 10^{-5}$ S, $h_{ie5} = 2.5$ kΩ, $R_C = 5$ kΩ, $R_E = 500$ Ω, $R_{E3} = 3.3$ k Ω, and $R_B = 100$ kΩ. Calculate numerical values for parts B–F above.

3.9 Two, matched, ***n***-channel JFETs are connected as shown in Figure P3.9. They are both characterized by the saturation-region, JFET drain current relation: $I_D = I_{DSS}(1 - V_{GS}/V_P)^2$. The capacitor, C_o, blocks DC from the output signal. The circuit input is the pure difference-mode signal, $v_{gd} = v_1$. *Find* an algebraic expression for I_L and the AC v_o.

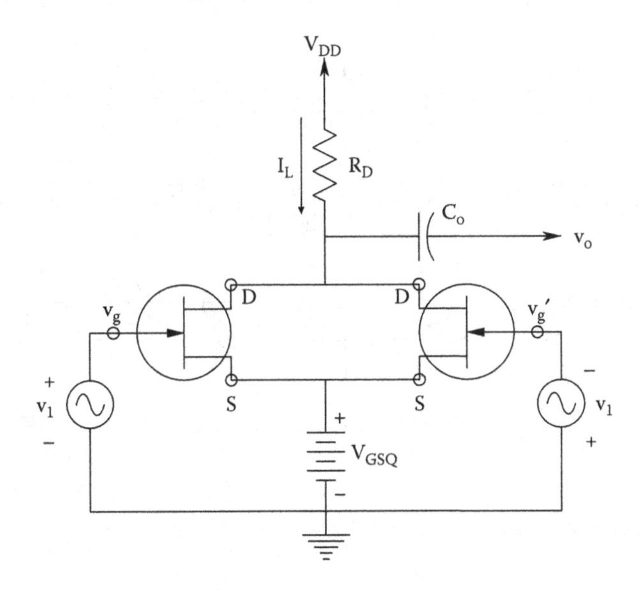

3.10 Two, matched 2N2222A BJTs are used to make a BJT DA shown in Figure P3.10.

(A) *Simu*late the circuit under CM excitation and make a Bode plot of $\mathbf{A}_c = \mathbf{V}_o/\mathbf{V}_{1c}$. Let 1k Hz ≤ f ≤ 0.1 GHz

(B) Now make a Bode plot of the DM gain, $\mathbf{A}_d = \mathbf{V}_o/\mathbf{V}_{1d}$.

(C) Plot the DA's CMRR in dB over 1 kHz to 0.1 GHz.

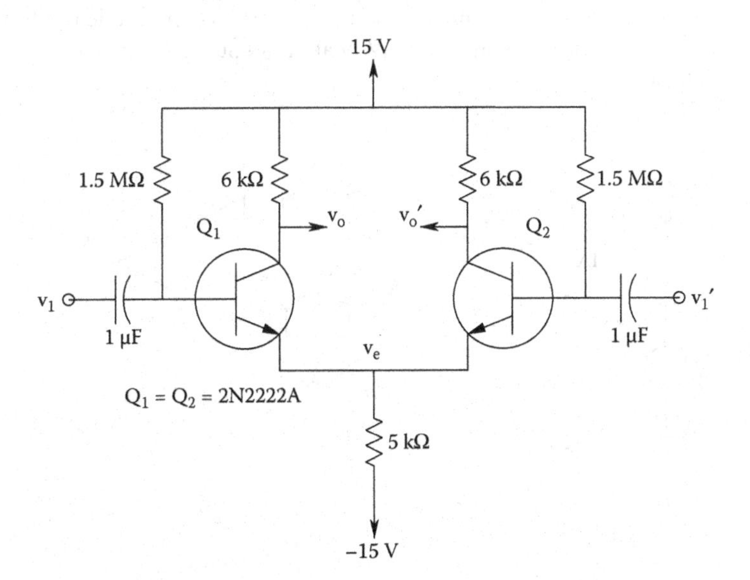

3.11 A BJT DA is shown in Figure P3.11. The circuit is symmetrical. $R_E = 10^5\ \Omega$, $R_S = 500\ \Omega$, $R_C = 6.8\ k\Omega$, $R_B = 1\ M\Omega$, BJTs: $h_{oe} = h_{re} = 0$, hfe = 100, $h_{ie} = 2.5\ k\Omega$. Assume C_c is a small-signal short circuit.

(A) Use MFSS analysis and the bisection theorem to find numerical values for A_D, A_C and the CMRR. $A_D \equiv v_o/v_{1d}$, $A_C \equiv v_o/v_{1c}$.

(B) Now the v_o output is coupled to a 10 kΩ load resistance, R_L, making the DA circuit asymmetrical, so the bisection theorem no longer can be used (Repeat A).

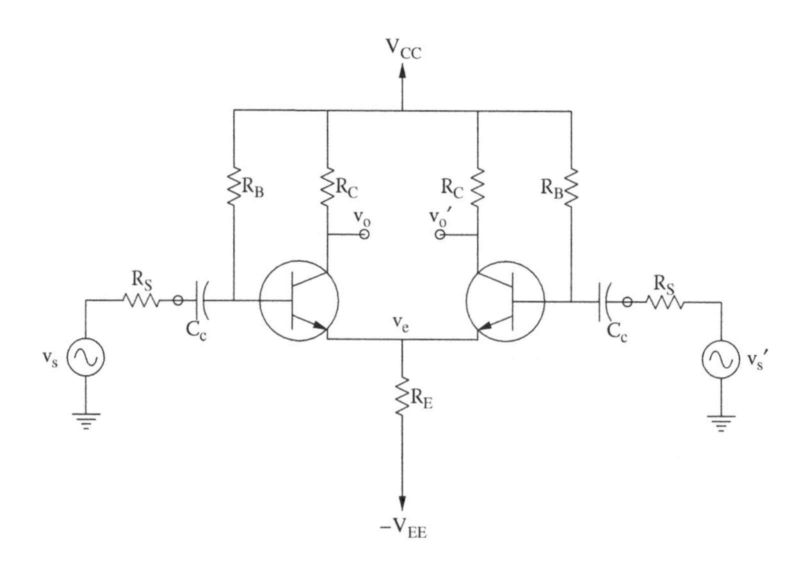

3.12 It is desired to *measure* the CMRR of a student-built differential amplifier. See Figure P3.12. First, the two inputs are shorted together and connected to a 100 Hz sinusoidal source. The source amplitude is adjusted so that when the peak output signal is 1.0 V, the input is 10 V peak. Then the negative input to the amplifier is grounded, and the source is connected to the + input. Its amplitude is adjusted so that $V_o = 10$ V peak when the input is 20 mV peak. Find numerical values for A_D, A_C, and the CMRR in dB.

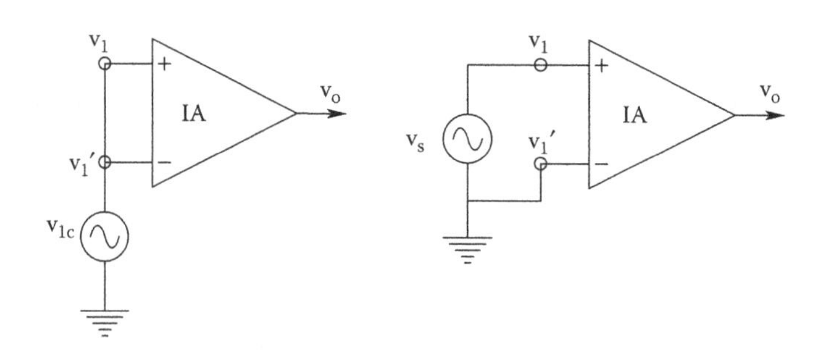

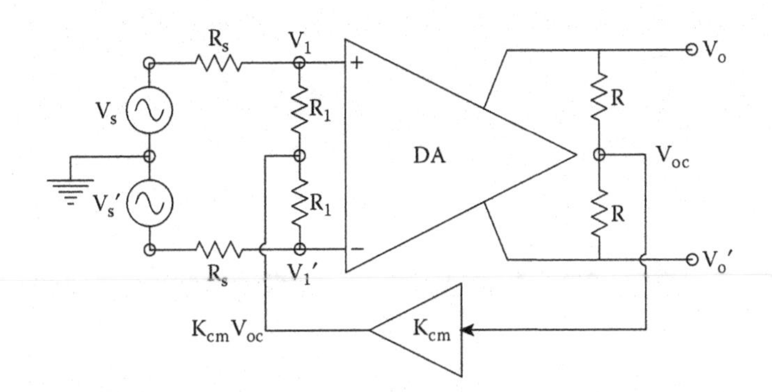

3.13 *Common-mode negative feedback* is applied around a DA having a differential output, shown in Figure P3.13. The amplifier follows the relations $V_o = A_D V_{1d} + A_C V_{1c}$, $V'_o = -A_D V_{1d} + A_C V_{1c}$. Also, $V_{1c} = A_C V_{1c}$, and let $\alpha \equiv R_1/(R_1 + R_s)$ and $\beta = R_s/(R_1 + R_s)$.

(A) Use superposition to find expressions for V_1 and V'_1.

(B) Find an expression for V_{1c} when V_s and V'_s are such that the input is pure V_{sc}.

(C) Find an expression for V_{1d} when the input is pure V_{sd}.

(D) Find an expression for the CMNF amplifier's CMRR. Compare it to the CMRR of the DA alone. Let $R_1 = R_2 = 10^6\ \Omega$, $K_{cm} = -10^3$, $A_C = 1$, $A_D = 10^3$. Evaluate the system's CMRR numerically.

4 General Properties of Electronic, Single-Loop Feedback Systems

4.1 INTRODUCTION

In electronic circuits and systems, *feedback* will be defined as a process whereby a signal proportional to the system's output is combined with a signal proportional to the input to form an error signal which affects the output. Nearly, all analog electronic circuits use feedback; either implicitly as the result of circuit design (e.g., from an unbypassed BJT emitter resistor) or explicitly by a specific circuit network between the output and the input nodes. A circuit can have one or more specific *feedback loops.* However, in the interest of simplicity, we will consider the effects of a single feedback loop on circuits with single inputs. There are four categories of electronic feedback; feedback can make an electronic system unstable (deliberately, as in the design of oscillators), or make it stable and change certain signal conditioning characteristics. The effects of feedback on amplifier *frequency response, gain, noise, output and input impedance, linearity,* and *noise* are described in the following sections.

Op amps are used to illustrate many properties of single-input single-output (SISO) feedback systems because all op amp circuits use external feedback, and they have relatively simple dynamic characteristics. A systems approach will be used in discussing amplifier performance with feedback, and little attention will be paid to the details of the internal electronic components. Block diagrams will be used, as well as signal flow graphs and Mason's rule (see the Appendix of this Text), to describe the systems under consideration, and the *root locus technique* will be used to explore feedback amplifier performance in the frequency domain (see Chapter 5 in this Text).

4.2 CLASSIFICATION OF ELECTRONIC FEEDBACK SYSTEMS

Examine Figure 4.1, which illustrates the general architecture of a simple, SISO feedback system, both as a linear signal flow graph (SFG) and a block diagram. Reduction of either the signal flow graph or the block diagram yields the well-known transfer function:

$$\frac{V_o}{V_s} = \frac{\alpha K_v}{1 - \beta K_v} \tag{4.1}$$

From this simple result, the following important quantities describing feedback systems can be defined:

$$\text{Forward gain} = \text{open} - \text{loop gain} \equiv \alpha K_v \tag{4.2a}$$

$$\text{Loop gain} = A_L \equiv \beta K_v \tag{4.2b}$$

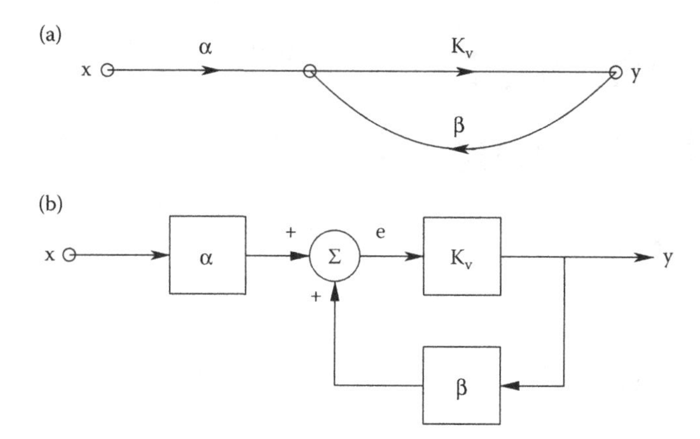

FIGURE 4.1 Two alternate representations for a single-input single-output (SISO) linear feedback system. (a) Signal flow graph notation. (b) Block diagram notation.

$$\text{Return difference} = \text{RD} \equiv 1 - A_L \tag{4.2c}$$

$$\text{dB of feedback} \equiv -20 \log |1 - A_L| \tag{4.2d}$$

Note that $\boldsymbol{\alpha}$, $\boldsymbol{\beta}$, $\mathbf{K_v}$, and $\mathbf{A_L}$ can be scalars or *vectors* (complex functions of frequency).

A SISO system is said to have negative feedback (NFB) if it has a minus sign associated with either $\mathbf{K_v}$, $\boldsymbol{\beta}$, or the summer, or all three elements in the block diagram. Control systems generally use NFB, and it is usual to assume a *vector subtraction* of $\boldsymbol{\beta}\mathbf{V_o}$ at the summer. Electronic systems do not necessarily have a subtraction at the summer; it depends on circuit design. To see if a SISO electronic feedback system has negative feedback, one must inspect its entire loop gain. $\mathbf{A_L}(j0)$ will have a minus sign (be a negative number) if the feedback amplifier is a *direct-coupled* (d-c), negative feedback system. If the amplifier is *reactively coupled* (r-c), then $\mathbf{A_L}(j\omega)$ will have a minus sign at midfrequencies (its phase angle will be –180°). A feedback amplifier is generally described in terms of voltages, but VCCSs are encountered. Considering that electronic feedback can have either sign and the fed-back quantity can be voltage or current, it is clear that four major types of feedback exist in active electronic circuits:

- Negative voltage feedback (NVFB)
- Negative current feedback (NCFB)
- Positive voltage feedback (PVFB)
- Positive current feedback (PCFB)

Negative voltage feedback is encountered most frequently in electronic engineering practice. We will examine its properties in the following section.

4.3 SOME EFFECTS OF NEGATIVE VOLTAGE FEEDBACK

4.3.1 Reduction of Output Resistance

Figure 4.2 illustrates a simple Thevenin amplifier circuit having NVFB applied to its summing junction (input node). We assume that the amplifier's input resistor, $R_i >> R_F$ and R_s, so R_i can be ignored in writing the node equation for V_i. Also, in finding the NVFB amplifier's open-circuit

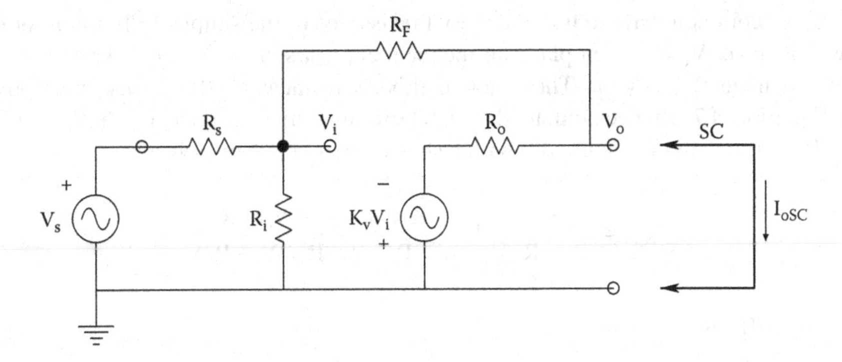

FIGURE 4.2 Schematic of a simple Thevenin VCVS with negative feedback. See Text for analysis.

voltage gain, assume that $R_o << R_F$, so that there is negligible voltage drop across R_o. Thus, the node equation is

$$V_i[G_s + G_F] - V_oG_F = V_sG_s \tag{4.3}$$

Also,

$$V_o \cong -K_vV_i \tag{4.4}$$

Hence,

$$V_i = -V_o / K_v \tag{4.5}$$

and

$$-(V_o/K_v)(G_s + G_F) - V_oG_F = V_sG_s \tag{4.6}$$

Thus, Equation 4.6 can be used to write the closed-loop system's scalar transfer function (voltage gain):

$$\frac{V_o}{V_s} = \frac{-K_vG_s}{G_s + G_F + K_vG_F} = \frac{-K_vR_F/(R_F + R_s)}{1 + K_vR_s/(R_F + R_s)} = A_v \tag{4.7}$$

In Equation 4.7, we note by comparison to Equation 4.1 that

$$A_L = -K_v[R_s/(R_F + R_s)] \text{ (note system has NFB)} \tag{4.8}$$

$$\alpha = R_F/(R_F + R_s) \tag{4.9}$$

$$\beta = R_s/(R_F + R_s) \tag{4.10}$$

In op amps, K_v is numerically very large, so Equation 4.7 reduces to the well-known gain relation for the ideal op amp inverter: $V_o/V_s = -R_F/R_s$.

There are two common ways to find the output resistance of the simple NFB amplifier of Figure 4.2: One way is to set $V_s = 0$, then place an independent test source, V_t, between the V_o node and ground and calculate $R_{out} = V_t / I_t$. The other method is to measure the open-circuit output voltage using Equation 4.7, then calculate the short-circuit output current (with $V_o = 0$). Clearly, $R_{out} = V_{OC}/I_{oSC}$. Inspection of Figure 4.2 with a shorted output lets one write

$$I_{oSC} = \frac{V_s}{(R_s + R_F)}\left[1 - \frac{K_v R_F}{R_o}\right] \cong \frac{-V_s K_v R_F}{R_o(R_F + R_s)} \tag{4.11}$$

Now R_{out} with NFB can be found:

$$R_{out} = \frac{\dfrac{-K_v R_F/(R_F + R_s)}{1 + K_v R_s/(R_F + R_s)}}{\dfrac{-V_s K_v R_F}{R_o(R_F + R_s)}} = \frac{R_o}{1 + K_v R_s/(R_F + R_s)} = \frac{R_o}{1 + \beta K_v} = \frac{R_o}{1 - A_L} \tag{4.12}$$

In general, the NFB amplifier's output impedance can be written as a vector function of frequency:

$$\mathbf{Z}_{out}(j\omega) = R_o / RD(j\omega) \tag{4.13}$$

We note that in general, $|\mathbf{Z}_{out}(j\omega)|$ is very small (e.g., milliohms) at DC and low frequencies, then gradually increases with ω. This property can be demonstrated by assuming K_v to have a frequency response of the form

$$K_v(j\omega) = \frac{K_{vo}}{j\omega\tau + 1} \tag{4.14}$$

Now from Equation 4.12, we have,

$$Z_o(j\omega) = \frac{R_o}{1 + \beta K_{vo}/(j\omega\tau + 1)} = \frac{R_o(j\omega\tau + 1)}{j\omega\tau + (1 + \beta K_{vo})} = \frac{[R_o/(1 + \beta K_{vo})](j\omega\tau + 1)}{j\omega\tau/(1 + \beta K_{vo}) + 1} \tag{4.15}$$

From Equation 4.15, it is clear that $|\mathbf{Z}_o| \cong R_o/\beta K_{vo}$ at DC and increases with frequency to $|\mathbf{Z}_o| = R_o$ at frequencies above $\beta K_{vo}/\tau$ r/s.

4.3.2 Reduction of Total Harmonic Distortion

A very important property of NFB is the reduction of *total harmonic distortion* (THD) at the output of amplifiers, in particular, power amplifiers. First, it is necessary to examine what we mean by THD. Assume that a certain amplifier has a single-valued, soft saturation, input/output nonlinearity modeled by

$$y = ax + bx^2 + cx^3 + dx^4 + ex^5 + \ldots \tag{4.16}$$

Clearly, $a = K_v$, the linear gain. The real b, c, d, e, … terms can be zero or have either sign. They give rise to the harmonic distortion which can be the result of transistor cut-off or saturation, or power supply saturation. If $x(t) = X_o \sin(\omega_o t)$, the output y(t) will contain the desired fundamental frequency from the a-term, as well as unwanted harmonics. For example,

$$y(t) = aX_o \sin(\omega_o t) + (bX_o^2 / 2)[1 - \cos(2\omega_o t)] + (cX_o^3 / 4)[3\sin(\omega_o t) - \sin(3\omega_o t)] + \ldots \quad (4.17)$$

The power terms approximating the nonlinear transfer characteristic of the amplifier generate in addition to the desired fundamental frequency, DC, fundamental, and harmonics of the order of the nonlinear term. These can be summarized by the expression 4.18 in which we assume the DC term is filtered out:

$$y(t) = K_v X_o \sin(\omega_o t) + H_2 \sin(2\omega_o t) + H_3 \sin(3\omega_o t) + H_4 \sin(1\omega_o t) + \ldots \quad (4.18)$$

The total RMS harmonic distortion is defined as

$$\text{THD} \equiv \sqrt{H_2^2/2 + H_3^2/2 + H_4^2/2 + \ldots} = \sqrt{\sum_{k=2}^{\infty} (H_k^2/2)} = v_d(v_{osl}) \quad (4.19)$$

Note that $H_k^2/2$ is the mean squared value of the kth harmonic; $(K_v^2 X_o^2 / 2)$ is the MS value of the fundamental frequency (desired) component of the output. In general, the larger X_o, the larger will be the THD.

Figure 4.3a illustrates a block diagram showing how the RMS THD generated in the output (power) stage of an amplifier can be added to the output of a NFB amplifier. Distortion is assumed to occur in the last stage. If there were no feedback ($\beta = 0$), $V_o = V_s \alpha K_v + v_d(V_s \alpha K_v)$. V_s is adjusted so the RMS output signal is v_{osl}.

$$V_o = \overset{v_{osl}}{\frac{V_s \alpha\, K_v}{1 + \beta\, K_v}} + \overset{\text{THD}}{\frac{v_d(V_{osl})}{1 + \beta\, K_v}} \quad (4.20)$$

With NFB, the output RMS THD is reduced by a factor of $1/(1 + \beta K_v)$, given that the signal output is the same in both the nonfeedback and the feedback cases. This result has important implications in the design of nearly distortion-free audio power amplifiers, and linear signal conditioning systems in general which use op amps. v_{dk} in Figure 4.3b is simply the kth RMS harmonic voltage; i.e., $v_{dk} = H_k/\sqrt{2}$. In Figure 4.3c, we see how the RMS THD increases as the signal output is made larger. At $v_{os} = V_{CL}$, the level of distortion increases abruptly because the amplifier begins to saturate and clip the output signal waveform.

In good, low-distortion amplifier design the input stages are made linear as possible, and the amplifier is designed so that the output (power) stage saturates before the input and intermediate gain stages do. This allows the THD voltages to effectively be added in the last stage, and thus the RMS THD is reduced by a factor of $1/(1 - \mathbf{A_L}) = 1/\mathbf{RD}$.

4.3.3 Increase of NFB Amplifier Bandwidth at the Cost of Gain

It is axiomatic in the design of electronic circuits that negative feedback allows one to extend closed-loop amplifier bandwidth (BW) at the expense of DC or midband gain. Another way of looking at the effect of NFB on BW is to observe that every amplifier is endowed with some gain*bandwidth product (GBWP); as a figure of merit; larger is better and more expensive. GBWP remains relatively constant as feedback is applied, so when NFB reduces gain, it increases BW. The

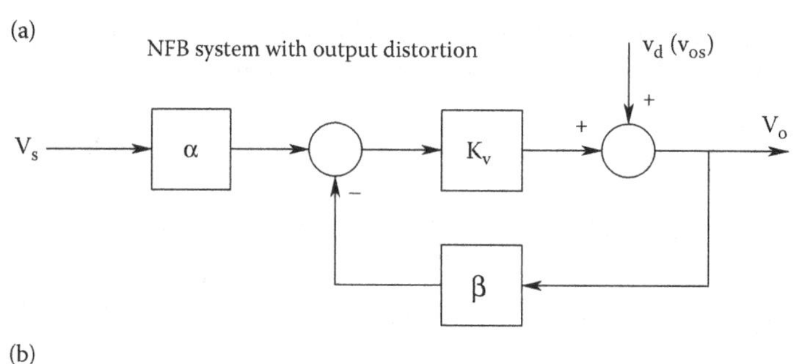

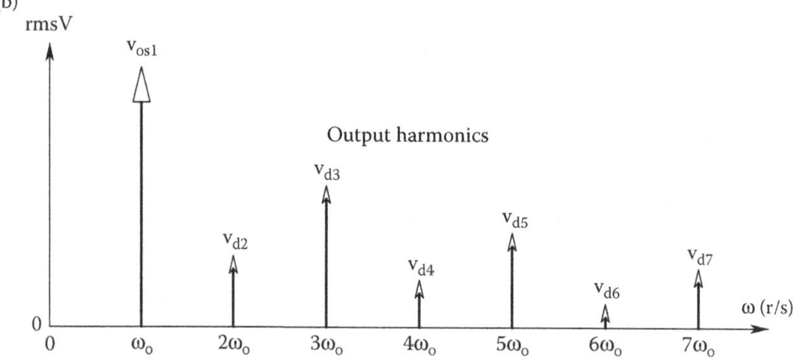

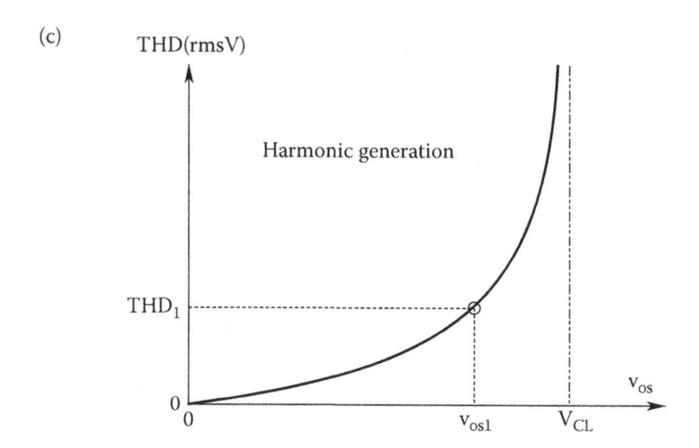

FIGURE 4.3 (a) Block diagram of a SISO negative voltage feedback system with output harmonic distortion voltage introduced in the last (power) stage. A sinusoidal input of frequency ω_o is assumed. (b) RMS power spectrum of the feedback amplifier output. v_{os1} is the RMS amplitude of the fundamental frequency output, the $\{v_{dk}\}$ are the RMS amplitudes of the harmonics caused by distortion. (c) A plot of how total harmonic distortion typically varies as a function of the amplitude of the fundamental output voltage.

frequency-compensated (FC) op amp makes an excellent example of GBWP constancy. The open-loop gain of a FC op amp can be given by

$$\frac{V_o}{V_i - V_i'} = \frac{K_{vo}}{s\tau_a + 1} \tag{4.21}$$

We note that the op amp is a difference amplifier and has a gain*bandwidth product:

$$GBWP_{oa} = K_{vo} / (2\pi\tau_a) \text{ Hz} \tag{4.22}$$

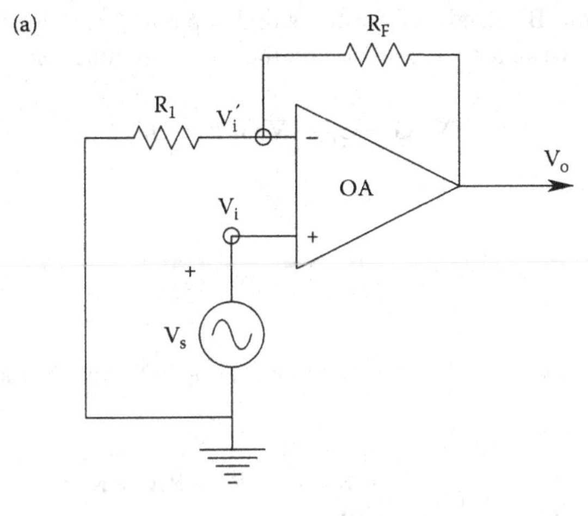

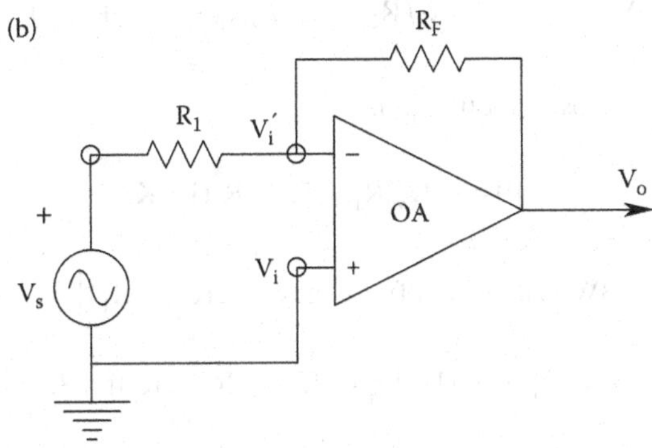

FIGURE 4.4 (a) An op amp connected as a noninverting amplifier. (b) An op amp connected as an inverting amplifier.

Now connect the OA as a simple noninverting amplifier, as shown in Figure 4.4a. The amplifier's output is

$$V_o = (V_s - \beta V_o) K_{vo} / (s\tau_a + 1) \tag{4.23}$$

$$\textit{Where}: \ \beta \equiv R_1 / (R_1 + R_F) \tag{4.24}$$

Solving for the voltage gain, we find

$$\frac{V_o}{V_s} = A_v(s) = \frac{K_{vo} / (1 + \beta K_{vo})}{s\tau_a / (1 + \beta K_{vo}) + 1} \tag{4.25}$$

The GBWP for this closed-loop amplifier is simply

$$GBWP_{amp} = \frac{K_{vo}}{(1 + \beta K_{vo})} \frac{(1 + \beta K_{vo})}{2\pi\tau_a} = GBWP_{oa} \tag{4.26}$$

For the closed-loop feedback amplifier to have *exactly* the same GBWP as the open-loop op amp is a special case. Note that the closed-loop gain is divided by the RD, and the closed-loop BW is multiplied by the RD.

Next, consider the gain, BW, and GBWP of a simple op amp inverter, shown in Figure 4.4b. To address this problem, we write a node equation on the summing junction (V_i') node:

$$V_i'(G_1 + G_F) - V_o G_F = V_s G_1 \tag{4.27}$$

We note that

$$V_o = -V_i' K_{vo}/(s\tau_a + 1) \tag{4.28}$$

Equation 4.28 is solved for V_i', and substituted into Equation 4.27, and the closed-loop transfer function is found:

$$\frac{V_o}{V_s} = A_v(s) = \frac{-K_{vo}R_F / [R_F + R_1(1 + K_v)]}{s\tau_a(R_F + R_1)/[R_F + R_1(1 + K_v)]} \tag{4.29}$$

The low- and midfrequency closed-loop gain is

$$A_v(0) = -K_{vo}R_F / [R_F + R_1(1 + K_v)] \tag{4.30}$$

The closed-loop amplifier's BW is its –3 dB frequency where $|\mathbf{A}_v(f_b)| = |\mathbf{A}_v(0)|/\sqrt{2}$. This is simply

$$f_b = [R_F + R_1(1 + K_v)] / [2\pi\tau_a(R_F + R_1)] \quad \text{Hz} \tag{4.31}$$

Thus, its gain bandwidth product is

$$GBWP_{amp} = \frac{K_{vo}R_F[R_F + R_1(1 + K_{vo})]}{[R_F + R_1(1 + K_{vo})]\,[2\pi t_a(R_F + R_1)]} = \frac{K_{vo}}{2\pi\tau_a}\frac{R_F}{(R_F + R_1)} = GBWP_{oa}\alpha \tag{4.32}$$

where α is the feed-forward attenuation of the op amp's feedback circuit. Thus, the inverting gain op amp circuit with feedback has a GBWP that is lower than the GBWP of the op amp itself. As R_F is increased, so $\mathbf{A}_v(0)$ increases, and $GBWP_{amp} \rightarrow GBWP_{oa}$. *In all cases, the use of NFB extends the high-frequency half-power frequency at the expense of gain.*

4.3.4 Decrease in Gain Sensitivity

Gain sensitivity is the fractional change in closed-loop gain resulting from changes in amplifier circuit component values. In the case of the basic SISO feedback system of Figure 4.3a, the closed-loop gain is

$$\frac{V_o}{V_s} = A_v = \frac{\alpha K_v}{1 + \beta K_v} \tag{4.33}$$

The gain *sensitivity* of A_v with respect to the gain K_v is defined by

$$S_{Kv}^{Av} \equiv \frac{\Delta A_v / A_v}{\Delta K_v / K_v} \tag{4.34}$$

so now,

$$\Delta A_v = \left(\frac{\partial Av}{\partial K_v}\right)\Delta K_v \tag{4.35}$$

and the partial derivative is

$$\frac{\partial A_v}{\partial K_v} = \frac{\alpha[(1+\beta K_v)-\beta K_v]}{(1+\beta K_v)^2} = \frac{\alpha K_v}{(1+\beta K_v)}\frac{K_v^{-1}}{RD} \tag{4.36}$$

Thus,

$$\Delta A_v = \frac{A_v \Delta K_v}{K_v[RD]} \tag{4.37}$$

And, the gain sensitivity is

$$S_{Kv}^{Av} \equiv \frac{\Delta A_v / A_v}{\Delta K_v / K_v} = \frac{A_v \Delta K_v / A_v}{K_v[RD]\Delta K_v / K_v} = \frac{1}{[RD]} \tag{4.38}$$

In op amps, 1/[RD] is on the order of 10^{-4} to 10^{-7}, so a circuit with NFB is generally quite insensitive to variations in its DC, open-loop gain, K_{vo}.

It is also of interest to see how sensitivity varies as a function of frequency in NFB circuits. Note that complex algebra must be used in the calculation of such sensitivities, because the closed-loop gain (frequency response) is complex. Here, one can express the closed-loop gain in polar form for convenience:

$$A_v(j\omega) = |A_v(j\omega)|\, e^{j\theta(\omega)} \tag{4.39}$$

The amplifier's parameter sensitivity can also be written as

$$S_p^{Av} = \frac{dA_v / A_v}{dp/p} = \frac{d(\ln A_v)}{d(\ln p)} \tag{4.40}$$

where p is a parameter in the NFB circuit. From Equation 4.39 we can write

$$\ln[A_v(j\omega)] = \ln|\mathbf{A}_v(j\omega)| + j\theta(\omega) \tag{4.41}$$

Substitution of Equation 4.41 into Equation 4.40 yields

$$S_p^{Av} = \frac{d(\ln|\mathbf{A}_v(j\omega)|)}{dp/p} + j\frac{d\theta(\omega)}{dp/p} \tag{4.42}$$

The *real part* of S_p^{Av} is called the parameter *magnitude sensitivity*; the *imaginary part* of S_p^{Av} is the parameter *phase sensitivity*. Generally, p will be a real number, which simplifies the calculation of Equation 4.42. Sensitivity analysis using Equation 4.42 can be utilized to evaluate active filter designs.

4.4 EFFECTS OF NEGATIVE CURRENT FEEDBACK

The purpose of negative current feedback (NCF) is to create an approximation to a voltage-controlled current source (VCCS) so that the output current, I_L, is proportional to V_s, regardless of the load, which can be nonlinear.

In NCF amplifiers, the signal which is fed back is proportional to the current through the load, I_L. NCF, like NVF, extends the bandwidth of the amplifier within the feedback loop. Unlike NVF, NCF raises the output resistance of the amplifier within the loop. The properties of a single op amp circuit with NCF, illustrated in Figure 4.5, will be investigated; frequency dependence will not be treated in this example. A VCCS is characterized by a transconductance, G_M, and a Norton shunt conductance, G_o.

First, it is necessary to find an expression for the circuit's $G_M \equiv I_L/V_s$. Note that the current is given by Ohm's law:

$$I_L = \frac{V_i' K_{vo}}{R_o + R_L + R_c} \tag{4.43}$$

The summing junction node voltage is found:

$$V_i'[G_1 + G_F] - (-I_L R_c G_F) = G_1 V_s \tag{4.44}$$

$$\downarrow$$

$$V_i' = \frac{G_1 V_s - I_L R_c G_F}{G_1 + G_F} \tag{4.45}$$

Substituting Equation 4.45 into Equation 4.43, one can solve for G_M:

$$\frac{I_L}{V_s} = G_M = \frac{K_{vo} G_1}{(R_o + R_L + R_c)(G_1 + G_F) + K_{vo} R_c G_F} \tag{4.46}$$

Now in general, $K_{vo} R_c G_F >> (R_o + R_L + R_c)(G_1 + G_F)$, so

$$G_M \cong R_F / R_c R_1 \quad \text{Siemens} \tag{4.47}$$

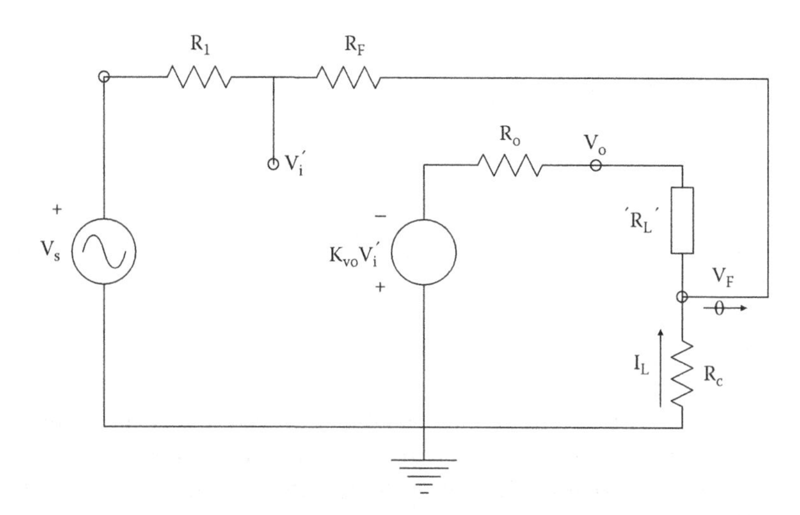

FIGURE 4.5 Schematic of a simple Thevenin VCVS with negative current feedback (NCFB).

The next step is to address how NCF affects the VCCS's *Norton output conductance*. First, one calculates the circuit's OCV, given $R_L \to \infty$. This condition also makes $I_L = V_F = 0$. Now the summing junction voltage is

$$V_i' = V_s \frac{R_F}{R_F + R_1} \tag{4.48}$$

And the OCV is

$$OCV = V_s \frac{R_F}{R_F + R_1} K_{vo} \quad \text{Volts} \tag{4.49}$$

Next, find the short-circuit current (SCC); i.e., the I_{Lsc} when $R_L = 0$. This condition also makes $V_F = V_o$.

The SCC is

$$I_{Lsc} = \frac{V_i' K_{vo}}{R_o + R_c} \tag{4.50}$$

here V_i' is found from

$$V_i'[G_1 + G_F] - (-I_{Lsc} R_c) G_F = V_s G_1 \tag{4.51}$$

$$\downarrow \quad V_i' = \frac{V_s G_1 - I_{Lsc} G_F}{G_1 + G_F} \tag{4.52}$$

Equation 4.52 is substituted into Equation 4.50 and I_{Lsc} is found:

$$I_{Lsc} = \frac{V_s G_1 K_{vo}}{(R_o + R_c)(G_1 + G_F) + K_{vo} R_c G_F} \tag{4.53}$$

Now the Norton G_{out} of the amplifier with NCF is simply the ratio of I_{Lsc} to the OCV:

$$G_{out} = \frac{\dfrac{V_s G_1 K_{vo}}{(R_o + R_c)(G_1 + G_F) + K_{vo} R_c G_F}}{\dfrac{V_s R_F K_{vo}}{(R_F + R_1)}} = \frac{G_o}{(1 + R_c G_o) + K_{vo} G_o R_c R_1 / (R_F + R_1)} \quad \text{Siemens} \tag{4.54}$$

It is seen that the second term in the denominator of Equation 4.54 makes $G_{out} \ll G_o$, which is desirable in making an effective VCCS.

In order to see how the closed-loop, VCCS's frequency response is affected by NCF, we only need to replace the op amp's open-circuit, VCVS with $K_{vo}/(j\omega\tau_a + 1)$. The transconductance is now found to be

$$G_M(j\omega) = \frac{\dfrac{K_{vo} R_F}{(R_1 + R_F)(R_o + R_c + R_L) + K_{vo} R_c R_1}}{j\omega \dfrac{\tau_a}{\left\{ \dfrac{K_{vo} R_c R_1}{(R_1 + R_F)(R_o + R_c + R_L)} + 1 \right\}} + 1} \cong \frac{R_F / (R_1 R_c)}{j\omega \dfrac{\tau_a (R_1 + R_F)(R_o + R_c + R_L)}{K_{vo} R_c R_1} + 1} \tag{4.55}$$

Now the approximate $\mathbf{G_M}(0) \cong R_F/(R_1 R_c)$, and the –3 dB frequency is given by

$$f_b \cong \frac{K_{vo} R_c R_1}{2\,\pi\,\tau_a (R_1 + R_F)(R_o + R_c + R_L)} \text{ Hz} \tag{4.56}$$

In the relations 4.55 and 4.56, it was assumed that $K_{vo}R_cR_1 >> (R_1 + R_F)(R_o + R_c + R_L)$. Note that the closed-loop system's bandwidth is extended by the NCF. The NVF circuit of Figure 4.5 is simple, but suffers the disadvantage of having the R_L "floating" between V_o and R_c. Also, the peak current is limited by the op amp used.

In Section 2.6.7 on laser diodes, it was determined that an effective VCCS using NCF can be made from three op amps. The op amp that drives R_L can be made a power op amp, and the load can be grounded. Figure 4.6 illustrates this NCF circuit. As in the example above, the VCCS's $\mathbf{G_M}(j\omega)$ and $\mathbf{Z_{out}}(j\omega)$ will be found. Because the two feedback amplifiers are unity gain, they have –3 dB frequencies approaching their op amp's f_T, and thus can be treated as pure gains (+1 and –1, respectively). The node equation for the summing junction is written as

$$V_i'[3G] - V_oG - (-V_L)G = V_sG \tag{4.57}$$

Two auxiliary equations are used:

$$V_o = -I_L(R_F + \text{“}R_L\text{”}) \tag{4.58}$$

$$V_i' = \frac{V_o(j\omega\tau_a + 1)}{K_{vo}} \tag{4.59}$$

When Equations 4.58 and 4.59 are substituted in Equation 4.57, and terms are rearranged, we obtain

$$\frac{I_L}{V_s} = G_M(j\omega) = \frac{\dfrac{K_{vo}}{3(R_F + R_L) + K_{vo}R_F}}{j\omega\dfrac{\tau_a 3(R_F + R_L)}{3(R_F + R_L) + K_{vo}R_F} + 1} \tag{4.60}$$

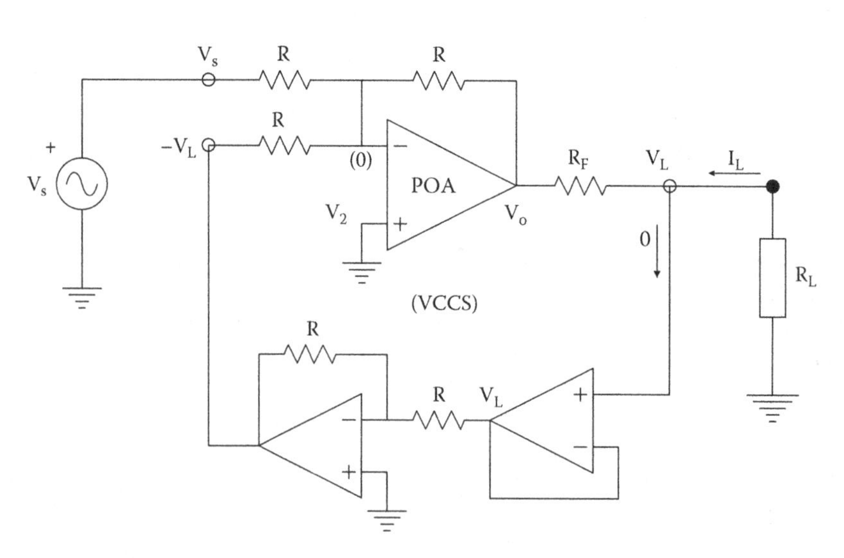

FIGURE 4.6 A three-op amp VCCS in which the load is grounded. POA = power op amp. Analysis is in the Text.

In practical cases, $K_{vo} R_F >> 3(R_F + R_L)$, so it is possible to approximate the VCCS's transconductance by

$$\mathbf{G_M}(j\omega) \cong \frac{G_F}{j\omega\tau_a 3(R_F + R_L)/(K_{vo}R_F) + 1} \tag{4.61}$$

So, it is clear that $\mathbf{G_M}(0) \cong G_F$, and the break frequency is

$$f_b = \frac{K_{vo}R_F}{2\pi\tau_a 3(R_F + R_L)} \tag{4.62}$$

which is certainly greater than the op amp's f_T.

The VCCS's $\mathbf{Z_{out}}(j\omega)$ is now of interest. Ideally, it should approach infinity. To find it, one will take the ratio of the circuit's OCV to SCC. Under OCV conditions, $I_L = 0$ and $V_L = V_o$. Using the node equation for V_i', it is easy to write

$$OCV = \frac{-V_s K_{vo}}{3(j\omega\tau_a + 1)} \tag{4.63}$$

Next we find the VCCS's SCC. Under SCC conditions, $R_L = 0$ and $V_L = 0$. The node equation for V_i' yields

$$\mathbf{Z_{out}}(j\omega) = \frac{R_F(K_{vo} + 3)[j\omega 3\tau_a/(K_{vo} + 3) + 1]}{3\ (j\omega\tau_a + 1)} \cong \frac{R_F K_{vo}[j\omega 3\tau_a/K_{vo} + 1]}{3(j\omega\tau_a + 1)} \tag{4.64}$$

From Equation 4.64, it can be seen that at low frequencies, $\mathbf{Z_{out}}(0) = R_F K_{vo}/3$. At frequencies above $K_{vo}/3\tau_a$ r/s, $Z_{out}(hi) \cong R_F$, which is not very high, making a poor VCCS at high frequencies.

4.5 POSITIVE VOLTAGE FEEDBACK

4.5.1 Introduction

Positive voltage feedback (PVF) is seldom used in SISO feedback amplifiers. PVF *increases* the closed-loop gain, *decreases* the closed-loop bandwidth, *increases* the R_{out} of the system, and *increases* harmonic distortion at a given output level. These actions are based on the simple fact that the loop gain in a simple SISO feedback amplifier with PVF is $A_L = +\beta K_v$, so that for $+\beta K_v >> 1$, the return difference $(1 - \mathbf{A_L})$ is < 1. PVF can be used to deliberately make a feedback system unstable so that it oscillates.

The following section illustrates the exceptional use of PVF to increase the bandwidth of an amplifier used to couple intracellular glass micropipette electrodes used in neurophysiology to further signal conditioning stages.

4.5.2 Amplifier with Capacitance Neutralization

Glass micropipette electrodes (GMEs) are used to penetrate cell membranes, allowing the measurement of the DC resting potential across the membrane and, in the case of nerve and muscle cells, the transient action potentials associated with these cells. GMEs are made by heating and pulling small-diameter, borosilicate class capillary tubing to a small diameter tip, which can range from 0.25 to 1 μm ID. The GMEs are then artfully filled with a conductive electrolyte solution such as 3M KCl, or potassium citrate, etc. A Ag|AgCl fine wire electrode is inserted in the outer (large) end of the filled GME to make conductive contact with the filling electrolyte. Using a micromanipulator, the GME tip is caused to penetrate the membrane of a cell under investigation. The cell membrane generally forms a tight seal around the fine tip of the GME after penetration.

A standalone GME with its tip immersed in a beaker of normal saline, in which a large Ag|AgCl reference electrode is also located, allows one to measure the impedance of the filled GME. At DC and very low frequencies, the resistance of the GME can be on the order of 10 to 500 MΩ, depending on the GME's tip geometry and the filling electrolyte. There is also distributed stray capacitance between the tip lumen and the external electrolyte, the glass serving as the dielectric. Thus, the immersed tip appears as a short section of nonuniform, RC transmission line giving distributed-parameter, low-pass filtering to any time-varying potential seen at the tip (Webster 1992, Chapter 5, La Valeé et al. 1969).

Rather than deal with the complexity of a transmission-line low-pass filter, and include the AC characteristics of the AgCl coupling and reference electrodes, we shall oversimplify the GME *in situ* by a simple R-C low-pass filter; R_μ is the GME's total DC resistance, and C_μ represents the total *effective* shunting capacitance of the GME's tip. Figure 4.7 shows the GME attached to the PVF amplifier. The amplifier uses an electrometer op amp that has a DC input bias current on the order of 10s of femptoamps. It is thus characterized by an input resistance on the order of 10^{13} Ω, and an input capacitance to ground, C_{in}, on the order of a single pF. The PVF is applied through a variable "neutralizing" capacitor, C_N. The noninverting gain of the amplifier, A_{vo}, is on the order 2 to 5, and is set by resistors R_F and R_1. To begin the analysis of this PVF amplifier, we consider the gain between the non-inverting node and the output, V_o/V_i. This gain is found by writing the node equation for the V_i' node:

$$V_i'[G_F + G_1] - V_o G_F = 0 \tag{4.65}$$

and

$$V_o = (V_i - V_i')\frac{K_{vo}}{j\omega\tau_a + 1} \tag{4.66}$$

Substituting Equation 4.66 into Equation 4.65, and assuming $R_1K_{vo}/(R_1 + R_F) >> 1$, one can find the frequency response function:

$$\frac{V_o}{V_i} = \frac{(1 + R_F / R_1)}{j\omega\tau_a(1 + R_F / R_1) / K_{vo} + 1} \tag{4.67}$$

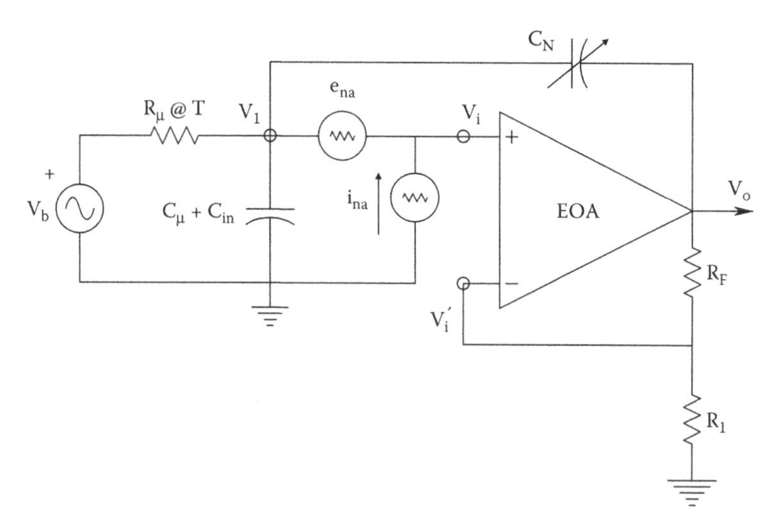

FIGURE 4.7 Schematic of a noninverting electrometer op amp (EOA) with positive voltage feedback through a small neutralizing capacitor, C_N. This circuit is used with glass micropipette microelectrodes to increase system bandwidth at the expense of noise.

We next examine the simple low-pass frequency response function of the GME alone:

$$\frac{V_i}{V_b} = \frac{1}{j\omega R_\mu (C_\mu + C_{in}) + 1} \tag{4.68}$$

To find the frequency response of the amplifier with PVF through C_N, one writes the node equation for V_i:

$$V_i[G_\mu + j\omega(C_T + C_N)] - V_o j\omega C_N = V_b G_\mu \tag{4.69}$$

Note that

$$C_T = C_\mu + C_{in} \tag{4.70}$$

and

$$\frac{V_o}{V_i} = \frac{A_{vo}}{j\omega\tau_a A_{vo} / K_{vo} + 1} \tag{4.71}$$

where $A_{vo} \equiv (1 + R_F/R_1)$.

Substituting from the equations above, the node equation can be written as

$$V_o \frac{(j\omega\tau_a A_{vo} / K_{vo} + 1)}{A_{vo}} [G_\mu + j\omega(C_T + C_N)] - V_o j\omega C_N = V_b G_\mu \tag{4.72}$$

Equation 4.72 can be wrestled algebraically into the transfer function of the capacitance-neutralized, GME amplifier:

$$\frac{V_o}{V_b} = \frac{A_{vo}}{(j\omega)^2 \tau_a A_{vo}(C_T + C_N)R_\mu / K_{vo} + j\omega\,[\tau_a A_{vo} / K_{vo} + R_\mu C_T - R_\mu C_N (A_{vo} - 1)] + 1} \tag{4.73}$$

From the standard quadratic form, the closed-loop amplifier's undamped natural frequency squared is

$$\omega_n^2 = \frac{K_{vo}}{\tau_o A_{vo}(C_T + C_N)R_\mu} \quad (\text{r/s})^2 \tag{4.74}$$

The amplifier's damping factor is found from the second term in the denominator of Equation 4.73:

$$\xi = (\omega_n / 2)[\tau_a A_{vo} / K_{vo} + R_\mu C_T - R_\mu C_N (A_{vo} - 1)] \tag{4.75}$$

It is now useful to illustrate how the capacitance-neutralized, PVF amplifier works with typical numbers. Let: $K_{vo} = 10^5$, $\tau_a = 10^{-2}$ sec, $A_{vo} = 2$, $R_\mu = 10^8\ \Omega$, $C_T = 3.05$ pF, $C_N = 2.95$ pF. From these numbers, one finds that $\omega_n = 9.129 \times 10^4$ r/s, and $\xi = 0.464$ (an underdamped, second-order system with good transient response). Note that if $C_N = C_T$, the system is highly underdamped, and if C_N is slightly greater than C_T, the amplifier's closed-loop poles lie in the right-half s-plane, making the amplifier oscillate! The price paid for extending the system's bandwidth can be shown to be excess noise (see Section 9.8.4).

4.6 CHAPTER SUMMARY

Most electronic amplifiers use negative voltage feedback (NVF), which has the effects listed below. *NVF:*

1. Reduces midband gain
2. Reduces total harmonic distortion at the output at a given signal output power level
3. Reduces Z_{out} at low and midfrequencies
4. Decreases gain sensitivity to certain circuit parameters
5. Decreases the output signal-to-noise ratio slightly
6. Increases the closed-loop amplifier's bandwidth
7. Can either increase or decrease R_{in}, depending on the circuit
8. Can make a system unstable if incorrectly applied.

Negative current feedback (NCF) was shown to be useful in making a VCCS out of an amplifier with normally low R_{out}. NCF is used to raise the Thevenin R_{out} so that the NCF amplifier appears to be a current source. Otherwise, its properties are similar to those resulting from NVF. Positive voltage feedback (PVF) reverses properties 1–4 and 6 in the list above for NVF. PVF does have use in capacitance neutralization, and it is used in the design of certain oscillators because it can make systems unstable more easily than NVF.

CHAPTER 4 HOME PROBLEMS

4.1 Negative current feedback is used in a VCCS circuit used to power a laser diode (LAD), as shown in Figure P4.1. The LAD presents a nonlinear load to the VCCS. We wish the diode current to be independent of the LAD's nonlinear resistance.

(A) Assume the op amp is ideal, and the differential amplifier (DA) is a VCVS in which $V_2 = K_D(V_o - V_L)$. Derive an expression for the VCVS's transconductance, $G_M = I_L/V_s$.

(B) Now assume that the power op amp is non-ideal, so $V_o = K_{vo}(V_i - V_i')$. Derive an expression for the Norton output conductance seen by the LAD. (*Hint:* Set $V_s = 0$ and replace the LAD by a test voltage source, v_T. Find $G_{out} = i_T/v_T$.)

4.2 Negative voltage feedback is used to make an electronically-regulated, DC voltage source, shown in Figure P4.2. The design output voltage is 15 V at 1 A. load. The power *npn* BJT can be modeled by a mid-frequency h-parameter model with: $h_{fe} = 19$, $h_{oe} = 2 \times 10^{-5}$ S, $h_{re} = 0$, $h_{ie} = V_T/I_{BQ}$, $V_T = 0.026$ V, $I_{EQ} = 1$ A, DA gain is $K_D = 1 \times 10^4$, $R_L = 15\ \Omega$, neglect current through $R_F + R_1$, $V_R = 6.2$ V, feedback attenuation $\beta = R_1/(R_1 + R_2) = 6.2/15$. The raw DC has a ripple voltage, v_r, added to it. $R_S = 50\ \Omega$.

(A) Find an algebraic expression for and evaluate numerically the regulator's ripple gain, $A_R = v_o/v_r$. Use the MFSSM for the BJT (e.g., DC sources → ground).

(B) Now let $v_r = h_{oe} = 0$. Find an expression for and evaluate numerically the regulator's output resistance, R_{out}, seen by R_L. You can find $R_{out} = v_t/i_t$ by replacing R_L with a small-signal test voltage source, v_t.

(C) Evaluate the regulator's *regulation,* $\rho = \Delta V_o/\Delta R_L$.

4.3 An op amp is ideal except for a finite differential voltage gain: $v_o = K_{vo}(v_i - v_i')$. In the circuit of Figure P4.3, the op amp is connected to make a VCCS for R_L.

(A) What kind of feedback is used? NVFB, PVFB, NCFB, or PCFB?

(B) Give an expression for $G_M = I_L/V_s$. Show what happens to G_M as $K_{vo} \to \infty$.

(C) Find an expression for the Thevenin R_{out} that R_L 'sees'.

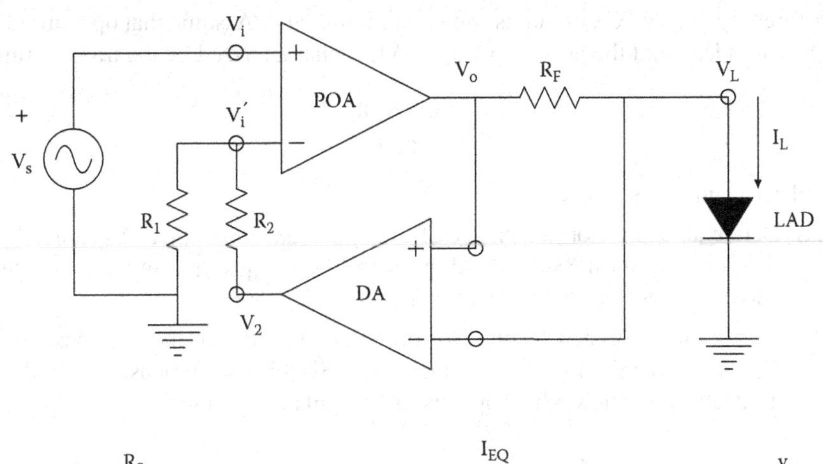

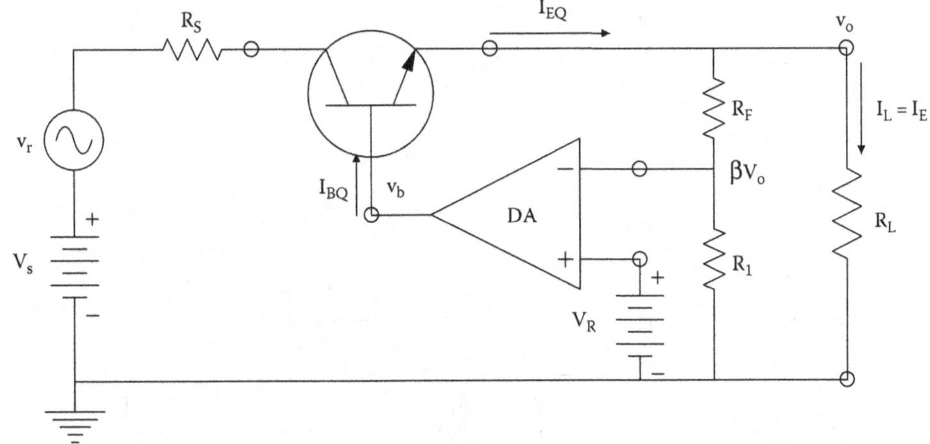

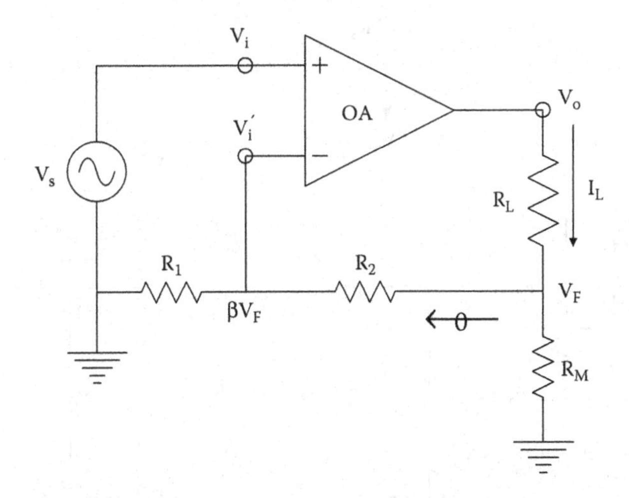

4.4 Figure P4.4 illustrates a source-follower/grounded gate JFET amplifier with feedback. Both JFETs are identical with the same MFSSM in which $g_m > 0$ and $g_d = 0$. The feedback voltage, $V_o = -K_D V_2$, is applied through resistor R_F to the common source node.

(A) Derive an expression for $A_v = V_2/V_1$ with no feedback (set $R_F = \infty$).

(B) Find an expression for $A_v = V_o/V_1$ with feedback. Let $K_D \rightarrow \infty$; give A_v.

4.5 A three-op amp VCCS circuit is shown in Figure P4.5. Assume that op amps OA2 and OA3 are ideal, and the power op amp, OA1, is characterized by the transfer function:

$$V_o = \frac{(V_1 - V_1')K_{vo}}{(\tau s + 1)}$$

and zero output resistance.

(A) Derive an expression for the VCCS's *output transadmittance*, $\mathbf{Y_M}(j\omega) = \mathbf{I_L}/\mathbf{V_s}$, in time-constant form. Sketch and dimension $20 \log|\mathbf{Y_M}(j\omega)|$ vs ω and $\angle\, Y_M(j\omega)$ vs ω (Bode plot). Show what happens to $\mathbf{Y_M}(j\omega)$ as $K_{vo} \to \infty$.

(B) Derive an expression for the Norton output admittance the nonlinear load sees, $\mathbf{Y_{out}}(j\omega) = \mathbf{I_L}/\mathbf{V_L}$, in time-constant form. Sketch and dimension a Bode plot of $\mathbf{Y_{out}}(j\omega)$ vs ω. Show what happens to $\mathbf{Y_{out}}(j\omega)$ as $K_{vo} \to \infty$.

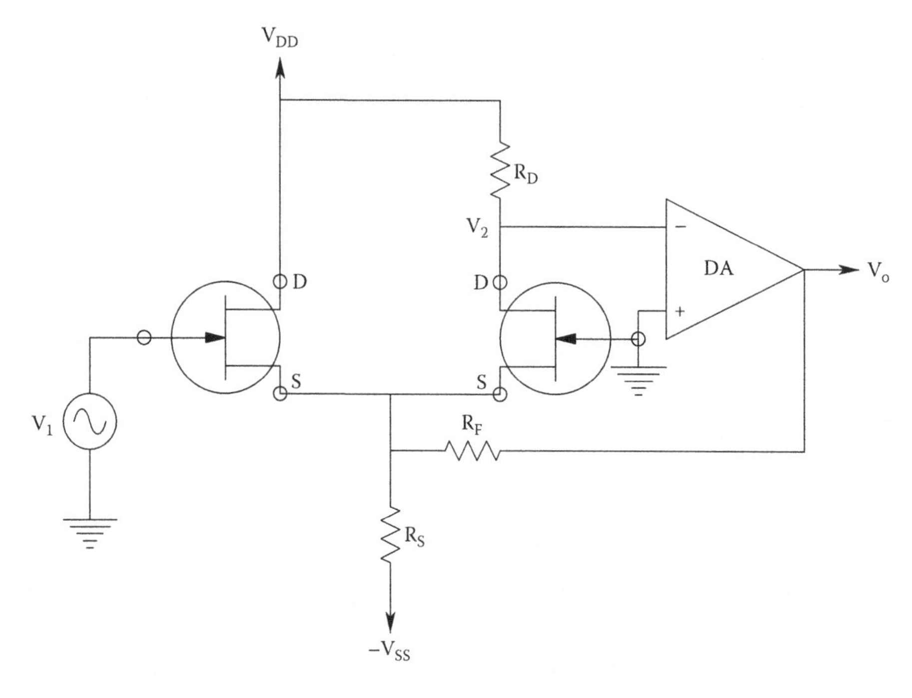

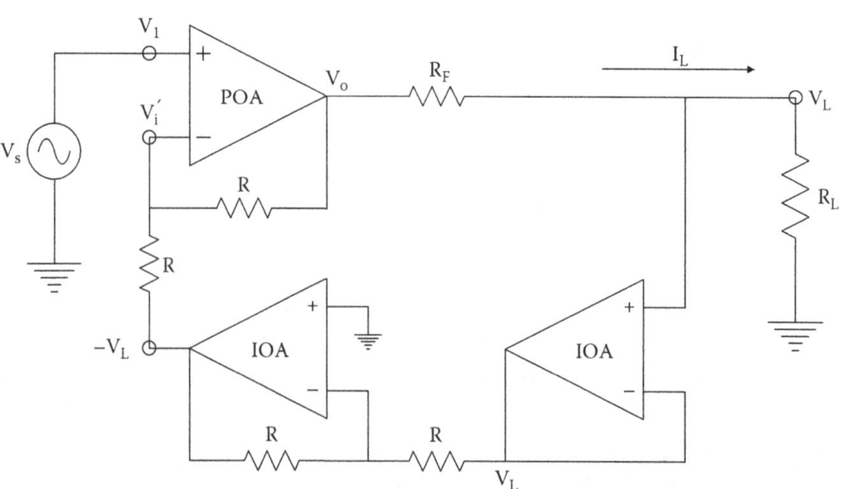

4.6 A DA is given a form of *common-mode negative feedback* (CMNF), as shown in Figure P4.6. The DA has a differential output from which v_{oc} is derived by a voltage divider. The amplifier is described by the scalar equations:

$v_o = A_D v_{1c} + A_C v_{1c}$ $v_o' = -A_D v_{1c} + A_C v_{1c}$ Also, it is clear that $v_{oc} = A_C v_{1c}$. Define $\alpha = R_1/(R_1 + R_s)$ and $\beta = R_s/(R_1 + R_s)$.

(A) Find expressions for v_{1c} and v_{1d} in terms of v_{sc} and v_{sd}, and α, β, K, A_D, and A_C.

(B) Give an expression for v_o in terms of v_{sc} and v_{sd} and circuit parameters.

(C) Find an expression for the system's single-ended CMRR.

(D) Let $A_D = 100$, $A_C = 0.01$, $\alpha \cong 1$, $\beta = 0.01$, and $K = 10^4$. Evaluate the single-ended CMRR numerically, and compare it to the CMRR of the DA.

4.7 The op amp circuit shown in Figure P4.7 is a form of *current mirror.* The BJT can be modeled by its MFSSM with $h_{re} = h_{oe} = 0$. The op amp is ideal except for the gain:

$$v_o = \frac{K_v(v_i - v_i')}{(\tau s + 1)}$$

Find an expression for $I_2/I_1(jw)$ in time constant form.

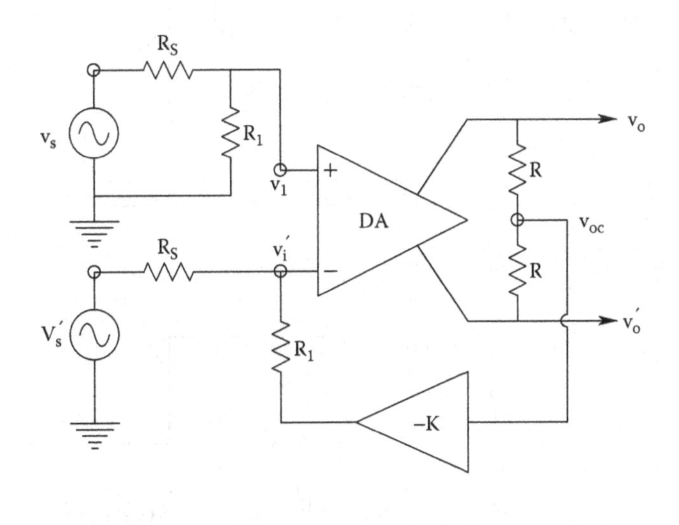

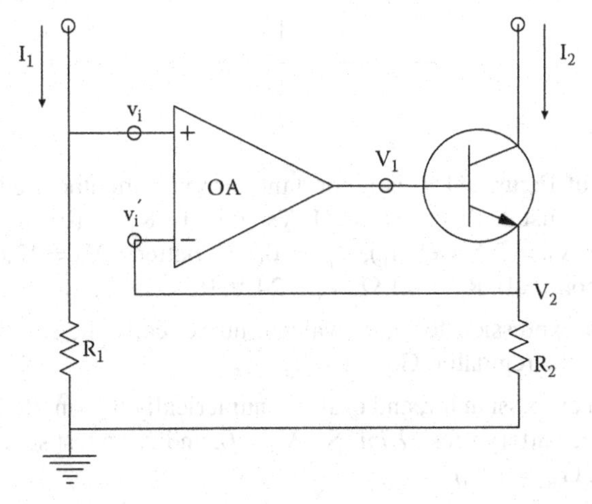

4.8 Negative current feedback is used to make an op amp/FET VCCS, shown in Figure P4.8. MFSS analysis will be used. The FET is characterized by (g_m, g_d), and the op amp has a finite voltage gain so $v_g = K_V (v_1 - v_s)$. Assume V_{DS} is large enough to keep the FET in channel saturation.

(A) Find an expression for the VCCS's small-signal transconductance, $G_M = i_d/v_1$.

(B) Find an expression for the VCCS's Norton output conductance, G_{out}.

(C) Let $K_v = 10^4$, $g_m = 10^{-3}$ S, $g_d = 10^{-5}$ S, and $R_S = 1$ kΩ. Find numerical values for G_M and G_{out}.

4.9 A certain power op amp (POA) has an open-loop gain of $V_o/V_i' = -5 \times 10^4$. When it is connected as a gain of −250 amplifier, it has a total harmonic distortion (THD) of 0.5% of the RMS fundamental output signal voltage, V_{os}, when the rms $V_{os} = 10.0$ V. *Find* the % THD when the amplifier is given a gain of −1 (unit inverter) and the V_{os} is again made 10.0 VRMS. See Figure P4.9.

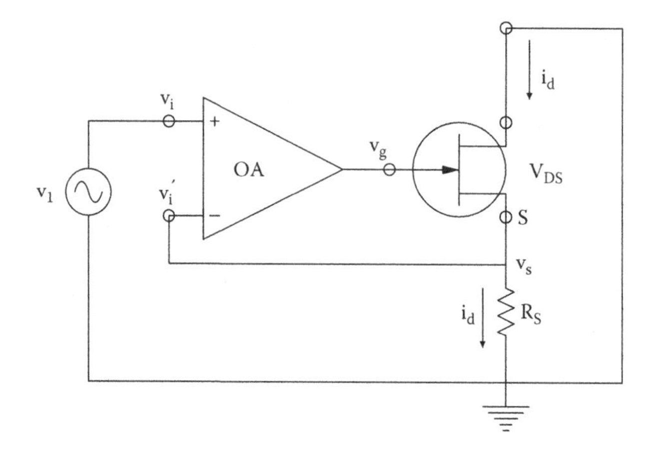

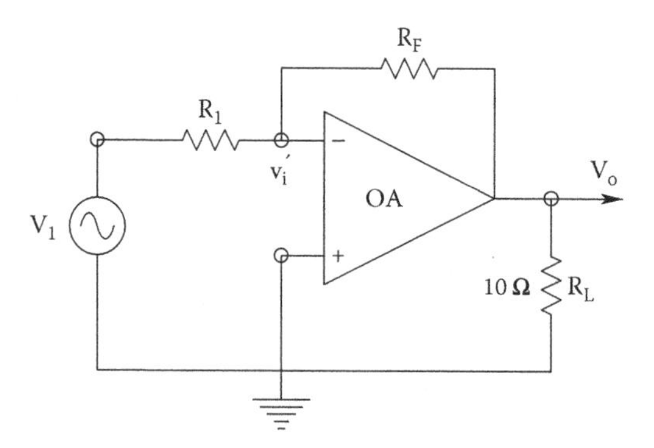

4.10 The circuit of Figure P4.10 is a constant-current regulator used for charging batteries. NCFB is used. *Assume:* the DA's gain is $K_D = 10^5$, $h_{oe} = h_{re} = 0$, $h_{fe} = 19$, $R_m = 1.0$ Ω, $V_R = 5$ V (sets I_L), $V_{BE} = 0.7$ V, Battery: $V_B = 12.6$ V (nominal), series resistance (nominal), $R_B = 0.1$ Ω, $V_S = 24$ V, $R_S = 13$ Ω.

(A) Find an expression for, and evaluate numerically the small-signal transconductance of the regulator, $G_M = I_L/V_R$.

(B) Find an expression for, and evaluate numerically the small-signal Norton conductance the battery sees. (*Hint:* Set $V_R = 0$, and use a test source, v_t, in place of the battery. $G_{out} = i_t/v_t$).

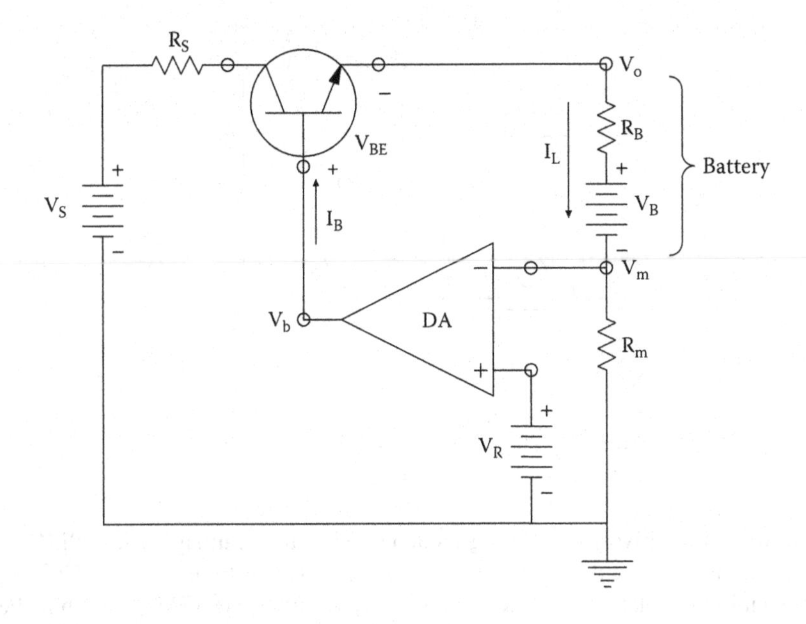

4.11 We have shown that NVFB reduces amplifier output impedance. In this problem, you will investigate how NVFB affects input impedance. In the schematic of Fig. P4.11 below, an amplifier is given negative feedback as shown. *Find* the input resistance with feedback, $R_{in} = V_s/I_s$.

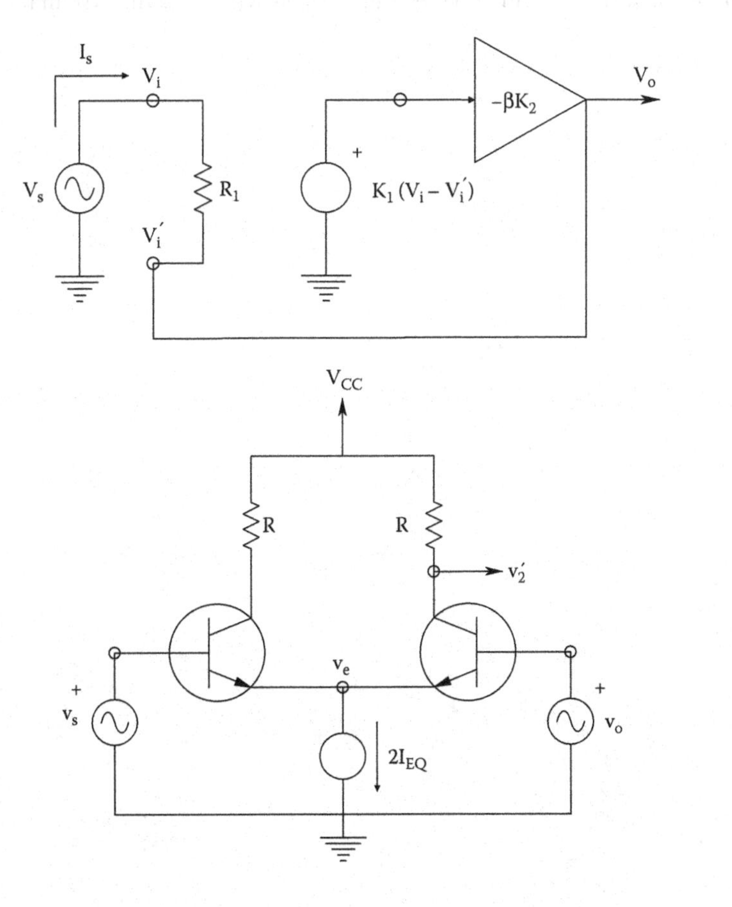

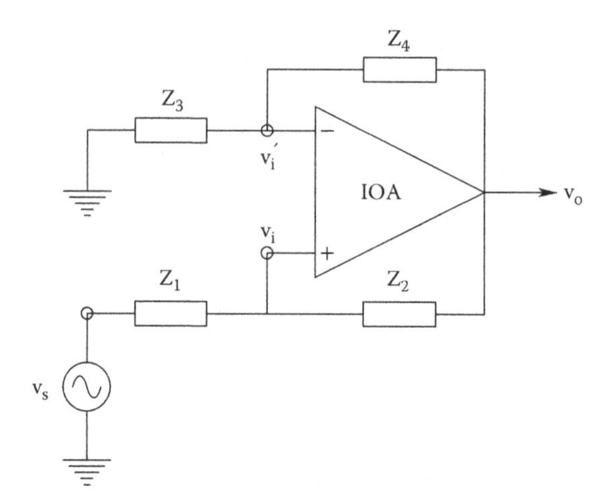

4.12 One way of additively combining feedback with the input signal in a SISO feedback amplifier is to use a difference amplifier, illustrated in Figure P4.12. The output, v_2', is given by the relation: $v_2' = K_F(v_s - v_o)$. Use a simple MFSSM for the matched BJTs in which $h_{re} = h_{oe} = 0$, and h_{fe} and $h_{ie} > 0$. A dc current source supplies the emitter currents of the two BJTs. *Derive* an expression for K_F in terms of circuit parameters.

4.13 Both positive and negative feedback are used on an ideal op amp, shown in Figure P4.13.

(A) Derive an expression for V_o/V_s in terms of the circuit parameters.

(B) What vector condition on the impedances will make the system unstable?

5 Feedback, Frequency Response, and Amplifier Stability

5.1 INTRODUCTION

This chapter describes the details of how feedback changes an open-loop amplifier's frequency response and examines how negative voltage feedback (NVF) and positive voltage feedback (PVF) can lead to amplifier instability. Practical use can be made of instability; we can design tunable sinusoidal oscillators using the same analytical techniques used in the design of linear feedback amplifiers.

Over the years, there have been many analytical techniques used to analyze and design feedback systems. In the author's opinion, the *root locus technique* is one of the more useful techniques. It allows the s-plane location of the closed-loop (CL) system's poles to be found, given the system's DC- or midfrequency loop gain, and the location of the poles and zeros of the system's loop gain, $A_L(s)$. Once one knows the closed-loop poles and zeros, it is simple to find the CL system's frequency response, or its output in time, given a transient input.

5.2 REVIEW OF AMPLIFIER FREQUENCY RESPONSE

5.2.1 INTRODUCTION

The steady-state, sinusoidal frequency response has long been a performance criterion for linear signal conditioning systems. For example, an amplifier is given a continuous sinusoidal input of known frequency and amplitude, which does not saturate the amplifier. At the output, one measures a sinusoidal output of the same frequency, but which, in general, will have a different amplitude from the input, and a phase shifted from the input sinusoid. Both the amplitude and phase shift of the output are frequency dependent. The frequency response measured experimentally can be used to define the *frequency response function* of the amplifier. This is the 2-D vector gain, $\mathbf{H}(j\omega)$. In polar form

$$\mathbf{H}(j\omega) \equiv \frac{|\mathbf{V}_o|}{|\mathbf{V}_s|}(\omega)\angle\theta(\omega) \tag{5.1}$$

The frequency-dependent ratio of output voltage to input voltage magnitudes is called the *amplitude response* (AR), and $\theta(\omega)$ is the phase angle between the output and the input sine waves. The frequency response function, $\mathbf{H}(j\omega)$, whether measured or calculated, is in general a 2-D vector [it has a magnitude and an angle as shown in Equation 5.1, or equivalently, real and imaginary parts, $\mathbf{H}(j\omega) = h_r(\omega) + jh_i(\omega)$].

There are two major ways of presenting frequency response data: (1) by a *Bode plot* and (2) by a *polar (Nyquist) plot*. Bode plots are much more widely used to characterize analog electronic signal conditioning systems used in biomedicine and will be considered here. Both Bode and Nyquist plots are considered in detail in Section 2.4.6 of Northrop (2010).

5.2.2 Bode Plots

A Bode plot is a system's frequency response plot done on *log-linear graph paper.* The (horizontal) frequency axis has a logarithmic scale; $20\log_{10}|\mathbf{H}(f)|$ is plotted on the linear vertical axis, which has the units of decibels (dB), and the phase angle of **H**(f), (θ(f)), which is the phase angle between the output and input sinusoids ($f = \omega/2\pi$). One advantage of plotting $20\log_{10}|H(f)|$ vs f on semilog paper is that plots are made easier by the use of asymptotes giving the frequency-response behavior relative to the system's break frequencies or natural frequencies. Also by using a logarithmic function, products of terms appear graphically as sums. Perhaps the best way to introduce the art of Bode plotting is by example.

Example 1

A simple low-pass system: Let us assume a system is described by the first-order frequency response function:

$$\frac{\mathbf{Y}}{\mathbf{U}}(j\omega) = \frac{C}{j\omega(a) + b} = \mathbf{H}(j\omega) \tag{5.2}$$

It is algebraically more convenient when doing a Bode plot to have the frequency response function in a *time-constant form.* That is, the 0th power of $s = j\omega$ is given a coefficient of 1, in both numerator and denominator, sic:

$$\frac{\mathbf{Y}}{\mathbf{U}}(j\omega) = \frac{C/b}{j\omega(a/b) + 1} = \mathbf{H}(j\omega) \text{ (time-constant from)} \tag{5.3}$$

The quantity (a/b) is the system's *time constant,* which has the units of time. One advantage of the time-constant format is that when **U** is DC, $\omega = 0$, and the DC gain of the system is simply $K_{vo} = (C/b)$. The vector *magnitude* of the frequency response vector function is just

$$|\mathbf{H}(j\omega)| = \frac{C/b}{\sqrt{\omega^2(a/b)^2 + 1}} \tag{5.4}$$

And its dB logarithmic value is just

$$dB = 20\log(C/b) - 10\log[\omega^2(a/b+1)^2 + 1] \tag{5.5}$$

For $\omega = 0$, dB = 20 log(c/b). For $\omega = (a/b)^{-1}$ r/s, dB = 20 log(C/b) − 10 log[2], or the DC level minus 3 dB. $\omega_o = (a/b)^{-1}$ r/s is the system's break frequency. For $\omega \geq 10\omega_o$, the AR is given by

$$dB = 20\log(c/b) - 20\log[\omega] - 20\log[a/b] \tag{5.6}$$

From Equation 5.6, one sees that the asymptote has a slope of −20 dB/decade of radian frequency, or equivalently, −6 dB/octave (a doubling of frequency). The phase of this system is given by

$$\theta(\omega) = -\tan^{-1}(\omega\, a/b) \tag{5.7}$$

The minus sign is because the complex portion of Equation 5.3 is in its denominator. Thus, the phase goes from 0° at $\omega = 0$ to −90° as $\omega \to \infty$. Figure 5.1 illustrates the complete Bode plot for the simple first-order, low-pass system, plotted with (normalized radian frequency).

Example 2

This is an underdamped, second-order, low-pass system described by the frequency response vector function:

$$\frac{\mathbf{Y}}{\mathbf{U}}(j\omega) = \frac{D}{a(j\omega)^2 + b(j\omega) + c} = \frac{B}{A}\angle\theta = \mathbf{H}(j\omega) \tag{5.8}$$

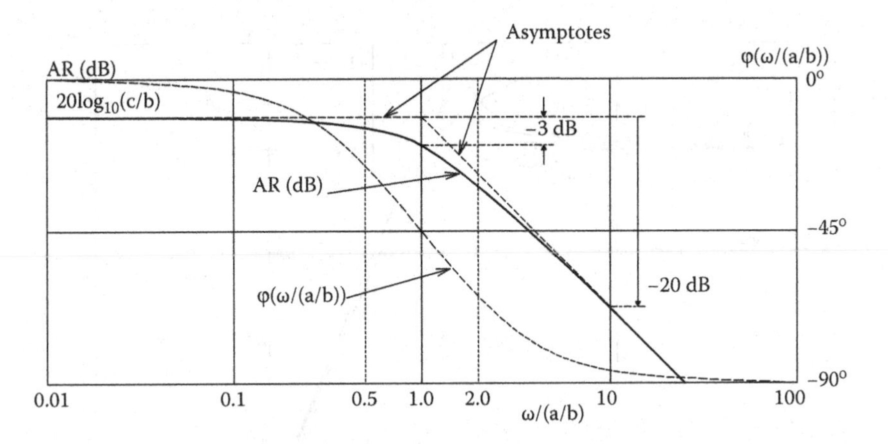

FIGURE 5.1 Normalized Bode plot for a real-pole low-pass filter. Asymptotes, AR, and phase are shown.

To put this frequency response function in time-constant form to facilitate Bode plotting, it is necessary to divide the numerator and denominator by c:

$$\frac{\mathbf{Y}}{\mathbf{U}}(j\omega) = \frac{D/c}{(a/c)(j\omega)^2 + (b/c)(j\omega) + 1} = \frac{D/c}{(j\omega)^2/\omega_n{}^2 + (2\xi/\omega_n)(j\omega) + 1} \tag{5.9}$$

where $c/a \equiv \omega_n{}^2$, the system's *undamped natural radian frequency* squared, and $b/c \equiv 2\xi/\omega_n$, and ξ is the system's *damping factor.*
The system has complex-conjugate roots to the characteristic equation of its ODE if $0 < \xi < 1$. In this *second example,* assume that the system is underdamped, i.e., $0 < \xi < 1$. Now the Bode magnitude plot is found from

$$dB = 20\log(d/c) - 10\log\{[1 - \omega^2/\omega_n{}^2]^2 + [2\xi/\omega_n)\omega]^2\} \tag{5.10}$$

At DC and $\omega << \omega_n$ and $\omega_n/2\xi$, dB $\cong$ 20 log(d/c). The undamped natural frequency is $\omega_n = \sqrt{c/a}$ r/s. When $\omega = \omega_n$, dB = 20 log(d/c) − 20 log[(2ξ/ωn) ωn] = 20 log(d/c) − 20 log[2ξ], and when $\omega >> \omega_n$, dB = 20 log(d/c) − 40 log[ω/ωn]. Thus, for $\omega = \omega_n$ and $\xi < 0.5$, the dB curve rises to a peak above the intersection of the asymptotes. The high-frequency asymptote has a slope of −40 dB/decade of radian frequency or −12 dB/octave (doubling) of radian frequency. These features are shown schematically in Figure 5.2. The phase of the second-order low-pass system can be found by inspection of the frequency response function of Equation 5.9. It is simply

$$\theta = -\tan^{-1}\left(\frac{\omega(2\xi/\omega_n)}{1 - \omega^2/\omega_n{}^2}\right) \tag{5.11}$$

It can be shown (Ogata 1970) that the magnitude of the resonant peak normalized with respect to the system's DC gain is

$$M_p = \frac{|\mathbf{H}(j\omega)|_{max}}{|\mathbf{H}(j0)|} = \frac{1}{2\xi\sqrt{1-\xi^2}} \quad \text{for } 0.707 \geq \xi \geq 0. \tag{5.12}$$

And the frequency at which the peak AR occurs is given by

$$\omega_p = \omega_n\sqrt{1 - 2\xi^2} \ \text{r/s}. \tag{5.13}$$

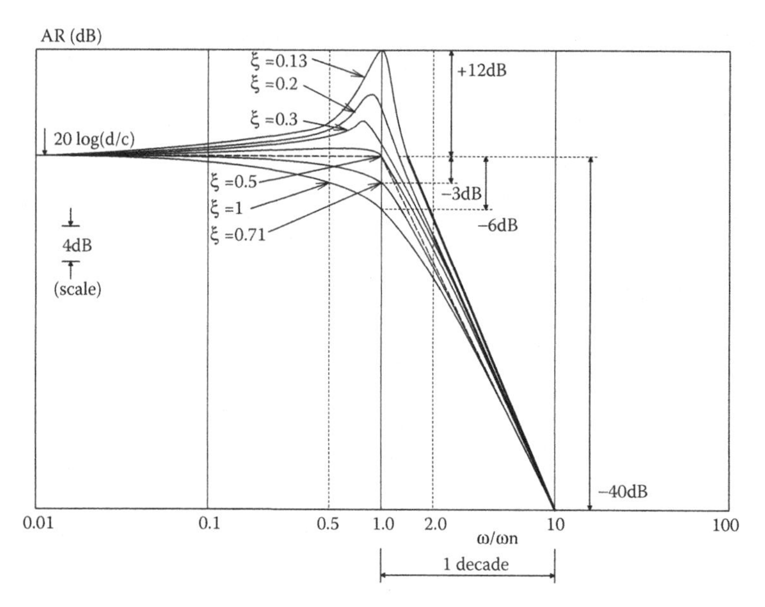

FIGURE 5.2 Normalized Bode magnitude plots of a typical underdamped, quadratic low-pass filter with various damping factors.

Example 3

A *lead/lag* filter is described by the frequency response function:

$$\frac{\mathbf{Y}}{\mathbf{X}} = \frac{j\omega/\omega_1 1}{j\omega/\omega_2 + 1} = H(j\omega), \quad \omega_2 > \omega_1 \tag{5.14}$$

For the Bode plot, at $\omega = 0$, dB $= 20\log|\mathbf{H}(j\omega)| = 0$ dB. At $\omega = \omega_1$, dB $\cong 20\log(\sqrt{2}) - 20\log(1) = +3$ dB. For $\omega >> \omega_2$, dB $\cong 20\log(\omega_2/\omega_1)$. The phase of the lead/lag filter is given by

$$\theta = \tan^{-1}(\omega/\omega_1) - \tan^{-1}(\omega/\omega_2) \tag{5.15}$$

The Bode magnitude response and phase of the lead/lag filter are shown in Figure 5.3.

Example 4

In this final example, we consider the frequency response of an RC amplifier with four real poles and two zeros at the origin of the s-plane. Its transfer function in Laplace format is

$$H(s) = \frac{s^2 K_v}{(s+\omega_1)(s+\omega_2)(s+\omega_3)(s+\omega_4)} \tag{5.16}$$

Now write the transfer function in factored time constant form for Bode plotting, and let $\mathbf{s} \rightarrow j\omega$:

$$\mathbf{H}(j\omega) = \frac{(j\omega)^2[K_v/(\omega_1\ \omega_2\ \omega_3\ \omega_4)]}{(j\omega\tau_1+1)(j\omega\tau_2+1)(j\omega\tau_3+1)(j\omega\tau_4+1)} \tag{5.17}$$

where $\tau_k = 1/\omega_k$. The algebraic expression for the Bode AR is

$$\begin{aligned} AR = {} & 20\log[K_v/(\omega_1\ \omega_2\ \omega_3\ \omega_4)] + 40\log(\omega) - 10\log[(\omega\tau_2)^2+1] \\ & - 10\log[(\omega\tau_2)^2+1] - 10\log[(\omega\tau_3)^2+1] - 10\log[(\omega\tau_4)^2+1] \end{aligned} \tag{5.18}$$

At $\omega << 1/\tau_1$, the AR $\cong 20\log[K_v/(\omega_1\ \omega_2\ \omega_3\ \omega_4)] + 40\log(\omega)$, the asymptote slope is + 40 dB/decade up to $\omega = \omega_1$. For $\omega_1 \le \omega \le \omega_2$, the asymptote slope is + 20 dB/decade,

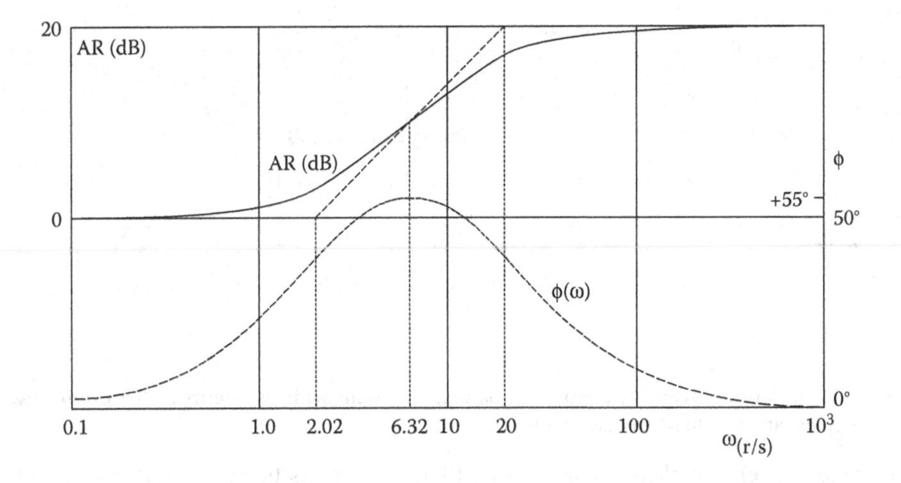

FIGURE 5.3 Bode plot of a lead-lag filter with one real pole and one real zero, magnitude and phase.

and for $\omega_2 \le \omega \le \omega_3$, the slope is 0; this is the midfrequency range of the plot. The midfrequency gain is

$$AR_{mid} \cong 20\log[K_v/(\omega_1\,\omega_2\,\omega_3\,\omega_4)] + 40\log(\omega) - 10\log[(\omega\tau_1)^2] - 10\log[(\omega\tau_2)^2] \quad (5.19a)$$

$$\downarrow$$

$$AR_{mid} \cong 20\log[K_v/(\omega_1\,\omega_2\,\omega_3\,\omega_4)] + 40\log(\omega) - 20\log(\omega) + 20\log(\omega_1) - 20\log(\omega) + 20\log(\omega_2) \quad (5.19b)$$

$$\downarrow$$

$$AR_{mid} \cong 20\log[K_v/(\omega_3\,\omega_4)] \quad (5.19c)$$

The AR asymptote then goes down at −20 dB/decade for $\omega_3 \le \omega \le \omega_4$, and at −40 dB/decade for $\omega > \omega_4$.

Figure 5.4 shows the AR plot for this amplifier. Its phase response is given by

$$\theta(\omega) = +180^\circ - \tan^{-1}[\omega\tau_1] - \tan^{-1}[\omega\tau_2] - \tan^{-1}[\omega\tau_3] - \tan^{-1}[\omega\tau_3] \quad (5.20)$$

$\theta(\omega)$ starts at + 180° at low ω and approaches −180° as $\omega \to \infty$.

Because frequency response has traditionally been used as a descriptor for electronic amplifiers and feedback control systems, many texts on electronic circuits and control systems have introductory sections on this topic with examples (see, for example, Northrop 1990; Ogata 1990, Section 6-2; Schilling and Belove 1989, Section 9.1-2; Nise 1995, Chapter 10). Modern circuit simulation software applications such as Spectrum Software's Micro-Cap10™, various versions of SPICE and PSPICE™ 9.1, and National Instruments' NI Multisim™ compute Bode plots for active and passive circuits, and MATLAB®, Simulink®, and Simnon® will provide them for general linear systems described by ODEs or state equations.

5.3 WHAT IS MEANT BY FEEDBACK SYSTEM STABILITY

An unstable amplifier either spontaneously oscillates or produces a saturated DC output. The oscillations ideally would be sinusoidal, but they grow in amplitude until the transistors in the amplifier are cutoff and/or saturate, producing a clipped, distorted output at the oscillation frequency.

There are two ways a feedback amplifier can be unstable. (1) If one (or more) closed-loop pole lies in the right-half s-plane *on the real axis,* there will be no oscillation, just a saturated output.

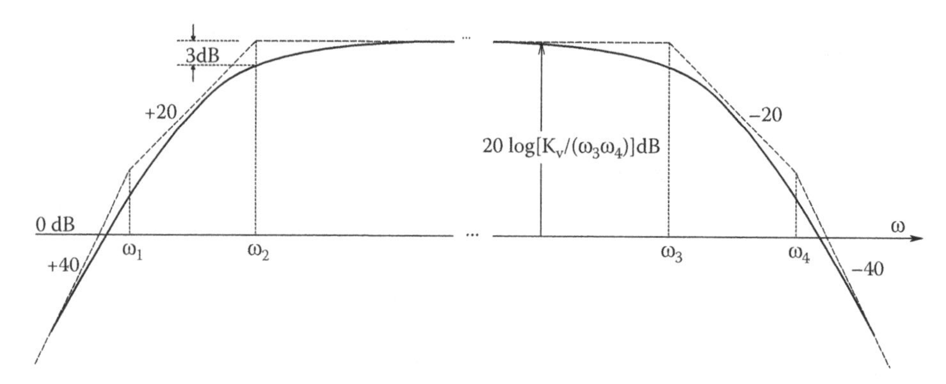

FIGURE 5.4 Typical Bode magnitude plot of a bandpass system with two zeros at the origin, two low-frequency real poles, and two high-frequency real poles.

(2) When two (or more), complex-conjugate closed-loop pole-pairs lie in the right-half s-plane, the amplifier will begin oscillating spontaneously; and the oscillations will grow in amplitude until the amplifier saturates and clips the output sine wave's peaks. Use of the *root locus* (RL) *technique* indicates at once if a feedback amplifier will be unstable at a given gain because the RL branches locate the system's closed-loop poles as a function of the scalar loop gain.

The *describing function method* (Ogata 1970; Northrop 2000, Chapter 3) of analyzing *nonlinear feedback systems* can predict if a *nonlinear feedback system* will oscillate, as well as give its frequency and stable amplitude. Nonlinear systems can generate a stable periodic output known as a limit cycle (an example is a home heating system). Describing function analysis is more appropriate to control systems and will not be treated here.

Two other classic methods of testing feedback amplifier stability are the *Routh-Hurwitz test* and the *Nyquist test.* The Routh-Hurwitz test (Dorf 1967; Northrop 2000) uses an algebraic protocol to examine the roots of the numerator polynomial of the *return difference* (RD) of the closed-loop transfer function. Recall that the zeros of the RD are the poles of the closed-loop system. If any of the roots of the RD have positive real parts (e.g., lie in the right-half s-plane), the closed-loop system will be unstable. It is easy today, given a linear feedback system's RD(s), to apply the *ROOTS* utility of MATLAB™ to the numerator polynomial and examine the roots for positive real values, if any. The Routh-Hurwitz test appears to be obsolete.

When doing electronic system design, useful information about the closed-loop behavior of a feedback system may be obtained from the *Nyquist test,* which is based on the steady-state, sinusoidal frequency response of the system's loop gain function. The Nyquist test is well-suited for design and stability analysis based on *experimental* frequency response data. To introduce the Nyquist test for closed-loop system stability, we call attention to the conventional, single-input, single-output linear feedback system shown in Figure 5.5. In this system, no minus sign assumption is made at the summing point. The closed-loop system transfer function is simply

$$\frac{Y}{X}(s) = \frac{G(s)}{[1 - A_L(s)]} = \frac{G(s)}{RD(s)} \tag{5.21}$$

In a negative feedback system, the loop gain, $A_L(s) = -G(s)H(s)$, so we finally have

$$\frac{Y}{X}(s) = \frac{G(s)}{[1 + G(s)H(s)]} \tag{5.22}$$

The denominator of the closed-loop transfer function is called the *return difference,* $RD(s) \equiv [1 + G(s)H(s)]$. If RD(s) is a rational polynomial, as stated earlier, then *its zeros are the*

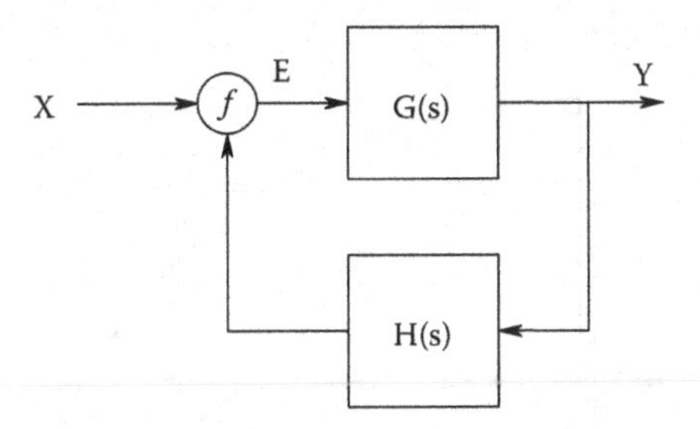

FIGURE 5.5 A simple, two-block, SISO feedback system.

poles of the closed-loop system function. The Nyquist test effectively examines the zeros of RD(s) to see if any lie in the right-half s-plane. Poles of the closed-loop system in the right-half s-plane produce unstable behavior. In practice, it is more convenient to work with $\mathbf{A_L(s)} = 1 - \mathbf{RD(s)}$, and see if there are complex (vector) **s** values that make $\mathbf{A_L(s)} \to 1\angle 0°$. The Nyquist test uses a process known as *conformal mapping* to examine the poles and zeros of $A_L(s)$, hence the zeros of RD(s). In the conformal mapping process used in the Nyquist test, the vector **s** lies on the contour C_1 shown in Figure 5.6. This contour encloses the entire right-half s-plane. The infinitesimal semicircle to the left of the origin is to avoid any poles of $A_L(s)$ at the origin. Because the test is a vector test, $A_L(s)$ must be written in vector difference form. For example

$$A_L(s) = \frac{K(s+a)}{(s+b)(s+c)} \to A_L(s) = \frac{-K(s-s_1)}{(s-s_2)(s-s_3)} = \frac{K|A|}{|B||C|}\angle -\pi + \theta_a - \theta_b - \theta_c \tag{5.23}$$

Factored Laplace form Vector difference form Vector polar form

The convention used in this text places a (net) minus sign in the numerator of the loop gain when the feedback system uses negative feedback. The root vectors $\mathbf{s_1} = -a$, $\mathbf{s_2} = -b$ and $\mathbf{s_3} = -c$ are negative real numbers. In practice, **s** has values lying on the contour shown in Figure 5.6. The vector differences $(\mathbf{s} - \mathbf{s_1}) = \mathbf{A}$, $(\mathbf{s} - \mathbf{s_2}) = \mathbf{B}$ and $(\mathbf{s} - \mathbf{s_3}) = \mathbf{C}$ are shown for $\mathbf{s} = j\omega_1$ in Figure 5.7. For each **s** value on the contour C_1, there is a corresponding vector value, $\mathbf{A_L(s)}$.

A fundamental theorem in conformal mapping says that if the tip of the vector **s** assumes values on the closed contour, C_1, then the tip of the $\mathbf{A_L(s)}$ vector will also generate a closed contour, the nature of which depends on its poles and zeros.

Before continuing with the treatment of the vector loop gain, it is necessary to go back to the vector return difference, $\mathbf{RD(s)} = \mathbf{1} - \mathbf{A_L(s)}$, and examine the Nyquist test done on the RD(s) of an obviously *unstable system.* Assume

$$RD(s) = \frac{K(s-1)}{(s+1)(s+1)} \to RD(s) = \frac{K(s-s_1)}{(s-s_2)(s-s_3)} \tag{5.24}$$

Recall that a right-half s-plane zero of **RD(s)** is a right-half (unstable) pole of the closed-loop system. The vector **s** assumes values on the contour C_1' in Figure 5.8. Note that C_1' does not need the infinitesimal semicircle around the origin of the s-plane because in this case, RD(s) has no poles or zeros at the origin. Note that as **s** goes from $\mathbf{s} = j0+$ to $\mathbf{s} = +j\infty$, the angle of the **RD(s)** vector goes from +180° to −90°, and $|\mathbf{RD(s)}|$ goes from K/2 to 0. When $|\mathbf{s}| = \infty$, $|\mathbf{RD(s)}| = 0$ and its angle goes from −90° to +90° at $\mathbf{s} = -j\infty$. The **RD(s)** vector contour (locus) in the **RD(s)** plane is shown in Figure 5.9. Note that the vector locus for $\mathbf{s} = -j\omega$ values is the mirror image of the locus for $\mathbf{s} = +j\omega$ values. It can also be seen in this case that the complete **RD(s)** locus (for all **s** values on C_1' traversed in a *clockwise* direction in the s-plane) makes one net clockwise encirclement of the origin in the **RD(s)** vector plane. This encirclement is the result of the contour C_1' having enclosed

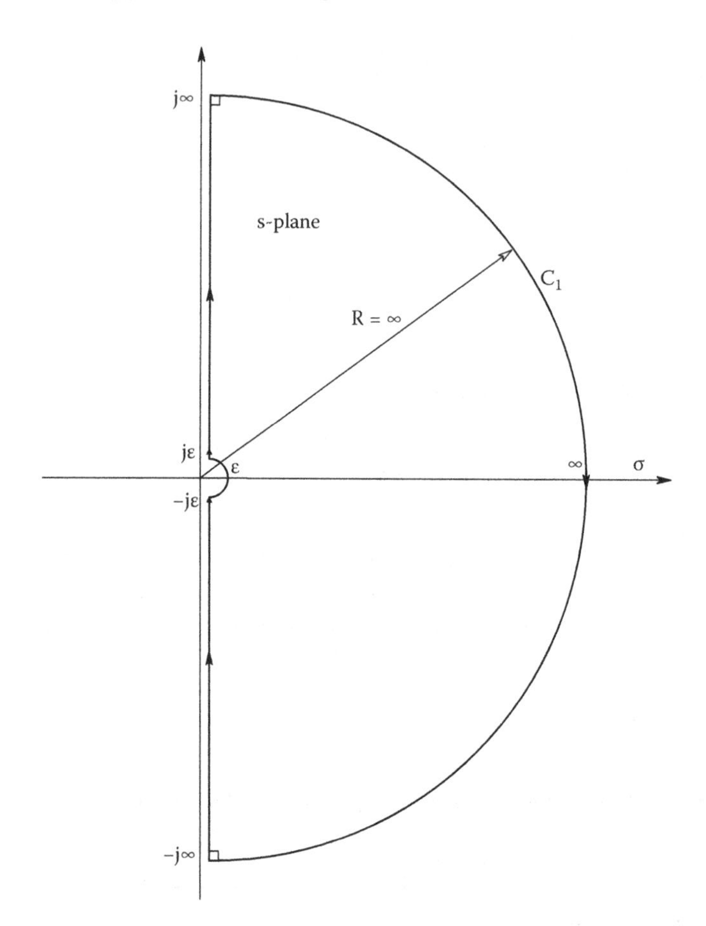

FIGURE 5.6 The contour C_1 containing (complex) s values, traversed clockwise in the s-plane.

the right-half s-plane zero of RD(s). The encirclement is the basis for the Nyquist test relation for the return difference:

$$Z = N_{cw} + P \tag{5.25}$$

where Z is the number of right-half s-plane zeros of **RD(s)**, *or* right-half s-plane poles of the closed loop system's transfer function.

Obviously, Z is desired to be zero. N_{CW} is the *observed* total number of clockwise encirclements of the origin by the **RD**(s) contour. P is the *known* number of right-half s-plane poles of **RD(s)** (usually zero).

Now return to the consideration of the more useful loop gain transfer function. Recall that when **RD(s)** = 0, $\mathbf{A_L}$(s) = +1. *For the first example,* we take

$$A_L(s) = \frac{-K(s-2)}{(s+5)^2(s+2)} \rightarrow A_L(s) = \frac{-K(s-s_1)}{(s-s_2)^2(s-s_3)} \tag{5.26}$$

Figure 5.10 shows the s-plane with the poles and zeros of $A_L(s)$, the contour C_1', and the vector differences used in calculating $\mathbf{A_L}$**(s)** as **s** traverses C_1' clockwise. Table 5.1 gives values of $|\mathbf{A_L}(s)|$ and $\angle\, \mathbf{A_L}(s)$ for **s** values on contour C_1'.

The polar plot of $\mathbf{A_L}$(s) is shown in Figure 5.11. Because $\mathbf{A_L}$(s) is used instead of **RD**(s), the point $\mathbf{A_L}$(s) = +1 is critical for encirclements, rather than the origin. The positive, real point of

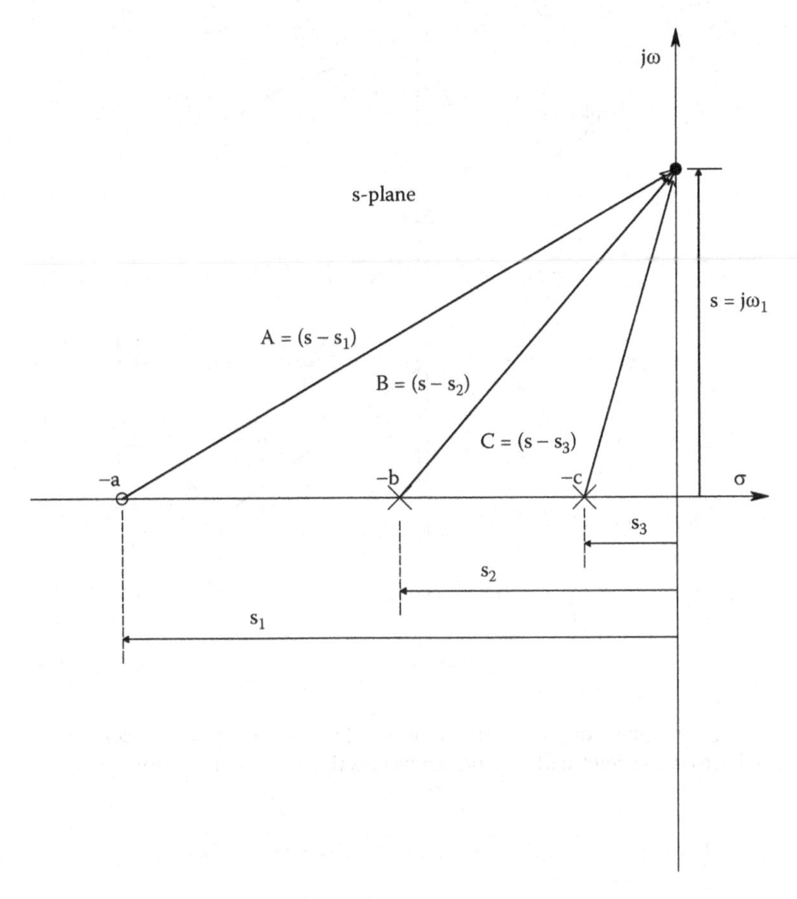

FIGURE 5.7 The s-plane showing vector differences from the real zero and two real poles of a lowpass filter to $\mathbf{s} = j\omega_1$.

intersection occurs for $\mathbf{s} = j0$. It is easily seen that if $K > 25$, there will be one net CW encirclement of the +1 point. The Nyquist conformal equation can be modified to

$$P_{CL} = N_{cw} + P \tag{5.27}$$

P_{CL} is the number of closed-loop system poles in the right-half s-plane. N_{CW} is the total number of clockwise encirclements of +1 in the $\mathbf{A}_L(\mathbf{s})$ plane as $\mathbf{s}$ traverses the contour C_1' clockwise. P is the number of poles of $A_L(s)$ known *a priori* to be in the right-half s-plane. Thus, for the system of the first example, $P = 0$, and $N_{CW} = 1$ only if $K > 25$. The closed-loop system is seen to be unstable with one pole in the right-half s-plane when $K > 25$.

In the second example, the system of Example 1 is given positive feedback. Thus,

$$A_L(s) = \frac{+K(s-2)}{(s+5)^2(s+2)} \tag{5.28}$$

Figure 5.12 shows the polar plot of the positive feedback system's $\mathbf{A}_L(\mathbf{s})$ as $\mathbf{s}$ traverses the contour C_1'. Now one sees that if K exceeds a critical value, there will be *two* clockwise encirclements of +1; hence, two closed-loop system poles will be in the right-half s-plane. Under these conditions, the instability will be a sinusoidal oscillation with an exponentially growing amplitude. To find the

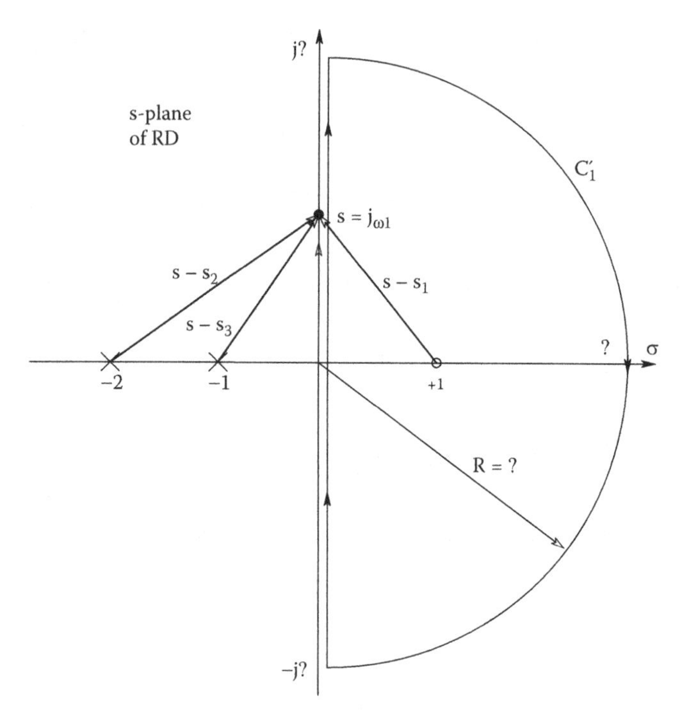

FIGURE 5.8 The vector s-plane of the return difference showing vector differences and contour C_1' for an RD(s) having a real zero in the right-half s-plane. s traverses the contour clockwise.

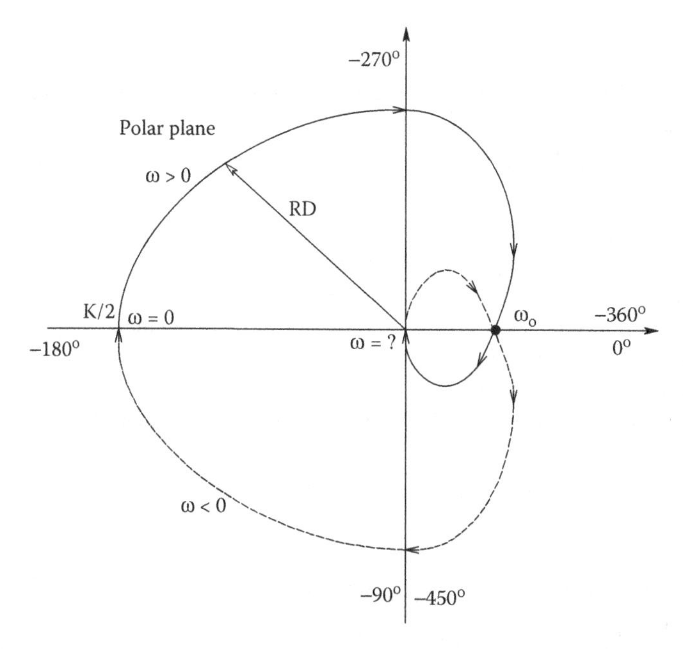

FIGURE 5.9 The vector contour in the polar (complex) plane of the **RD(s)** of Equation 5.24 as s traverses C_1' clockwise.

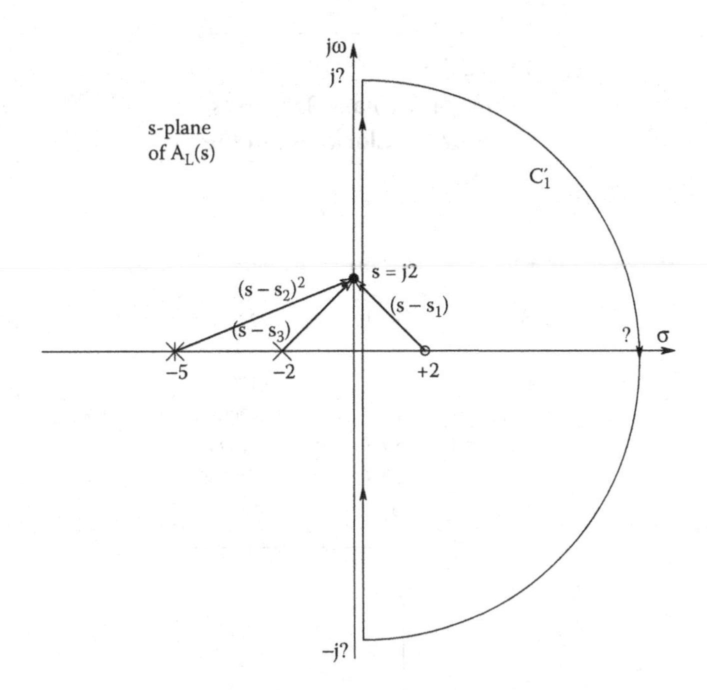

FIGURE 5.10 The vector s-plane of the loop gain showing vector differences and contour C_1' for a negative feedback system's $\mathbf{A_L(s)}$ having a real zero in the right-half s-plane. **s** traverses the contour clockwise.

critical value of K for instability, it is convenient to first find the $s = j\omega_o$ value at which the system will oscillate by examining the phase of $\mathbf{A_L}(j\omega_o)$ where $\mathbf{A_L}$ crosses the positive real axis:

$$-2\tan^{-1}(\omega_o/5) - \tan^{-1}(\omega_o/2) + [180° - \tan^{-1}(\omega_o/2)] = 0° \tag{5.29a}$$

$$\downarrow$$

$$-2\tan^{-1}(\omega_o/5) - 2\tan^{-1}(\omega_o/2) = 180° \tag{5.29b}$$

$$\downarrow$$

$$\tan^{-1}(\omega_o/5) + \tan^{-1}(\omega_o/2)] = 90° \tag{5.29c}$$

Trial and error solution of Equation 5.29C above yields $\omega_o = 3.162$ r/s. Substitution of this ω_o value into $|\mathbf{A_L}(j\omega_o)| = +1$, and solving for K we get K = 35.00. Therefore, if K > 35, the positive feedback system is unstable, having two, net CW encirclements of +1 and thus a complex-conjugate pole pair in the right-half s-plane. Furthermore, the frequency of oscillation at the threshold of instability is $\omega_o = 3.162$ r/s.

As the third and final example of the Nyquist stability criterion, examine the Nyquist plot of a third-order, negative feedback system with loop gain:

$$A_L(s) = \frac{-K\beta}{s(s+5)(s+2)} \tag{5.30}$$

This system has a pole at the origin, so in examining $\mathbf{A_L(s)}$, **s** must follow the contour C_1 having the infinitesimal semicircle of radius ε avoiding the origin. Start at **s** = jε and go to **s** = j∞. At **s** = jε, $|\mathbf{A_L(s)}| \to \infty$, and $\angle \mathbf{A_L} = -270°$. As **s** → j∞, $|\mathbf{A_L(s)}| \to 0$ and $\angle \mathbf{A_L} \to -450°$. Now when **s** traverses

TABLE 5.1
Values of $A_L(s)$ as s Traverses Contour C_1' Clockwise in the S-plane

S	$\lvert A_L(s) \rvert$	$\angle A_L(s)$
± j0	+ K/25	0°
j2	K/29	–133.6°
j5	K/50	–226.4°
j∞	0	–360°
+∞	0	–180°
– j∞	0	+ 360°
– j2	K/29	+ 133.6°
– j5	K/50	+ 226.4°
– j∞	0	+ 360°

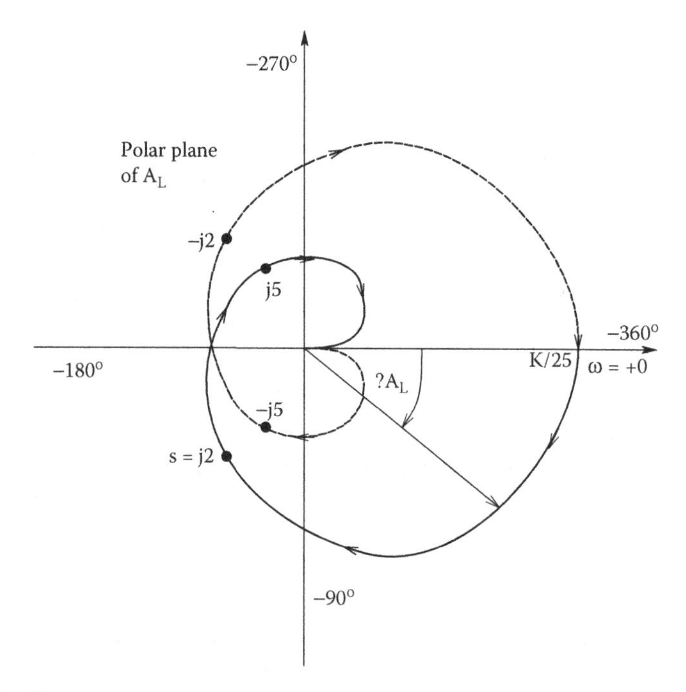

FIGURE 5.11 The Nyquist vector contour of the SISO *negative feedback* system's $\mathbf{A_L(s)}$ as s traverses C_1'. Note that this type of contour is always symmetrical around the real axis, and is closed because C_1' is also closed. See Text for discussion of stability.

the ∞ radius semicircle on C_1, $|\mathbf{A_L(s)}| = 0$ and the phase goes through 0°, thence to +90°, all with $|\mathbf{A_L(s)}| = 0$. Now as **s** goes from $-j\infty$ to $-j\varepsilon$, $|\mathbf{A_L(s)}|$ grows larger, and its phase goes from +90° to –90° (or +270°). As **s** traverses the small semicircle part of C_1, $|\mathbf{A_L(s)}| \rightarrow \infty$, and the phase goes from –90° to –180° at $\mathbf{s} = \varepsilon$, thence to –270° at $\mathbf{s} = j\varepsilon$. The complete contour, $\mathbf{A_L(s)}$, is shown in Figure 5.13. Note that if Kβ is large enough, there are two, CW encirclements of +1 by the $\mathbf{A_L(s)}$ locus, signifying that there are two closed-loop system poles in the right-hand s-plane, hence oscillatory instability. Because $\mathbf{A_L}(j\omega_o)$ is real, we can set the imaginary terms in the denominator of $\mathbf{A_L}(j\omega_o) = 0$, and solve for ω_o. Thus,

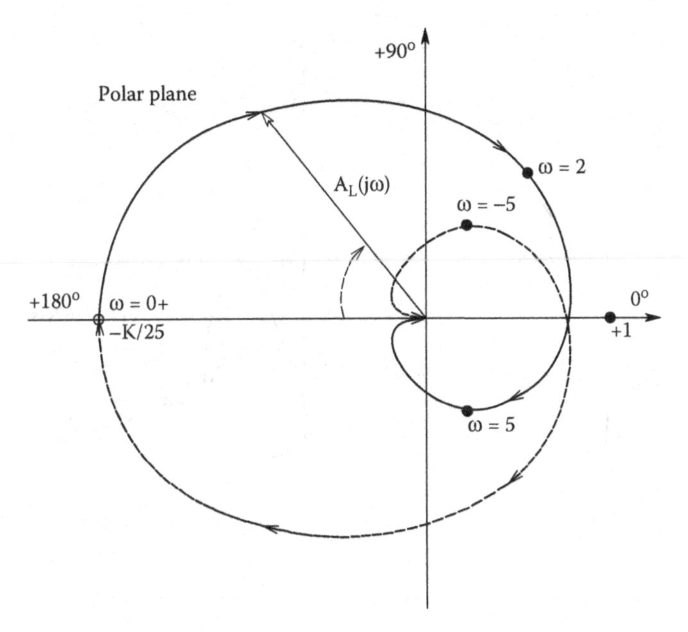

FIGURE 5.12 The Nyquist vector contour of the SISO *positive feedback system's* $\mathbf{A_L(s)}$ as s traverses C_1'. This is the same system as in Figure 5.11, except it has PFB.

$$j\omega_o(j\omega_o + 5)(j\omega_o + 2) = -j\omega_o^3 - 7\omega_o^2 + 10\,j\omega_o = \text{Real} \tag{5.31}$$

Thus, $(-j\omega_o^3 + 10\,j\omega_o)$ must $= 0$, which leads to $\omega_o = 3.162$ r/s, and $K\beta > 7\omega_o^2 = 70$ for instability.

5.4 USE OF ROOT LOCUS IN FEEDBACK AMPLIFIER DESIGN

Given the knowledge of the positions of the poles and zeros of the loop gain of a linear, SISO, single-loop, feedback system, the root locus technique allows us to predict precisely where the closed-loop poles of the system will be as a function of system gain. Thus, root locus (RL) can be used to predict the conditions for instability, as well as to design for a desired, closed-loop transient response. Many texts on linear control systems treat the generation and interpretation of root locus plots in detail (Kuo 1982; Ogata 1990). Root locus has also been used in the design of electronic feedback amplifiers, including sinusoidal oscillators (Northrop 1990).

It is often tedious to construct root locus diagrams by hand on paper, except in certain simple cases described below. Detailed, quantitative RL plots can be generated using the MATLAB® subroutine, "RLOCUS." Several of the examples in this section are from MATLAB plots.

The concept behind the root locus diagram is simple: Figure 5.14 shows a simple one-loop, linear, SISO feedback system. The closed-loop gain is

$$\frac{Y}{X}(s) = \frac{C(s)G_P(s)}{1 - A_L(s)} = \frac{C(s)G_p(s)}{1 + C(s)G_p(s)H(s)} = F(s) \tag{5.32}$$

C(s) is the controller transfer function acting on E(s), $G_p(s)$ is the plant transfer function (input U(s), output Y(s)), and H(s) is the feedback path transfer function. The system loop gain is

$$A_L(s) = -C(s)G_p(s)H(s) \tag{5.33}$$

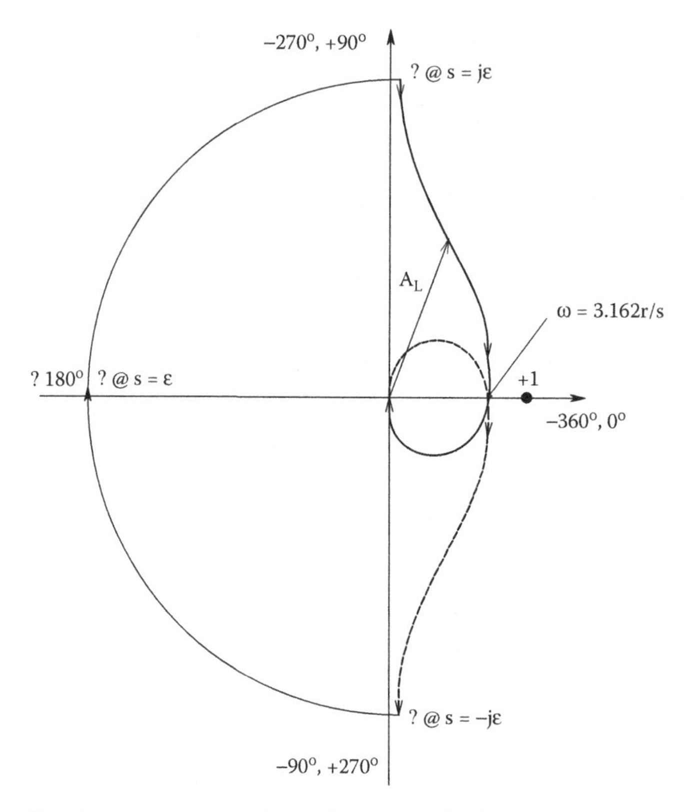

FIGURE 5.13 The Nyquist vector contour plot of the NFB $\mathbf{A_L(s)}$ of Equation 5.30. This $\mathbf{A_L(s)}$ has a pole at the origin.

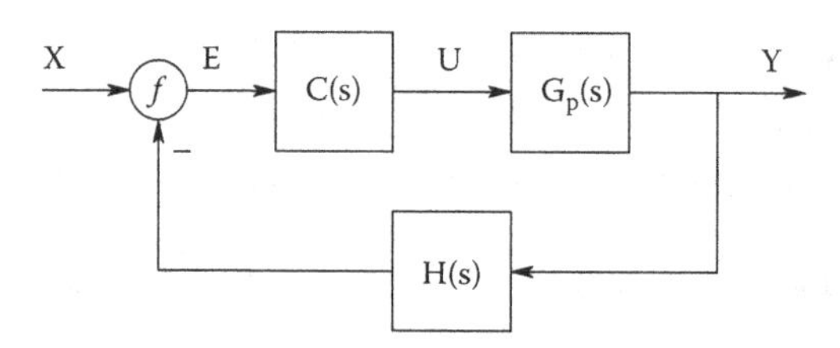

FIGURE 5.14 A three-block, SISO system with negative feedback.

(The minus sign indicates that the system uses negative feedback.) The RL technique allows one to plot in the s-plane those complex **s** values that make the return difference → 0, thus making the closed-loop transfer function, $|\mathbf{F(s)}| \rightarrow \infty$. The **s** values that make $|\mathbf{F(s)}| \rightarrow \infty$ are of course, by definition, the poles of $\mathbf{F(s)}$. These poles move in the s-plane as a function of a gain parameter in a predictable, continuous manner as the gain is changed. Since finding **s** values that set $\mathbf{A_L(s)} = 1\angle 0°$ is the same as setting $|\mathbf{F(s)}| = \infty$, the root locus plotting rules are based on finding **s** values that cause the angle of $-\mathbf{A_L(s)} = -180°$, and $|-\mathbf{A_L(s)}| = 1$. The root locus plotting rules are based on satisfying either the *angle* or *magnitude condition* on $-\mathbf{A_L(s)}$. The vector format of $-\mathbf{A_L(s)}$ is used to derive the RL plotting rules.

An example of how this is done is given below. First, assume a negative feedback system with the loop gain, $A_L(s)$, given below. Note that there are three, equivalent ways of writing $A_L(s)$:

$$A_L(s) = \frac{-K\beta(s\tau_1 + 1)}{(s\tau_2 + 1)(s\tau_3 + 1)} \quad \text{(time constant form)} \tag{5.34a}$$

$$A_L(s) = \frac{-K\beta\tau_1}{\tau_2\ \tau_3} \frac{(s+1/\tau_1)}{(s+1/\tau_2)(s+1/\tau_3)} \quad \text{(Laplace form)} \tag{5.34b}$$

$$-A_L(s) = \frac{K\beta\tau_1}{\tau_2\ \tau_3} \frac{(s-s_1)}{(s-s_2)(s-s_3)} \quad \text{(vector difference from)} \tag{5.34c}$$

where $s_1 = -1/\tau_1$, $s_2 = -1/\tau_2$, and $s_3 = -1/\tau_3$.

For the *magnitude criterion,* **s** must satisfy

$$\frac{|s-s_1|}{|s-s_2||s-s_3|} = \frac{\tau_2\tau_3}{K\beta\tau_1} \tag{5.35a}$$

For the *angle criterion,* **s** must satisfy

$$\theta_1 - (\theta_2 + \theta_3) = -180^\circ . \tag{5.35b}$$

The Nine basic root locus plotting rules are derived from the preceding angle and magnitude conditions and are used for pencil and paper construction of RL diagrams. They are

(1) *Number of Branches:* There is one branch for each pole of $A_L(s)$.
(2) *Branch Starting Points:* Locus branches start at the poles of $A_L(s)$ for $K\beta = 0$.
(3) *Branch End Points:* The branches end at the finite zeros of $A_L(s)$ for $K\beta \to \infty$. Some zeros of $A_L(s)$ can be at $|s| = \infty$.
(4) *Behavior of the Loci on the Real Axis:* (From the angle criterion.) For a negative feedback system, on-real axis locus branches exist to the left of an odd number of on-axis poles and zeros of $A_L(s)$. If the feedback for some reason is positive, then on-axis locus branches are found to the right of a total odd number of poles and zeros of $A_L(s)$. See examples below.
(5) *Symmetry:* Root locus plots are symmetrical around the real axis in the s-plane.
(6) *Magnitude of Gain at a Point on a Valid Locus Branch:* From the magnitude criterion, at a vector point **s** on a valid locus branch we have:

$$K\beta = \frac{|s-s_2||s-s_3|\tau_2\tau_3}{|s-s_1|\tau_1} \tag{5.36}$$

(7) *Points Where Locus Branches Leave or Join the Real Axis:* The breakaway or reentry point is algebraically complicated to find, also, there are methods based on both the angle and magnitude criteria. For example, in a negative feedback system loop gain function with three real poles, two locus branches leave the two poles closest to the origin and travel toward each other along the real axis as Kβ is raised. At some critical Kβ, the branches break away from the real axis, one at + 90° and the other at –90°. If we examine the angle criterion at the breakaway point, as shown in Figure 5.15, it is clear that

$$-(\theta_1 + \theta_2 + \theta_3) = -180^\circ \tag{5.37}$$

From the geometry on the figure, the angles can be written as arctangents:

$$\tan^{-1}[\varepsilon/(\omega_1 - P)] + \tan^{-1}[\varepsilon/(\omega_2 - P)] + \{\pi - \tan^{-1}[\varepsilon/(P-\omega_3)]\} = \pi \tag{5.38}$$

For small arguments, $\tan^{-1}(x) \cong x$, so

$$[\varepsilon/(\omega_1 - P)] + [\varepsilon/(\omega_2 - P)] - [\varepsilon/(P-\omega_3)] = 0 \tag{5.39}$$

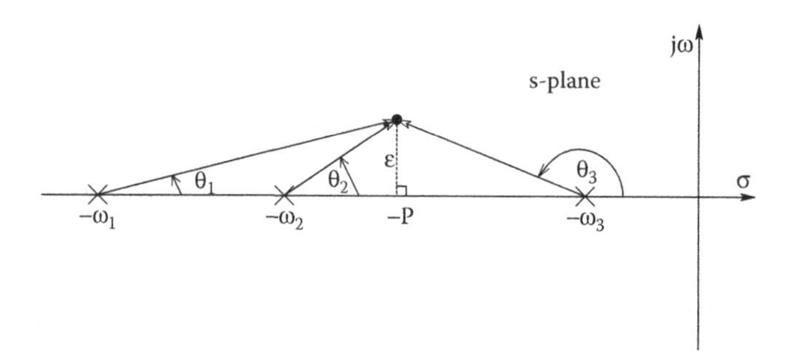

FIGURE 5.15 S-plane vector diagram illustrating the vectors and angles required in calculating the breakaway point of complex conjugate root locus branches when they leave the real axis. (See Part 7 of the *Nine Basic Root Locus Plotting Rules* in the Text.)

TABLE 5.2
Asymptote Angles with the Real Axis in the S-plane

Negative Feedback		Positive Feedback	
N − M	φ_k	N − M	φ_k
1	180°	1	0°
2	90°, 270°	2	0°, 180°
3	60°, 180°, 300°	3	0°, ± 120°
4	45°, 135°, 225°, 315°	4	0°, 90°, 180°, 270°

This equation can be written as a quadratic in P:

$$3P^2 - 2(\omega_1 + \omega_2 + \omega_3)P + (\omega_2\omega_3 + \omega_1\omega_2 + \omega_1\omega_3) = 0 \tag{5.40}$$

The desired P-root of course lies between $-\omega_2$ and $-\omega_3$.

(8) *Breakaway or Reentry Angles of Branches With the Real Axis:* The loci are separated by angles of 180° /n, where n is the number of branches intersecting the real axis. In most cases, n = 2, so the branches approach the axis perpendicular to it.

(9) *Asymptotic Behavior of the Branches for* Kb → ∞:

(a) The number of asymptotes along which branches approach zeros at $|s| = \infty$ is $N_A = N - M$, where N is the number of finite poles and M is the number of finite zeros of $A_L(s)$.

(b) The angles of the asymptotes with the real axis are φ_k, where k = 1 ... N − M. φ_k is given in Table 5.2.

(c) The intersections of the asymptotes with the real axis is a value I_A along the real axis. It is given by

$$I_A = \frac{\Sigma(\text{real parts of finite poles}) - \Sigma(\text{real parts of finite zeros})}{N - M} \tag{5.41}$$

An example of finding the asymptotes and I_A is shown in Figure 5.16. This negative feedback system has a loop gain with four poles at s = 0, s = − 3, and a complex-conjugate pair at s = − 1 ± j2. There are no finite zeros. Thus, $I_A = [(-3 - 1 - 1) - (0)]/4 = -5/4$. From the table, the angles are, ± 45° and ± 135°. This RL plot was done with MATLAB™.

To get a feeling for plotting RL diagrams on paper with the rules above, it is necessary to examine several more representative examples:

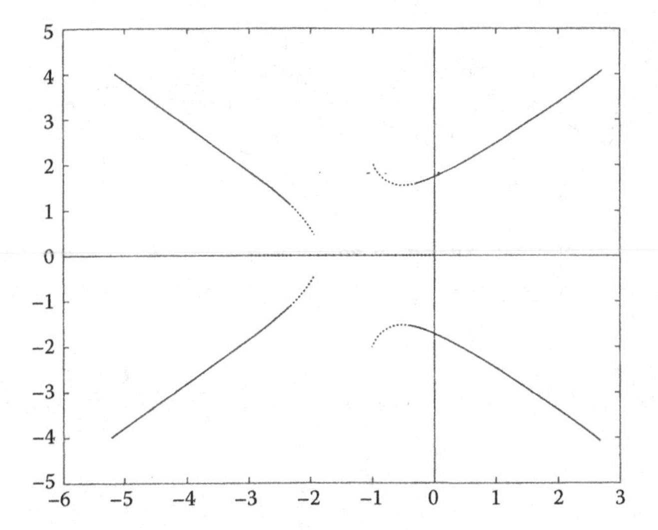

FIGURE 5.16 A MATLAB™ RLOCUS plot for a negative feedback loop gain with a pole at the origin, a real pole, and a pair of C-C poles.

Example 1

Examines the use of root locus in the design of a feedback amplifier using two op amp gain stages as shown in Figure 5.17a. This feedback amplifier can never be unstable, but its closed-loop poles can have so little damping that the system is useless. Stage 1's gain is given by

$$K_{v1}(s) = \frac{V_2}{(V_1 - V_1')} = \frac{10^5}{10^{-3}s+1} = \frac{10^8}{s+1000} \tag{5.42}$$

Stage 2's gain is given by

$$K_{v2}(s) = \frac{V_o}{V_2} = \frac{-10^4}{4\times10^{-3}s+1} = \frac{-2.5\times10^6}{s+2.5\times10^2} \tag{5.43}$$

The NVF system's loop gain is therefore

$$A_L(s) = -\frac{\beta\, 2.5\times10^{14}}{(s+10^3)(s+2.5\times10^2)} \tag{5.44}$$

The system's root locus diagram is shown in Figure 5.17b. The locus branches begin on the loop gain poles and move parallel to the jω axis in the s-plane to ±j∞ as β increases. The locus branches meet on the negative real axis at $\mathbf{s} = I_A$, where they become complex-conjugate:

$$\begin{aligned} I_A &= \frac{\Sigma(\text{real parts of finite poles}) - \Sigma(\text{real parts of finite zeros})}{N-M} \\ &= \frac{-10^3 - 2.5\times10^2}{2} = -6.25\times10^2 \end{aligned} \tag{5.45}$$

It is desired to have the closed-loop system poles at **P** and **P***, so its damping factor will be $\xi = 0.7071$.

From the geometry of the RL plot, the closed-loop $\omega_n = 6.25\times10^2\times\sqrt{2} = 8.84\times10^2$ r/s. From the RL magnitude criterion, one finds the β value to place the closed-loop poles at **P** and **P***:

$$|-A_L(s=P)| = 1 = \frac{\beta_P 2.5\times10^{14}}{|A||B|} \tag{5.46}$$

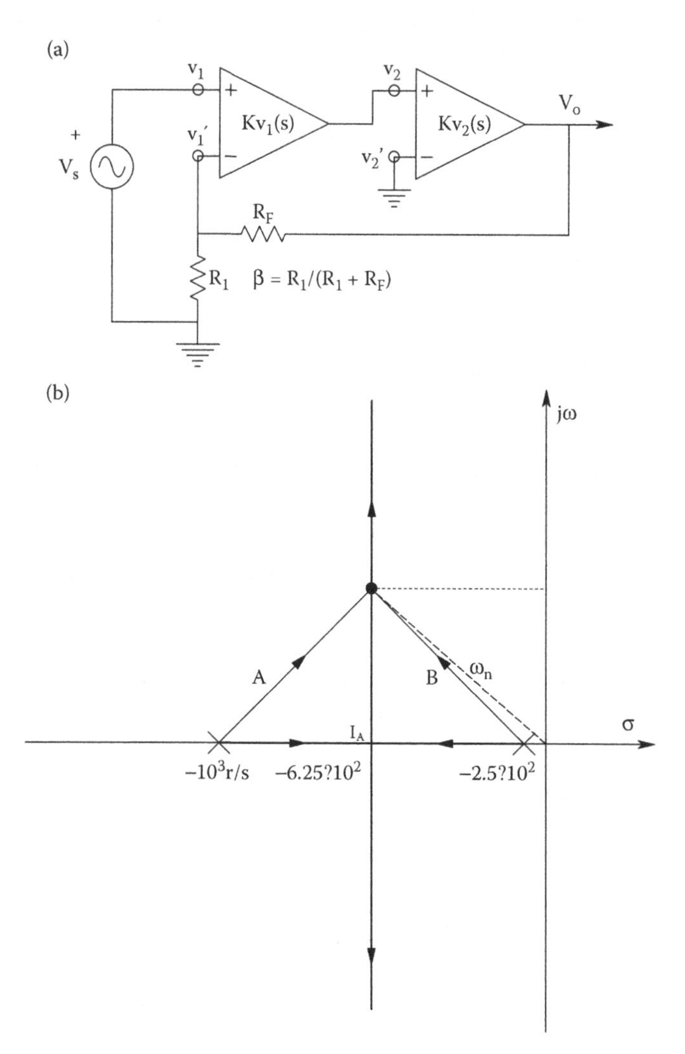

FIGURE 5.17 (a) Two op amps connected as a noninverting amplifier with overall NVFB. (b) Root locus diagram for the amplifier. Note that unless a sharply tuned closed-loop frequency response is desired, the feedback gain, b, must be very small to realize a closed-loop system with a damping factor of 0.7071.

The vectors **A** and **B** are defined in the figure, and the Pythagorean theorem tells us

$$|A| = |B| = \sqrt{(6.25\times 10^2)^2 + (3.75\times 10^2)^2} = 7.289\times 10^2 \tag{5.47}$$

Thus, the value

$$\beta_p = \frac{(7.289\times 10^2)^2}{2.5\times 10^{14}} = 2.125\times 10^{-9}, \tag{5.48}$$

will give the closed-loop system a damping factor of 0.707. The feedback amplifier's closed-loop, DC gain is

$$A_r(0) = +\frac{10^9}{1+2.125\times 10^{-9}\times 10^9} = 3.20\times 10^8 \tag{5.49}$$

In summary, the cascading of two compensated op amps, with a single feedback loop, gives a closed-loop amplifier with high gain but relatively poor bandwidth. As an exercise, consider the –3 dB bandwidth possible if you cascade two, noninverting op amp amplifiers, each with its own NVF such that their combined DC gain is 3.20×10^8.

Example 2

Examines the commonly encountered circle root locus. The negative feedback system's loop gain transfer function has two real poles and a real zero:

$$A_L(s) = \frac{-K_p\beta(s+a)}{(s+b)(s+c)} \tag{5.50}$$

where $a > b > c > 0$. Angelo (1969) gave an elegant proof that this system's root locus does indeed contain a circle centered on the zero of AL(s). The circle's radius R was shown to be the geometrical mean distance from the zero to the poles. That is,

$$R = \sqrt{(a-b)(a-c)} \tag{5.51}$$

The break away and reentry points are easily found from a knowledge that the circle has a radius **R** and is centered at **s** = –a. The circle root locus is shown in Figure 5.18a.

If the loop gain's poles are complex-conjugate, the root locus is an interrupted circle, shown in Figure 5.18b. The circle is still centered on the zero at **s** = – a. The poles are at **s** = $-\alpha \pm j\gamma$. The $A_L(s)$ is

$$A_L(s) = \frac{-K_p\beta(s+a)}{s^2 + s(2\alpha) + (\alpha^2 + \gamma^2)} \tag{5.52}$$

The circle's radius is now found from the Pythagorean theorem:

$$R = \sqrt{(a-\alpha)^2 + \gamma^2} \tag{5.53}$$

Note that as the gain, $K_p\,\beta$, is increased, the closed-loop system poles become more and more damped, until they both become real, one approaching the zero at **s** = –a, the other going to $-\infty$.

The damping of a *complex-conjugate* (CC) *pole-pair* in the s-plane can be determined quantitatively by drawing a line from the origin to the upper-half plane pole. The damping factor, ζ, associated with the CC poles can be shown to be the cosine of the angle the line from the origin to the CC pole makes with the negative real axis. That is, $\xi = \cos(\phi)$. If the poles lie close to the $j\omega$ axis, $\phi \rightarrow 90°$, and $\xi \rightarrow 0$. The length of the line from the origin to one of the CC poles is the undamped natural frequency, ω_n, of that CC pole-pair. Recall that the CC pole pair is the result of factoring the quadratic term, $[s^2 + s(2\xi\omega_n) + \omega_n^2]$. By way of example, the damping of the open-loop, CC pole pair in Figure 5.18b is $\xi = \cos[\tan^{-1}(\gamma/\alpha)] = \alpha/\omega_n$.

Many other interesting examples of root locus plots are to be found in the control systems texts by Kuo (1982) and Ogata (1970) and the electronic circuits text by Gray and Meyer (1984). We have seen that circle root locus plots are easy to construct graphically by hand. More complex root locus plots should be done by computer. In closing, it should be stressed that root locus plots show the closed-loop systems *poles*. Closed-loop zeros can be found algebraically. They are generally fixed (not functions of gain) and do affect system transient response. Merely locating the closed-loop poles in what appear to be a good position does not necessarily guarantee a step response without an objectionable overshoot.

Figure 5.19a–l illustrate typical root locus diagrams for linear, SISO, feedback systems. Locus branches for loop gains with NFB (left column) and for PFB (right column) are shown. The unstable

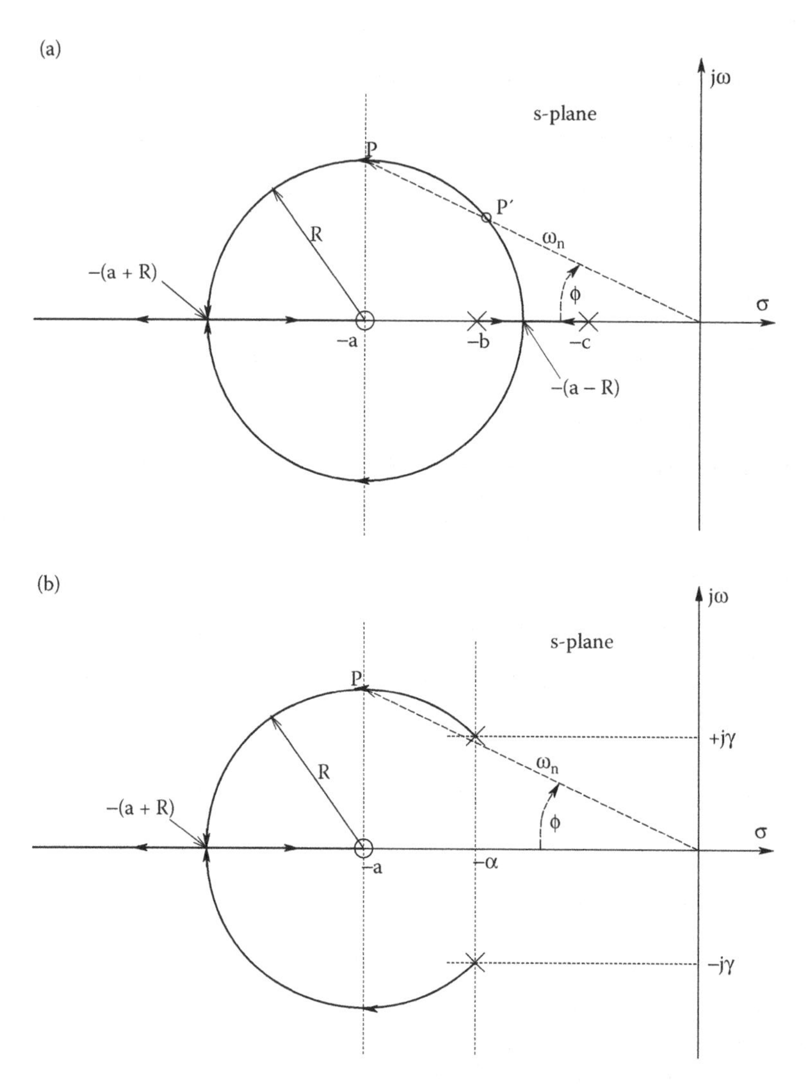

FIGURE 5.18 (a) The well-known circle root locus for a NFB system with two real poles an a high-frequency real zero. See Text for discussion. (b) Interrupted circle root locus for the same NFB system with complex-conjugate poles at $s = -\alpha \pm j\gamma$.

systems oscillate when complex-conjugate closed-loop pole pairs move into the right-half s-plane, and they saturate when one closed-loop pole moves into the right-half s-plane.

5.5 USE OF ROOT LOCUS IN THE DESIGN OF "LINEAR" OSCILLATORS

5.5.1 Introduction

"Linear" oscillators are used to generate sinusoidal signals for many applications; probably the most important is testing the steady-state sinusoidal frequency response of amplifiers; they are also used in measurements as the signal source for AC bridges used to measure the values of circuit components R, L & C, as well as circuit **Z**(jω) and **Y**(jω). Still another oscillator application is a signal source in acoustic measurements. In biomedicine, oscillators are used to power AC current sources in impedance pneumography and plethysmography (Northrop 2002), to power Doppler ultrasound probes, for ultrasonic imaging, and for hearing tests, etc.

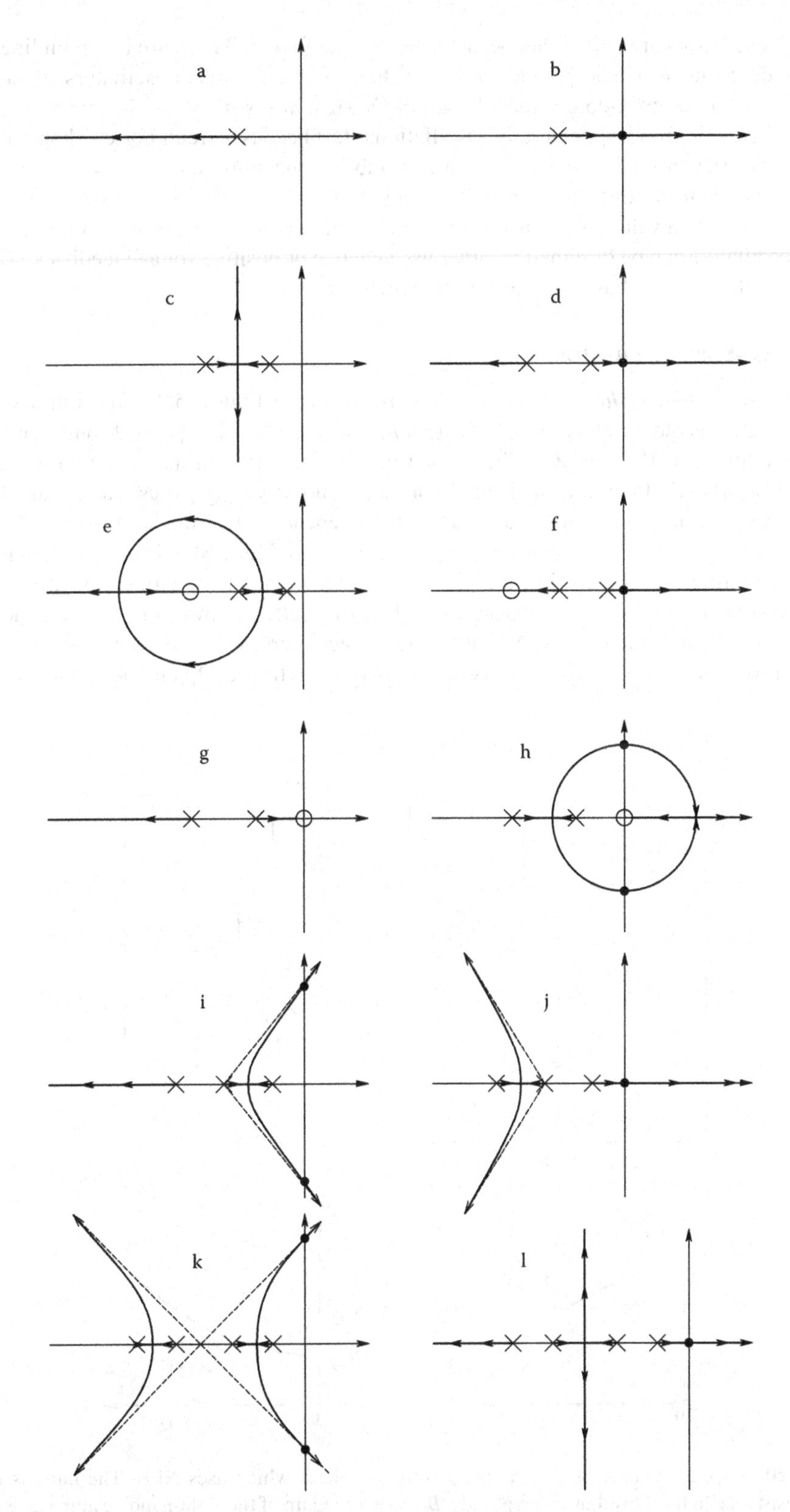

FIGURE 5.19 (a)–(h) Representative root locus plots for four loop gain configurations for both NFB and PFB conditions. PFB root locus plots are on the right. (i)–(l) R-L plots of systems with 3 and 4 real-pole loop gains.

"Linear" oscillators are called that because the criteria for oscillation are based on linear circuit theory and root locus, which is applied to linear systems. In reality, linear oscillators are designed to have a closed-loop, complex-conjugate pole pair *in the right half s-plane,* so that output oscillations, when they start, will grow exponentially. Oscillations start because circuit noise voltages or turn-on transients excite the unstable system. To limit and stabilize the amplitude of the output oscillations, a *nonlinear mechanism* must be used to effectively lower the oscillator's loop gain in an output-dependent manner to a value that will sustain stable oscillations at some design output amplitude.

Linear oscillators can be designed to either use negative or positive voltage feedback. The first to be analyzed below in the phase-shift oscillator which uses NVF.

5.5.2 Phase-Shift Oscillator

A schematic for a *phase-shift oscillator* (PSO) is shown in Figure 5.20. To simplify analysis, the op amps are treated as ideal. The PSO uses *negative feedback* applied through an R-C filter with transfer function, $V_i/V_o = \beta(s)$. The second op amp provides an automatic gain control that reduces the oscillator's loop gain as a function of its output voltage, thus stabilizing the output amplitude. A small tungsten lamp is used as voltage-dependent resistance. As the voltage across the lamp, V_b, increases, its filament heats up (becomes brighter). Metals such as tungsten have positive temperature coefficients, i.e., the filament resistance increases with temperature. Filament temperature is approximately proportional to the lamp's electrical power input, hence the curve of $R_b(V_b)$ is approximately square-law. As the lamp's voltage increases, so does its resistance, and the gain of the inverting op amp stage decreases as shown in the figure. Op amp #2's gain is

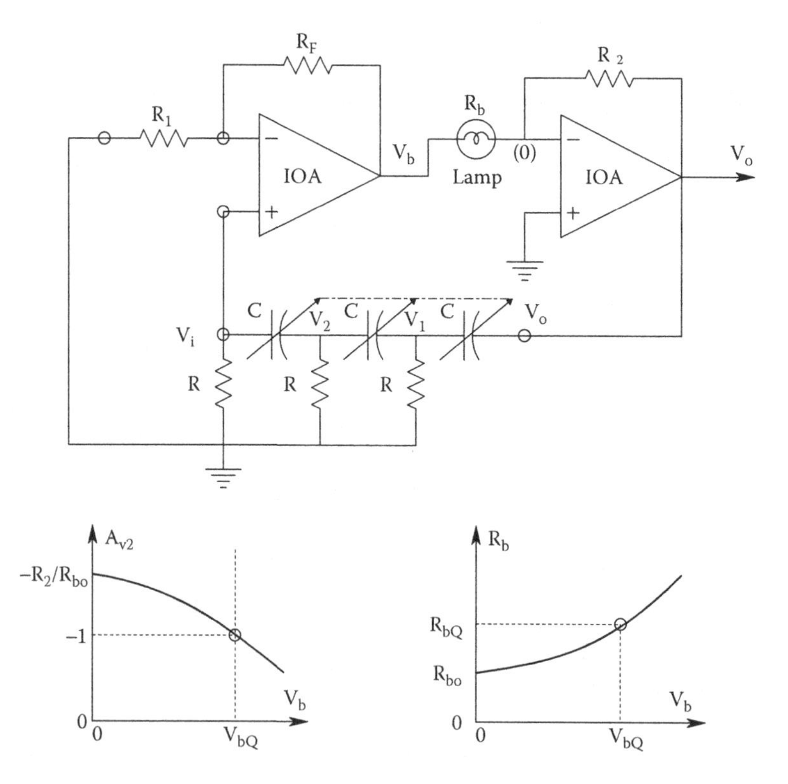

FIGURE 5.20 *Top:* Schematic of an R-C phase-shift oscillator which uses NFB. The lamp is used as a nonlinear resistance to limit oscillation amplitude. *Bottom left:* Gain of the right-hand op amp stage as a function of the RMS V_b across the bulb. *Bottom right:* Resistance of the lamp as a function of the RMS V_b. The resistance increase is due to the tungsten filament heating.

$$\frac{V_o}{V_b} = A_{v2} = -\frac{R_2}{R_b(V_b)} \tag{5.54}$$

R_2 is made equal to the desired $R_b = R_{bQ}$ at the desired $V_b = V_{bQ}$, so $A_{v2} = -1$ when $V_b = V_{bQ}$. If $V_b > V_{bQ}$, then $|A_{v2}| < 1$. The gain of the first (non-inverting) op amp stage is simply $V_b/V_i = (1 + R_F/R_1) = A_{v1}$.

The gain of the feedback circuit is found by writing the three node equations for the circuit:

$$V_1(s2C + G) - V_2 sC + 0 = V_o sC \tag{5.55a}$$

$$-V_1 sC + V_2(s2C + G) - V_i sC = 0 \tag{5.55b}$$

$$0 - V_2 sC + V_i(sC + G) = 0 \tag{5.55c}$$

Using Cramer's rule, we solve for $\beta(s) = V_i/V_o$:

$$\beta(s) = \frac{V_i}{V_o} = \frac{s^3}{s^3 + s^2 6/(RC) + s\ 5/(RC)^2 + 1/(RC)^3} \tag{5.56}$$

The three roots (poles) of $\beta(s)$ are real and negative, i.e., they lie on the negative real axis in the s-plane. Their vector values are found with MATLAB™'s ROOTS utility: $\mathbf{s_1} = -5.0489/(RC)$, $\mathbf{s_2} = -0.6431/(RC)$ & $\mathbf{s_3} = -0.3080/(RC)$. The PS oscillator's loop gain as a function of frequency, in vector form is

$$A_L(s) = \frac{-s^3(1 + R_F/R_1)(R_2/R_b)}{(s - s_1)(s - s_2)(s - s_3)} = \frac{-s^3(1 + R_F/R_1)(R_2/R_b)}{BCD} \tag{5.57}$$

Alternately, $\mathbf{A_L}$ can be written as an unfactored frequency response polynomial:

$$\mathbf{A_L}(j\omega) = \frac{(-j\omega^3)(1 + R_F/R_1)(R_2/R_b)}{[1/(RC)^3 - \omega^2 6/(RC)] + j[\omega\ 5/(RC)^2\ j\omega^3]} \tag{5.58}$$

The *Barkhausen criterion* can be used to find the frequency of oscillation, ω_o, and the critical gain required for a pair of the oscillator's closed-loop, complex-conjugate poles to lie on the $j\omega$ axis in the s-plane. To apply the algebraic Barkhausen criterion, set $\mathbf{A_L}(j\omega_o) = 1\angle 0°$, and note that for $\mathbf{A_L}(j\omega_o)$ to be *real, the real part of its denominator must* = 0. From this condition,

$$-\omega_o^2 6/(RC) + 1/(RC)^3 = 0, \tag{5.59}$$

The oscillation frequency is thus

$$\omega_o = 1/(\sqrt{6}RC) = 0.40825/(RC)\ \text{r/s} \tag{5.60}$$

The critical gain is found by setting

$$\mathbf{A_L}(j\omega_o) = \frac{(-j\omega_o^3)(1 + R_F/R_1)(R_2/R_b)}{-j\omega_o^3 + j\omega_o 5/(RC)^2} = 1 + j0 \tag{5.61}$$

and solving for $(1 + R_F/R_1)(R_2/R_b)$. Thus,

$$(1+R_F/R_1)(R_2/R_b) = 29 \tag{5.62}$$

For oscillations to start, for $V_b \cong 0$, and $(1 + R_F/R_1)(R_2/R_{bo})$ must be >29, so that the system's poles will lie in the right-half s-plane and the oscillations (and V_b) will start and grow exponentially. When V_b reaches V_{bQ}, $R_2/R_b = R_2/R_{bQ} = 1$, and $(1 + R_F/R_1)(R_2/R_b) = 1$, and the PSO's poles are at $\mathbf{s} = \pm j\omega_o$, giving stable oscillations with $V_o = V_{bQ}$.

Although the root locus diagram can be used to find the frequency of oscillation and the critical DC gain (29), in this case, application of the Barkhausen criterion saves the work of having to plot the root locus to-scale and doing a graphical solution. We need not factor the cubic polynomial when using the Barkhausen method. Figure 5.21 illustrates the root locus diagram for the NVF phase-shift oscillator. Pole positions and locus break point from real axis are not to scale. In practice, a PSO can be tuned by varying a triple-ganged parallel-plate capacitor. Oscillator range can be changed by switching the three resistors in the β filter. In the early 1950s, the Hewlett-Packard 200CD audio oscillator used a PSO with this tuning scheme, and also a tungsten filament lamp for amplitude control. Of course, the 200CD oscillator used vacuum tubes, not op amps.

5.5.3 Wien Bridge Oscillator

Another commonly used oscillator that is effective in the millihertz to 100s of kHz range is the Wien bridge oscillator, shown in Figure 5.22. This oscillator uses PVF through a simple R-C filter. The filter's transfer function is

$$\beta(s) = \frac{V_1}{V_o} = \frac{1/(G+sC)}{1/sC + R + 1/(G+sC)} = \frac{s/(RC)}{s^2 + s^3/(RC) + 1/(RC)^2} \tag{5.63}$$

The quadratic denominator of β(s) is easily factored. The roots are at: $\mathbf{s_1} = -2.618/(RC)$ & $\mathbf{s_2} = -0.382/(RC)$. Now the gain of the second op amp is simply $A_v = V_o/V_1 = (1 + R_F/R_{bo})$ for very small V_1. When V_1 increases as the oscillations grow, R_b increases, decreasing A_v to the critical value that balances the oscillator's poles on the jω axis at $\pm j\omega_o$; $A_{vcrit} = (1 + R_F/R_{bQ})$.

The Wien bridge oscillator's loop gain in vector form is

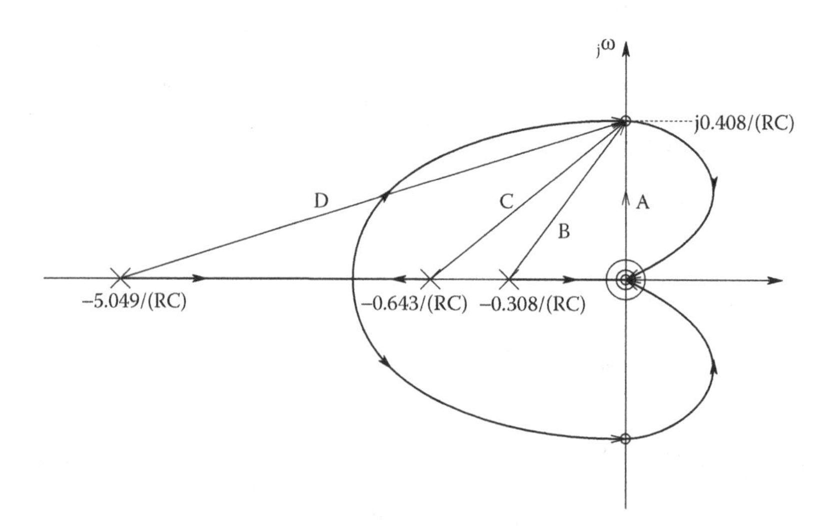

FIGURE 5.21 Root locus diagram of the NFB phase-shift oscillator. Note that the oscillation frequency is *ca.* 0.408/RC r/s.

$$A_L(s) = \frac{+s\,A_v/(RC)}{(s - s_1)(s - s_2)} \tag{5.64}$$

The WB oscillator's root locus diagram is, strangely, a circle, as shown in Figure 5.23. From the RL magnitude criterion, it is possible to write

$$|A_L(j\omega_o)| = \frac{|C|A_v/(RC)}{|A||B|} = 1 = \frac{1/(RC)\ A_v\ 1/(RC)}{\sqrt{[2.618/(RC)]^2 + 1/(RC)^2}\ \sqrt{[(0.382/(RC)]^2 + 1/(RC)^2}} \tag{5.65}$$

$$\downarrow$$

$$1 = \frac{1/(RC)^2 A_v}{1/(RC)^2\,2.80249 \times 1.07048} = A_v/3 \tag{5.66}$$

Thus, when $A_{vcrit} = 3$, the WB oscillator's poles are on the $j\omega$ axis at $s = \pm j/(RC)$, the condition that sustains steady-state output oscillations of amplitude $V_o = 3V_{1Q}$.

Both the Wien bridge and phase-shift oscillators described above have low total harmonic distortion (THD) in their outputs. The low distortion is the result of the use of the tungsten lamp in the automatic gain control nonlinearity. Other oscillators that use diode or zener diode clipping to regulate the oscillator's loop gain can have outputs with greater THD.

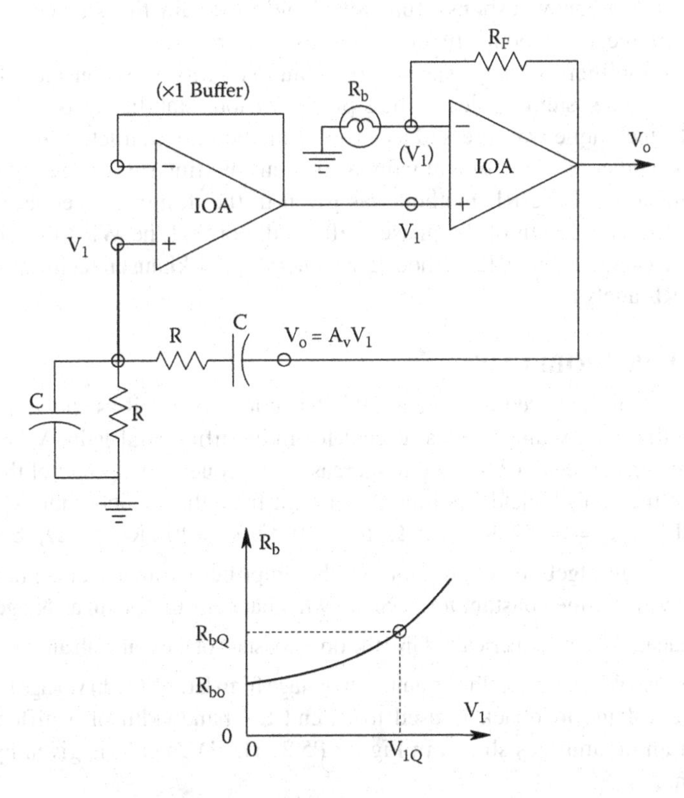

FIGURE 5.22 *Top:* schematic of a PFB, Wien bridge oscillator. The buffer amp is not really necessary if a high input resistance op amp is used for the output. As in the case of the phase-shift oscillator, the oscillation amplitude is regulated by nonlinear feedback from a lamp. *Bottom:* The lamp's resistance as a function of the RMS voltage, V_1, across it.

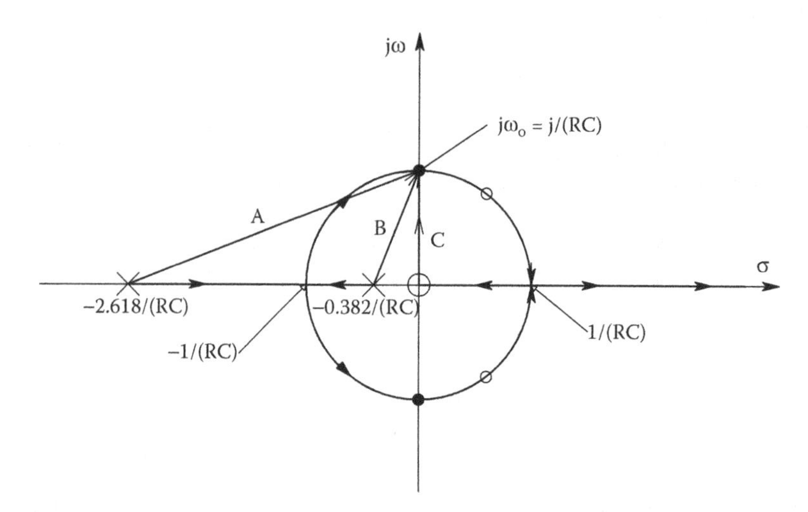

FIGURE 5.23 The Wien bridge oscillator's root locus diagram. Oscillation frequency is near 1/RC r/s.

5.6 CHAPTER SUMMARY

This chapter began with a review of the frequency response as a descriptor for linear amplifier performance. The basics of Bode plotting an amplifier's frequency response were examined, including the use of asymptotes to expedite pencil-and-paper Bode plots, given an amplifier's transfer function or frequency response function. How to obtain the frequency response phase function from the frequency response function was also covered.

The concept of amplifier stability was set forth, and stability was considered from the viewpoint of the location of a system's poles in the s-plane. Various stability tests were mentioned, and the root locus (RL) technique was stressed as a useful method for characterizing a linear feedback system's closed-loop poles as a function of gain. Root locus plotting rules were given with examples of RL plots. Application of the RL method was given in the design of feedback amplifiers with useful pole locations. The design of the phase-shift oscillator and the Wien bridge oscillator were shown to be made easier with the RL method. The venerable Barkhausen technique was introduced as an alternate to RL analysis.

CHAPTER 5 HOME PROBLEMS

5.1 A power op amp is used to drive a CRT deflection yoke coil as shown in Figure P5.1. Assume that the op amp is ideal except for finite differential gain: $V_o = K_v (V_i - V_i')$. Negative current feedback is used to increase the frequency response of the coil current, I_L, hence the coil's B field. Assume the current from the V_F node into R_F is negligible, $L = 0.01$ Hy, $R_L = 0.5\ \Omega$, $R_1 = 10^4\ \Omega$, $R_F = 10^4\ \Omega$, $K_v = 10^4$, $R_M = 1\ \Omega$, & R_F, $R_1 >> R_M$.

(A) Derive an algebraic expression for the amplifier's transfer admittance, $\mathbf{Y}_L(j\omega) = (I_L/V_L)$, in time constant form. Show what happens to $\mathbf{Y}_L(j\omega)$ as K_v. gets very large.

(B) Evaluate $Y_L(j\omega)$ numerically. Give the time constant of the coil with and without feedback.

(C) How would you protect the op amp output stage from large L(di/dt) voltage transient spikes?

5.2 Negative voltage feedback is used to extend the bandwidth of a differential amplifier (not an op amp), as shown in Figure P5.2. The DA's gain is given by the transfer function:

$$V_o = \frac{10^3(V_i - V_i')}{(10^{-3}s+1)(2\times10^{-4}s+1)}$$

(A) Draw the system's root locus diagram to scale. Let $\beta \equiv R_1/(R_1 + R_F)$.

(B) Find the numerical value of β required to give the closed-loop poles a damping factor $\xi = 0.707$.

(C) What is the system's dc gain with the β value found in part B)? Give the system's f_T with this β.

Compare this f_T to the f_T of the amplifier without feedback ($\beta = 0$).

(D) The same amplifier is compensated with a zero in the feedback path. Thus, $\beta = \beta_o (3.333 \times 10^{-5}\,s + 1)$.

Repeat parts A through C above.

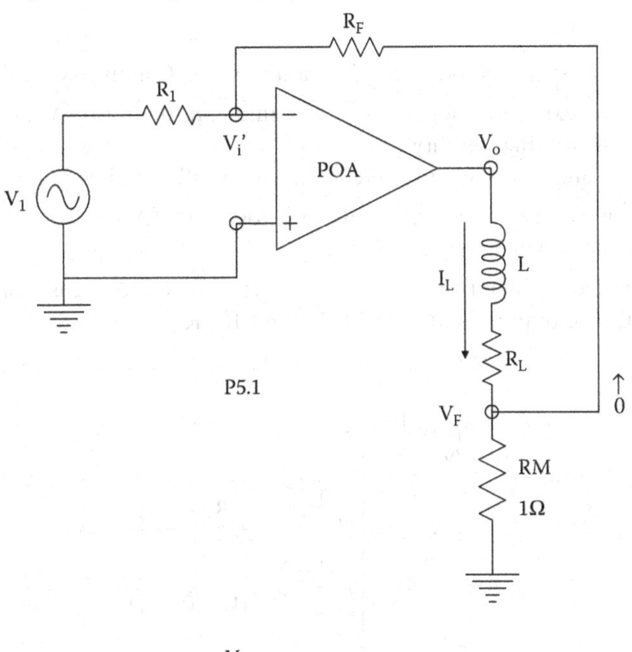

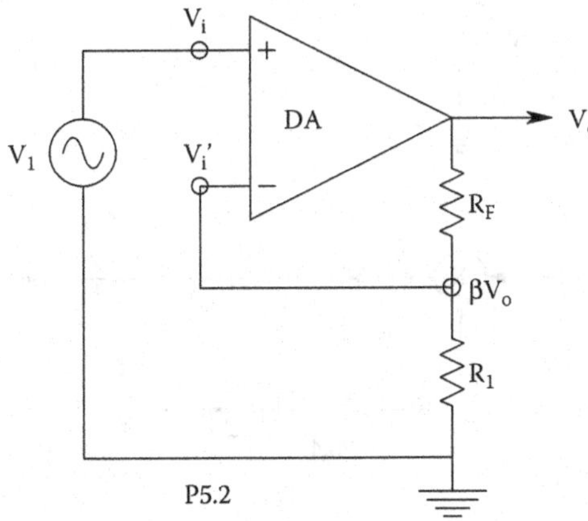

5.3 A nonideal op amp circuit is shown in Figure P5.3. The op amp's transfer function is

$$V_o = \frac{10^4(V_i - V_i')}{(10^{-3}s + 1)} = H_\infty(s)(V_i - V_i')$$

Assume: $R_1 = 10^4\ \Omega$, $R_F = 90\ k\Omega$, $R_o = 100\ \Omega$, & $\beta = R_1/(R_1 + R_F)$.

(A) Find an algebraic expression for the amplifier's Thevenin output impedance, $\mathbf{Z}_{out}(j\omega)$, at the V_o node, in time-constant form. (Neglect $R_F + R_1$ to ground at the output.)

(B) Sketch and dimension the Bode plot asymptotes for $|\mathbf{Z}_{out}(j\omega)|$.

5.4 (A) Use the root locus technique to find the range of feedback gain, β (+ and – values) over which the cubic system of Figure P5.4 is stable.

(B) What is the minimum value of β required for oscillation? At what Hz frequency, f_o, will the system first oscillate?

5.5 Positive voltage feedback is used around an op amp which is ideal except for its gain:

$$\frac{V_o}{V_i} = \frac{+K_v}{\tau_a s + 1}$$

See Figure P5.5.

(A) Sketch the system's root locus diagram to-scale. Can this system oscillate?

(B) Derive an expression for $(V_o/V_1)(s)$ in time-constant form. What conditions on R_1 and R_2 determine stability?

5.6 Two ideal op amps are used to make a "linear" oscillator, shown in Figure P5.6.

(A) Give an expression for the oscillator's loop gain, $A_L(s)$. Note that the oscillator uses positive voltage feedback.

(B) Design the oscillator to oscillate at 3.0 kHz. Use a root locus graphical approach. Specify the required numerical values for R_F, R_1, and C_1.

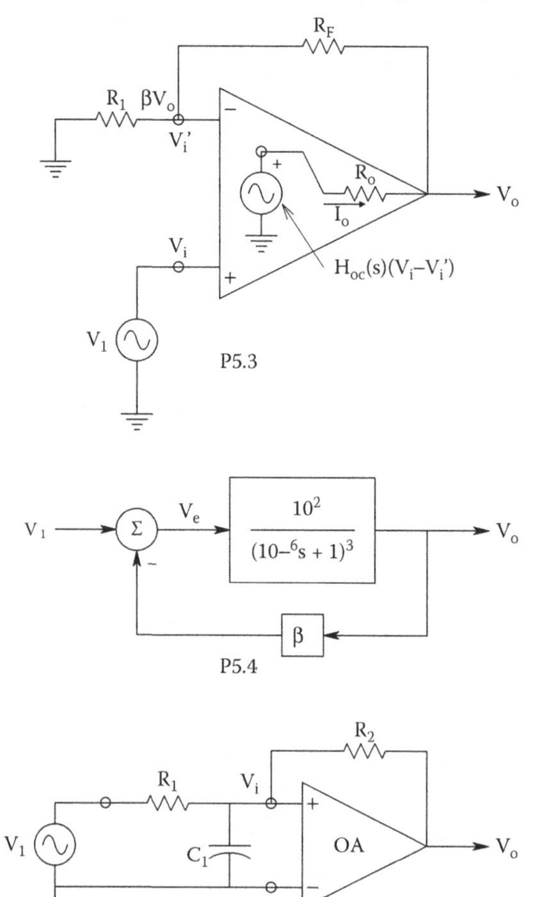

(C) Illustrate a nonlinear circuit means to limit the peak amplitude of V_o to 5.0 V.

5.7 A certain feedback amplifier has the loop gain:

$$A_L(s) = \frac{+K_a(s-400)}{s^2 + s(1000) + 10^6}$$

(A) Assume $K_a > 0$. Draw the system's root locus diagram to scale as a function of increasing K_a. Find the numerical of K_a at which the system is on the verge of oscillation. Find the oscillation frequency, ω_o r/s.

(B) Now assume K_a is < 0. Sketch the system's root locus to scale for increasingly negative K_a. Find the K_a value at which the system has two equal, real, negative poles. (Use MATLAB's™ *RLocus* program.)

5.8 A certain feedback amplifier has the loop gain:

$$A_L(s) = \frac{-K_v}{s^2 + s2\xi\omega_n + \omega_n^2}$$

(A) Plot and dimension the root locus for this system for $0 < Kv \leq \infty$.

(B) Plot and dimension the root locus for this system for $0 > K_v \geq -\infty$. Give an expression for the K_v value at which the system becomes unstable.

5.9 A prototype "linear" oscillator is shown in Figure P5.9. Assume the op amps are ideal.

(A) Find an expression for the transfer function, $(V_2/V_1)(s)$.

(B) Find an expression for the circuit's loop gain. Break the loop at the $V_1 - V_1'$ link. $\mathbf{A_L(j\omega) = V_1'/V_1}$.

(C) Use MATLAB's *RLocus* program to draw the oscillator's root locus diagram as a function of β for positive β. $0 < \beta \leq 1$.

(D) Use the *Barkhausen criterion* to find an expression for the oscillation frequency, ω_o r/s, and the critical gain, β, required for oscillation.

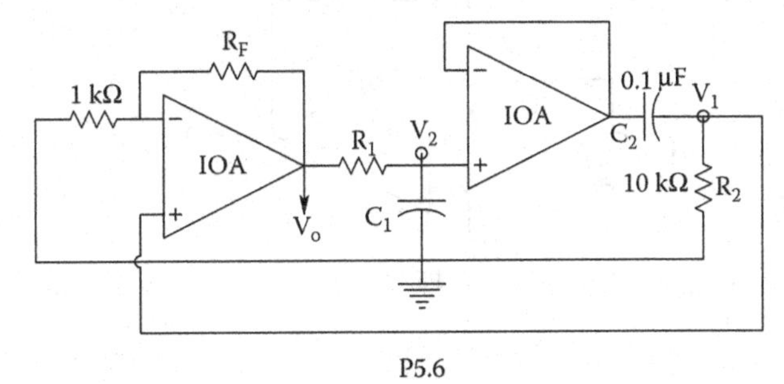

P5.6

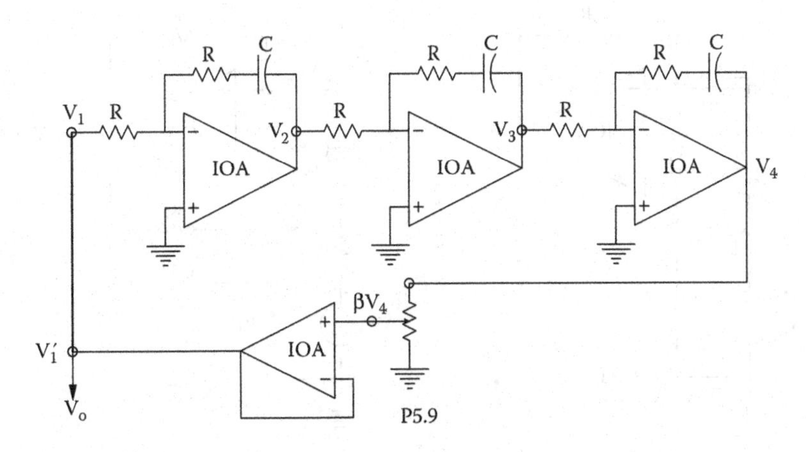

P5.9

5.10 An otherwise ideal op amp has the gain:

$$\frac{V_o}{V_i'}(s) = \frac{-10^5}{10^{-2}s+1}$$

The op amp is connected as a simple inverting gain amplifier, as shown in Figure P5.10.

(A) Find the maximum DC gain the amplifier can have and have a –3 dB frequency of 50 kHz.

That is, find the R_F required.

(B) For the R_F of part (A), find the inverting amplifier's f_T.

5.11 Figure P5.11B illustrates a "Regenerative Magnetic Pickup Circuit" as described in *NASA Tech Briefs #GSC-13309.* The purpose of the circuit is to present a multiturn magnetic search coil with a negative terminating impedance that when summed with the series impedance of the coil itself forms a very low Thevenin impedance, allowing more current, I_s, to flow from the open-circuit induced voltage, $V_s = N\dot{\Phi}$, where N is the number of turns of the search coil, and $\dot{\Phi}$ is the time rate of change of the magnetic flux linking the coil's area. The op amp, less search coil, forms what is called a negative impedance converter circuit (NIC) (Ghaussi 1971, Chapter 8). Assume the op amp is ideal in this analysis.

(A) Refer to Figure P5.11A. Find an expression for the transfer function, $(V_o/V_s)(s)$. Let $L_s = 0.01$ Hy, $R_s = 100\ \Omega$, $R_3 = 10^4$. Also evaluate the transfer function's break frequency, $f_b = \omega_b/2\pi$, and its DC gain.

(B) Refer to Figure P5.11B. Replace the search coil (L_s, R_s) with just the voltage source, V_s. Find expressions for the input current, I_s, and the input impedance looking into the V_i' node. (Note that it emulates a negative inductance.)

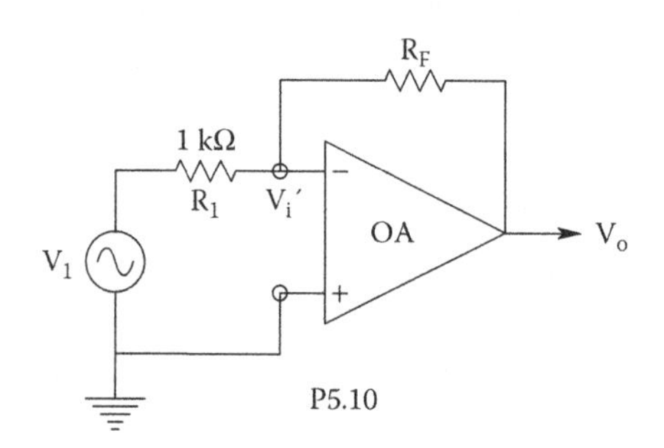

P5.10

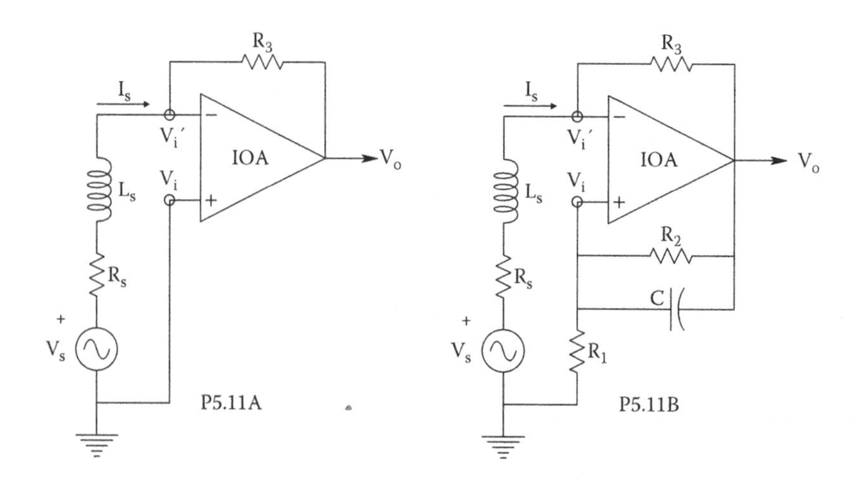

P5.11A

P5.11B

(C) Now consider the search coil in place with open-circuit, induced EMF, V_s. Derive an expression for $(V_o/V_s)(s)$ in time-constant form. Comment on the conditions on the circuit parameters (R_1, R_2, R_3, and C) that will make the circuit unstable or the DC gain infinite.

5.12 Both negative voltage feedback *and* positive current feedback are used on a power op amp circuit, shown in Figure P5.12. The op amp is ideal except for the differential gain:

$$V_o = \frac{K_{vo}(V_i - V_i')}{\tau s + 1}$$

Assume: $(R_1 + R_2) >> (R_3 + R_4)$, $\alpha \equiv R_2 /(R_1 + R_2)$, $\beta \equiv R_1 /(R_1 + R_2)$, $\gamma \equiv R_4/(R_3 + R_4)$.

(A) Assume op amp $R_{out} = 0$. Find an expression for V_o /V_1 in time-constant form. Comment how the PVFB affects the DC gain, corner frequency and gain-bandwidth product.

(B) Now let $R_{out} > 0$. Replace the load resistor, R_3, with a test voltage source, v_t, to find an expression for the Thevenin output resistance R_3 "sees."

5.13 It is desired to physically measure the slew rate of a prototype op amp design. The linear, open-loop, small-signal behavior of the op amp is known to be: $V_o = (V_i - V_i')10^5/(10^{-3}\ s + 1)$. The op amp is connected as a unity-gain follower, as shown in Figure P5.13A.

(A) Find $(V_o/V_s)(s)$ in Laplace form. What is the follower's time constant?

(B) A step input of 100 mV is given, i.e., $V_s(s) = 0.1$ /s. Sketch and dimension $v_o(t)$ at the follower output.

What is the maximum slope of $v_o(t)$?

(C) The follower's response to a 10 V input step, $V_s(s) = 10$/s, is shown in Figure P5.13B. Estimate the op amp's slew rate, η, in V/μs. Sketch and dimension $v_o(t)$ to the 10 V step when the slew rate is assumed to be infinite.

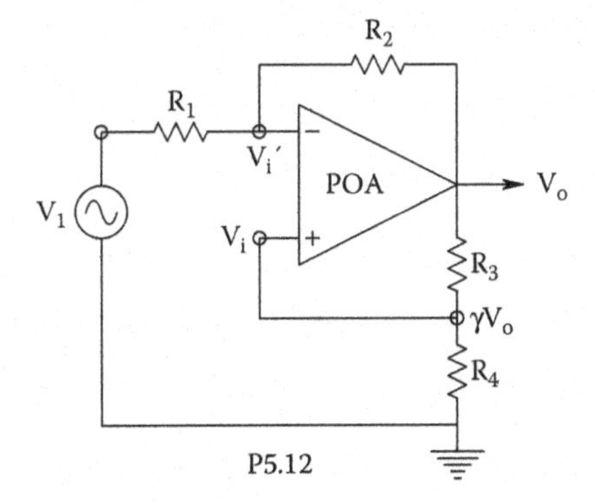

P5.12

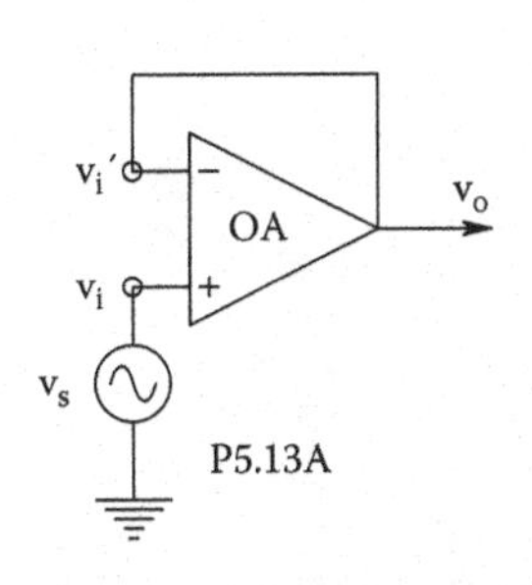

P5.13A

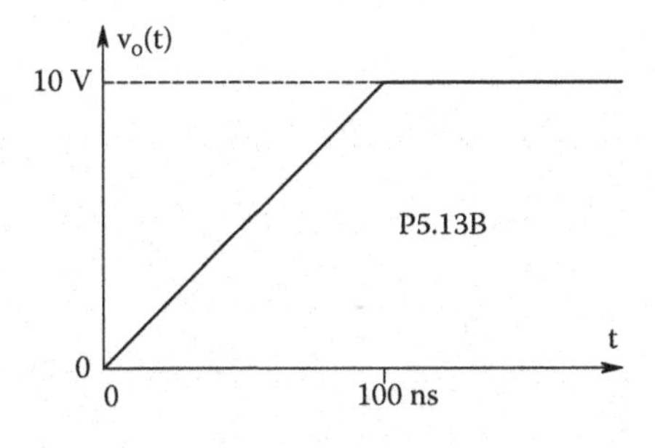

P5.13B

5.14 A certain op amp has open-loop poles at $f_1 = 100$ Hz and at $f_2 = 100$ kHz, and a negative real zero at $f_o = 110$ kHz. Its DC gain is 10^5. The op amp is connected as a non-inverting amplifier (see Text Figure 6.1C). Plot and dimension the amplifier's root locus diagram as a function of the closed-loop DC gain:

$V_o/V_s = (R_1 + R_F)/R_1$. Let V_o/V_s range from 1 to 10^3.

6 Operational Amplifiers and Comparators

6.1 IDEAL OP AMP

6.1.1 INTRODUCTION

The operational amplifier (op amp) had its origins back in the 1940–1960 era of electronics where its principal use was as an active element in analog computer systems. Early op amp circuits used vacuum tubes; op amps were used as summers, subtractors, integrators, filters, etc. in analog computer systems designed to model dynamic, electromechanical feedback systems such as autopilots, bombsights, and motor speed controls. With the rise of digital computers in the 1960s, analog computers were largely replaced for simulations by digital computers using software numerical methods such as IBM's CSMP™, also Tutsim™, Simnon™, MATLAB™, etc. However, electrical engineers found that the basic linear and nonlinear op amp building blocks could be used for analog signal conditioning in other systems. With the advent of semiconductors, op amps were designed with transistors as gain elements, instead of bulky vacuum tubes. The next step, of course, was to design integrated circuit (IC) op amps, one of the first of which was the venerable (but now obsolete) LM741. (Why, you might ask, is the LM741 obsolete? Newer op amps with better gain-bandwidth products have lower DC bias currents (I_B and I_B'), lower DC offset voltages (V_{OS}) and V_{OS} tempco, lower noise, higher DC gains, higher CMRRs, higher Z_{in}s, etc., and are often less expensive.)

At present, operational amplifiers (op amps) are used for a wide spectrum of linear biomedical signal conditioning applications, including *differential instrumentation amplifiers, electrometer amplifiers, low-drift DC signal conditioning, active filters, summers,* etc. Nonlinear op amp applications have expanded to include *true-RMS to DC conversion, precision rectifiers, phase-sensitive rectifiers, peak detectors, log converters,* etc.

Practical op amps come with a variety of specifications from the manufacturer, including, but not limited to

- DC gain, K_{V0}
- Common-mode rejection ratio (CMRR)
- Open-loop DM frequency response
- Gain-bandwidth product (f_T)
- Slew rate (η)
- Output resistance
- Difference-mode input resistance
- Common-mode input resistance
- Input DC bias current (I_B)
- Input short-circuit DC offset voltage (V_{OS})
- Input current noise root power spectrum (i_{na})
- Input short-circuit voltage noise root power spectrum (e_{na})
- Temperature coefficients (tempcos) of certain parameters, such as V_{OS} and I_B.

These specifications generally are included in any simulation program's op amp library and are used for detailed computer simulations of op amp–based, signal conditioning circuits used for design and/or performance analysis. However, it is often expedient for quick, pencil-and-paper analysis to use the parsimonious, *ideal op amp* (IOA) *model,* as described in the next section.

6.1.2 Properties of Ideal Op Amps

The IOA model makes use of the following assumptions: It is a differential voltage amplifier with a single-ended output. It has *infinite* input impedance, gain, CMRR, and bandwidth, as well as *zero* output impedance, noise, I_B, and V_{OS}. The IOA output is from an ideal, differential, voltage-controlled voltage source. As a consequence of the infinite differential gain assumption, a general principle of closed-loop IOA operation (with negative feedback) is that both input signals are equal. Putting it in another way, $(v_i - v_i') = 0$; hence, a finite output is obtained when the product of zero input and infinite differential gain is considered. In mathematical terms,

$$|(v_i - v_i')\, K_v| = |(0)\infty| = |v_o| < \infty \tag{6.1}$$

6.1.3 Some Examples of Op Amp Circuits Analyzed Using IOAs

The best way to appreciate how the IOA model is used is to consider some examples. In the first example, consider the simple inverting amplifier shown in Figure 6.1a. By the zero input voltage criterion described earlier, because the noninverting input is at ground potential, so must be the inverting input. This means that the inverting input (also called the op amp's summing junction) is a virtual ground; it is forced to be at 0 V by the negative feedback through the $R_F - R_1$ voltage divider. Because the *summing junction* (SJ) is at 0 V, the current in R_1 is by Ohm's law, $i_1 = v_s/R_1$. i_1 enters

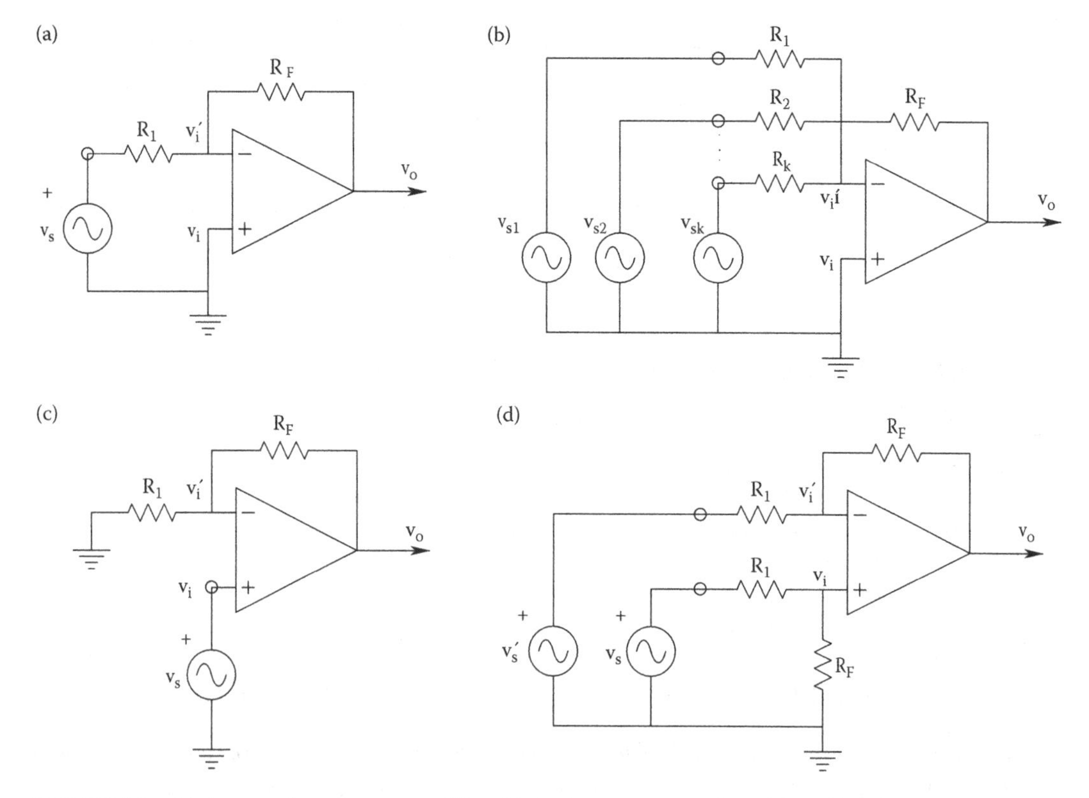

FIGURE 6.1 (a) An inverting op amp amplifier. (b) An inverting amplifier with multiple inputs. (c) A noninverting op amp amplifier. (d) An op amp difference amplifier.

the SJ and leaves through R_F. (No current flows into the IOA's inverting input because it has infinite input resistance.) By Ohm's law, the IOA's output voltage must be

$$v_o = -i_1 R_F = v_s(-R_F / R_1) \tag{6.2}$$

Thus, the simple inverting op amp's gain is $v_o/v_s = (-R_F/R_1)$. The minus sign comes from the fact that the SJ end of R_F is at 0 V.

In the second example, k input voltage signals are added in the inverting configuration; see Figure 6.1b. Currents through each of R_1, R_2, R_3, . . . R_k are added at the SJ. The net current is again found from Ohm's law and Kirchoff's current law:

$$i_{net} = v_{s1} / R_1 + v_{s2} / R_2 + \ . \ . \ . + v_{sk} / R_k \tag{6.3}$$

i_{net} flows through R_F, giving the output voltage

$$v_o = -R_F[v_{s1}G_1 + v_{s2}G_2 + . . . + v_{sk}G_k] \tag{6.4}$$

where it is obvious that $G_k = 1/R_k$, and $k = 3, 4, \ldots$.

In the third example, consider the basic, *noninverting IOA circuit*, shown in Figure 6.1c. In this case, the noninverting input is forced to be v_s by the source. Thus, the voltage at the SJ is also v_s. Now it is seen that resistors R_1 and R_F form a voltage divider, the input of which is some v_o which will force $v_i' = v_s$. The voltage divider relation

$$v_s = v_o \frac{R_1}{R_1 + R_F} \tag{6.5}$$

can be easily solved for v_o:

$$v_o = v_s(1 + R_F / R_1) \tag{6.6}$$

Thus, the noninverting IOA's gain is $(1 + R_F/R_1)$. If the output of the IOA is connected directly to the SJ (i.e. $R_F = 0$), clearly, $v_o/v_s = +1$, resulting in a unity-gain buffer amplifier with infinite R_{in} and zero R_{out}.

In example four, Figure 6.1d illustrates an IOA circuit configured to make a *differential amplifier.* To illustrate how this circuit works, we use *superposition.* The output from each source considered alone with the other sources set to zero is summed to give the net output. From the *first example,* $v_o' = v_s'(-R_F/R_1)$. (v_i remains zero because no current flows in the lower voltage divider with v_s set to zero.) Now set $v_s' = 0$, and consider v_i due to v_s. From the voltage divider at the noninverting input, $v_i = v_s R_F/(R_1 + R_F)$. Because the OA is ideal, $v_i' = v_i = v_s R_F/(R_1 + R_F)$. Using the noninverting gain relation derived in example three, v_o appears to be

$$v_o = [v_s R_F/(R_1 + R_F)](1 + R_F/R_1) = v_s(R_F/R_1) \tag{6.7}$$

Thus, the output voltage from both sources together is

$$v_o = [v_s - v_s'](R_F / R_1) \tag{6.8}$$

That is, the circuit appears as an ideal DA with a differential gain of (R_F/R_1). There are several reasons why a simple DA circuit like this is impractical in the real world. First, to get ideal DA performance, the actual DA must have an infinite CMRR, and second, the congruent resistors in the circuit must be *perfectly* matched. Also, the IOA analysis we have shown assumes ideal voltage sources in v_s and v_s'. Any finite, Thevenin source resistance associated with either source will add to either R_1, destroying the match and degrading the DA's CMRR.

As the fifth example of the use of the IOA assumption in analyzing OA circuits, consider the *full-wave rectifier circuit* shown in Figure 6.2. This is a nonlinear circuit because it uses diodes. The volt–ampere behavior of a *pn* junction diode is often approximated by the nonlinear equation:

$$i_D = I_{RS}[\exp(v_D / \eta V_T) - 1] \tag{6.9}$$

However, in this example, we will invoke the *ideal diode approximation* in which $i_D = 0$ for $v_D < 0$, and $v_D = 0$ for $i_D > 0$. This relation is shown in Figure 6.3a, and the diode equation is plotted in Figure 6.3b. Needless to say, an ideal diode compliments other electrical engineering idealizations, such as the ideal voltage source, current source, op amp, transformer, resistor, capacitor, and inductor.

To see how this circuit works, consider the voltages V_2 and V_3 as V_s is varied. First, it is obvious that if $V_s = 0$, then $V_2 = V_3 = 0$. Now let $V_s > 0$: The SJ voltage remains zero, and current i_s flows inward through the SJ. It cannot exit through D_1 because current cannot flow though an ideal diode in the reverse direction. The current, i_s, however, does flow through R_F and D_1. By Ohm's law, the voltage $V_2 = (V_s/R_1)(-R_F) = -V_s\,(R_F/R_1)$. V_3 is infinitesimally more negative than V_2 so D_2 will conduct.

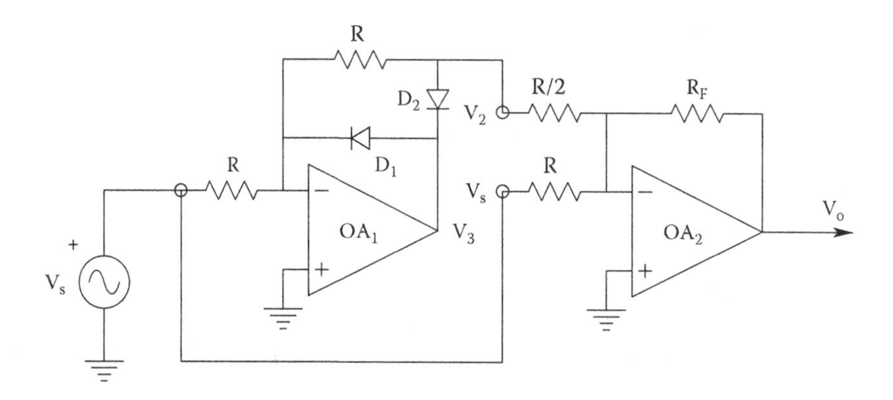

FIGURE 6.2 A full-wave rectifier (or absolute value circuit) using two op amps.

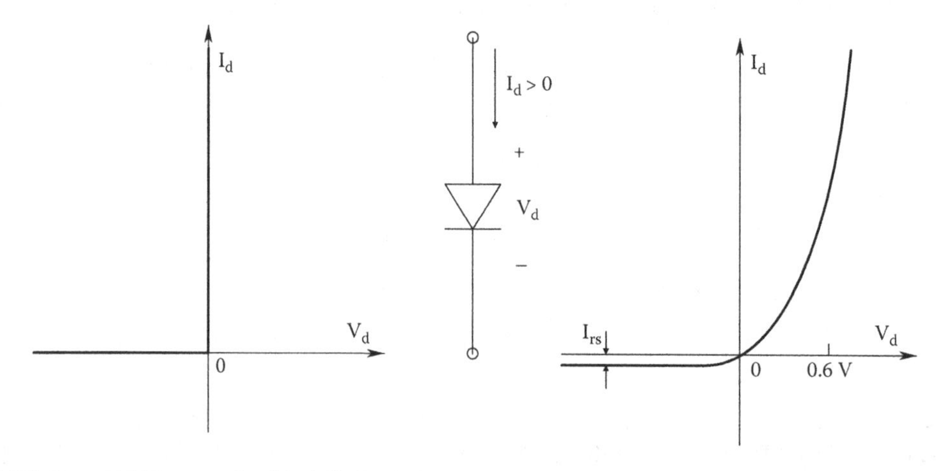

FIGURE 6.3 (a) I-V curve of an ideal diode. (b) I-V curve of a practical diode in which $i_D = I_{rs}[\exp(v_D/v_T) - 1]$.

Now consider $V_s < 0$: A current V_s/R_1 leaves the SJ; D_2 does not conduct, hence $V_3 = 0 + \varepsilon$. If no current flows through R_F, V_2 equals the SJ voltage, 0. In other words, V_2 sees a Thevenin OCV = 0 through a Thevenin resistor, R_F. To summarize: When $V_s > 0$, V_2 appears as an OCV of $-V_s(R_F/R_1)$ through a Thevenin series resistance of R_F ohms. When $V_s < 0$, the diodes cause the OCV, $V_2 = 0$ to appear through a Thevenin series R of R_F ohms.

V_o of the output IOA is given by

$$V_o = -R_F[V_s G + V_2 2G] \tag{6.10}$$

When the relations between V_2 and V_s above are combined in Equation 6.10, and R_1 and R_F are set equal to R, It is easy to show that in the ideal case.

$$V_o = (R_F / R)|V_s| \tag{6.11}$$

As the sixth example, consider the IOA representation of a *voltage-controlled current source* (VCCS) circuit. Figure 6.4 illustrates one version of the VCCS. (This circuit is found in several examples in this text.) The load, R_L, has one end tied to ground, and can be either linear (a resistance) or nonlinear (e.g., a laser diode). It is clear from Ohm's law that $(V_o - V_L)/R_F = i_L$, thus $V_L = V_o - i_L R_F$. It is also known from IOA behavior that the SJ voltage will be held at V_s by the feedback. Now one writes a node equation summing the currents *leaving* the SJ:

$$V_s[2G] - V_L[G] - V_o[G] = 0 \tag{6.12}$$

The conductances cancel, and we substitute $V_L = V_o - i_L R_F$ into Equation 6.12. The final result is simply

$$i_L = V_s G_F \tag{6.13}$$

The transconductance of the VCCS is simply G_F of the feedback resistor. Note that the unity-gain buffer is used so that all of i_L flows into R_L to ground. (This is especially important if R_L is a glass micropipette electrode with R_L on the order of hundreds of megohms.) The inverting IOA_3 is required so that the voltage difference across R_F is sensed to give current feedback. IOA_1 supplying

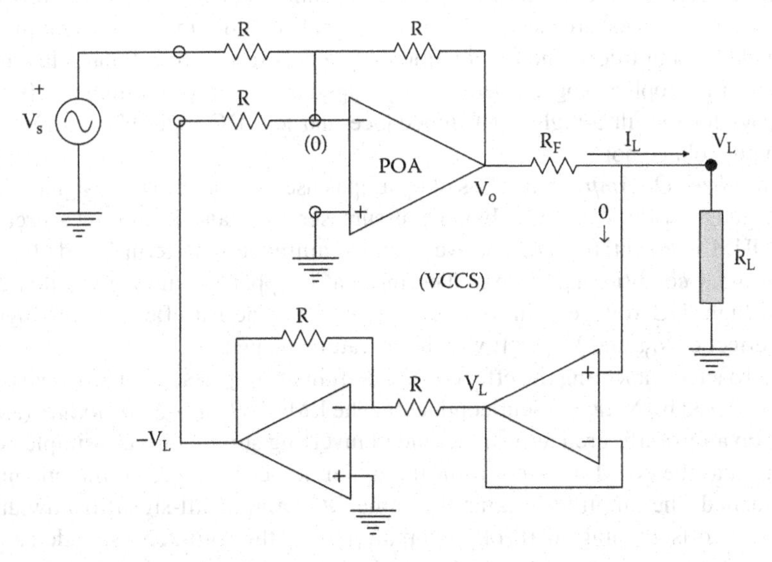

FIGURE 6.4 The three op amp VCCS.

i_L in a practical VCCS of this architecture can be a high-voltage output type, or a power op amp if high i_L is required.

Many more examples of IOA circuits can be considered. There are a number of them in the chapter home problems.

6.2 PRACTICAL OP AMPS

6.2.1 Introduction

Practical op amps are characterized by a set of parameters that were listed above in Section 6.1.1. In addition, the drift temperature (tempcos) coefficients are generally given for (V_{OS}), and the input DC bias currents (I_B, I_B'). Changes in these parameters can affect an op amp's DC output voltage. In the sections below, we will examine how a practical OA's parameters determine its behavior.

6.2.2 Functional Categories of Real Op Amps

Engineers and manufacturers group op amps into functional categories each of which has a set of unique features that makes them suitable for a unique design application. Six of these categories are described below.

Low-Noise Op Amps: Signal conditioning system design with low-noise op amps in the headstage is mandatory for maximum SNR_{out}. Low noise op amps can be characterized by low values of their equivalent short-circuit input voltage noise root spectrum, e_{na} nVrms/√Hz. In the author's experience, any op amp with an $e_{na} < 4$ nVrms/√Hz should be categorized as low noise. Some op amps with FET input transistors (head-stages) have exceptionally low equivalent input current noise, i_{na}, as well as low e_{na}. However, some of the lowest-noise op amps have BJT headstages, and boast e_{na}s in the order of 1 nVrms/√Hz. For example, the venerable OP-27 op amp has $e_{na} = 3.1$ nV/√Hz, and $i_{na} = 1$ pA/√Hz at 30 Hz. It uses a BJT headstage architecture and has $I_B = 12$ nA.

Electrometer Op Amps: The two salient properties of electrometer amplifiers are their ultra-low DC input bias currents, and their extra-high input resistances. For example, the Analog Devices' AD549 is an electrometer-grade, JFET headstage OA. Its I_B is rated from 60 to 200 fA (10^{15} A), but in selected units, can approach ±10 fA. R_{in} is on the order of 10^{13}–$10^{14}\,\Omega$, $e_{na} = 35$ nV/√Hz, $i_{na} = 0.16$ fArms/√Hz at 1 kHz, and there is 4 μVppk short-circuit input voltage noise in the 0.1–10 Hz band. Electrometer op amps (EOAs) are used to design d-c signal conditioning systems for pH meter glass electrodes, for charge amplifiers, and for conditioning signals from intracellular, glass micropipette electrodes used in neurophysiology, where source impedances can be as high as $10^9\,\Omega$. With the AD549, one pays for the ultra-high input impedance and low DC input bias current with a high short-circuit input voltage noise, e_{na}.

Chopper-Stabilized Op Amps: This class of op amp is used to condition DC signals from devices such as strain gauge bridges (used in blood pressure sensors), and in any measurement system in which the QUM is essentially DC and we wish to minimize long-term DC drift at the output of the analog signal conditioning system. The internal chopper circuitry gives this class of OA an exceptional high, DC voltage gain, on the order of 10^8. The net effect of this high gain is to minimize the effect of V_{OS} and V_{OS} drift with temperature change.

Another approach to canceling the effect of V_{OS} drift in op amps used in DC signal conditioning applications is offered by National Semiconductor. The LMC669 *auto-zero module* (AZM) can be used with any op amp configured as a single-ended inverting summer or as a simple noninverting amplifier. Note that the AZM does not limit the dynamic performance of the op amp circuit to which it is attached; the amplifier retains the same DC gain, small-signal bandwidth and slew rate. The effective offset voltage drift of any op amp using the auto-zero is made ca. 100 nV/°C. The maximum offset voltage using the AZM is ± 5 μV. The auto-zero's bias currents are ca. 5 pA (these must be added to the op amp's I_B in the inverting architecture); its clock frequency can be set from 100 Hz to 100 kHz. The National LMC669 auto-zero module is very useful to compensate for DC drift in circuits using special-purpose op amps, such as electrometers which normally have large offset voltages (≥200 μV) and large V_{OS} tempcos (≥5 μV/°C). The auto-zero does contribute to an increase in the circuit's equivalent input voltage noise. However, choice of sampling rate and step size, and the use of low-pass filtering in the feedback path can minimize this effect.

Wide-Band and High Slew Rate Op Amps: Wide-band and high slew-rate op amps are used for conditioning signals such as ultrasound (CW and pulsed) at frequencies in the 10s of MHz, as well as pulsed signals acquired in PET and SPECT imaging systems. A measure of op amp *small-signal bandwidth* is its unity gain bandwidth, f_T. In many op amps, f_T is also the device's gain-bandwidth product. As illustrated in some detail below, under closed-loop conditions there is a trade-off between op amp amplifier gain and bandwidth. For example, the Comlinear CLC440 voltage feedback op amp has $f_T = 750$ MHz. This means that when given a noninverting gain of 5, the –3 dB frequency will be 150 MHz using this amplifier, and 75 MHz when the gain is 10, etc. The CLC440 op amp has a relatively low $e_{na} = 4.5\ \text{nV}/\sqrt{\text{Hz}}$ at 1 kHz.

The *slew rate*, η, is the maximum rate of change of the output voltage; it is a nonlinear, large-signal parameter. If the input voltage is a high-frequency sine wave, the output, if slew-rate-limited, will appear triangular (except for the rounded tips) if its slope magnitude ($2\pi f V_{pk}$) exceeds the slew rate. The slew rate is defined mathematically as

$$\eta = \left|\frac{dV_o}{dt}\right|_{max} \tag{6.14}$$

The slew rate of the wide-bandwidth, CLC440 op amp is η = 1500 V/μs. High f_T op amps all have high ηs.

The AD549 electrometer op amp described above has $f_T = 0.7$ MHz and η = 2 V/μs; definitely not a wide-band op amp. There is no need to pay for high f_T and η if an op amp circuit is not required to amplify high frequencies at high amplitudes, or condition narrow, short rise-time pulses.

Current Feedback Op Amps: Figure 6.5 illustrates the circuit architecture of a CFOA connected as a noninverting amplifier. Note that internally, it uses a current-controlled voltage source (CCVS) to make its output Thevenin open-circuit voltage. The output voltage is given by

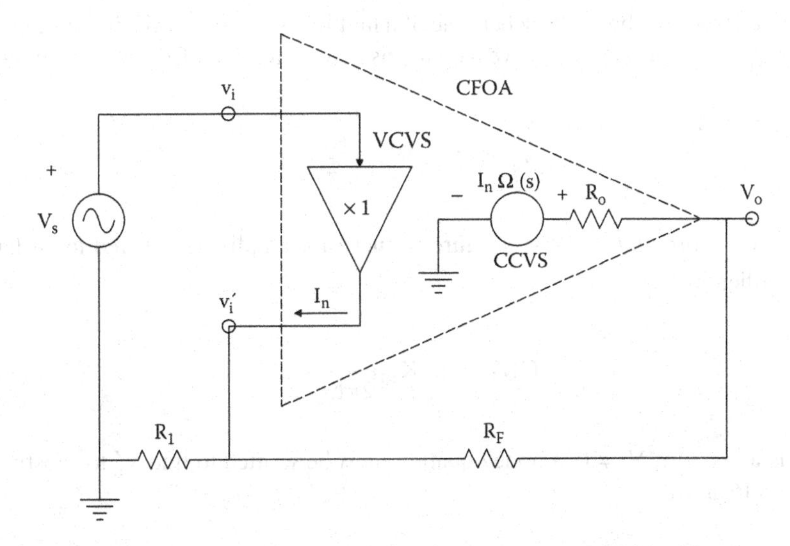

FIGURE 6.5 Simplified internal circuitry of a current-feedback op amp (CFOA). The output current of the unity gain VCVS controls the output of the Thevenin CCVS.

$$V_o = I_c \frac{\Omega_o}{\tau_s + 1} \tag{6.15}$$

Ω_o is the CFOA's *DC transresistance*. The input to the CFOA is a unity-gain, voltage-controlled voltage source (VCVS). The noninverting input (v_i) has a very high input resistance. The resistance looking into the inverting input (v_i') node is generally < 50 Ω; it is the Thevenin output resistance of the unity-gain, VCVS.

The output current of the VCVS, I_n, is determined by Kirchoff's current law (a node equation) written on the low-impedance, inverting (v_i') node. The R_{out} of the CCVS is also <50 Ω and generally can be neglected in pencil-and-paper analysis. The CFOA has many interesting properties which are described in Section 6.4 below. One interesting property is that unlike a voltage-input OA, the CFOA connected as a noninverting amplifier does not trade off bandwidth for closed-loop gain. Its gain can be shown to be set by R_1, while its closed-loop corner frequency is set by R_F. Its closed-loop DC gain is $(1 + R_F/R_1)$, similar to that of a conventional, noninverting, voltage feedback OA.

Power Op Amps: Power op amps are typically used as audio power amplifiers, drivers for small DC servo motors, powering ultrasound transducers, and as drivers for LEDs and laser diodes (as VCCSs). Most conventional op amps can source no more than about ±10 mA, also their output voltages saturate at slightly below their DC supply voltages, usually no more than ±15 V. The most robust power op amps (e.g., the Apex PA03) typically can source as much as ±30 A, given a supply voltage range of ±15 to ±75 V, and dissipate 500 W maximum. The PA03 has a slew rate of $\eta = 8$ V/μs and an $f_T = 1$ MHz. Other POAs such as the Apex PA85 have extraordinary dynamic properties: Namely, $I_{omax} = \pm$ 350 mA(peak), a supply voltage range of ±75/600 V, a power dissipation of 40 W, a slew rate of 1000 V/μs, and $f_T = 100$ MHz. The PA85 is well-suited to drive ultrasound transducers.

See Section 12.3 in this text for additional description of power op amps and their uses in biomedicine.

6.3 GAIN-BANDWIDTH RELATIONS FOR VOLTAGE-FEEDBACK OAS

6.3.1 GBWP of an Inverting Summer

Refer to Figure 6.1b which shows the schematic of a multiple (k)-input, inverting summer amplifier. The open loop op amp is assumed to have a compensated, differential frequency response modeled by

$$V_o = (V_i - V_i') \frac{K_{vo}}{j\omega\, \tau_a + 1} \tag{6.16}$$

The *gain-bandwidth product* (GBWP, a figure of merit for amplifiers, desired to be large) of the open-loop amplifier is

$$GBWP_{ol} \equiv K_{vo} \frac{1}{2\pi\tau_a} \text{ Hz} \tag{6.17}$$

Because this is a real OA, $V_i' \neq 0$, a node equation must be written to find V_i' to substitute into the gain Equation 6.16 above.

$$(V_i' - V_{s1})G_1 + (V_i' - V_{s2})G_2 + \ldots + (V_i' - V_{sk})G_k + (V_i' - V_o)G_F = 0 \tag{6.18}$$

$$\downarrow$$

$$V_i' = \frac{\left(\sum_{j=1}^{k} V_{sj} G_j\right) + V_o G_F}{G_F + \left(\sum_{j=1}^{k} G_j\right)} \tag{6.19}$$

Let us define: $\Sigma G \equiv \left[G_F + \sum_{j=1}^{k} G_j\right]$, and note that: $V_i' = \dfrac{-V_o(j\omega\tau_a + 1)}{K_{vo}}$ (6.20)

Hence, we can solve Equation 6.19 for V_o:

$$V_o = \frac{\dfrac{-K_{vo}\sum_{j=1}^{k} V_{sj} G_j}{\Sigma G + G_F K_{vo}}}{\dfrac{j\omega\tau_a \Sigma G}{\Sigma G + G_F K_{vo}} + 1} \tag{6.21}$$

The DC gain of the closed-loop frequency response function above for V_{sj} is simply

$$K_{dcj} = \frac{-G_j K_{vo}}{\Sigma G + G_F K_{vo}} \tag{6.22}$$

The closed-loop bandwidth for *all* V_{sj} is f_b:

$$f_b = \frac{\Sigma G + G_F K_{vo}}{2\pi\tau_a \Sigma G} \text{Hz} \tag{6.23}$$

The gain-bandwidth product for the jth input is

$$GBWP_j = \frac{K_{vo} G_j}{2\pi\tau_a \Sigma G} = \frac{GBWP_{OA} G_j}{\Sigma G} \tag{6.24}$$

where $(K_{vo}/2\pi\tau_a)$ is the GBWP of the open-loop OA, and $\Sigma G \equiv G_F + G_1 + G_2 + \ldots + G_k$.

Thus, the GBWP of the inverting OA summer is always slightly less than the GBWP of the OA alone, and depends on the circuit's gains.

6.3.2 GBWP of a Noninverting Voltage-Feedback OA

From Figure 6.1c, we see that the output of the noninverting amplifier can be written as

$$V_o = (V_s - V_i') \frac{K_{vo}}{j\omega\tau_a + 1} \tag{6.25}$$

As it was shown above, the OA alone has a GBWP given by $GBWP_{ol} = K_{vo}/(2\pi\tau_a)$. The summing junction voltage is found from the node equation:

$$(V_i' - V_o)G_F + V_i'G_1 = 0 \tag{6.26}$$

$$\downarrow$$

$$V_i' = V_oG_F/(G_1 + G_F) \tag{6.27}$$

Equation 6.27 for V_i' is substituted into Equation 6.25 to yield the noninverting amplifier's closed-loop frequency response:

$$\frac{V_o}{V_S} = \frac{\dfrac{K_{vo}(R_F + R_1)}{R_1(1 + K_{vo}) + R_F}}{\dfrac{j\omega\tau_a(R_F + R_1)}{R_1(1 + K_{vo}) + R_F} + 1} \tag{6.28}$$

The noninverting amplifier's DC gain is the numerator of Equation 6.28. In the limit, for very large K_{vo}, (where $K_{vo}R_1 >> R_F$), the DC gain is simply

$$K_{dc} \cong 1 + R_F/R_1 \tag{6.29}$$

which is the same as for an *IOA*. The closed-loop break frequency is

$$f_b = \frac{R_1(1 + K_{vo}) + R_F}{2\pi\tau_a(R_F + R_1)} \text{ Hz} \tag{6.30}$$

The noninverting amplifier's GBWP is thus

$$GBWP_{ni} = [Kvo / (2\pi\tau)] \text{ Hz} \tag{6.31}$$

Thus, $GBWP_{ni}$ *is the same as the op amp itself, and is independent of gain.* So, there is an ideal hyperbolic relation between closed-loop –3 dB frequency (f_{bcl}) and closed-loop gain. Thus,

$$f_{bcl} = [K_{vo} / (2\pi\tau_a)] / (1 + R_F / R_1) \text{ Hz} \tag{6.32}$$

The noninverting op amp amplifier is unique in this property.

6.4 GAIN-BANDWIDTH RELATIONS IN CURRENT FEEDBACK AMPLIFIERS

6.4.1 Noninverting Amplifier Using a CFOA

Refer to Figure 6.5. Assume that the CCVS has a transimpedance with frequency response

$$\frac{V_o}{I_C} = \frac{\Omega_o}{j\omega\tau_a + 1} \tag{6.33}$$

The gain-bandwidth product of the CCVS is simply $\Omega_o/(2\pi\tau_a)$ Ω Hz (note units).

A small, Thevenin source resistance appears in series with V_o from the CCVS. This R_o is << R_F, so we will neglect it. There is also a small, Thevenin R_o in series with the VCVS at the CFOA's input which we will neglect. We write a node equation at the V_i' node. Note that $V_i' = V_s$.

$$(V_s - V_o)G_F + V_sG_1 = I_c \tag{6.34}$$

Substituting Equation 6.34 for I_c into Equation 6.33, we obtain

$$V_o = \frac{[(V_s - V_o)G_F + V_sG_1]\Omega_o}{j\omega\tau_a + 1} \tag{6.35}$$

Equation 6.35 is solved for the frequency response of the closed-loop system:

$$\frac{V_o}{V_s}(j\omega) = \frac{(G_F + G_1)\Omega_o/(1 + G_F\Omega_o)}{j\omega\tau_a/(1 + G_F\Omega_o) + 1} \tag{6.36}$$

The closed-loop amplifier's break frequency is f_{bcl}:

$$f_{bcl} = \frac{1 + G_F\Omega_o}{2\pi\tau_a} = \frac{\Omega_o + R_F}{2\pi\tau_aR_F} \cong \frac{\Omega_o}{2\pi\tau_aR_F}, \text{because } \Omega_o >> R_F. \tag{6.37}$$

The closed-loop break frequency is solely a function of R_F; *it is independent of gain*. The closed-loop gain-bandwidth product of the noninverting, CFOA amplifier is easily found to be

$$\text{GBWP} = \frac{\Omega_o}{2\pi\tau_aR_F}(1 + R_F/R_1) = \frac{\Omega_o}{2\pi\tau_a}(G_F + G_1) \text{ Hz} \tag{6.38}$$

Curiously, the GBWP depends on the absolute values of the gain-determining resistors.

6.4.2 Inverting Amplifier Using a CFOA

Next, let us examine the gain-bandwidth relations in a CFOA connected as a simple inverter. Figure 6.6 shows the circuit. Note that the noninverting input node is grounded, so $v_i = v_i' = 0$. A node equation can still be written on the v_i' node:

$$(0 - V_s)G_1 + (0 - V_o)G_F - I_c = 0 \tag{6.39}$$

$$\downarrow$$

$$I_c = -(V_sG_1 + V_oG_F) \tag{6.40}$$

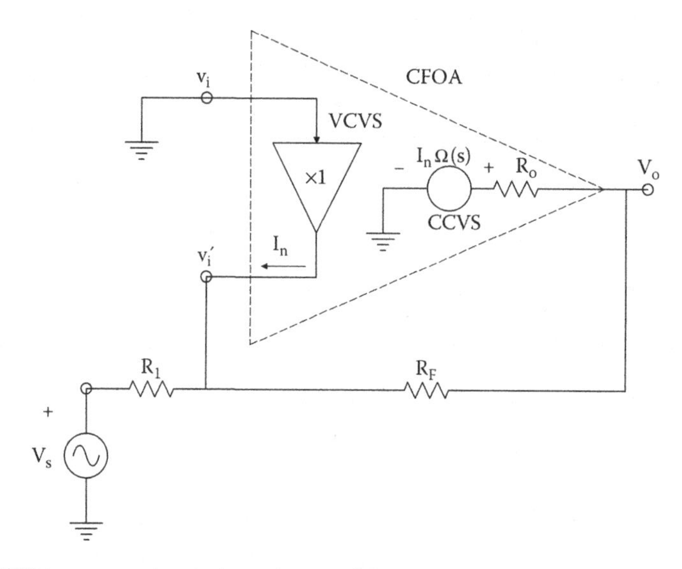

FIGURE 6.6 A CFOA connected as an inverting amplifier.

Equation 6.40 is substituted into Equation 6.33 to find the frequency response of the closed-loop amplifier:

$$V_o = -(V_s G_1 + V_o G_F)\frac{\Omega_o}{j\omega\tau_a + 1} \tag{6.41}$$

$$\downarrow$$

$$\frac{V_o}{V_s} = \frac{-G_1\Omega_o/(1+G_F\Omega_o)}{j\omega\tau_a/(1+G_F\Omega_o)+1} \tag{6.42}$$

Note that again, the closed-loop break frequency depends on the size of R_F:

$$f_{bcl} = \frac{1+G_F\Omega_o}{2\pi\tau_a} \cong \frac{\Omega_o}{2\pi\tau_a R_F} \text{ Hz} \tag{6.43}$$

The GBWP is

$$\text{GBWP} = \frac{(1+G_F\Omega_o)}{2\pi\tau_a}[G_1\Omega_o/(1+G_F\Omega_o)] = \frac{\Omega_o}{2\pi\tau_a R_1} \text{ Hz} \tag{6.44}$$

Curiously, the closed-loop break frequency depends only on R_1, and the closed-loop, DC gain is

$$V_o/V_s \cong -R_F/R_1 \tag{6.45}$$

6.4.3 Limitations of CFOAs

CFOAs cannot be directly substituted into most conventional voltage feedback OA circuits. For example, consider the CFOA "integrator" circuit shown in Figure 6.7a. The node equation on the v_i' node is written as

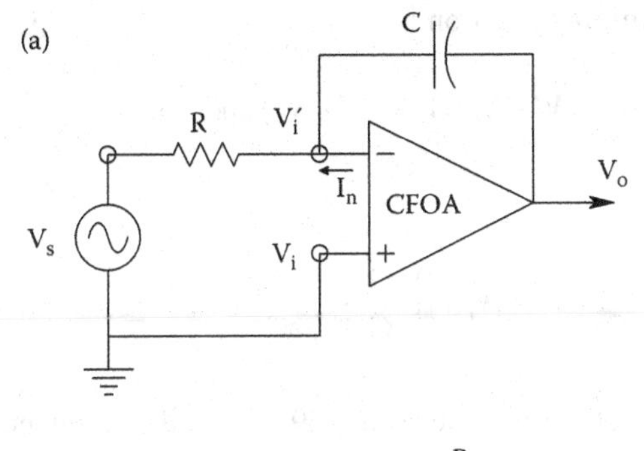

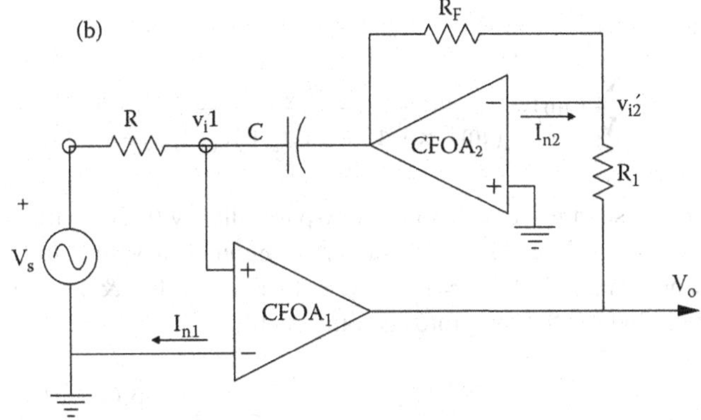

FIGURE 6.7 (a) A CFOA connected as a conventional integrator. The circuit does not integrate. (b) Two CFOAs connected to make a near ideal inverting integrator.

$$\mathbf{I_c} = (0 - \mathbf{V_s})G_1 + (0 - \mathbf{V_o})j\omega C \tag{6.46}$$

Equation 6.46 for I_c is substituted into Equation 6.33 for V_o:

$$\mathbf{V_o} = -(\mathbf{V_s}G_1 + \mathbf{V_o}j\omega C)\frac{\Omega_o}{j\omega\tau_a + 1} \tag{6.47}$$

$$\downarrow$$

$$\frac{\mathbf{V_o}}{\mathbf{V_s}} = \frac{-G_1\Omega_o}{j\omega(\tau_a + \Omega_o C) + 1} \tag{6.48}$$

Clearly, Equation 6.48 is the frequency response of a low-pass filter, not that of an operational integrator. The closed-loop time constant will be long, however. If $\Omega_o = 10^7$ ohms, and $C = 10^{-6}$ F, the closed-loop time constant will be ca. 10 s, which means that only signals with frequencies above ca. 40 mHz will be "integrated." This is a poor integrator.

By way of comparison, let us find the frequency response of a conventional voltage-feedback OA integrator. The VCVS op amp's open-loop gain is given by

$$\mathbf{V_o}/\mathbf{V_i'} = -\frac{K_{vo}}{j\omega\tau_a + 1} \tag{6.49}$$

The node equation for the summing junction is

$$(\mathbf{V}_i' - \mathbf{V}_s)G_1 + (\mathbf{V}_i' - \mathbf{V}_o)j\omega C = 0 \tag{6.50}$$

From which one finds

$$\mathbf{V}_i' = \frac{\mathbf{V}_s G_1 + \mathbf{V}_o j\omega C}{G_1 + j\omega C} \tag{6.51}$$

Equation 6.51 for $\mathbf{V}_i'$ is substituted into Equation 6.49 to find the frequency response function for the OA integrator:

$$\frac{\mathbf{V}_o}{\mathbf{V}_s}(j\omega) = \frac{-K_{vo}}{(j\omega)^2 R_1 C\tau_a + j\omega(\tau_a + K_{vo}R_1C) + 1} \tag{6.52}$$

The practical integrator is seen to be a two-pole low-pass filter with DC gain, $-K_{vo}$. To appreciate what happens to the integrator's poles, let us substitute numerical values for the parameters and factor the quadratic denominator. Let: $R_1 = 10^6\,\Omega$, $C = 1\,\mu F$, $K_{vo} = 10^5$, & $\tau_a = 15$ ms. The numerical frequency response function for the integrator is found to be

$$\frac{\mathbf{V}_o}{\mathbf{V}_s}(j\omega) = \frac{-1\text{ E5}}{(j\omega)^2 0.015 + j\omega(0.015 + 1\text{E5}) + 1} = \frac{-6.667\text{ E6}}{(j\omega)^2 + j\omega\ 6.667\text{ E6} + 66.667} \tag{6.53}$$

The right-hand fraction of the frequency response function is in Laplace form and is most easily factored to find its roots (poles). Thus, the integrator's frequency response function can be written in factored form:

$$\frac{\mathbf{V}_o}{\mathbf{V}_s}(j\omega) = \frac{-6.667\text{ E6}}{(j\omega + 3\text{E}-12)(j\omega + 6.667\text{E6})} = \frac{-3\text{E11}}{(j\omega 3.333\text{E11} + 1)(j\omega 1.5\text{E}-7 + 1)} \tag{6.54}$$

Note that in this case, the integrator time constant is *enormous* (3.333 E11 sec. = 1.0657E4 years), and the high-frequency pole is at 6.667 E6 r/s, which is the GBWP of this voltage feedback OA.

As a closing note, it is possible to design an effective integrator using two CFOAs, as shown in Figure 6.7b. This integrator is noninverting, however. If R is replaced with impedance $\mathbf{Z}_1$, and C with impedance $\mathbf{Z}_2$, then it can be shown that the circuit's transfer function is

$$\frac{V_o}{V_s}(s) = \frac{Z_2(s)R_A}{Z_1(s)R_F} \tag{6.55}$$

providing that $\Omega_{o1} = \Omega_{o2}$, $\tau_{a1} = \tau_{a2} \to 0$, $\Omega_{o1}G_{o1} >> 1$, and $R_F > R_A$.

6.5 ANALOG VOLTAGE COMPARATORS

6.5.1 Introduction

The integrated circuit, *analog voltage comparator* (AVC) is a useful circuit element with many applications in biomedical instrumentation, as well as in flash ADCs. The AVC is a simple analog-to-digital interface element; its input is an analog voltage difference, and its output is either a logic

HI or LO, depending on whether the input voltage difference is positive or negative. An *ideal* AVC performs the operation shown in Figure 6.8. That is, its output is logic HI when $(v_i - v_i') > 0$, and LO when $(v_i - v_i') \leq 0$. v_i or v_i' can be a DC reference (threshold) voltage, V_ϕ.

An actual AVC circuit combines the front end of a high-gain, analog differential amplifier (cf. Chapter 3 in this Text), with the output stage of an open-collector logic gate. Similar to an op amp, the differential front end of an AVC can be described in terms of its *difference-mode gain,* its *common-mode gain,* its *common-mode rejection ratio,* its *slew rate,* its *DC input offset voltage,* and its *input DC bias currents.* Figure 6.9 illustrates the *output stage* of the well-known LM311 AVC (or RCA CA311). Note that the analog DA front end has a symmetrical, push–pull output which is coupled to the driving transistors, Q_8 and Q_9, of the output stage. To heuristically examine how this circuit works, let us assume that $(v_i - v_i') > 0$. Assuming a large DM gain for the DA, v_o' goes negative turning off Q_8 and allowing v_{b10} to go positive. Positive-going v_{b10} makes v_{b11} go positive, turning off Q_{11}. Q_{11} turning off turns off Q_{15}, allowing V_o at its collector to go toward V_{LL} (+5 V), or logic HI. Also, $(v_i - v_i') > 0$ causes v_o to go positive, causing Q_9 to turn on. Q_9's emitter goes positive, forcing Q_8's emitter positive, further turning it off, etc. All this action can be summarized in Figure 6.10. v_i' is the DC reference voltage, V_ϕ. Note that the static transfer curve of the comparator in Figure 6.10 shows a narrow range of finite differential voltage gain (e.g., $K_D = 2 \times 10^5$ for the AD CMP04). Note that some AVCs also have complimentary, $(\overline{Q})$ outputs for design versatility (e.g., the AD9696 TTL output AVC).

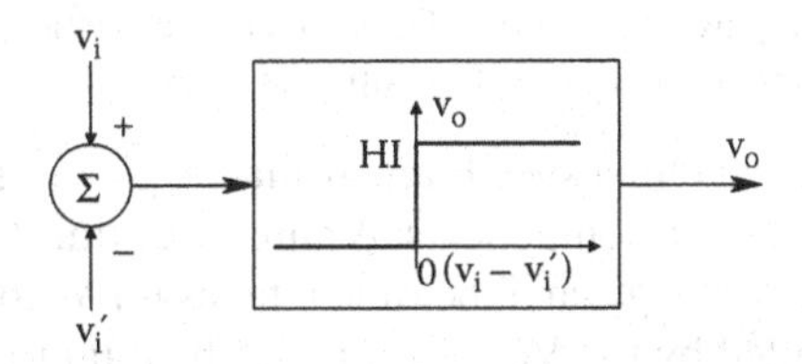

FIGURE 6.8 Block diagram of an ideal comparator I/O characteristic.

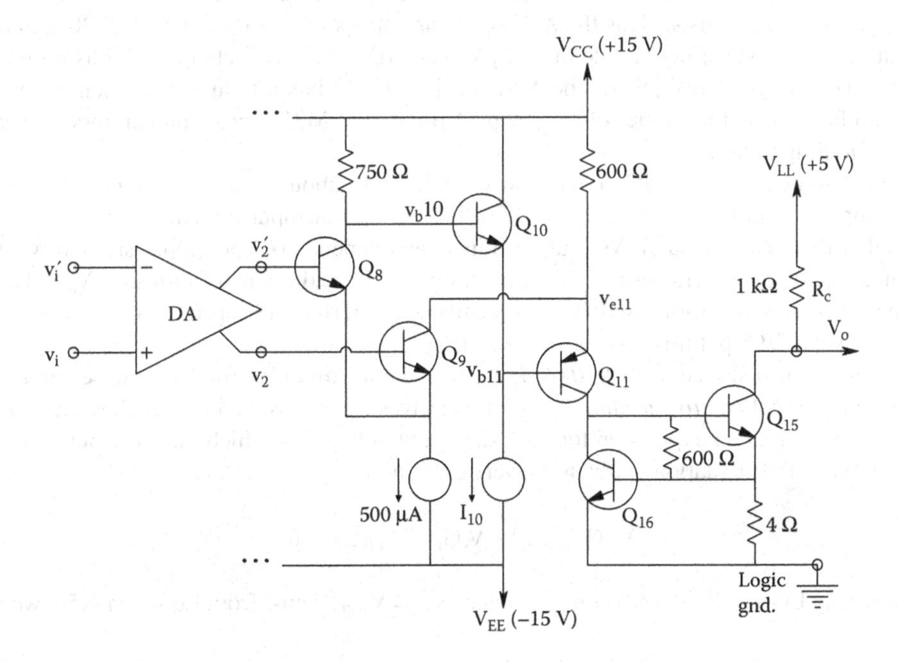

FIGURE 6.9 Partial (output circuit) schematic of an LM311 analog comparator. Note that an analog DA stage output is converted to an open-collector, TTL output BJT.

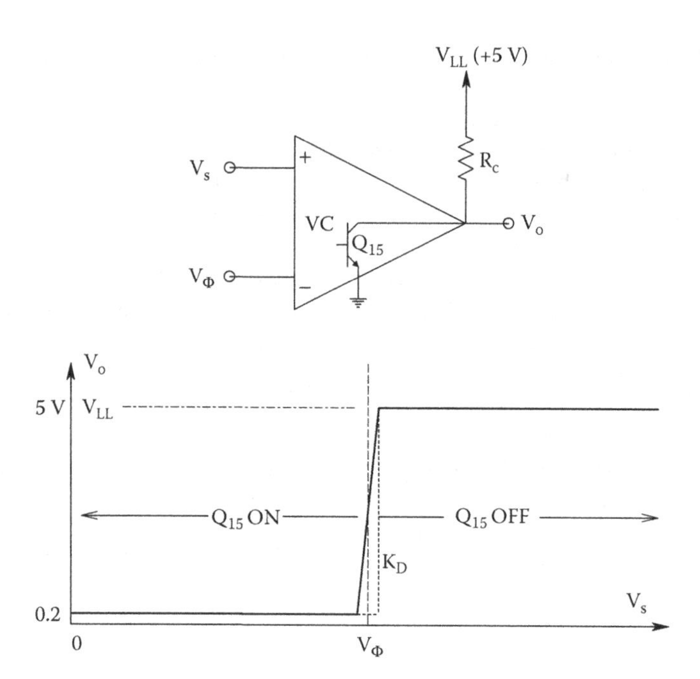

FIGURE 6.10 *Top:* Analog comparator. *Bottom:* Transfer characteristic of the comparator. Comparator gain, K_D, in the linear region is as high as an open-loop op amp.

A wide range of comparator switching speeds are available, given a step change in the polarity of $(v_i - v_i')$. AVC switching speed has two components: A pure delay time between the input step change and the beginning of output state change, and the time it takes for V_o to swing from LO to HI (or HI to LO). This latter delay is limited by the VC's slew rate. The total time for a comparator to reach its new output state following an input step change in $(v_i - v_i')$ polarity is called the *propagation delay time,* t_{PD}. The LM311 comparator output changes state in about 200 ns following the input step change. Newer designs such as the AD790 change states in ca. 40 ns. The AD790 also claims a maximum offset voltage magnitude of 250 μV. The AD96685 AVC claims a 2.5 ns propagation delay, and has a large, 1 mV $|V_{os}|$. The National LMH7322 has a total propagation delay of ca. 700 ps with fast rise and fall times of ca. 160 ps. Unlike the LM311, most comparators *do not* have a means of nulling their V_{OS}.

The input impedance of AVCs is generally fairly high, about what one might expect from a fast, BJT-input op amp. For example, the AD790 AVC has an input impedance given as 20 MΩ in parallel with 2 pF to ground. VC output impedance depends on the output state; if V_o is LO, the open-collector output transistor is saturated, and R_o is in the tens of ohms. If V_o is HI, then the output transistor is cut-off, and R_o is basically the external pull-up resistance used with the comparator (some VCs put this resistor in the IC).

AVCs are often operated with *hysteresis* to give them immunity fro input noise. Figure 6.11 illustrates an external *positive feedback circuit* that gives hysteresis, and the ideal, static I/O curve for the circuit. To find an expression for the exact input voltages at which the VC's output changes state, we write a node equation on the noninverting, v_i node:

$$V_i[G_1 + G_F] - V_sG_1 - V_{oLO}G_F = 0 \tag{6.56}$$

At switching LO → HI, V_i is assumed to equal $V_i' = V_{REF}$. Thus, from Equation 6.56, we have

$$V_{sHI} = \frac{V_R(G_1 + G_F) - V_{oLO}G_F}{G_1} = V_R(1 + R_1/R_F) - V_{oLO}(R_1/R_F) \tag{6.57}$$

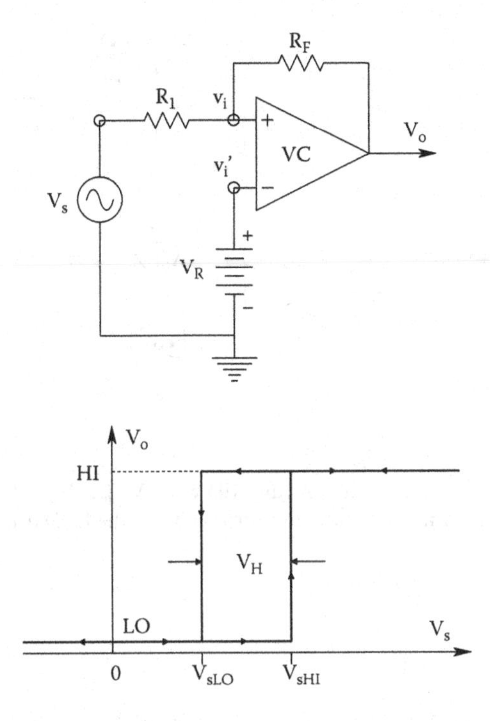

FIGURE 6.11 *Top:* A voltage comparator connected to have hysteresis. Note PFB. *Bottom:* Dimensions of the hysteresis I/O characteristic. See text for analysis.

When $V_s > V_{sHI}$, $V_o = V_{oHI} = +5$ V. Now V_s must decrease to V_{sLO} before $V_o = V_{oLO} = 0.2$ V again. Calculation of V_{sLO} uses the approach above, except V_{oHI} is used in the Equation 6.57 above, sic:

$$V_{sLO} = V_R(1 + R_1 / R_R) - V_{oHI}(R_1 / R_R) \tag{6.58}$$

Let us work a numerical example. Let: $R_1 = 10$ kΩ, $R_F = 100$ kΩ, $V_R = +1.0$ V, $V_{oHI} = +5.0$ V, and $V_{oLO} = +0.2$ V. From these values we find: $V_{sHI} = 1.08$ V, $V_{sLO} = 0.60$ V, and the width of the hysteresis can easily be shown to be

$$V_H = (V_{oHI} - V_{oLO})(R_1/R_F) = 0.48 \text{ V} \tag{6.59}$$

Note that the feedback around the comparator is PVF (cf. Chapter 4). The AVC with PFV not only has hysteresis for noise immunity, but the AVC with hysteresis can also be used as a simple, limit-cycling, ON–OFF controller for a switched control system such as an oven heater (Franco 1988, Chapter 7). It is also possible to reverse the positions of the DC reference voltage, V_R, and the input signal, V_s, in Figure 6.11, and still have hysteresis. It is left as an exercise for the reader to find expressions for V_{sLO}, V_{sHI}, and V_H under these conditions.

6.5.2 Applications of Voltage Comparators

Analog comparators find many applications in biomedical engineering. They are used in bar-graph (LED) display meters, very high-speed (flash) ADC converters (cf. Section 10.5.5), over- and under-range alarms, static window circuits, ON–OFF controllers, and dynamic pulse-height discriminators ("windows") used in nuclear medicine and in neurophysiology.

In a first example, examine a simple battery *overvoltage alarm* which is used to indicate that charging should cease. This circuit is shown in Figure 6.12. When $V_{Batt} > V_{REF}$, the output (open

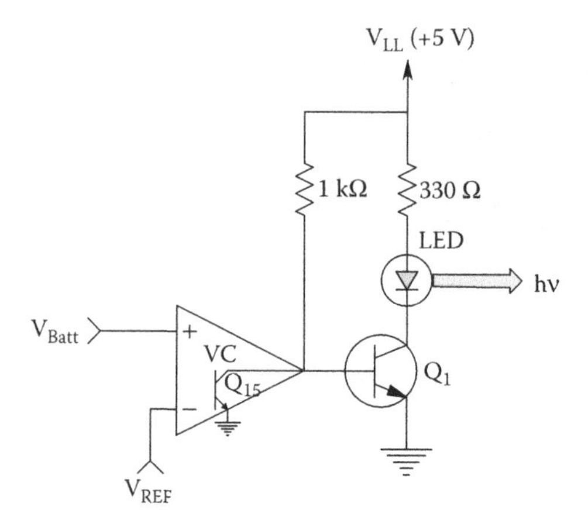

FIGURE 6.12 A comparator circuit that will light an LED when $V_{Batt} > V_{REF}$. If $V_{Batt} < V_{REF}$, then Q_{15} of the comparator is on and saturated pulling Q_1's base low, turning it and the LED off.

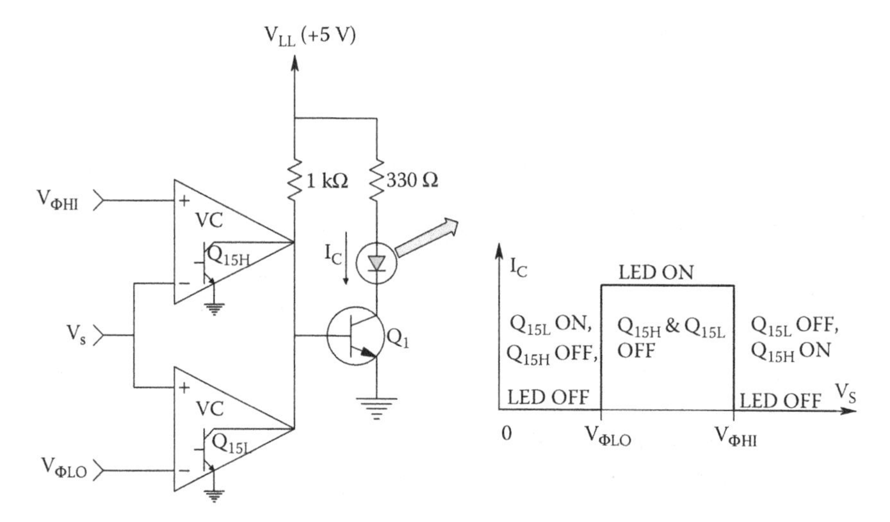

FIGURE 6.13 A comparator voltage range window that turns the LED on when V_s lies between V_{fLO} and V_{fHI}.

collector) transistor (Q_{15}) in the VC is turned off, allowing the base of Q_1 to conduct through the 1 kΩ pull-up resistor, saturating Q_1. The current through the lit LED is approximately (5 – 0.2 – 1.5)/330 = 10 mA. If $V_{Batt} < V_{REF}$, Q_{15} is ON and saturated, pulling the base of Q_1 down to ca. 0.2 V, keeping it off, and the LED unlit.

The second example of the use of AVCs is a *static window comparator* circuit that lights a LED while the input voltage falls in a certain range, or window, of values. The circuit is shown in Figure 6.13. (Note that tying the two open collector output transistors together to a common pull-up resistor effectively makes an AND gate.) Both comparator outputs must be HI (Q_{15L} and Q_{15H} are both cut-off) to light the LED. If either Q_{15} is ON, the base of Q_1 is pulled down to that Q_{15}'s V_{csat}, and Q_1 is cut-off (no light).

In a third and final example of using VCs, consider the circuit of a simple nerve spike pulse-height discriminator designed by the author (Northrop and Grossman 1974). This circuit is used in neurophysiological recording; it selects only those nerve impulses recorded with extracellular microelectrodes whose amplitudes fall within a narrow range of voltages (the window). This processing enables other, simultaneously recorded, very large (or small) action potentials to be ignored while the desired pulses can be counted, processed, and their instantaneous frequency calculated, etc. Figure 6.14 illustrates the schematic for this window circuit. Note this circuit involves sequential as well as combinational logic. Critical waveforms of this window circuit are shown in Figure 6.15. Note that three, one-shot multivibrators are used to generate narrow (e.g., 500 ns) output pulses given input logic state transitions. The NAND gate RS flip-flop serves as a "memory" that a rising V_s has exceeded $V_{\phi LO}$. Note that if V_s exceeds $V_{\phi LO}$, the output of VC-2, C_H, goes HI. This event triggers OS-3 to reset the RSFF Q output to LO, disabling the output AND gate. Now when the large input again falls below $V_{\phi LO}$, the P2 pulse does not produce an output. Note that it is only the falling edge of VC-1's output, C_L, that can produce an output. The second V_s pulse in Figure 6.15 lies in the window. The rising edge of C_L sets the RSFF Q output high, enabling the AND gate. When V_s falls below $V_{\phi LO}$, OS-2 produces a positive pulse which appears at V_o, signaling a pulse that occurred inside the window.

6.5.3 Discussion

In the sections above, the basic behavior of analog voltage comparators are described. We note that comparators are intended to signal analog input voltage inequalities to appropriate logic circuits or transistor switches. Op amps are for conditioning analog signals, giving an analog output. An important point should be made that an open-loop op amp (one without feedback) makes a poor comparator. Yes, op amps generally have very high gain differential input gains, and high CMRRs, but rapid changes in V_o are limited by the op amps' slew rate, η. η is typically on the order of 20 V/μs, which means it takes V_o roughly 250 ns to slew 5 V. Op amp outputs are generally not logic-level compatible; they swing to $\pm(V_{CC} - V_\delta)$, where V_δ is a fixed voltage by which a saturated V_o fails to reach the supply voltage. V_δ is different for different designs of op amps. *It is poor design practice to use op amps for comparator applications.*

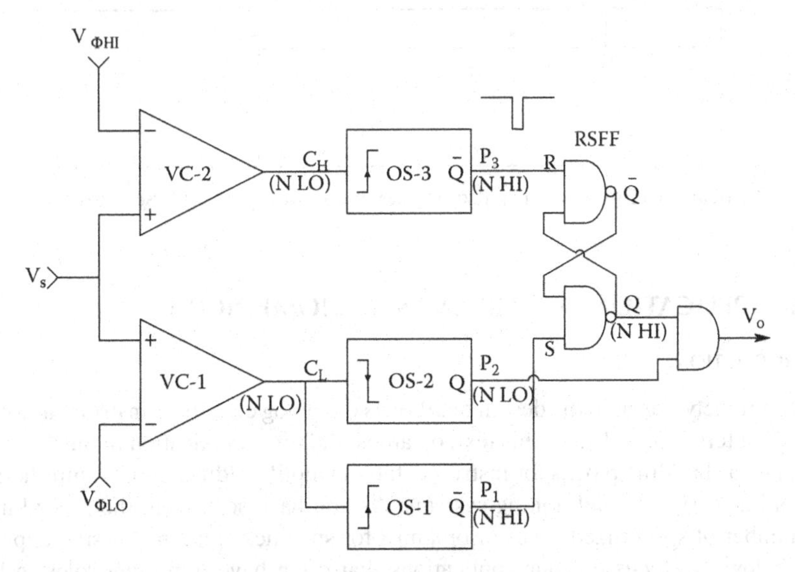

FIGURE 6.14 A nerve spike pulse-height window that produces an output pulse *only if* an input spike rises to its peak inside the window and then falls below the lower "sill." No output pulse is produced if an input spike rises through the window and exceeds the upper level, then falls below the sill.

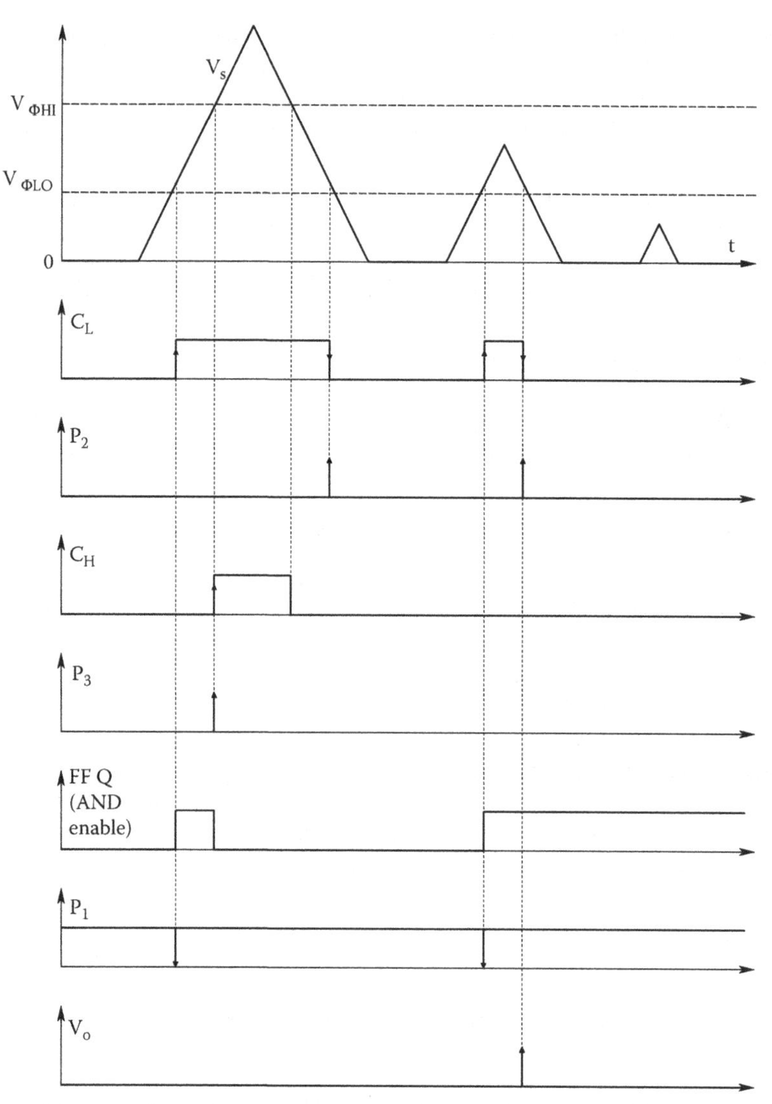

FIGURE 6.15 Critical waveforms for the pulse-height window of Figure 6.14. See Text for description.

6.6 SOME APPLICATIONS OF OP AMPS IN BIOMEDICINE

6.6.1 Introduction

Op amps are extremely useful in the design of all sorts of analog electronic instrumentation systems. As shown in Chapters 7, 8, and 15 of this text, op amps find great application in the design of analog active filters, and as building blocks for instrumentation amplifier (differential) amplifiers and other linear and nonlinear signal conditioning systems. As you have seen from the preceding sections, there are a number of specialized types of op amps for specific, signal processing applications. In the sections below, we focus on four applications that often have important roles in biomedical signal processing: Integrators, differentiators, charge amplifiers, and an isolated, two-op amp instrumentation DA useful for measuring biopotentials. This amplifier also includes a bandpass filter, and an analog photooptic coupler for galvanic isolation.

6.6.2 Analog Integrators and Differentiators

A simple op amp analog integrator is shown in Figure 6.16. An op amp integrator is hardly ever used as a standalone component; it is usually incorporated as part of a feedback loop to obtain some desired dynamic characteristic for the closed-loop system. The reason for not using it alone is that it integrates its own dc bias current and offset voltage, causing its output, in the absence of an input signal, to slowly and linearly drift into saturation. In the circuit of Figure 6.16, we set $V_s = 0$ and consider the op amp ideal so $v_i' = 0$. Thus, the node voltage V_1 must equal V_{OS}. Using superposition, and considering I_B and V_{OS} to be steps applied at t = 0, the integrator's time-domain output can be written as

$$V_o(t) = -\, t\, I_B / CF + V_{OS}(1 + t / RC_F) \tag{6.60}$$

I_B and V_{OS} can have either sign, depending on the op amp design and its temperature. V_{OS} magnitude is typically in the range of hundreds of μV, and I_B can range from 10s of fA to μA, again depending on OA design and temperature. If standalone analog integration must be done, the integrator drift must be considered. Op amps with low V_{OS} and I_B are used, and a means of shorting out C_F is used to ensure zero initial conditions at the start of integration. Digital integration is no panacea; it will integrate small analog offset voltages present in the antialiasing filter, the sample and hold, and the ADC itself.

Often when an integrator is used in a closed-loop system, it is desired to give its transfer function a real zero, as well as the pole at the origin. The zero is used to give the system better closed-loop dynamic performance. The zero is easily obtained by placing a resistance, R_F, in series with C_F. Assuming anIOA, the transfer function is

$$\frac{V_o}{V_s}(s) = -\frac{R_F + 1/sC_F}{R} = -\frac{(sR_FC_F + 1)}{s\,RC_F} = -\frac{K_i(s\tau_f + 1)}{s} \tag{6.61}$$

which is what is desired.

Figure 6.17 illustrates a conventional *op amp analog differentiator.* If we treat the op amp as ideal, and neglect C_F, then the transfer function is

$$\frac{V_o}{V_s}(s) = -sRC \tag{6.62}$$

which is the transfer function of an ideal time-domain differentiator with gain –RC.

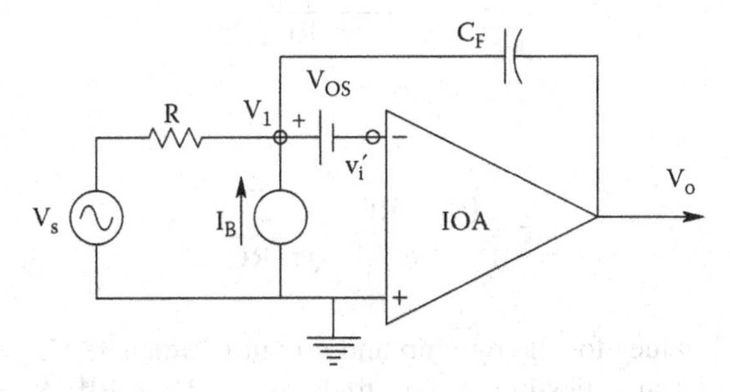

FIGURE 6.16 DC model of a voltage op amp integrator. The op amp is assumed ideal, and its offset voltage and bias current are externalized to its inverting (v_i') node. The integrator's behavior is analyzed in the Text.

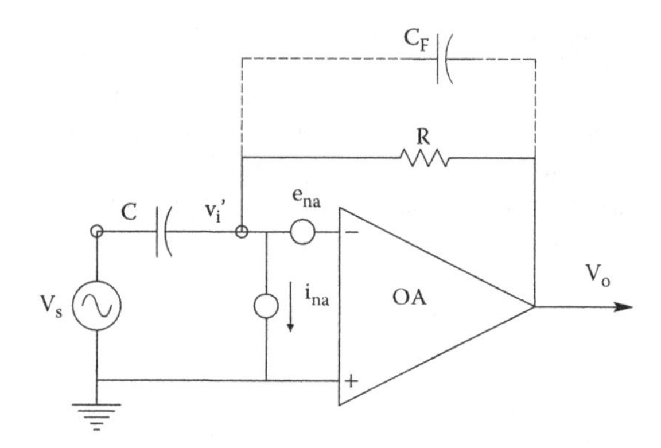

FIGURE 6.17 Circuit for an op amp differentiator. In this problem, the op amp's frequency response is considered, as well as its short-circuit input voltage noise root power spectrum, and input current noise root spectrum.

Now we consider what happens to the differentiator's transfer function when a real frequency-compensated op amp is modeled by the open-loop gain:

$$\frac{V_o}{V_i{}'}(s) = \frac{-K_{vo}}{\tau_A s + 1} \tag{6.63}$$

Now the node equation on the V_i' node is

$$V_i'(G + sC) - V_o G = V_s sC \tag{6.64}$$

Using Equation 6.63, V_i' can be eliminated in Equation 6.64, and the overall transfer function becomes

$$\frac{V_o}{V_s}(s) = \frac{-sRCK_{vo}/(1/K_{vo})}{s^2\tau_A RC/(1+K_{vo}) + s(\tau_A + RC)/(1+K_{vo}) + 1} \cong \frac{-sRC}{s^2\tau_A RC/K_{vo} + s(\tau_A + RC)/K_{vo} + 1} \tag{6.65}$$

Note that Equation 6.65 has the form of the transfer function of a quadratic bandpass filter shown in

$$\frac{V_o}{V_s}(s) = \frac{-s\,K}{s^2/\omega_n^2 + s2\xi/\omega + 1} \tag{6.66}$$

From Equations 6.66 and 6.65, we see that the resonant frequency is

$$\omega_n \cong \sqrt{K_{vo}/(\tau_A RC)} \text{ r/s} \tag{6.67}$$

The damping factor is

$$\xi = \frac{(\tau_A + RC)}{2\,K_{vo}} \frac{\sqrt{K_{vo}}}{\sqrt{\tau_A RC}} \tag{6.68}$$

When typical numerical values for the op amp and circuit parameters ($K_{vo} = 10^6$, $\tau_A = 0.001$ sec, $R = 10^6\ \Omega$, & $C = 10^{-6}$ F) are substituted, one finds $\omega_n = 3.16 \times 10^4$ r/s, and $\xi = 1.597 \times 10^{-2}$. This damping is equivalent to a quadratic BPF $Q = 1/(2\xi) = 31.3$, which is a sharply tuned filter. Thus, any fast transients in V_s will excite a poorly damped sinusoidal transient at the differentiator's output. This is not a good result.

Another problem with the simple R-C differentiator is the differentiation of the op amp's short-circuit, equivalent voltage noise, e_{na}. The transfer function for e_{na} is easily shown to be

$$V_o = E_{na}(1 + s\,RC) \tag{6.69}$$

Because e_{na} has a broadband spectrum, the differentiator's output noise has a spectrum that increases with frequency, making the output very noisy. (Note that the i_{na} component in V_o is not differentiated.)

When a feedback capacitor, C_F, is added in parallel with R, the differentiator's frequency response is found from the new node equation:

$$V_i'[G + s(C + C_F)] - V_o(G + sC_F) = V_s sC \tag{6.70}$$

Using Equation 6.63, V_i' in Equation 6.70 can be eliminated and the transfer function written as

$$\frac{V_o}{V_s}(s) = \frac{-sRC}{s^2\tau_A R(C + C_F)/K_{vo} + s[(\tau_A + RC)/K_{vo} + RC_F] + 1} \tag{6.71}$$

The differentiator transfer function still has the format of a BPF. Let's examine its ω_n and damping. All parameters are the same as above, and $C_F = 6.7 \times 10^{-11}$ F (67 pF).

$$\omega_n^{\,2} = \frac{K_{vo}}{\tau_A R(C + C_F)} = \frac{10^6}{10^{-3} \times 10^6 \times (10^{-6} + 6.7 \times 10^{-11})} = 9.99933 \times 10^8 \tag{6.72}$$

$$\downarrow$$

$$\omega_n = 3.1622 \times 10^4 \text{ r/s} \tag{6.73}$$

The damping factor is now found from

$$2\xi/\omega_n = \frac{\tau_A + RC}{K_{vo}} + RC_F \tag{6.74}$$

$$\xi = 0.5 \times 3.1622 \times 10^4 \left(\frac{10^{-3} + 1}{10^6} + 6.7 \times 10^{-11} \times 10^6\right) = 1.075 \tag{6.75}$$

Note that ω_n has changed little, but now the system is slightly overdamped, i.e., the poles are close to each other on the negative real axis in the s-plane. Now the differentiator's frequency response is still bandpass with its peak gain at the same frequency, but no longer is severely underdamped. Making C_F larger will make the system more overdamped, it will have two real poles, one below ω_n and the other above it.

Thus, we see that for practical reasons, an op amp, analog differentiator should have a small feedback capacitor in parallel with the feedback R to limit its bandwidth and give it reasonable damping so that input noise spikes will not excite "ringing" in its output.

6.6.3 Charge Amplifiers

A *charge amplifier* is used to condition the output of a piezoelectric transducer used in such applications as *accelerometers, dynamic pressure sensors, microphones,* and *ultrasonic receivers.* Figure 6.18 illustrates the schematic of an electrometer op amp used as a charge amplifier. The shunt capacitance, C_T, includes the capacitance of the piezotransducer, the connecting coax (if any), and

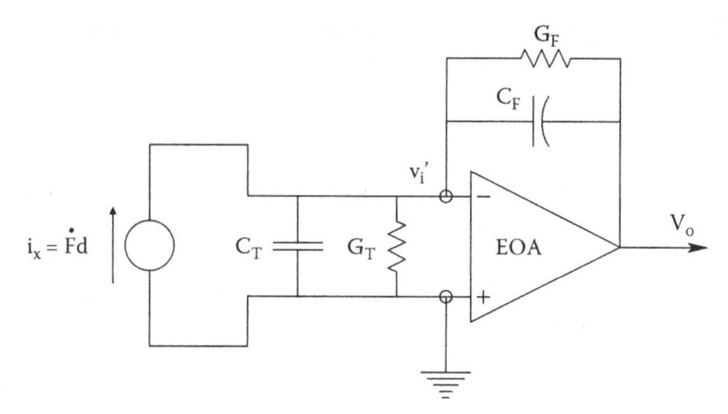

FIGURE 6.18 An electrometer op amp is used to make a charge amplifier to condition the output of a piezoelectric force transducer. See Text for analysis.

the input capacitance of the op amp. Similarly, the conductance G_T includes the leakage conductance of the transducer, the connecting cable, and the op amp's input conductance. The op amp is assumed to have a finite gain and frequency response, i.e., it is nonideal in this respect. Thus, the summing junction voltage, v_i', is finite. The op amp's gain is modeled by

$$V_o = -V_i' \frac{K_{vo}}{\tau s + 1} \tag{6.76}$$

The node equation for the summing junction is

$$V_i'[s(C_F + C_T) + G_T + G_F] - V_o[sC_F + G_F] = \dot{F}(s)d = sF(s)d \tag{6.72}$$

From which we obtain

$$V_i' = \frac{sF(s)d + V_o(sC_F + G_F)}{[s(C_F + C_T) + G_T + G_F]} \tag{6.58}$$

$$\downarrow$$

$$V_o(\tau s + 1) = -K_{vo} \frac{sF(s)d + V_o(sC_F + G_F)}{[s(C_F + C_T) + G_T + G_F]} \tag{6.79}$$

$$\downarrow$$

$$\frac{V_o}{F}(s) = \frac{-s\, K_{vo} d}{s^2\tau(C_F + C_T) + s[\tau(G_F + G_T) + C_F + C_T + K_{vo}C_F] + K_{vo}G_F} \tag{6.80}$$

To put Equation 6.80 into time-constant format, divide top and bottom by $K_{vo}\,G_F$, and note that certain terms in the denominator are negligibly small. We let $\mathbf{s} = j\omega$ in order to write the charge amplifier's frequency response:

$$\frac{V_o}{F}(s) \cong \frac{-j\omega dR_F}{(j\omega)^2\tau(C_F + C_T)R_F / K_{vo} + j\omega C_F R_F + 1} \tag{6.81}$$

The frequency response function of Equation 6.81 is bandpass with two real poles. The low-frequency one is set by the feedback R and C and is: $\mathbf{s_1} \cong -1/(R_F C_F)$ r/s. The high-frequency pole can be shown to be approximately: $\mathbf{s_2} \cong -(K_{vo}/\tau)[C_F/(C_F + C_T)] = \omega_T C_F/(C_F + C_T)$ r/s. ω_T is the op amp's *radian* gain-bandwidth product. For example, set $K_{vo} = 10^6$, $\tau = 10^{-3}$ sec, $C_F = 10^{-9}$ F, $C_T = 10^{-9}$ F,

$G_F = 10^{-10}$ S, and $G_T = 10^{-12}$ S. Now the low break frequency is at $f_{lo} = 1.59 \times 10^{-2}$ Hz, and the high break frequency is at $f_{hi} = 80$ MHz, which is adequate for conditioning 5 MHz ultrasound.

6.6.4 A Two-Op Amp, ECG Amplifier

Op amps can be used to make high-gain differential amplifiers with high common-mode rejection ratios, as described in Section 3.7.2 of this text. The 2-op amp DA of Figure 3.15 was found to have the DM gain:

$$V_o = (V_s - V_s')2(1 + R/R_F) \quad (6.82)$$

R and R_F should be chosen so the amplifier's DM gain is 10^3. To use this amplifier as an ECG system front-end, we must define the ECG bandpass with a high- and low-pass filter. An easy design is to cascade the Sallen & Key high- and lowpass filters, as shown in Figure 6.19 The HPF is given complex-conjugate poles with an $f_n = 0.1$ Hz, and a damping factor of $\xi = 0.707$. Using the design formulas given in Section 7.2.2, one sees that $C_1 = C_2 = C$, and for $\xi = 0.707$, $R_1 = 2\,R_2$. $f_n = 1/(2\pi C\sqrt{R_1 R_2})$, so we can solve for R_1 and R_2 after choosing C = 3.3 μF. A little algebra gives $R_2 = 3.31 \times 10^5$ and $R_1 = 6.821 \times 10^5\ \Omega$.

The parameters for the S&K LPF are found from: $\xi = \sqrt{C_2/C_1} = 0.707$ and $f_n = 1/(2\pi R\sqrt{C_1 C_2}) = 100$ Hz. Clearly, $C_2 = 2C_1$ for the desired damping. Let us choose $C_1 = 0.1$ μF, so $C_2 = 0.2$ μF. Using the f_n relation, $R = 1.125 \times 10^4\ \Omega$. The op amps need not be special low-noise or high f_T designs, the ECG signal has limited bandwidth, and the noise performance is set by the differential front-end amplifier having the gain of 10^3.

Now that the ECG signal has been amplified and its bandwidth defined, it is necessary to consider *patient galvanic isolation.* One easy way to achieve isolation is to run the DA and filter op amps on an isolated battery power supply with no ground connection common with the power line mains. A pair of 12 V batteries can be used with IC voltage regulators to give ±8 V to run the four signal conditioning op amps. One cannot simply connect the output of the filter to an oscilloscope or computer to view the ECG, because *the common ground from the oscilloscope or computer destroys patient galvanic isolation.* Thus, some means of coupling the signal without the necessity of a common ground must be used. One means is to sample the isolated ECG and convert it with a serial output, isolated ADC, and then couple the digitized ECG to the outside using a *photo-optic coupler* (POC) (a transformer can also be used). The digitized ECG must then be converted to analog form with a serial input DAC to be viewed on an oscilloscope or be an input to a strip-chart recorder.

A simpler form of galvanic isolation that uses POCs and gives an analog output is shown in Figure 6.20. OA1 is run from the isolated battery power supply of the signal conditioner. The top LED in the dual POC IC is biased on with the 3 mA DC current source, causing an average light intensity I_{lo} to be emitted. The isolated, conditioned, ECG output, V_3, causes the light intensity to vary proportionally around the average level, I_{lo}. The light from LED_1 is transmitted through a plastic light guide to photo-diode, PD_1. An increase in the light hitting the photojunction of PD_1 causes a proportional increase in its (reverse) photocurrent. PD_1's increased photo-current is the base current

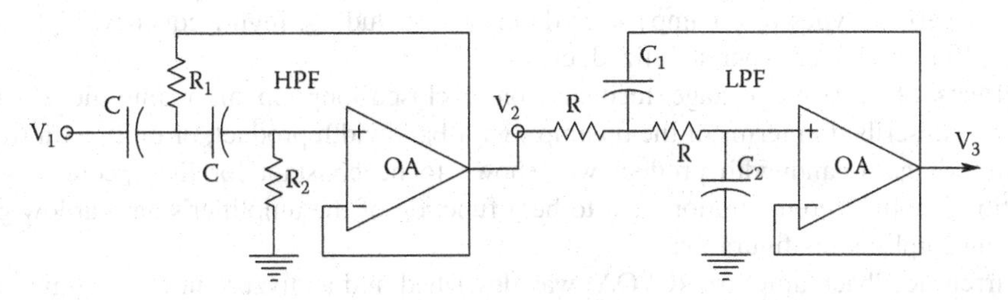

FIGURE 6.19 A bandpass filter for electrocardiography made from cascaded Sallen & Key high- and low-pass filters.

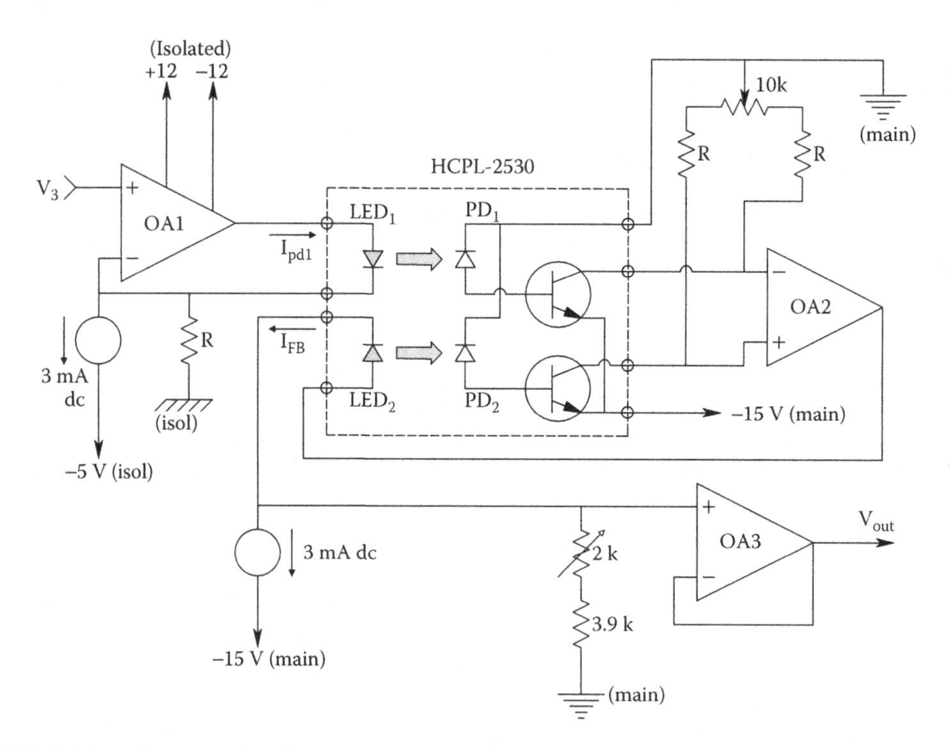

FIGURE 6.20 A linear, analog photo-optic coupler used to provide galvanic isolation between the battery-operated ECG measurement differential amplifier and bandpass filter, and the output recording and display systems.

of the top *npn* BJT, so its collector current increases, causing the inverting input of op amp OA2 to go negative, making OA2's output go positive. The positive increment on OA2's output increases the current in LED_2 above its 3 mA bias, increasing its light output, in turn increasing the photocurrent in PD_2, increasing the base current in its BJT, causing the + input of OA2 to go negative, closing a negative feedback path that compensates for LED and PD nonlinearities. Note that the ECG ground is completely isolated from the output ground as is the analog ECG signal, V_3, from V_{out}. The output of the feedback POC system is taken as the voltage across the 2k + 3.9k resistors.

6.7 CHAPTER SUMMARY

This chapter has been about op amps and comparators. We began by reviewing the properties of the IOA and showing how it can be used to facilitate heuristic analysis of op amp circuits.

Practical, conventional op amps were shown to be characterized by finite, frequency-dependent difference-mode gains, and finite input and output resistances. Their inputs were also characterized by two DC bias currents, a DC offset voltage, a short-circuit input noise voltage, and an input noise current. The various types of op amps were described, including: high-frequency, high slew rate, low-noise, electrometer, chopper-stabilized, etc.

The effects of negative voltage feedback on a closed-loop op amp amplifier's frequency response was described in terms of the op amp's gain-bandwidth product, or unity gain frequency. The amplifier's gain-bandwidth product was shown to be constant for the special case of the noninverting amplifier configuration, and to be a function of the amplifier's gain at low gains for the inverting amplifier configuration.

The current feedback amplifier (CFOA) was described and analyzed; in the noninverting gain configuration, the closed-loop amplifier's break frequency was found to be independent of the closed-loop gain, and only depend on the absolute value of the feedback resistance. The same situation obtains for the inverting amplifier configuration using the CFOA. CFOAs were also shown to be unsuitable for integrators unless a special, 2-CFOA circuit is used.

Voltage comparators were described and shown to have DA front ends and TTL or ECL logic outputs. Comparators are useful in biomedical applications including pulse height windows used in neurophysiology and in nuclear medicine.

Finally, applications of op amps as differentiators, integrators, charge amplifiers, and in ECG signal conditioning were examined.

CHAPTER 6 HOME PROBLEMS

6.1 An Apex™ PA08A high-voltage power op amp is used to drive a resistive load. This op amp can output up to ±150 mA, and swing its output voltage up to ±145 V. Its slew rate is 30 V/μs. What is the maximum Hz frequency of a sinusoidal input it can amplify to get a 100 VRMS sinusoidal output without slew-rate distortion?

6.2 Figures P6.2A and B illustrate a commutating auto-zero (CAZ) op amp connected as a noninverting amplifier with voltage gain, $(1 + R_F/R_1)$. This is an Intersil ICL7605/7606 CAZ amplifier intended for nondrifting, DC amplification applications, such as strain gauge bridges and electronic scales. The overall bandwidth is made about 10 Hz. Note that the CAZ op amp has two, matched op amps internally, and a number of analog MOS switches to periodically change its input circuitry and switch its output. Two, matched external capacitors are used to store dc offset voltages. Assume the two internal op amps are ideal except for their offset voltages. *Describe* how this circuit works to realize an amazing overall offset voltage tempco of ±10 nV/°C.

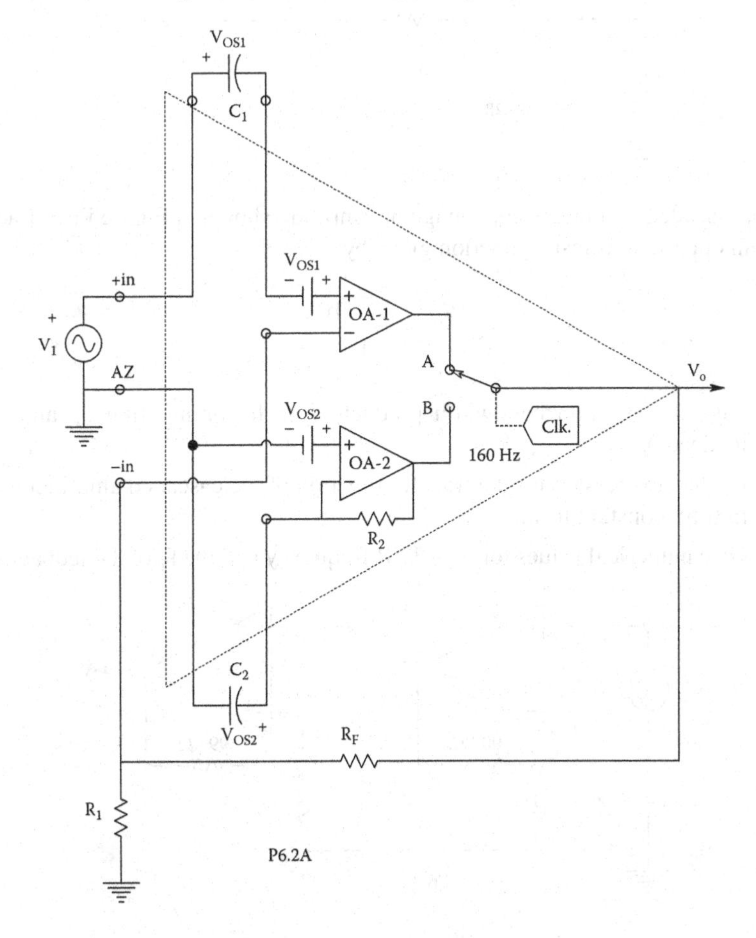

P6.2A

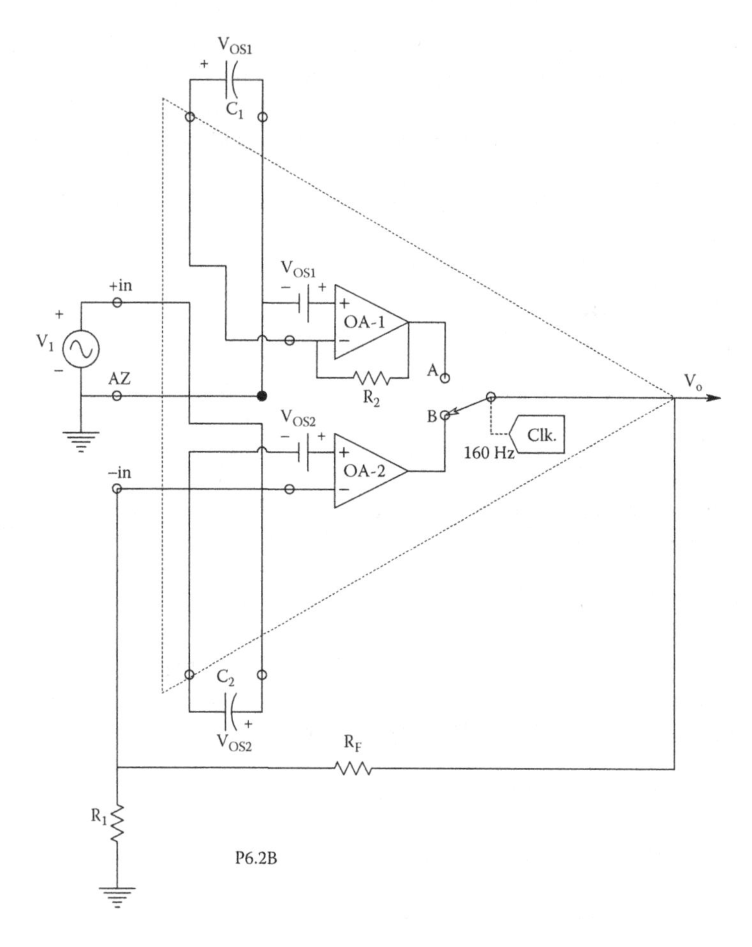

P6.2B

6.3 Two, cascaded, noninverting, voltage op amps are shown in Figure P6.3. Each op amp has an open-loop transfer function given by

$$\frac{V_o}{(V_i - V_i')} = \frac{10^5}{10^{-3}s + 1}$$

(A) Give the Hz gain*bandwidth product of each noninverting op amp alone (no feedback).

(B) Find an expression for the transfer function of the cascaded amplifiers $(V_3/V_1)(s)$ in time-constant form.

(C) Give numerical values for the –3 dB frequency and the f_T of the fedback amplifier.

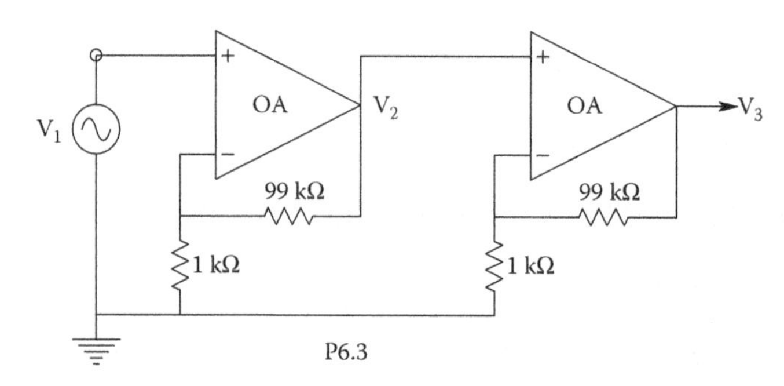

P6.3

6.4 Use an ECAP to simulate the response of a simple inverting op amp amplifier with a gain of –100 to a 1.0 kHz, 10 mV peak square wave. A TI TL071 op amp is used.

6.5 In this problem, you will examine the frequency dependence of a noninverting op amp amplifier's output impedance, $Z_o(j\omega)$. The circuit is shown in Figure P6.5. Let: $R_o = 50\ \Omega$, $R_F = 99\ k\Omega$, $R_1 = 1\ k\Omega$, & $V_{oc} = (V_i - V_i')\ 10^4/(10^{-3}\, j\omega + 1)$.

(A) Write an expression for $Z_o(j\omega) = I_t/V_t$ in time-constant form.

(B) Make a dimensioned bode plot of $Z_o(j\omega)$ (magnitude and phase).

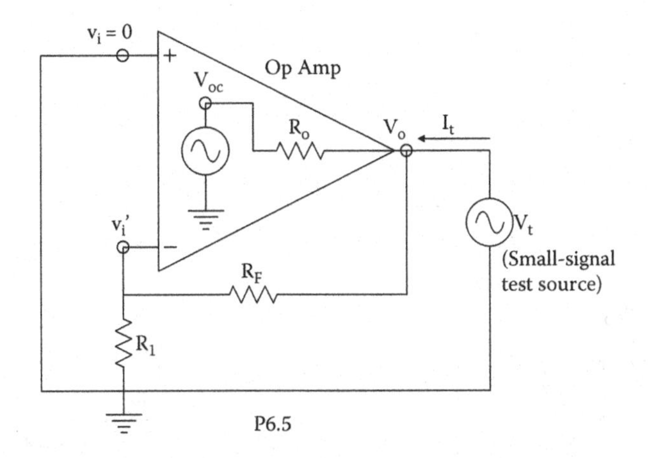

P6.5

6.6 A 6.2 V zener diode is used in the feedback path of an IOA as shown in Figure P6.6. A simplified ZD I-V curve is shown. $R_1 = 1\ k\Omega$. Plot and dimension $V_o = f(V_1)$.

6.7 A version of a diode bridge is shown in Figure P6.7. Assume $v_1(t) = 1.4\sin(377t)$, and $R_L = 1\ k\Omega$. Plot and dimension several cycles of $V_o(t)$ and $V_2(t)$. Assume the diodes have the I-V characteristic shown.

6.8 Another precision rectifier bridge is shown in Figure P6.8. $v_1(t)$ and the diodes are the same as in Prob. 6.7.

6.7 Plot and dimension several cycles of $V_o(t)$ and $V_2(t)$.

6.9 An ***npn*** BJT is used in the feedback path of an IOA as shown in Figure P6.9. The BJT is forward-biased; its collector current can be modeled by:

$$I_C \cong I_s \exp(V_{BE} / V_T)$$

where I_s is the collector saturation current = 0.25 pA, V_{BE} is the base-emitter voltage, and $V_T = \eta kT/q \cong 26$ mV at room temperature. Plot and dimension $V_o = f(V_1)$.

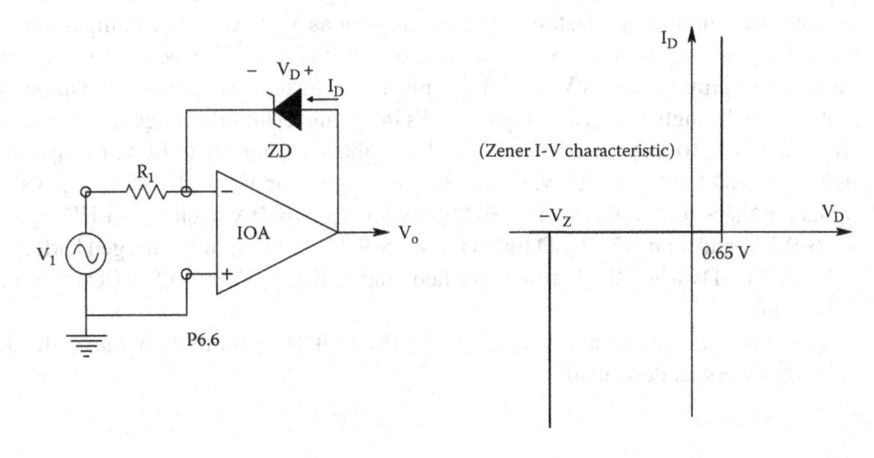

P6.6

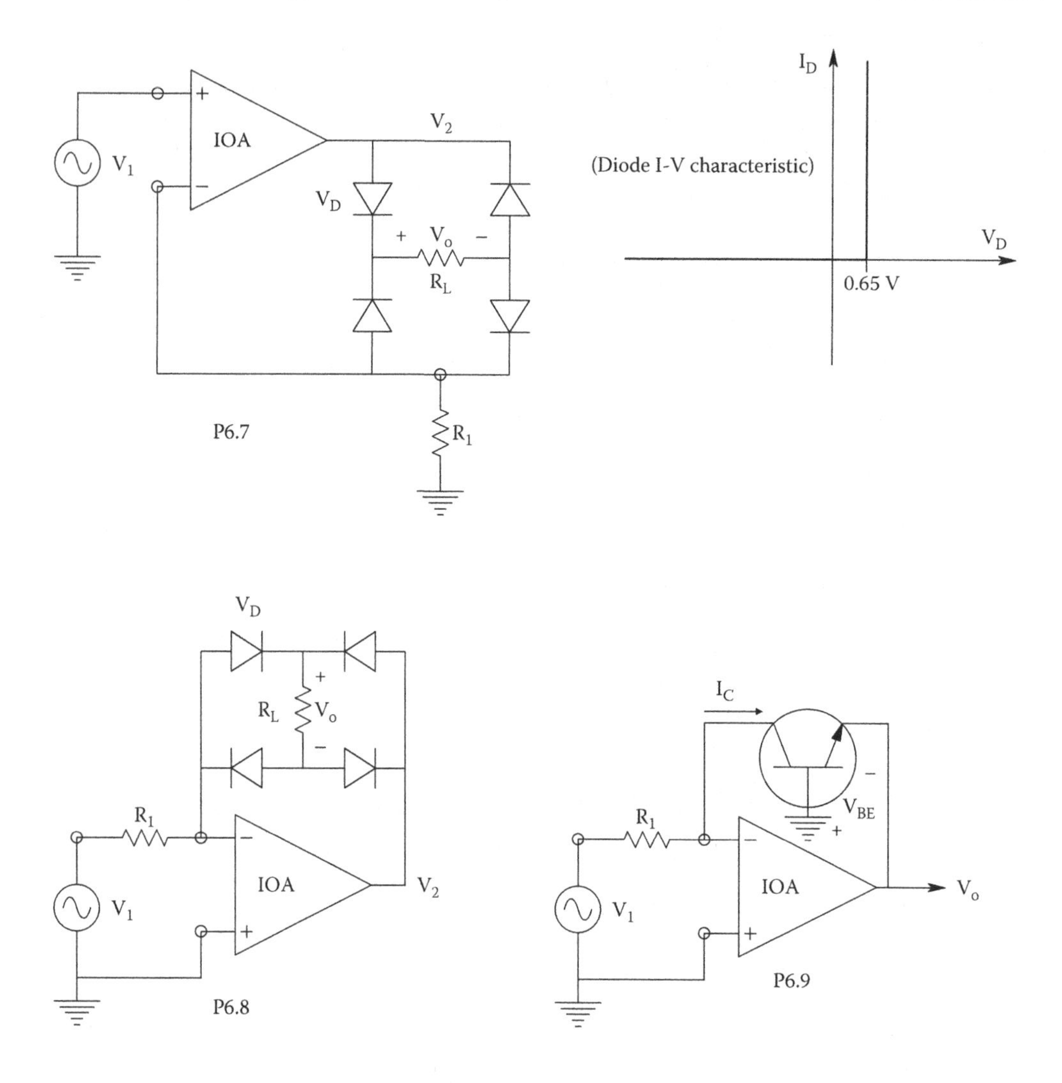

6.10 A laptop computer uses a nominal 12 V battery. It is desired to design a bargraph-type LED voltmeter display that will measure the battery voltage over the range of 9 to 12 V. A partial schematic of the voltmeter is shown in Figure P6.10. An LM336 IC reference voltage chip supplies a constant 2.5 VDC as long as $V_B > 6$ V. The comparators also run off V_B as long as $V_B > 6$ V. Comparator 1 lights its LED when the voltage at its inverting terminal exceeds $V_R = 2.5$ V. This makes its logic output low and allows current to flow through its LED. Comparator 1's inverting terminal voltage is $\alpha_1 V_B$. $\alpha_1 = R/(R + R_{1a})$. $R \equiv 10\ k\Omega$. Comparator 1's LED lights only for $V_B > 12$ V. Comparator 2 lights its LED for $V_B > 11.5$ V, Comp 3's LED lights for $V_B > 11.0$ V, Comp 4's LED lights for $V_B > 10.5$ V, Comp 5's LED lights for $V_B > 10.0$ V, Comp 6's LED lights for $V_B > 9.5$ V, and Comp 7's LED lights for $V_B > 9.0$ V. Thus, a fully charged battery will light all 7 LEDs when the button is pushed, and if $10.0 < V_B < 10.5$, LEDs 5, 6, and 7 only light.

Calculate the necessary values of R_{1a} through R_{7a} required to make the LED voltmeter work as described.

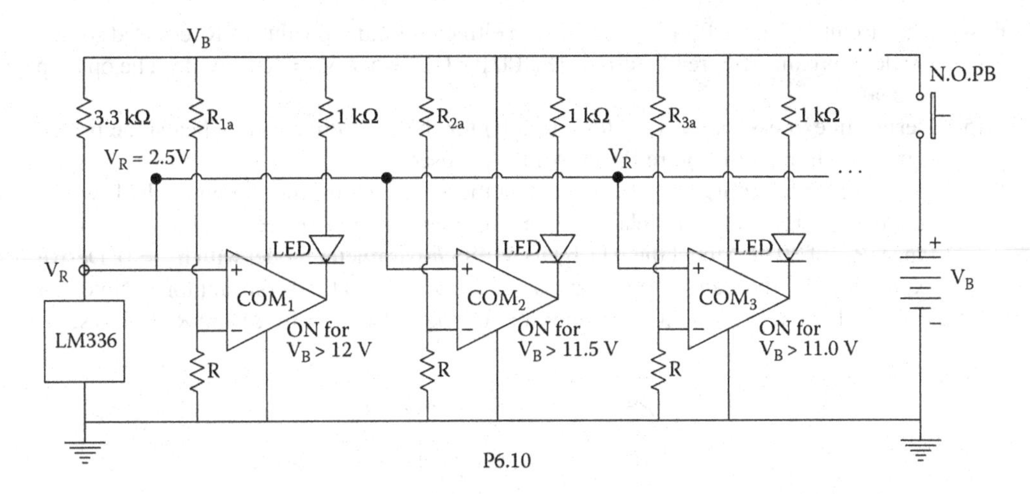

P6.10

6.11 Figure P6.11 shows a noninverting op amp amplifier, and its equivalent input resistance circuit. *Find an algebraic expression* for the input admittance, $G_{in} = I_s/V_s$ Siemens. Assume that $V_o = V_s(1 + R_F/R_1)$ for the amplifier. Assume that R_i and $R_{cm} >> R_F$ and R_1. Evaluate G_{in} numerically: Let $R_i = 10\ M\Omega$, $R_{cm} = 400\ M\Omega$, $R_F = R_1 = 3.3\ k\Omega$.

6.12 Find an expression for the transfer function of the filter of Figure P6.12 in time-constant form. The op amp is ideal.

6.13 Find an expression for the frequency response function of the filter of Figure P6.13 in time constant form. What function does this circuit perform on V_s?

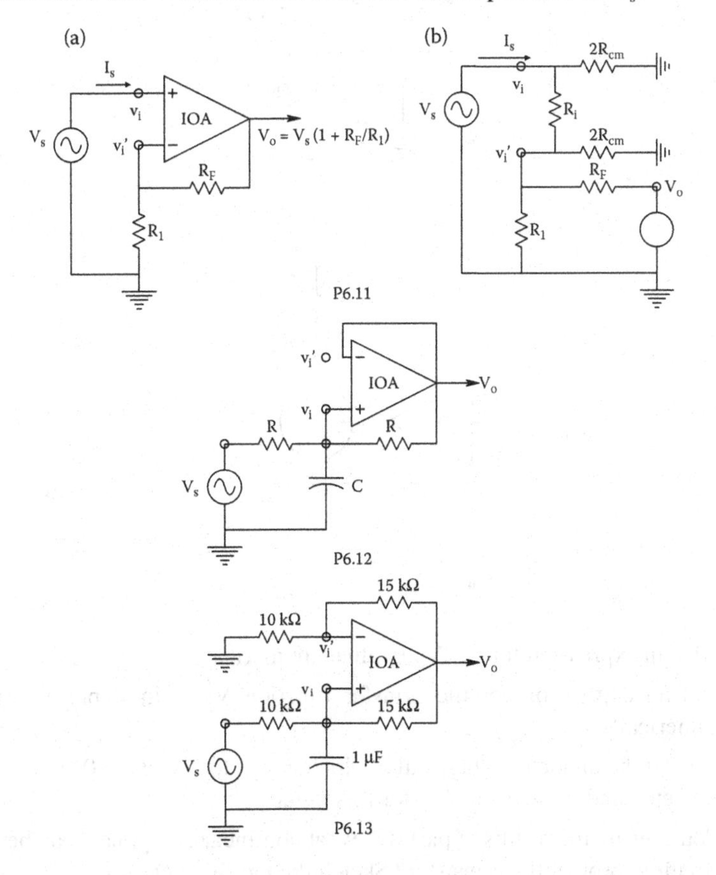

P6.11

P6.12

P6.13

6.14 The circuit of Figure P6.14 is a DC millivoltmeter. Find the value of R required so that the dc microammeter reads full-scale (100 μADC) when $V_s = 100$ mV dc. The op amp is ideal.

6.15 Derive an expression for $V_o = f(V_s, R, \Delta R)$ for the one active arm Wheatstone bridge signal conditioner of Figure P6.15. An IOA is used.

6.16 In Figure P6.16, an IOA is used to control the collector current of a power BJT, which supplies a relay coil. The relay coil has an inductance of 0.1 Hy, and a series resistance, R_L, of 30 Ω. Model the BJT by its MFSS *h*-parameter model with $h_{oe} = 0$. Derive expressions for the transfer functions, V_b/V_s, and V_c/V_s in time constant form. Note that $V_e/V_s = 1$ because of the IOA assumption. Let $h_{fe} = 19$, $h_{ie} = 10^3$ Ω and $R_E = 100$ Ω.

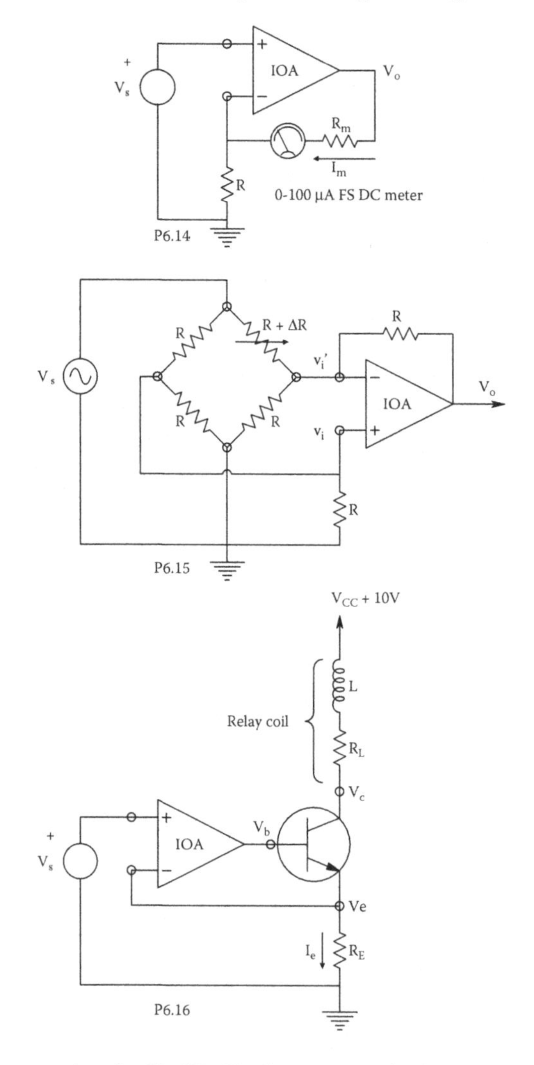

(A) Find an expression for V_b/V_s. Evaluate numerically.

(B) find an expression for the transfer function V_c/V_s in Laplace form. Evaluate numerically.

(C) Let $V_s(t)$ be an ideal voltage pulse which jumps to 2 V at t = 0, and to zero at t = 1 s. Sketch and dimension $V_c(t)$ for this input.

(D) Considering the results of part (C), what nonlinear component can be added to the circuit to protect the transistor? Sketch the modified circuit.

7 Introduction to Analog Active Filters

7.1 INTRODUCTION

Filter (*n.*) is an electrical engineering term having a broad meaning. Filters are generally considered to operate on signals in the frequency domain; that is, they attenuate, stop, pass, or boost certain frequency regions in the input signal's power density spectrum. These operations are called *filtering* (*v.*). Filter operations are classified as low-pass (LP), bandpass (BP), high-pass (HP), band-reject (BR), or notch. Bandpass and band-reject filters can have narrow (tuned) pass-bands or reject bands. One descriptor of such sharply tuned filters is their "Q." Q can be defined as the BP filter's center frequency, f_c, divided by its half-power bandwidth, Δf; the narrower the bandwidth, the higher the Q. (Δf is generally measured as the frequency span between half-power frequencies, where the filter's frequency response function is down to 0.7071 times the peak pass gain, or –3 dB from the peak gain.) Thus, mathematically, $Q \equiv f_c/\Delta f$.

Filter transfer functions can be expressed in general as rational polynomials in the complex variable, **s**. The rational polynomials can be factored to find the *poles and zeros* of the transfer function. The filter's poles are the roots of the denominator polynomial; its zeros are the roots of the numerator polynomial. Roots are the complex values of **s** that make a polynomial equal to zero. If the highest power of s in the denominator polynomial is n, there will be n poles in the complex s-plane. If the filter is stable (and all should be), all of the filter's poles will lie in the left-half s-plane. Likewise, if the highest power of s in the numerator polynomial is m, there will be m zeros in the s-plane. The zeros can lie anywhere in the s-plane; if some lie in the right-half s-plane, the filter is called *non-minimum phase.* If *all* the poles and zeros have negative real parts (i.e., lie in the left-half s-plane), the filter is called *minimum phase.* The poles and zeros can have real values, or occur in complex-conjugate pairs of the form, $\mathbf{s} = \alpha \pm j\beta$, where β is nonnegative and $-\infty < \alpha < \infty$. Conjugate zeros on the $j\omega$ axis are found in notch filters.

A filter's *frequency response* (Bode plot) is found by letting $\mathbf{s} = j\omega$ in the filter's transfer function, and then finding 20 times the log of the magnitude of the frequency response function vs $f = \omega/2\pi$ Hz, and also the angle of the frequency response function vector in degrees vs f.

Analog active filters use feedback around op amps to realize desired transfer functions for applications such as bandpass, low-pass, and notch filtering to improve signal-to-noise ratios. Active filters (AFs) use only capacitors and resistors in their circuits. Inductors are not used because they are generally large, heavy, and imperfect, i.e., they have significant losses from coil resistance and other factors. AFs are also used to realize sharp cutoff low-pass filters (LPFs) for antialiasing filtering of analog signals before periodic, analog-to-digital conversion (sampling). Active notch filters are often used to eliminate the coherent interference, which accompanies the recording of ECG, EMG, and EEG signals.

Some disconcerting news is that since EEs first discovered that op amps can be used to realize multipole filters, numerous different AF designs have been developed for each of the various filtering operations. In fact, many excellent texts have been written on the specialized art of active filter design, for example, Schaumann et al. (2009), Pactitis (2007), Williams and Taylor (2006), Irons (2005), Ghaussi and Laker (2003). In some AF designs, filter parameters such as midband gain, break frequency, Q, or damping factor cannot be designed for with unique R and C components. For example, all the filter's Rs and Cs interact, so no one component or set of components can independently determine midband gain, break frequency, damping factor, etc.

The good news is that now high-order active filters are generally designed on a modular, cascaded basis using certain preferred circuit architectures that allow exact pole and zero placement in the s-plane by single component value choices. Below we will examine some examples of these preferred AF architectures beginning with the simple controlled source, Sallen & Key (S&K), quadratic, low-pass filter.

7.2 ACTIVE FILTER APPLICATIONS

Most analog active filters used in biomedical signal conditioning are intended to restrict the amplifier passband to that of the signal spectrum, thereby cutting off broadband noise outside the signal spectrum and improving the signal-to-noise ratio at the filter output over that at the input of the signal conditioning system. Another major application of active filters is *antialiasing,* i.e., attenuating signal and noise power at the input to an analog-to-digital converter to a negligible level at frequencies of half the sampling frequency and greater.

In modern ECG and EEG data acquisition systems, one often finds an optional *notch filter,* which can be used to attenuate *coherent interference* (hum) at line frequency (60 Hz) picked up by the ECG leads.

All-pass filters are used to generate a phase shift between the input and output signal without attenuation. All-pass filters are used to adjust synchronization signal phase in lock-in amplifiers and synchronous rectifiers and to correct for phase lags inherent in data transmission on coaxial cables and other transmission lines.

7.3 TYPES OF ANALOG ACTIVE FILTERS

7.3.1 Introduction

In the AF designs described below, the op amps will be assumed to be *ideal.* For serious design evaluation, computer modeling must be used with op amp dynamic models. Note that a filter's *transient response* can be just as important as its frequency response. The bandpass filtering of an ECG signal is an example of a biomedical application of an active filter that is transient-response sensitive. The fidelity of the sharp QRS spike must be preserved for diagnosis; also, there must be little rounding of the R-peak, and no transient "ringing" following the QRS spike. The linear phase, *Bessel filter* is one class of filter architecture that is free from ringing and is suitable for conditioning ECG signals. The exact position of the poles of a high-order ($n > 2$) Bessel filter determines its characteristics.

7.3.2 Sallen & Key, Controlled-Source AFs

A basic, active filter building-block is the S&K, quadratic (two-pole), controlled source (VCVS) architecture. S&K AFs can be *cascaded* to make high-order low-, high-, or bandpass filters.

A low-pass S&K filter is shown in Figure 7.1. S&K AFs are quadratic filters, i.e., they generally have a pair of complex-conjugate (C-C) poles, as shown in Figure 7.2. Their transfer function denominators are of the form: $[s^2 + s2\xi\omega_n + \omega_n^2]$. The real part of the C-C poles is negative (at $\alpha = -\xi\omega_n$), and the imaginary parts are at $\pm j\omega_n\sqrt{1-\xi^2}$. ω_n is called the undamped natural frequency (in radians/s) and ξ is the damping factor. The poles are C-C when $0 < \xi < 1$. When $\xi > 1$, the poles are real. The damping factor is the cosine of the angle between the negative real axis in the s-plane and the vector connecting the origin with the upper pole. The closer the poles are to the $j\omega$ axis, the less damped is the output response of the filter to transient inputs. Also, LPFs with

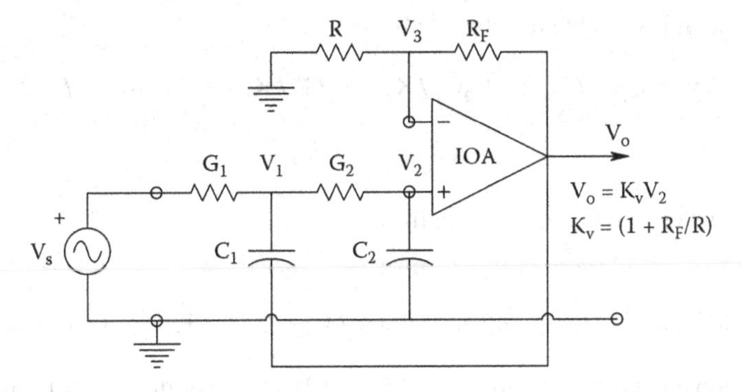

FIGURE 7.1 A Sallen & Key quadratic low-pass filter.

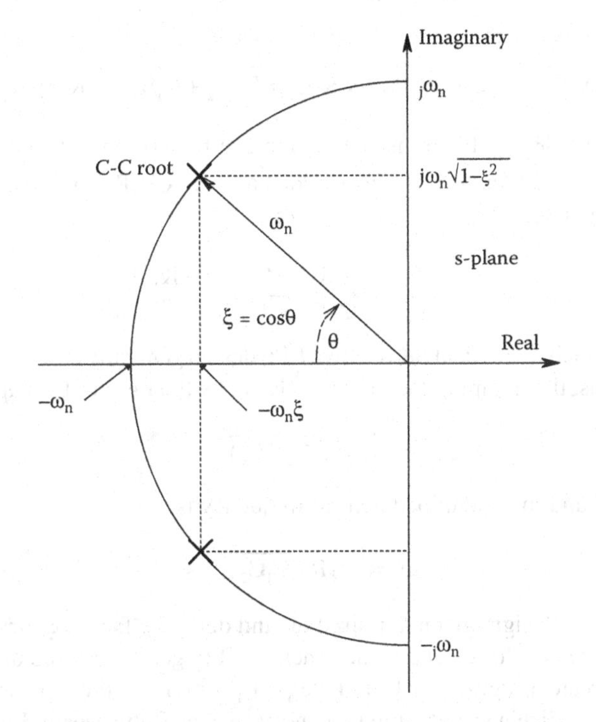

FIGURE 7.2 Complex-conjugate pole geometry in the s-plane, showing the relations between pole positions and the natural frequency and damping factor.

low damping exhibit a peak in their steady-state sinusoidal frequency response (Bode magnitude response) around ω_n.

To find the S&K LPF's transfer function, one writes the node equations for the V_1 and V_2 nodes:

$$V_1[G_1 + G_2 + sC_1] - V_2G_2 - V_0sC_1 = V_SG_1 \tag{7.1a}$$

$$-V_1G_2 + V_2[G_2 + sC_1] = 0 \tag{7.1b}$$

Now V_2 can be replaced with V_o/K_v, and the node equations rearranged:

$$V_1[G_1 + G_2 + sC_1] - V_o[sC_1 + G_2 / K_v] = V_sG_1 \tag{7.2a}$$

$$-V_1G_2 + V_o[G_2 + sC_2] / K_v = 0 \tag{7.2b}$$

Using Cramer's rule, it is possible to solve for V_o:

$$\Delta = s^2C_1C_2/K_v + s[C_2G_1/K_v + C_2G_2/K_v - C_1G_2] + G_2^2/K_v \tag{7.3}$$

$$\Delta V_o = +V_sG_1G_2 \tag{7.4}$$

Thus, the LPF's transfer function can be finally written as

$$\frac{V_o}{V_s}(s) = \frac{G_1G_2}{s^2C_1C_2/K_v + s[C_2G_1/K_v + C_2G_2/K_v + C_1G_2/K_v - C_1G_2] + G_1G_2/K_v} \tag{7.5}$$

Now multiply the top and bottom of Equation 7.5 by $R_1R_2K_v$ to put the filter's transfer function into time-constant form, used for Bode plotting:

$$\frac{V_o}{V_s}(s) = \frac{K_v}{s^2C_1C_2R_1R_2 + s[R_1C_2 + R_2C_2 + C_1R_1(1-K_v)] + 1} \tag{7.6}$$

The denominator of the S&K AF's transfer function can be written in the standard underdamped quadratic form: $s^2/\omega_n^2 + s\,2\xi/\omega_n + 1$. By inspection, $\omega_n = 1/\sqrt{R_1R_2C_1C_2}$ r/s. The filter's DC gain is K_v, and its damping factor is:

$$\xi = \frac{[C_2(R_1 + R_2) + C_1R_1(1-K_v)]}{2\sqrt{R_1R_2C_1C_2}} \tag{7.7}$$

For reasons of simplicity, practical S&K active LPF design generally sets $K_v = 1$ and $R_1 + R_2 = R$. Under these conditions, the damping factor is simply set by the ratio of the capacitor values:

$$\xi = \sqrt{(C_2/C_1)} \tag{7.8}$$

The DC gain is unity, and the undamped natural frequency is

$$\omega_n = 1/(R\sqrt{C_1C_2}) \text{ r/s} \tag{7.9}$$

To execute an S&K LPF design, given a desired ω_n and damping factor, ξ, first set the value of C_2/C_1, then pick absolute values for C_1 and C_2 and then set R to get the desired ω_n. Several S&K LPFs can be cascaded to create a high-order LPF. Pole pair positions in the s-plane can individually be controlled (ξ_k, ω_{nk}) to realize a specific filter category such as Butterworth, Bessel, Chebychev, etc.

Next, consider the design of the *Sallen & Key high-pass filter,* shown in Figure 7.3. Analysis proceeds in the same manner used for the S&K LPF, except $K_v = 1$ is assumed; thus $V_2 = V_o$. The node equations are

$$V_1[G_1 + s(C_1 + C_2)] - V_o[G_1 + sC_2] = V_s sC_1 \tag{7.10a}$$

$$-V_1 sC_2 + V_o[G_2 + sC_2] = 0 \tag{7.10b}$$

Thus,

$$\begin{aligned}\Delta &= G_1G_2 + sC_2G_1 + sC_1G_2 + sC_2G_2 + s^2C_1C_2 + s^2C_2^2 - sC_2G_1 - s^2C_2^2 \\ &= G_1G_2 + s[C_1G_2 + C_2G_2] + s^2[C_1C_2]\end{aligned} \tag{7.11}$$

and

$$\Delta V_0 = V_S S^2 C_1C_2 \tag{7.12}$$

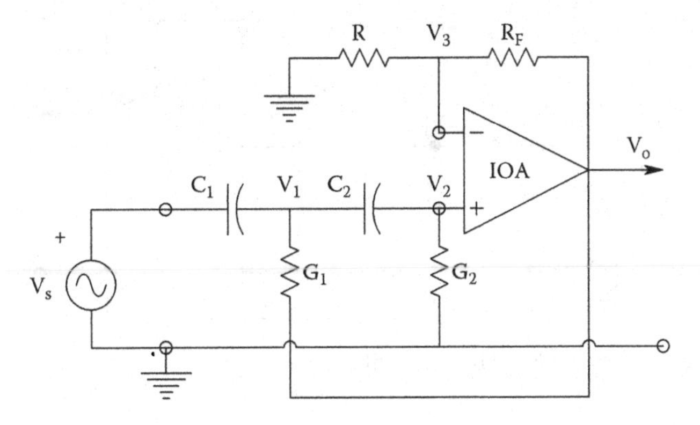

FIGURE 7.3 A Sallen & Key quadratic high-pass filter.

Thus, the S&K HPF transfer function is

$$\frac{V_o}{V_s}(s) = \frac{s^2C_1C_2}{s^2[C_1C_2] + s[C_1G_2 + C_2G_2] + G_1G_2} \tag{7.13}$$

By multiplying the top and bottom of Equation 7.13 by R_1R_2, the transfer function is put in time constant form:

$$\frac{V_o}{V_s}(s) = \frac{s^2C_1C_2R_1R_2}{s^2C_2C_1R_1R_2 + sR_1[C_1 + C_2] + 1} \tag{7.14}$$

Now let $C_1 = C_2 = C$ to obtain the final form of the HPF transfer function:

$$\frac{V_o}{V_s}(s) = \frac{s^2C^2R_1R_2}{s^2C^2R_1R_2 + sR_1 2C + 1} \tag{7.15}$$

where $\omega_{nh} = 1/[C\sqrt{R_1/R_2}]$ r/s, and $\xi_h = \sqrt{R_1/R_2}$.

If an S&K LPF is put in series with an S&K HPF, we obtain a *fourth-order bandpass filter* with two low-frequency, C-C poles at ω_{nlo}, a mid-band gain of 1, and a pair of C-C poles from the LPF at ω_{nhi}. Clearly, $\omega_{nlo} < \omega_{nhi}$. (The BPF is fourth-order because it has four poles.) The damping factors, ξ_h and ξ_{lo} determine the amount of ringing or transient settling time when the BPF is presented with a transient input such as an ECG QRS spike. ξ is usually set between 0.707 and 0.5.

A final S&K filter to consider is the quadratic BPF shown in Figure 7.4. The filter's transfer function is found by first writing the node equations on the V_1 and $V_2 = V_o$ nodes:

$$V_1[G_1 + G_3 + sC_1] - V_o[G_3 + sC_1] = V_sG_1 \tag{7.16a}$$

$$-V_1sC_1 + V_o[G_2 + s(C_1 + C_2)] = 0 \tag{7.16b}$$

The determinant is

$$\begin{aligned}\Delta &= G_1G_2 + sC_1G_1 + sC_2G_1 + G_3G_2 + sC_1G_3 + sC_2G_3 + sC_1G_2 + sC^2G_1^2 + \\ &= s^2C_1C_2 - sC_1G_3 - s^2C_1^2G_2(G_1 + G_3) + s[C_1(G_1 + G_2) + C_2(G_1 + G_3) + s^2C_1C_2\end{aligned} \tag{7.17}$$

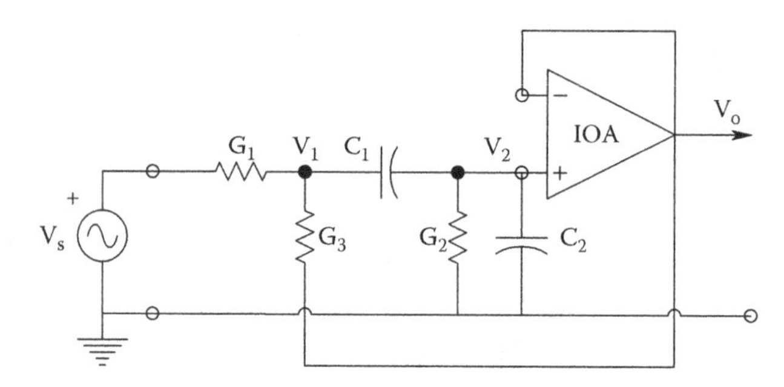

FIGURE 7.4 A Sallen & Key quadratic bandpass filter.

V_o is found from

$$\Delta V_o = V_s s C_1 G_1 \tag{7.18}$$

The BP transfer function is first written as

$$\frac{V_o}{V_s}(s) = \frac{sC_1G_1}{s^2C_1C_2 + s[C_1(G_1 + G_2) + C_2(G_1 + G_3)] + G_2(G_1 + G_3)} \tag{7.19}$$

To simplify, let $C_1 = C_2 = C$, and multiply top and bottom by $R_1\,R_2\,R_3$:

$$\frac{V_o}{V_s}(s) = \frac{sCR_2G_3}{s^2C^2R_1R_2R_3 + sCR_2[2R_3 + R_1] + (R_3 + R_1)} \tag{7.20}$$

Next, to put the transfer function in time-constant form, divide top and bottom by $(R_3 + R_1)$.

$$\frac{V_o}{V_s}(s) = \frac{sCR_2R_3 / (R_3 + R_1)}{s^2C^2R_1R_2R_3/(R_3 + R_1) + sCR_2[(2R_3 + R_1)(R_3 + R_1)] + 1} \tag{7.21}$$

The filter's undamped natural frequency is $\omega_n = 1/[C\sqrt{R_1R_2R_3(R_3 + R_1)}]$ r/s, its peak gain at $\omega = \omega_n$ is $R_3/(2\,R_3 + R_1)$, and the BPF's Q is

$$Q \equiv 1/2\xi = \frac{\sqrt{R_1R_2R_3(R_3 + R_1)}}{R_2(2R_3 + R_1)} \tag{7.22}$$

The S&K BPF's peak gain and Q are independent of C; C can be used to set ω_n once the three resistors are chosen to find the desired Q and peak gain. This is not as easy a filter to design as the separate S&K LPF and HPF which can be cascaded to form a broad-band BPF.

In closing this section on S&K, controlled (voltage) source quadratic filters, it is noted that the designer *must* simulate the filter's behavior with an accurate model of the op amp to be used in order to predict the filter's behavior at high frequencies (near the op amp's f_T), and how the filter behaves with transient inputs.

7.3.3 Biquad Active Filters

For many filter applications, the Biquad AF architecture offers ease in design when two-pole filters are desired; *independent* setting of ω_n, ξ, and midband gain, K_{vo}, are possible with few components (Rs and Cs). There are two Biquad AF architectures: the one- and two-loop. One cost of the biquad

AFs is that they use more than one op amp (3 or 4) to realize what an S&K AF can do with one op amp. The benefit of the biquad architecture is ease in design. Figure 7.5 shows the one- and two-loop configurations. The two-loop biquad filter's transfer functions will be analyzed at the V_3, V_4, and V_5 output nodes. *The output at the V_5 node is low-pass;* this can be shown by writing the transfer function using Mason's rule (see the Appendix of this text).

$$\frac{V_5}{V_s}(s) = \frac{(-R/R_1)(-R/R_2)(-1/sR_3C)(-1/sR_3C)}{1-[(-1)(-R/R_2)(-1/sR_3C)+(-1)(-1/sR_3C)^2]} \quad (7.23)$$

This LPF transfer function can be simplified algebraically to time-constant form:

$$\frac{V_5}{V_s}(s) = \frac{R^2/R_1R_2}{s^2R_3{}^2C^2 + s[RR_3C/R_2]+1} \quad (7.24)$$

By comparison with the standard quadratic polynomial form, one has

$$\omega_n = 1/(R_3C) \text{ r/s} \quad (\omega_n \text{ set by } R_3 \text{ and C}) \quad (7.25a)$$

$$\xi = R/2R_2 \quad (\text{damping factor set by } R_2) \quad (7.25b)$$

$$K_{vo} = R^2/R_1R_2 \quad (\text{DC gain set by } R_1, \text{ once } R_2 \text{ chosen}) \quad (7.25c)$$

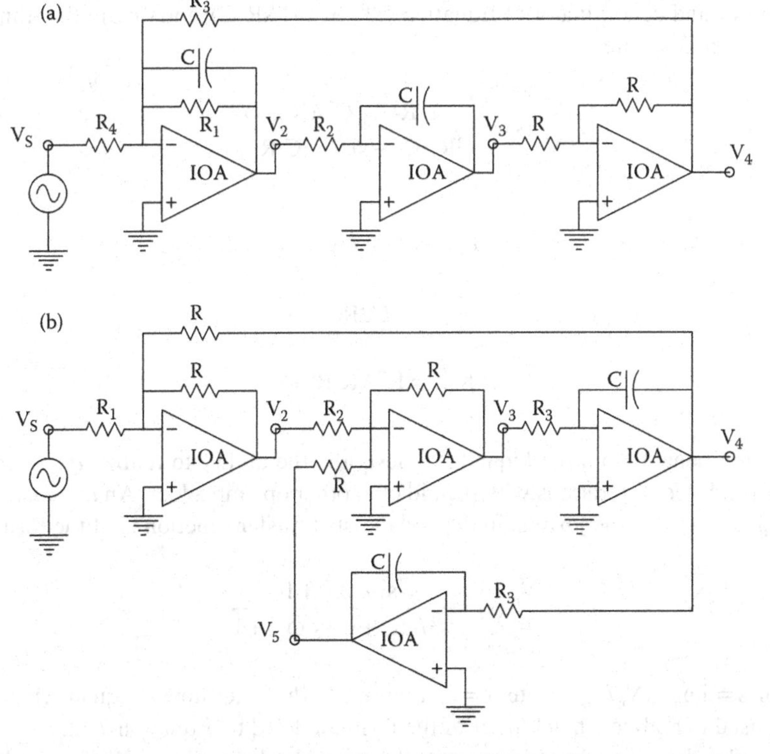

FIGURE 7.5 (a) The three-op amp, single-loop, biquad active filter. (b) The four-op amp, two-loop, biquad active filter.

Next, consider the transfer function for V_4. Note that the denominator is the same as for the V_5 transfer function.

$$\frac{V_4}{V_s}(s) = \frac{(-R/R_1)(-1/sR_3C) + (-1)(-1/sR_3C)}{1 - [(-1)(-R/R_2)(-1/sR_3C) + (-1)(-1/sR_3C)^2]} \tag{7.26}$$

When the numerator and denominator of Equation 7.26 are multiplied by $(-1/sR_3C)^2$, one gets

$$\frac{V_4}{V_s}(s) = \frac{-sR^2R_3C/(R_1R_2)}{s^2R_3{}^2C^2 + s[RR_3C/R_2] + 1} \tag{7.27}$$

which is an inverting, quadratic BPF. The filter parameters are

$$\omega_n = 1/(R_3C) \text{ r/s } (\omega_n \text{ set by } R_3 \text{ and } C) \tag{7.28a}$$

$$Q = R_2/R \text{ (Q set by } R_2\text{: } Q = 1/2\xi) \tag{7.28b}$$

$$K_{vo} = R/R_1 \quad \text{(peak gain at } \omega_n \text{ set by } R_1) \tag{7.28c}$$

Finally, examine the transfer function to the V_3 node. By Mason's rule,

$$\frac{V_3}{V_s}(s) = \frac{(-R/R_1)(-R/R_2)}{1 - [(-1)(-R/R_2)(-1/sR_3C) + (-1)(-1/sR_3C)^2]} \tag{7.29}$$

Divide numerator and denominator of Equation 7.29 by $(-1/sR_3C)^2$ and obtain the transfer function of a quadratic high-pass filter:

$$\frac{V_4}{V_s}(s) = \frac{s^2R^2R_3{}^2C^2/(R_1R_2)}{s^2R_3{}^2C^2 + s[RR_3C/R_2] + 1} \tag{7.30}$$

As before,

$$\omega_n = 1/(R_3C) \text{ r/s} \tag{7.31a}$$

$$\xi = R/2R_2 \tag{7.31b}$$

$$K_{vhi} = R^2/(R_1R_2) \tag{7.31c}$$

An interesting benefit from the biquad AF design is the ability to realize *quadratic notch* and *all-pass filter* (APF) configurations with the aid of another op amp adder. An *ideal notch filter* has a pair of conjugate zeros on the $j\omega$ axis in the s-plane; its transfer function is of the form

$$\frac{V_n}{V_s}(s) = \frac{s^2/\omega_n{}^2 + 1}{s^2/\omega_n{}^2 + s/(Q\,\omega_n) + 1} \tag{7.32}$$

Clearly, when $s = j\omega_n$, $|(V_n/V_s) \times (j\omega_n)| = 0$. Figure 7.6 illustrates how a biquad AF and an op amp adder can be used to realize a notch filter of the form modeled by Equation 7.32.

The biquad plus the op amp summer architecture can also be used to realize a *quadratic all-pass filter* in which a pair of complex-conjugate zeros is found in the right-half s-plane with positive real

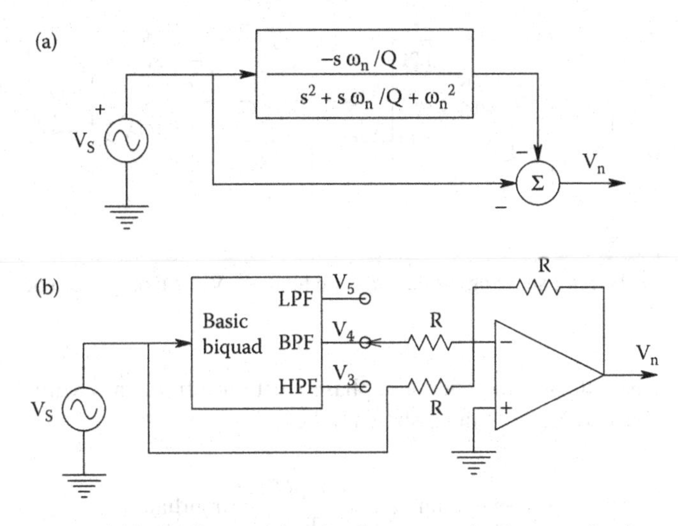

FIGURE 7.6 (a) A systems' block diagram showing how a notch filter can be formed from a quadratic BPF. (b) A practical circuit showing how a two-loop biquad's V_4 BPF output can be added to V_s to make the notch filter.

parts the same magnitude as the C-C poles in the left-half s-plane. The general form of this APF is given in Equation 7.33:

$$\frac{V_{ap}}{V_s}(s) = \frac{s^2/\omega_n^2 - s^2\xi/\omega_n + 1}{s^2/\omega_n^2 + s^2\xi/\omega_n + 1} \tag{7.33}$$

Figure 7.7 illustrates the circuit architecture which is used to realize a symmetrical APF. The APF output is given by

$$V_{ap} = -R_6[V_s/R_5 + V_4/R_4] \tag{7.34}$$

Now substitute the transfer function for the BPF into Equation 7.34 to get the APF transfer function:

$$\frac{V_{ap}}{V_s}(s) = -\left\{R_6/R_5 + \frac{(R_6/R_4)(-sR^2R_3C/(R_1R_2))}{s^2R_3{}^2C^2 + s[RR_3C/R_2] + 1}\right\}$$

$$= -\left\{\frac{s^2(R_6/R_5)R_3{}^2C^2 + s(R_6/R_5)[RR_3C/R_2] - s(R_6/R_4)R^2R_3C/(R_1R_2) + (R_6/R_5)}{s^2R_3{}^2C^2 + s[RR_3C/R_2] + 1}\right\} \tag{7.35}$$

To obtain the symmetric APF, let $R_1 = R$, $R_5 = 2R_4$, and $R_6 = R_5$. The desired transfer function is then

$$\frac{V_{ap}}{V_s}(s) = \frac{s^2R_3{}^2C^2 - sR_3CR/R_2 + 1}{s^2R_3{}^2C^2 + sR_3CR/R_2 + 1} \tag{7.36}$$

The natural frequency of both poles and zeros is

$$\omega_n = 1/(R_3C) \text{ r/s} \tag{7.37a}$$

$$\xi = R/2R_2 \tag{7.37b}$$

$$K_{vo} = -1, -\infty \le \omega \le \infty \tag{7.37c}$$

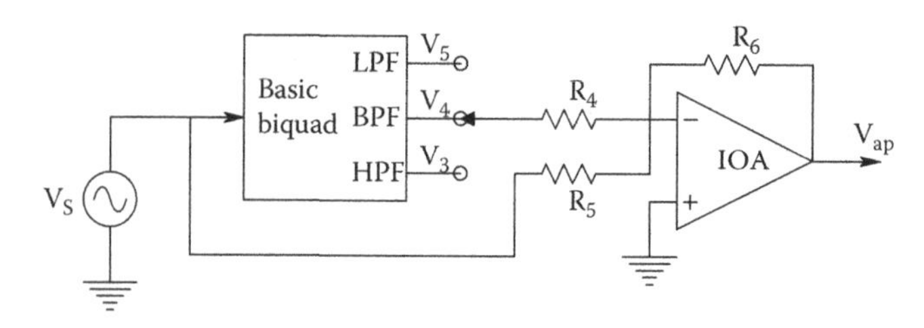

FIGURE 7.7 A practical circuit showing how a two-loop biquad's V_4 BPF output can be added to V_s to make a quadratic all-pass filter.

The purpose of all-pass filters is to generate a phase shift with frequency with no attenuation; the phase of the APF described earlier can be shown to be

$$\varphi = -\pi - 2\tan^{-1}\left[\frac{\omega(R_3C)R/R_2}{1-\omega^2 R_3 2C^2}\right] \text{ randians} \tag{7.38}$$

7.3.4 Generalized Impedance Converter AFs

Often it is desired to design AFs that work at very low frequencies, e.g., below 20 Hz. Such filters can find application in conditioning low-frequency physiological signals such as the ECG, EEG, and heart sounds. If a conventional biquad AF is used to make a high-pass filter whose $f_n = 1$ Hz, for example, it is necessary to use very large capacitors which are not only expensive, but take up excessive volume on a PC board. For example, the capacitor required for $f_n = 1$ Hz and $R_3 = 100$ kΩ is

$$C = \frac{1}{2\pi f_n R_3} = 1.59\ \mu F \tag{7.39}$$

The generalized impedance converter (GIC) circuit, shown in a general format in Figure 7.8, allows the size of a small capacitor, e.g., 0.001 μF, to be electronically magnified, or transformed into a large, equivalent, very *high-Q inductor,* or made into a *D-element* which can be shown to have the impedance, $Z_D(\omega) = 1/(\omega^2 D)$, where D is determined by certain R_s and C_s as shown below.

An expression for the driving point impedance of the general GIC circuit, $\mathbf{Z_{11}} = \mathbf{V_1/I_1}$, is now found. Clearly, from Ohm's law

$$Z_n = V_1/I_1 = \frac{V_1}{(V_1 - V_2)/Z_1} \tag{7.40}$$

Also, from the ideal op amp assumption and Ohm's law one can write the currents

$$I_2 = (V_2 - V_1)/Z_2 = I_3 = (V_1 - V_3)/Z_3 \tag{7.41}$$

$$I_4 = (V_3 - V_1)/Z_4 = I_5 = V_1/Z_5 \tag{7.42}$$

From the preceding three equations (7.40, 7.41, and 7.42), it is easy to show

$$V_3 = V_1(1 + Z_4/Z_5) \tag{7.43}$$

$$V_2 = V_1\left(\frac{Z_3Z_5 - Z_2Z_4}{Z_3Z_5}\right) \tag{7.44}$$

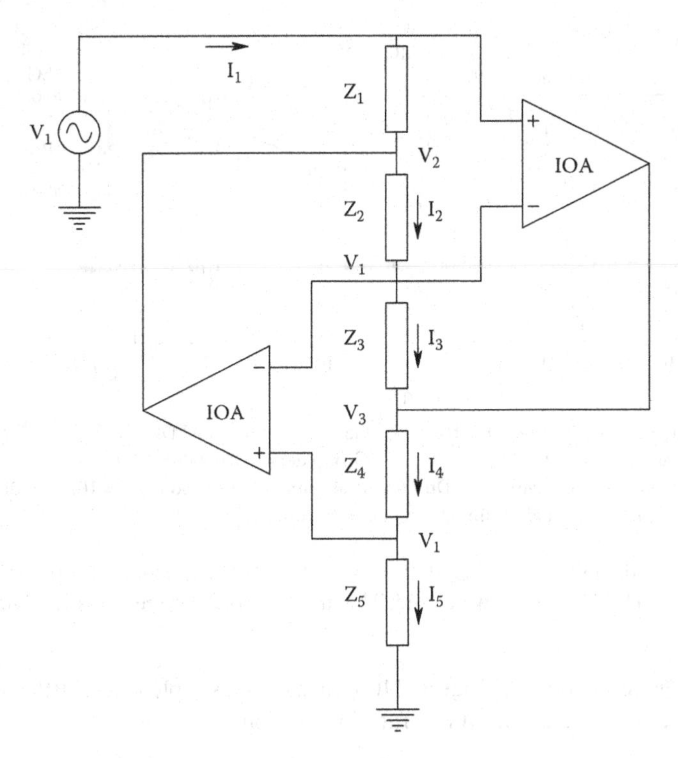

FIGURE 7.8 General architecture for a generalized impedance converter (GIC) circuit. The $\mathbf{Z}_k$ can either be resistances or capacitances ($1/j\omega C_k$), depending on the filter requirement.

And the GIC driving point impedance is given compactly as

$$Z_n = V_1/I_1 = Z_1 Z_3 Z_5/(Z_2 Z_4) \text{ (complex) ohms} \tag{7.45}$$

Now if $\mathbf{Z_2}$ or $\mathbf{Z_4} = 1/j\omega C$ (a capacitor), and the other elements are resistors, $\mathbf{Z_{11}}$ has the form

$$Z_n = j\omega[C_4 R_1 R_3 R_5/R_2] \text{ reactive (inductive) ohms} \tag{7.46}$$

That is, the GIC emulates a low-loss inductor over a wide range of frequency. The inductance of the emulated inductor is

$$L_{eq} = [C_4 R_1 R_3 R_5/R_2] \text{ Hy.} \tag{7.47}$$

Figure 7.9 illustrates the magnitude and phase response of an inductive $\mathbf{Z_{11}}$ vs frequency. $20 \log|\mathbf{Z_{11}}(f)|$ and $\angle\, \mathbf{Z_{11}}(f)$ vs f are plotted using MicroCap™. The circuit used in this simulation is the same as in Figure 7.8, with $\mathbf{Z_1} = \mathbf{Z_3} = \mathbf{Z_4} = \mathbf{Z_5} = 1$ kΩ, and $\mathbf{Z_2} = 1/j\omega C_2$; $C_2 = 0.1$ μF. From Equation 7.47, we see that the simulated inductance is 0.1 Hy. (Op amp output current saturation effects are not included in this simple simulation.) Note that $|\mathbf{Z_{11}}(f)|$ increases linearly with frequency until about 180 kHz, where its phase abruptly goes from the ideal +90° to −270°, and $20 \log|\mathbf{Z_{11}}(f)|$ exhibits a tall peak at *ca.* 1 MHz. Clearly, the circuit model emulates a 0.1 Hy inductor below 180 kHz. A simple, nonsaturating, two-time-constant model of the TL082 op amp was used in the MicroCap™ simulation.

Because the GIC inductive $\mathbf{Z_{11}}$ is referenced to ground, it must be used in active filter designs that require inductors with one end tied to ground. Figure 7.10a illustrates an inductive GIC used

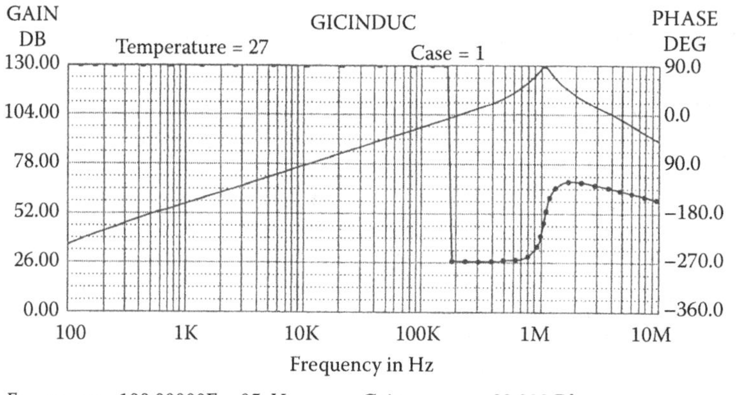

Frequency = 100.00000E + 05 Hz   Gain = 89.003 Db
Phase angle = −158.263 Degrees   Group delay = 0.00000E + 00
Gain slope = −114.36240E − 01 Db/Oct   Peak gain = 128.556 Db/F = 107.01700E + 04
1: Another run 2: Analysis limits 3: Quit 4: Dump

FIGURE 7.9 Magnitude and phase of $\mathbf{Z}_{11}(f)$ looking into a GIC emulation of a 0.1 HY inductor. In this MicroCap simulation, TL072 op amps were used. The inductor emulation remains valid up to ca. 160 kHz.

in a simple, high-Q, quadratic BPF. Figure 7.10b illustrates a simple R-L-C BPF suitable for circuit analysis. A node equation gives the BPF's transfer function:

$$\frac{V_o}{V_s}(s) = \frac{s\, L_{eq}/R}{s^2 C L_{eq} + s L_{eq}/R + 1} \tag{7.48}$$

In this filter,

$$\omega_n = 1/\sqrt{CL_{eq}} \ \text{r/s} \tag{7.49a}$$

$$Q = 1/(2\xi) = R\sqrt{C/L_{eq}} \tag{7.49b}$$

$$\frac{V_o}{V_s}(j\omega_n) = 1\angle 0^\circ \tag{7.49c}$$

L_{eq} is given by Equation 7.47.

The GIC "D element" $\mathbf{Z}_{11}$ is a *frequency-dependent negative resistance* (FDNR). It can be made by putting capacitors in the $\mathbf{Z}_1$ and $\mathbf{Z}_3$ positions in the GIC circuit. Thus, the driving point impedance is real and negative:

$$\mathbf{Z}_{11} = \frac{(1/j\omega C_1)(1/j\omega C_3)R_5}{R_2 R_4} = \frac{-R_5}{\omega^2 C_1 C_3 R_2 R_5} = \frac{-1}{\omega^2 D} \ \text{ohms} \tag{7.50}$$

$$D = C_1 C_3 R_2 R_4 / R_5 \tag{7.51}$$

Figure 7.11 shows how the D element can be used to make a quadratic LPF. Write the node equation for V_o in terms of the Laplace complex variable, s:

$$V_o[G + sC + s^2 D] = V_s G \tag{7.52}$$

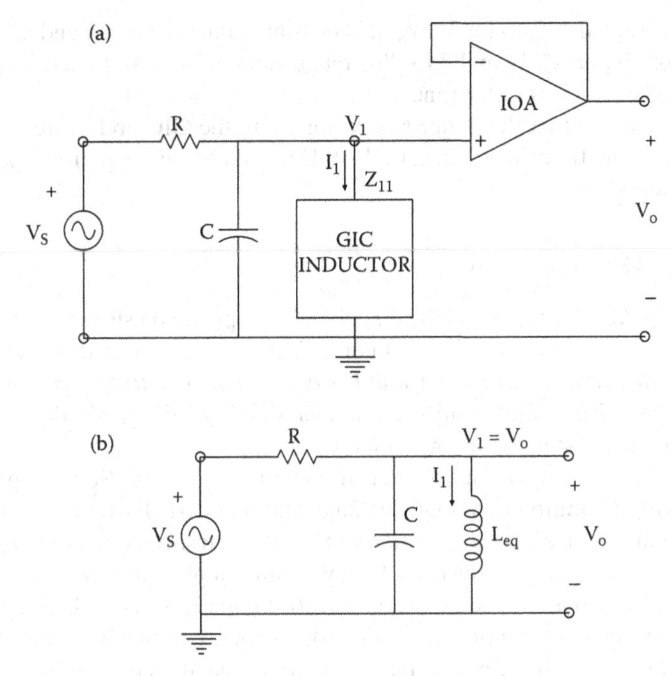

FIGURE 7.10 (a) Circuit of an RLC bandpass filter using a GIC inductor. The GIC circuit allows emulation of a very large, high-Q inductor over a wide range of frequencies, and is particularly well-suited for making filters in the sub-audio range of frequencies. (b) The actual BPF.

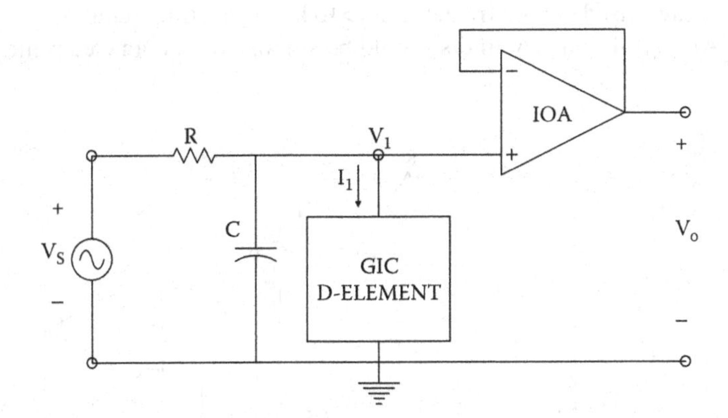

FIGURE 7.11 Circuit showing how a GIC "D" element can make a low-frequency, low-pass filter.

Solving for V_o yields

$$\frac{V_o}{V_s}(s) \equiv \frac{1}{s^2DR + sCR + 1} \tag{7.53}$$

Clearly, for the GIC FDNR LPF,

$$\omega_n = 1/\sqrt{DR}\ \text{r/s} \tag{7.54a}$$

and

$$\xi = \sqrt{R/D}(C/2) \tag{7.54b}$$

By using relation Equation 7.44 for V_2/V_S, it is possible to realize *notch* and *all-pass* filters from the basic GIC circuit. Figures 7.12 and 7.13 illustrate examples of these filters. It is left as exercises for the reader to develop their transfer functions.

In summary, note again that the major reason for using the GIC architecture is to realize AFs that are useful at very low frequencies, e.g., 0.01–10 Hz, without having to use expensive, very large capacitances or inductances.

7.3.5 Choice of AF Components

Because most analog AFs used in biomedical applications operate on signals in the 0–5 kHz range, overall filter high-frequency response is often not an important consideration. Instead, we are concerned with *noise, linearity, DC drift,* and *stability of parameter settings* (DC gain, ω_n, and damping, ξ). To minimize noise and maximize parameter stability, one generally chooses metal film resistors (or wirewound resistors) with low tempcos.

Choice of capacitors is important in determining filter linearity. Some capacitor dielectrics exhibit excessive losses, unidirectional DC leakage, and dielectric hysteresis and thus can distort filtered signals. In particular, *electrolytic and tantalum* dielectric capacitors *are not* recommended for AF components; they are usually used for bypassing applications where they are operated with a fixed DC voltage bias. Polycarbonate dielectric capacitors can also distort signals. The best capacitor dielectrics are air, mica, ceramic, oiled paper, and mylar. Again, low tempcos are desired. Do not be tempted to use electrolytic or tantalum capacitors in an AF designs that requires large capacitor values in order to realize a low ω_n. Instead, use a GIC design for the filter which uses smaller Cs.

Op amps used in AFs also must be chosen for DC stability (low offset voltage tempco), low noise, and high DC gain. Filters used at high frequencies (>10 kHz) generally require op amps with appropriately high f_Ts. All high-frequency filters should be simulated with an electronic circuit analysis

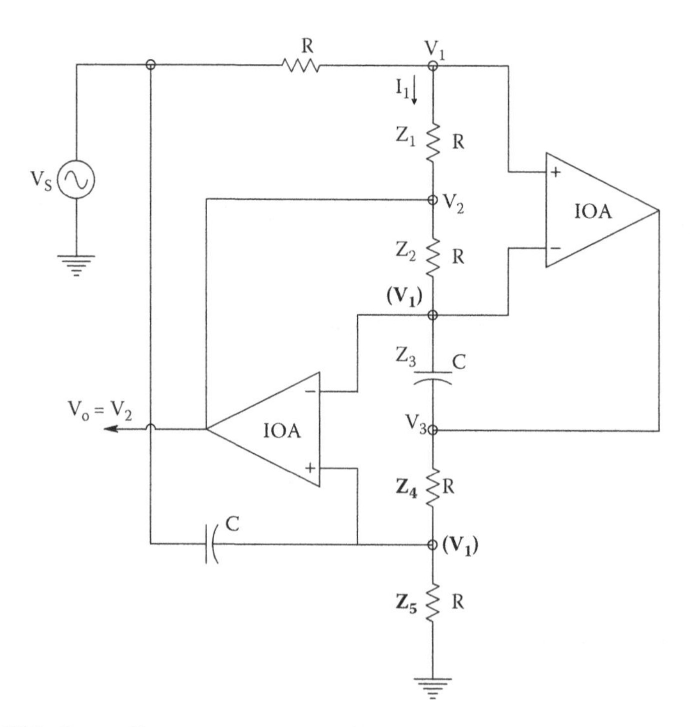

FIGURE 7.12 A GIC all-pass filter.

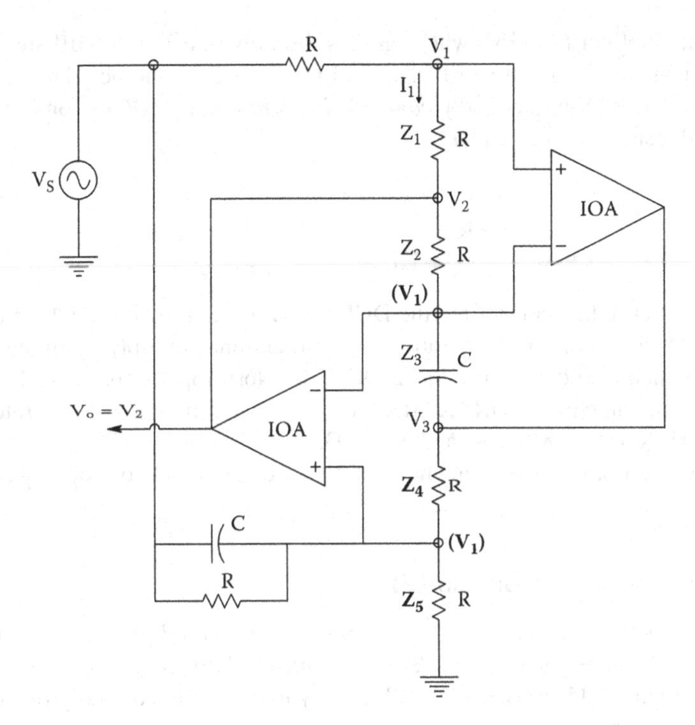

FIGURE 7.13 A GIC notch filter.

program such as MicroCap™ or SPICE™ to ensure that no surprises will occur at high frequencies near the op amps' f_Ts.

7.4 ELECTRONICALLY TUNABLE AFS

7.4.1 INTRODUCTION

In many biomedical instrumentation systems, a conditioned (by filtering) analog signal is periodically sampled and digitized. The digital number sequence is then further processed by certain digital algorithms which can include, but are not limited to: Signal averaging, computation of signal statistics (e.g., mean, RMS value), computation of the discrete Fourier transform, convolution with another signal or kernel, etc. Often it is desired to use the computer to change the analog input filter's parameters (half-power frequencies or center frequency, damping factor or Q of a tuned filter) to accommodate a new sampling rate or changes in the analog signal's power spectrum.

A particular application of a computer-controlled analog filter is the *antialiasing* (A-A) *low-pass filter.* To prevent aliasing and the problems this creates for the signal in digital form, the A-A filter must pass no significant signal spectral power to the analog-to-digital converter at frequencies above one-half the sampling frequency, f_s. $f_s/2$ is called the *Nyquist frequency,* f_n. (See Section 10.2 for a complete treatment of sampling and aliasing.)

The key to designing a digitally tuned active filter is the *variable gain element* (VGE) (Northrop 1990, Section 10.1). There are several approaches to the design of digitally controlled variable gain elements (DCVGEs): One can use a digital-to-analog converter (DAC) configured to produce 0–10 VDC output, V_C, which is the input to an *analog multiplier* IC. The other input to the analog multiplier is the time-variable analog signal, $v_k(t)$, whose amplitude is to be adjusted. The output of the analog multiplier is then: $v_k'(t) = v_k(t)V_C/10$. $V_C/10$ varies from 0 to 1 in steps determined by the quantization set by the number of binary bits input to the DAC. Another VGE is the digitally programmed gain amplifier (DPGA), whose gain is digitally selected in 6 dB steps (i.e., 1, 2, 4, 8, 16, 32, 64, 128) using a 3-bit input word (e.g., the MN2020). Still another class of DCVGE is represented by the AD8400, 8-bit, *digitally controlled potentiometer* (DCP) connected as a variable resistor. The DCP resistance is given by

$$V_j' = R_{total} \sum_{k=1}^{N} B_k 2^{k-(1+N)} = R_{total} A_k \tag{7.55}$$

where N is the number of bits controlling the DCP and B_k is the kth bit state (0 or 1).

Note that the DCP is similar in operation to a 2-quadrant, multiplying digital-to-analog converter (MDAC), which also can be used as a DCVGE (Northrop 1990). Other DCPs include, but are not limited to: the Intersil/XICOR® X0319, the Dallas/Maxim® DS1805, the Intersil® ISL22315, ISL23415, X9C102, X9C103, X0C104, and X9C503.

In the following sections, we examine how DCVGEs can tune a two-loop biquad A-A LPF's ω_n and Q.

7.4.2 A Tunable, Two-Loop Biquad LPF

Figure 7.14 illustrates the schematic of a 2-loop biquad LPF with digital control of its natural frequency at constant damping using 8-bit, *digitally controlled attenuators* (DCAs). (One form of a DCA is shown in Figure 7.15. It uses a DPP.) It is easy to derive this digitally tuned LPF's transfer function using Mason's rule:

$$\frac{V_o}{V_s}(s) = \frac{(-1/s\xi)(-2\xi)(\eta)(-1/sRC)(\eta)(-1/sRC)}{1-[(-1)(-2\xi)(\eta)(-1/sRC)+(-1)(\eta)(-1/sRC)(\eta)(-1/sRC)]} \tag{7.56a}$$

$$\downarrow$$

$$\frac{V_o}{V_s}(s) = \frac{1}{s^2(RC/\eta)^2 + s(RC/\eta)(2\xi)+1} \tag{7.56b}$$

From the standard quadratic format,

$$\omega_n = \eta/RC \quad r/s \tag{7.57}$$

The constant damping, ξ, is set by the size of the input resistor ($2\xi R$) and the resistor size V_2 sees ($R/2\xi$). Thus, with 1 LSB in, $W_n = \{0,0,0,0,0,0,0,1\}$, $\omega_n = (1/256)(1/RC)$ r/s; with $W_N = \{1,1,1,1,1,1,1,1\}$, $\omega_n = (255/256)(1/RC)$ r/s. The DC gain of the filter is +1.

As the second example, consider the digitally controlled bandpass filter shown in Figure 7.16 in which two, N-bit, serial binary words (W_{N1} and W_{N2}) are used to set the filter's natural frequency, ω_n, and a third variable gain element is used to adjust the filter's Q. In this example, *digitally controlled amplifier gains are used.* Using Mason's rule as before, one can write the transfer function as

$$\frac{V_4}{V_s}(s) = \frac{(-1)A_1(-1/128)A_2(-1/sRC)}{1-[(-1)A_1(-1/128)A_2(-1/sRC)+(-1)A_2(-1/sRC)A_2(-/sRC)]} \tag{7.58}$$

$$\downarrow$$

$$\frac{V_4}{V_s}(s) = \frac{-s(A_1/A_2)RC/128}{s^2(RC/A_2)^2 + sRC(A_1/A_2)/128+1} \tag{7.59}$$

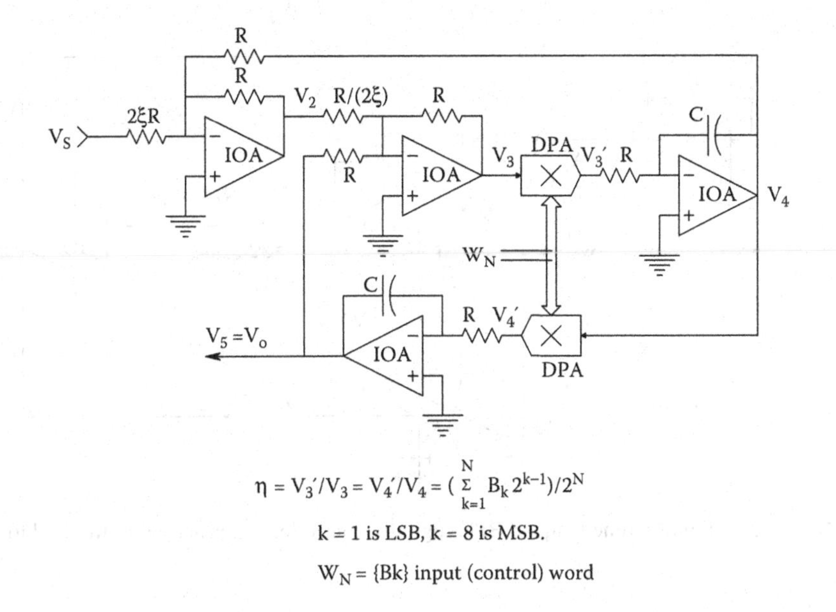

FIGURE 7.14 The use of two, parallel digitally controlled attenuators to tune the break frequency of a two-loop biquad low-pass filter at constant damping. See Text for analysis.

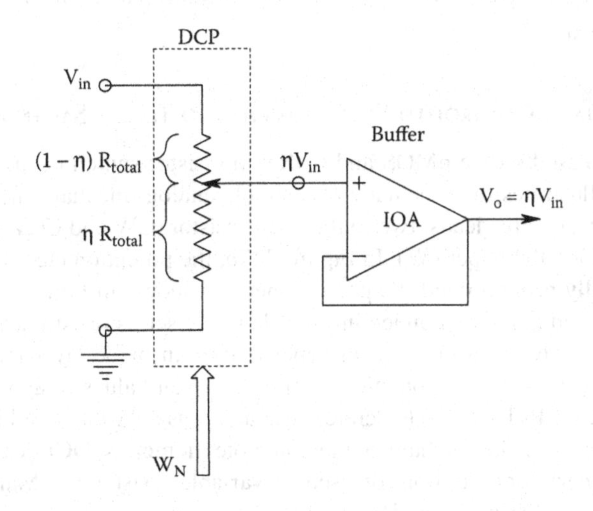

FIGURE 7.15 Schematic of a digitally controlled attenuator (DCA).

where the resonant frequency is set by $\mathbf{A_2}$, and the Q by $1/\mathbf{A_1}$:

$$\omega_n = A_2/RC \text{ r/s} \tag{7.60a}$$

$$Q = 128/A_1 \tag{7.60b}$$

$$\frac{\mathbf{V_4}}{\mathbf{V_s}}(\omega_n) = -1(\text{peak gain}) \tag{7.60b}$$

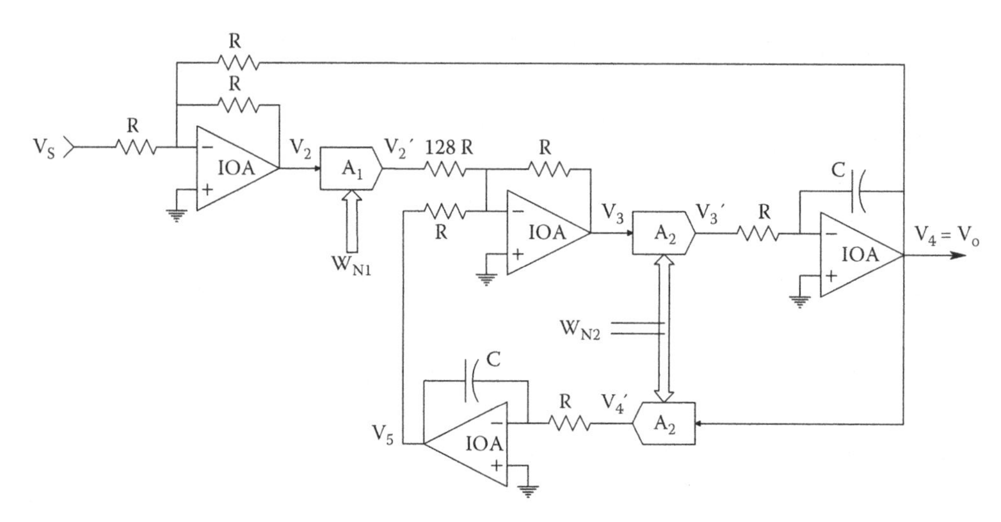

FIGURE 7.16 In this digitally tuned biquad BPF, digitally controlled amplifier gains are used to set ω_n and the Q.

Note that the $\mathbf{A_1}$ digitally controlled, variable gain amplifier drives a resistor of 128R so that the effective gain from V_2 to V_3 is $(-\mathbf{A_1}/128)$. $\mathbf{A_1}$ values are typically (1, 2, 4, 8, 16, 32, 64, 128), so the BPF's Q values are (128, 64, 32, 16, 8, 4, 2, 1). Thus, the digital word, $\mathbf{W_{N2}}$, can be used to scan the filter's center frequency over a 1:128 range under constant Q conditions, or adjust the BPF's Q *independently* with $\mathbf{W_{N1}}$.

7.4.3 Use of Digitally Controlled Potentiometers to Tune a Sallen & Key LPF

DCPs are IC devices based on the nMOS and CMOS transistor switch technology used in certain ADCs. Figure 7.17a illustrates the schematic of a simple analog (mechanical) potentiometer. Note that the potentiometer has three leads; two to the fixed resistor (CW and CCW), and the third (variable) connection is called the wiper (W). In Figure 7.17b, the potentiometer is connected as a variable resistor. A digitally programmed, IC potentiometer is shown in Figure 7.17c. Only one MOS transistor switch is closed at a time connecting a node in the series resistor array to the wiper. The resistors are generally polycrystalline silicon deposited on an oxide layer for electrical isolation. They can have equal values (linear potentiometer) or be given values to approximate logarithmic attenuation. Typically, DCPs have 256 (discrete) taps, and thus an 8-bit, serial input word is needed to select the wiper position. Like mechanical (analog) potentiometers, DCPs can be given the potentiometer (voltage divider) configuration, or used as variable resistances. Manufacturers of DCPs include Analog Devices, Maxim, Intersil, and Xicor.

A DCP connected as a variable resistor can be used to set an AF's filtering parameters (ω_n, gain, and Q or damping). Figure 7.18 illustrates the use of two DCPs (with the same control input) to tune an S&K LPF at constant damping by varying R. Recall that the natural frequency of a, S&K LPF's poles is at $\omega_n = 1/(R\sqrt{C_1C_2})$ r/s, and its damping factor is solely determined by the square root of the ratio of the capacitors, *viz.*, $\xi = \sqrt{(C_2/C_1)}$. Hence, for this LPF, $\omega_n = 1/(R_{dp}\sqrt{C_1C_2})$ r/s. Note that ω_n varies hyperbolically with R_{dp}.

A number of examples exist of electronically tuned AFs (cf. Ch. 10 in Northrop 1990). Analog voltages or currents derived from DACs, or serial or parallel digital words can be used to set resistors or gains in digitally controlled variable gain elements (DCVGEs). (A classic example of adaptive filter design is the venerable Dolby B™ audio noise reduction system; this system was treated in detail in Chapter 10 of Northrop 1990.)

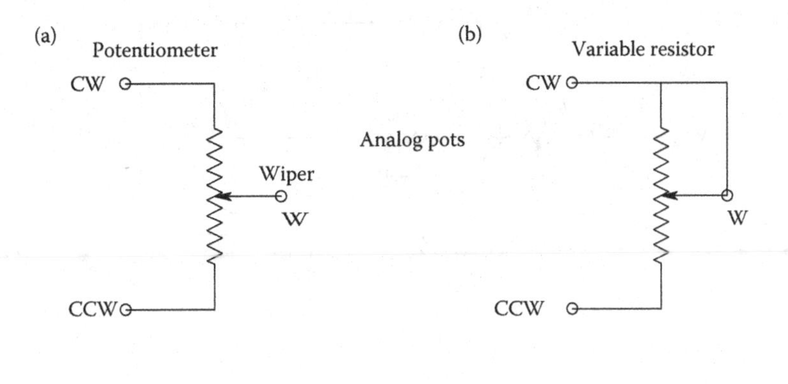

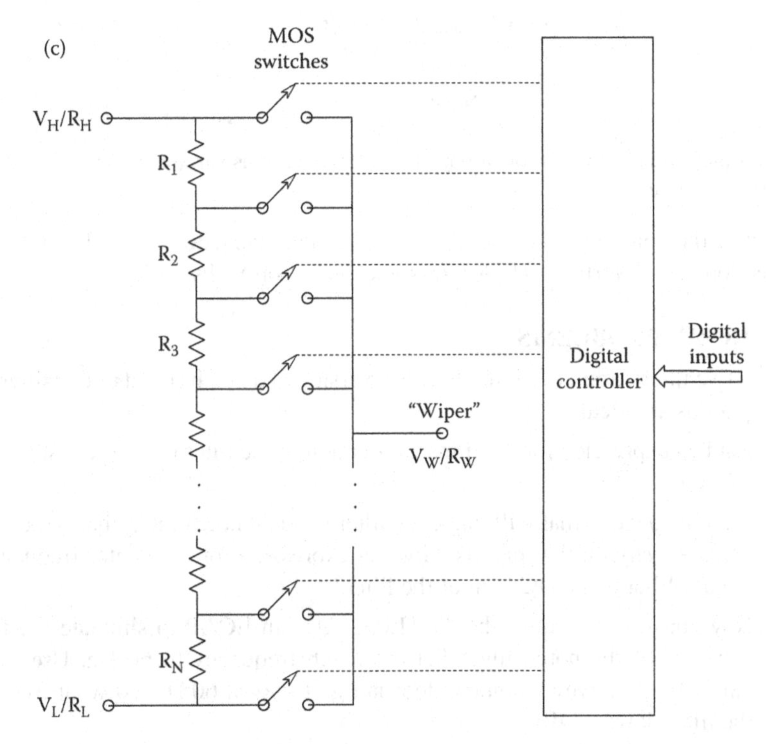

FIGURE 7.17 (a) Schematic of a conventional, mechanically tuned, analog potentiometer. (b) A potentiometer connected as a variable resistor. (c) A digitally programmed, analog potentiometer. Only one MOS switch is closed at a time. An 8-bit digital pot has 256 taps.

7.5 CHAPTER SUMMARY

There are many op amp active filter architectures. Some are easier to design with than others. This chapter focused on the easy ones: the controlled-source, S&K filters, the biquad active filter family, and the filters based on the GIC circuit. Also covered was the design and analysis of electronically tunable active filters using variable-gain elements such as analog multipliers, multiplying DACs, DCPs, and digitally controlled gain amplifiers. Electronically tuned filters have application as antialiasing filters and tuned filters that can track a coherent signal's frequency, to compensate for Doppler shift, for example.

Although not covered in this chapter, the reader should appreciate that there is a family of active filters called *switched-capacitor filters* (SCFs) that are primarily used in telecommunications. The SCFs use MOS switches to commute capacitors in what would otherwise be an op amp, R-C filter design. The switched capacitor can be shown to emulate a resistor of value $R_{eq} = T_c/C_s$, where

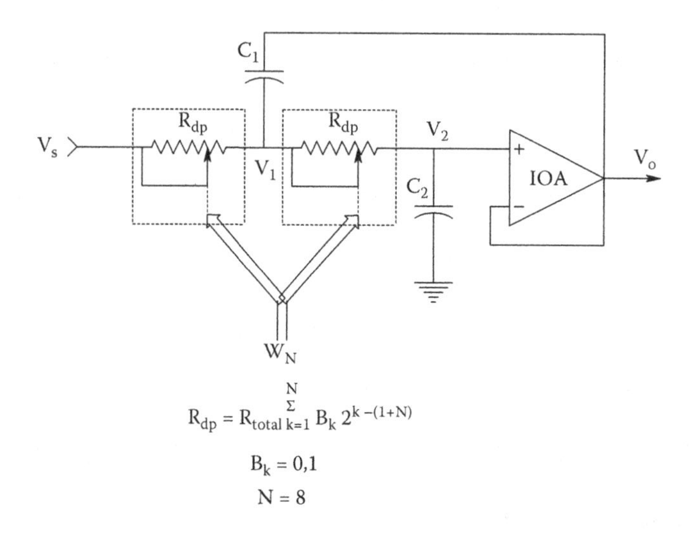

FIGURE 7.18 A pair of digitally controlled potentiometers is used as variable resistors in a digitally tuned, Sallen & Key low-pass filter.

T_c is the period of the commutation, and C_s is the switched capacitor value. The interested reader can consult Section 9.2 in Northrop (1990) for some details on SCFs.

CHAPTER 7 HOME PROBLEMS

7.1 The active filter circuit of Figure P7.1 is a version of a notch (band reject) filter. Assume the op amps are ideal.

(A) Find an expression for the transfer function of the filter in time-constant form. Let $RC = \tau$.

(B) Find the β value that will make the filter an ideal notch filter, that is, put conjugate zeros *exactly* on the $j\omega$ axis. Give an expression for the center frequency of the notch. What is the DC gain of the filter?

(C) Now make the op amps be TI TL072. Use an ECAP to simulate the frequency response of the notch filter. Set the notch frequency to 60 Hz. Use the ideal β value. Explain why the notch does not go to $-\infty$ at 60 Hz. At what frequencies is the filter down −3 dB?

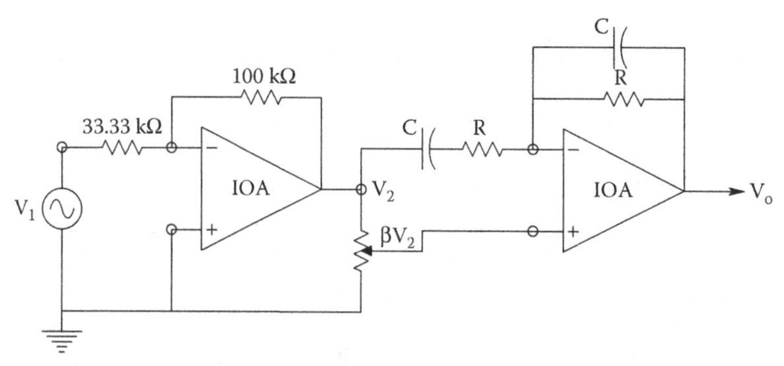

7.2 (A) Consider the S&K high-pass filter shown in Text Figure 7.3. Design an HPF with passband gain of unity, $f_n = 100$ Hz, and $\xi = 0.707$. Use a TL071 op amp. Specify circuit parameters.

(B) Use an ECAP Bode plot to verify your design. Give the −3 dB frequencies of the filter, and its high- and low-frequency f_Ts.

7.3 Derive an expression for the transfer function of the active filter of Figure P7.3 in time constant form. Give expressions for the filter's ω_n, DC gain, and damping factors of the numerator and denominator.

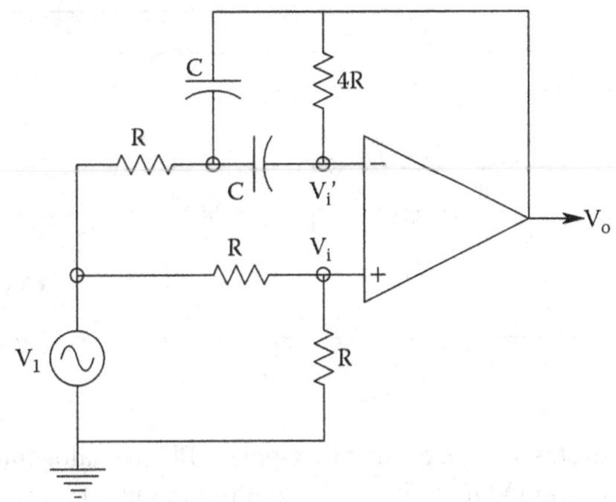

7.4 Design a bandpass filter for neural spike signal conditioning using two, cascaded, quadratic S&K active filters (1 LoP, 1 HiP) having the following specifications: Midband gain = 0 dB, −3 dB f_{LO} = 300 Hz, ξ_{LO} = 0.5, −3 dB f_{HI} = 4 kHz, ξ_{HI} = 0.5. (Note that the filter −3dB frequencies are not necessarily their f_ns.) Use OP-27 op amps. Specify the R & C values. Note: All Rs must be between 10^3 and 10^6 Ω, and C values must lie between 3 pF and 3 μF. Verify your design with an ECAP Bode plot.

7.5 Design a quadratic GIC bandpass filter for geophysical applications to condition a seismometer output having f_n = 1 HZ and Q = 10. Verify your design with an ECAP Bode plot. Use the same ranges of Rs and Cs as in Prob. 7.4.

7.6 (A) Write the transfer function, $\mathbf{V}_4/\mathbf{V}_1$ in time-constant form for the three-op amp biquad AF shown in Figure P7.6.

(B) Write the transfer function, $\mathbf{V}_2/\mathbf{V}_1$ for the AF in TC form. Give expressions for ω_n, Q, and $\mathbf{V}_2/\mathbf{V}_1$ at ω_n.

(C) Write an expression for the transfer function, $\mathbf{V}_5/\mathbf{V}_1$, in time constant form. Use an ECAP to make a Bode plot of $\mathbf{V}_5/\mathbf{V}_1$. Let R = 1 kΩ, R_1 = 10 kΩ, R_4 = 1 kΩ, C = 10 nF, and op amps are TL074s.

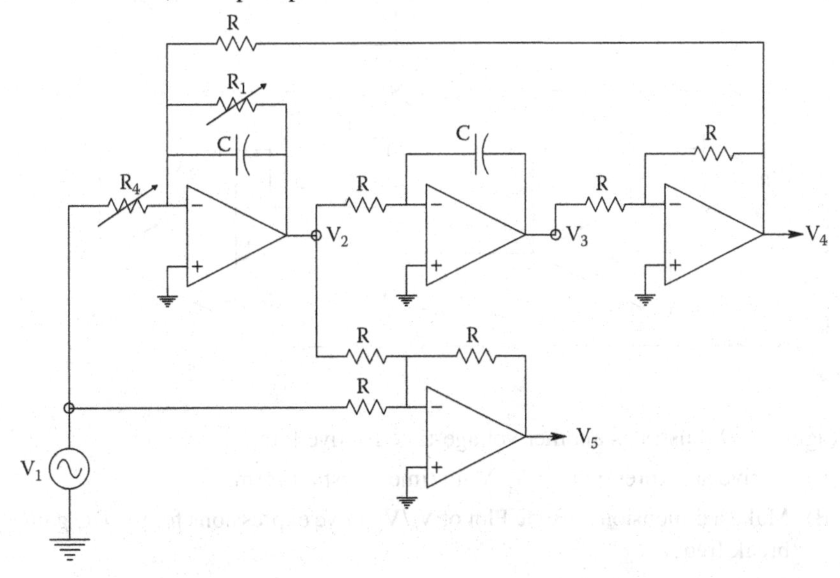

7.7 Find an expression for $\mathbf{V_4/V_1}$ in time-constant form for the biquad AF shown in Figure P7.7. Give expressions for ω_n, Q and $|\mathbf{V_4/V_1}|$ at ω_n. Assume ideal op amps.

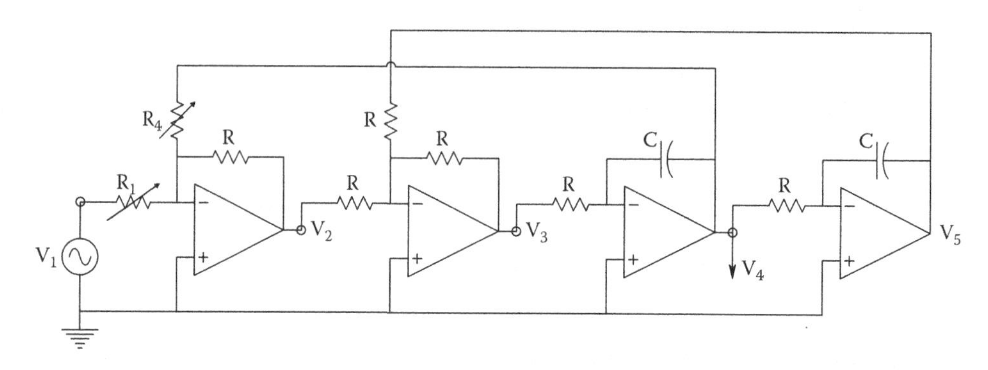

7.8 Figure P7.8 illustrates a voltage-tunable, 1-pole, LPF an analog multiplier is used as the variable-gain element (VGE). The analog multiplier output $V_3 = -V_2V_c/10$.

(A) Derive an expression for V_o/V_1 in time-constant form.

(B) Make a dimensioned Bode Plot of V_o/V_1. Give expressions for the dc gain and the break frequency.

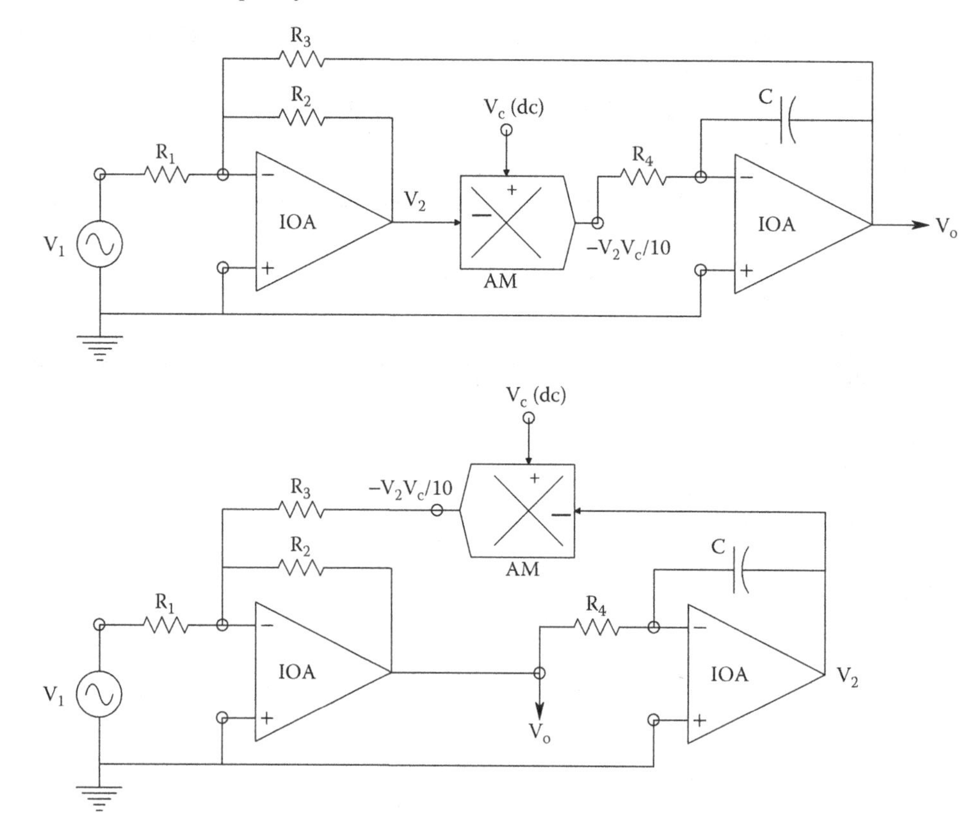

7.9 Figure P7.9 illustrates another voltage-tuned active filter.

(A) Derive an expression for V_o/V_1 in time-constant form.

(B) Make a dimensioned Bode Plot of V_o/V_1. Give expressions for the DC gain and the break frequency.

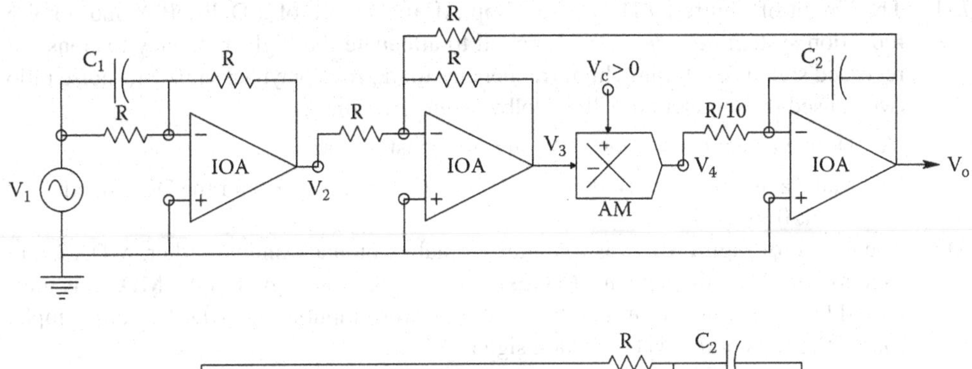

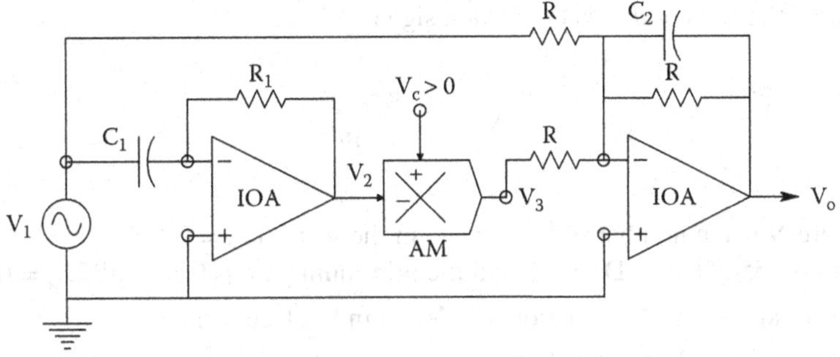

7.10 The circuit of Figure P7.10 is an op amp AF realization of a Dolby B™ audio noise reduction system recording *encoder*. It is designed to boost the high-frequency response of magnetic tape-recorded signals containing little power at high frequencies in order to improve playback signal-to-noise ratio (when used in conjunction with a Dolby B *decoder* filter). (Magnetic tape has an omnipresent high-frequency background "hiss" on playback, regardless of signal strength.)

(A) Derive an expression for V_o/V_1 in time-constant form.

(B) Make a dimensioned Bode Plot of V_o/V_1. Give expressions for the DC gain and the break frequencies.

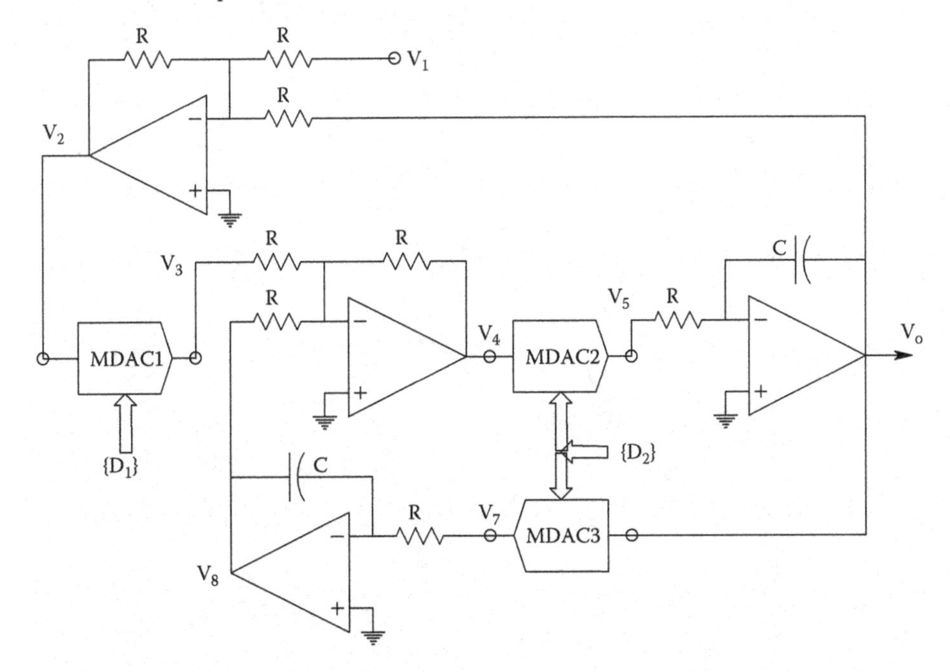

7.11 The circuit of Figure P7.11 is an op amp AF realization of a Dolby B™ audio noise reduction system *decoder*. It is designed to attenuate the high-frequency response of recorded signals containing high frequencies to improve playback signal-to-noise ratio (when used in conjunction with a Dolby B *encoder* filter).

(A) Derive an expression for V_o/V_1 in time-constant form.

(B) Make a dimensioned Bode Plot of V_o/V_1. Give expressions for the DC gain and the break frequencies.

7.12 The circuit of Figure P7.12 is a digitally tunable, biquad bandpass filter. MDACs are used as variable gain elements (VGEs). The analog input signal to the MDAC is multiplied by a fraction determined by the digital word input to the MDAC. For example, for MDAC1, its output is the analog signal:

$$V_3 = V_2 \frac{\sum^{N} D_{1k} 2^{k-1}}{2^N}$$

where N is the number of binary bits in the word, $D_{1k} = 0,1$, for $N = 8$, the maximum gain is 255/256 (All $D_{1k} = 1$), and the minimum gain is 0/256 (all $D_{1k} = 0$).

(A) Find the transfer function, $(V_o/V_1)(s)$ in Laplace format.

(B) Give expressions for the filter's ω_n, Q, and peak gain in terms of $\{D_{1k}\}$, $\{D_{2k}\}$, and system parameters.

What is the range of Q? Assume $N = 8$ bits and the op amps are ideal.

7.13 Derive the transfer function in time-constant form for the GIC all-pass filter of Text Figure 7.12.

7.14 Derive the transfer function in time-constant form for the GIC notch filter of Text Figure 7.13.

8 Instrumentation and Medical Isolation Amplifiers

8.1 INTRODUCTION

Instrumentation amplifiers (IAs) are basically IC differential amplifiers characterized by having very high input impedances, a very high common-mode rejection ratio (CMRR), and a midband differential gain generally in the range from × 1 to × 1000, set by a single resistor. In addition, IAs are also designed to have low noise, low offset voltage, low bias current, and offset current.

Medical isolation amplifiers (MIAs) are basically IAs that have an ultralow conductance pathway between the input (patient) terminals and the output terminals, the power supply, and ground. These ultralow conductance pathways provide what is called ohmic or galvanic isolation for a patient. In medical applications, this isolation is required for reasons of *patient safety*. The DC resistance between input and output terminals is typically on the order of gigaohms (thousands of megohms), and for AC, the capacitance between input and output terminals is on the order of single picoFarads (1 pF = 10^{-12} F).

There are *five* established isolation architectures which will be described. These include (1) *Transformer isolation* in which power is coupled to the (isolated) input stage by high-frequency current and signal is also coupled to the output stage by a transformer, by modulating the power supply oscillator "carrier." A new development in isolation coupling is the Analog Devices *i*Coupler® family of chip-scale, transformer technology, and signal couplers. For example, an ADuM1100BR *i*Coupler has a maximum data rate of 100 Mbps with an 18 ns propagation delay, while a fast optocoupler has a maximum data rate of 12.5 Mbps and a propagation delay of 40 ns. Miniature chip-scale transformer designs are possible when the switching frequencies are on the order of 300 MHz. The IC transformer coils are electrically isolated by 20 μm polyimide resin spacers, giving a primary-to-secondary HiV isolation of 5 kV. Because of their small size and low cost, we expect AD *i*Couplers to be incorporated in instrumentation isolation amplifiers and perhaps MIAs in the not-to-distant future. (2) *Photo-optic coupling* in which the isolated, conditioned input signal is coupled to the output by means of photo-optic couplers (using a LED and a photodiode or photoresistor). Power is still supplied through a high-frequency, isolation transformer. (3) *Capacitive coupling* of a signal-modulated, high-frequency digital carrier from the isolated input stage through a pair of 1 pF capacitors to a demodulator in the output stage. (4) *Magnetic coupling* using *giant magnetoresistive resistors* (GMRs) in a Wheatstone bridge. A GMR's resistance is altered by its local magnetic field. The isolated input signal is converted to a current which is passed through coils in close proximity to two GMRs in a bridge. The ΔRs unbalance the bridge, which is on the output side of the IA. The unbalance is detected by a DA, which generates a current that is used to renull the bridge. The renulling current is sensed and is proportional to the input voltage. Isolation is maintained by the ohmic isolation between the input coils and the GMR bridge resistors.

(5) The *flying capacitor chopper* circuit uses a small capacitor that is charged up by the signal voltage, and then switched by a high-speed, DPDT relay to an output amplifier that reads the voltage across the capacitor. Such switched-capacitor IAs have ohmic isolation set by the relay structure and are useful only for DC or very low-frequency signals.

8.2 INSTRUMENTATION AMPS

IAs, per se, are not suitable for medical applications because, as we described earlier, medical amplifiers require severe galvanic isolation. Several analog IC manufacturers make IAs, including, but not limited to, Analog Devices, Burr-Brown/Texas Instruments, and Linear Technologies.

We first examine some of the properties of a low-cost, low-power IA, the AD620. This amplifier can have its differential gain set from 1 to 10^3 by a single resistor. The −3 dB *bandwidth* (BW) varies with gain in accordance with the gain × bandwidth constancy relation. At $A_v = 10^3$, the −3 dB BW is ca. 10 kHz, at $A_v = 100$, the BW is ca. 120 kHz, at $A_v = 10$, the BW is ca. 400 kHz, and at $A_v = 1$, the BW is ca. 1 MHz.

The equivalent, short-circuit input voltage noise root power spectrum, e_{na}, also depends on A_v. For $A_v = 100, 10^3$, $e_{na} = 9\ \text{nV}/\sqrt{\text{Hz}}$ at 1 kHz. Unfortunately, the input noise *increases as the gain* A_v *decreases*. The input current noise, $i_{na} = 100$ fA rms/$\sqrt{\text{Hz}}$, regardless of gain. The AD620's CMRR varies with gain, ranging from 90 dB at $A_v = 1$ to 130 dB at $A_v = 10^3$. This IA's input bias current, $I_B = 0.5$ nA, the input offset voltage, V_{os}, is 15 μV. The input impedance is 10 GΩ||2 pF for both common-mode and difference-mode inputs (see Chapter 3).

A low-noise precision IA, the AMP01 by Analog Devices, offers slightly different specifications: The gain is set between 1 and 10^3 by a single resistor. The −3dB bandwidths are ca. 26, 82, 100, and 570 kHz for gains of 10^3, 10^2, 10, and 1, respectively. The short-circuit input voltage noise root spectrum is 5 nV/$\sqrt{\text{Hz}}$ at $A_v = 10^3$ and 1 kHz, and the current noise spectrum is 0.15 pA/$\sqrt{\text{Hz}}$ at $A_v = 10^3$ and 1 kHz. The AMP01's input resistance is 1 GΩ for difference-mode signals at $A_v = 10^3$, and 20 GΩ for common-mode inputs at $A_v = 10^3$. The input bias current is typically 1 nA (relatively high), and the input offset voltage is typically ±20 μV. The AMP01's CMRR is 130, 130, 120, and 100 dB for gains of 10^3, 10^2, 10, and 1, respectively.

The advantage of using a commercial IA instead of a "homebrew" IA made from three op amps (see Section 3.7.2) is that the designer does not need to meet the out-of-the-box CMRR specifications of the commercial IA, i.e., the designer does not need resistors matched to at least 0.02%, and matched input op amps. Components matched to 0.02% are expensive in terms of time and money. Figure 8.1 illustrates a simplified schematic of the AD620 IA from its data sheet supplied by Analog

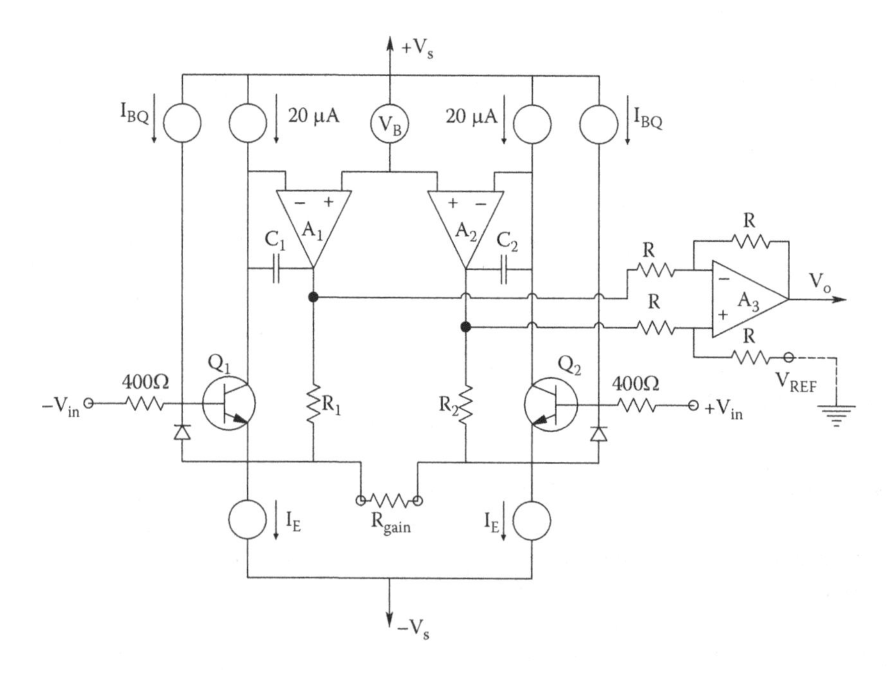

FIGURE 8.1 Simplified schematic of an Analog Devices' AD620 Instrumentation amplifier.

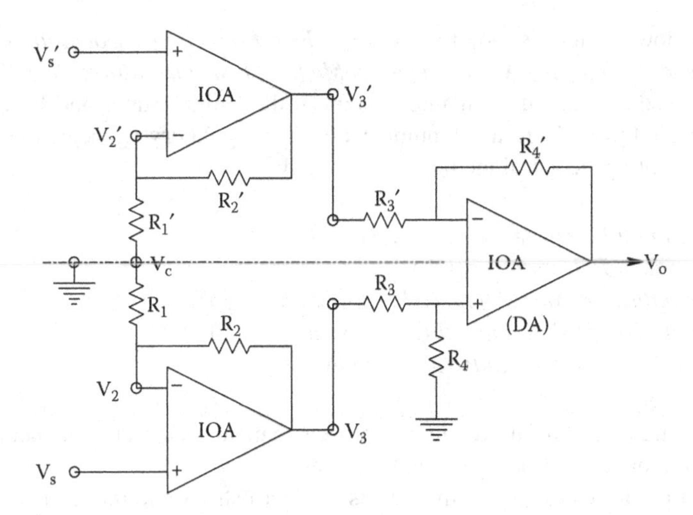

FIGURE 8.2 The "classic," three-op amp instrumentation amplifier.

Devices. Super-beta transistors Q_1 and Q_2 connected as differential pair are the input elements of this IA. The 400Ω resistors and diodes at each transistor base serve to protect the IA from transient overvoltages.

According to Analog Devices 1994:

> [Negative] Feedback through the Q1-A1-R1 loop and the Q2-A2-R2 loop maintains constant collector current of the input devices Q1, Q2 thereby impressing the input voltage across the external gain setting resistor R_{gain}. This creates a differential gain from the inputs to the A1/A2 outputs given by $G = (R_1 + R_2)/R_{gain} + 1$. The unity gain subtractor [DA] A3 removes any common-mode signal, yielding a single-ended output referred to the REF [V_{REF}] pin potential.
>
> The value of [R_{gain}] also determines the transconductance of the preamp stage. As [R_{gain}] is reduced for larger gains, the transconductance increases asymptotically to that of the input transistors. This has three important advantages: (a) Open-loop gain is boosted for increasing programmed gain, thus reducing gain-related errors. (b) The gain-bandwidth product (determined by C1, C2 and the preamp transconductance) increases with programmed gain, thus optimizing frequency response. (c) The input voltage noise is reduced to a value of 9 nV/√Hz, determined mainly by the collector current and base resistance of the input devices.

It is clear that the AD620 has many design features that make it outperform the simple 3-op amp IA shown in Figure 8.2. Given proper ohmic isolation, the AD620 can make an effective ECG amplifier. It can be run on batteries as low as ±2.3 V, and its output can modulate a voltage-to-frequency converter (VFC), also battery powered, generating NBFM. The VFC's digital output can be coupled to the nonisolated world through a photo-optic coupler, and thence be demodulated by conventional means, filtered, and further amplified.

8.3 MEDICAL ISOLATION AMPS

8.3.1 INTRODUCTION

All amplifiers used to record biopotential signals from humans (ECG, EEG, EMG, EOG, etc.) must meet certain safety standards for worst-case voltage breakdown and maximum leakage currents through their input leads which are attached to electrodes on the body, and maximum current through any driven output lead attached to the body. A variety of testing conditions or scenarios to ensure patient safety have been formulated by various regulatory agencies. The conservative leakage current and voltage breakdown criteria set by the *National Fire Protection Association* (NFPA) (Quincy, MA), and the *Association for the Advancement of Medical Instrumentation* (AAMI) have generally been adopted by medical equipment manufacturers in the United States and by US hospitals and other health-care facilities. There are a number of other regulatory agencies that are involved in formulating and adopting electrical medical safety standards:

- The *International Electrotechnical Commission* (IEC).
- The *Underwriters Laboratories* (UL).
- The *Health Industries Manufacturers' Association* (HEMA).
- The *National Electrical Manufacturers' Association* (NEMA).
- The *US Food and Drug Administration* (FDA).

Most of the standards have been adopted to prevent patient electrocution, including burns, the induction of fibrillation in the heart, pain, muscle spasms, etc.

Space does not permit us to go into the effects of electroshock and many of scenarios by which it can occur. Nor can the technology of safe grounding practices and ground fault interruption be explored. The interested reader should consult Chapter 14 in Webster (1992) for a comprehensive treatment of these details.

If the threshold, AC, heart surface current required to induce cardiac fibrillation in 50% of dogs tested is plotted vs frequency, it is seen that the least current is required between 40 and 100 Hz. From 80 to 600 μARMS of 60 Hz current will induce cardiac fibrillation when applied directly to the heart, as through a catheter (Webster 1992, 2009). Thus, the NFPA-ANSI/AAMI standard for ECG amplifier lead leakage is that *isolated* input lead current (at 60 Hz) must be <10 μA between any two leads shorted together, <10 μA for any input lead connected to the power plug ground (green wire) with and without the amplifier's case grounded. A more severe test is that isolation amplifier input lead leakage current must be <20 μA when any input lead is connected to the high side of the 120 VAC mains. The *medical isolation amplifier* (MIA) has evolved to meet these severe tests for leakage currents.

Isolation is accomplished by galvanically separating the input stage of the isolation amplifier (IA) from the output stage. That is, the input stage has a separate, floating power supply and a "ground" that is connected to the output side of the IA by a resistance of more than 1000 MΩ (R_L), and a parallel capacitance in the low picofarad range (C_L). The signal input terminals of the input stage are isolated from the IA's output by a similar very high impedance, although the Thevenin output resistance of the IA can range from milliohms to several hundred ohms.

A simplified, series leakage current pathway from the MIA's inputs to the patient's heart consists of: V_T, the high CM test voltage (several thousand volts RMS, 60 Hz) applied to the MIA's inputs and its power supply inputs. V_T is connected to a parallel R-C circuit consisting of R_L, the total equivalent leakage resistance of the MIA in parallel with C_L, the equivalent shunt leakage capacitance of the MIA. This low admittance parallel circuit is in series with R_L, the internal body resistance, including the heart tissue. I_H is the actual current though the heart that could cause ventricular fibrillation; $\mathbf{I_H} \cong \mathbf{V_T Y_L} = \mathbf{V_T}(G_L + j\omega C_L)$. Note that $|\mathbf{Y_L}| << G_H$.

8.3.2 Common Types of Medical Isolation Amplifiers

Current practice uses *three* major means of effecting the high galvanic isolation of the input and output stages of MIAs: *The first means* is to use a high-quality, toroidal transformer to magnetically couple regulated, high-frequency, AC power from the output side to the isolated, input stage (patient side) where it is rectified and filtered. AC power is also coupled to rectifiers and filters serving the output amplifiers. Power frequencies in the range of 50–500 kHz are typically used with transformer isolation MIAs. The output signal from the isolated headstage modulates an AC carrier, which is

TABLE 8.1
Comparison of Properties of Some Popular Medical Isolation Amplifiers

Amplifier	IA294	IA296	BB3652	BB ISO121	AD210
Isol. /Type	Transformer/ MIA	Transformer/ MIA	Optical/MIA	Capacitor/MIA	Transformer/MIA
Manufacturer	**Intronics**	**Intronics**	**Burr-Brown**	**Burr-Brown**	**Analog Devices**
CMV isolation	±5000 V cont. ±6500 V 10 ms pulse	±5000 V cont ±6500 V 10 ms pulse	±2000 V continuous ±5000 V, 10 s	3500 Vrms	2500 Vrms contin. 3500 Vpk contin.
CMRR @ 60 Hz	120 dB @ 60 Hz	160–170 dB	80 dB @ 60 Hz	115 dB IMR @ 60 Hz	100 dB
Gain range	10 (fixed)	1–100	1 to > 100, by formula	1 V/V (fixed)	1–100 V/V
Leakage to 120 Vac mains	10 μA max	0.5 μA	0.5 μA 1.8 pF leakage capacitance	I_{ac} = V2pfC C ≅ 2.21 pF	—
Noise	8 μV ppk 0.05–100 Hz	0.3 μV ppk 10–100 Hz BW	4 μV ppk 0.05 – 100 Hz BW	4 μVrms/√Hz	18 nV/√Hz @1 kHz
Bandwidth	0–1 kHz	0–1 kHz, −3 dB	0–15 kHz, ± 3 dB	0–60 kHz (c. 200 kHz clock)	20 kHz −3 dB
Slew-rate	—	—	1.2 V/μs	2 V/μs	—

coupled to a demodulator on the output side by a signal transformer. Transformer coupling can provide 12–16 bit resolution, and bandwidths up to 75 kHz. Galvanic isolation with transformers is excellent; their maximum breakdown voltage can be made as high as 10 kV, but is often lower.

A second means of isolation is to use photo-optic coupling of the amplified signal; usually pulse-width or delta-sigma modulation of the optical signal is used, although direct, linear, analog, photo-optic coupling can be used. In an optical type of IsoA, a separate, isolated, DC/DC converter must be used to power the input stage. Photo-optic couplers can be made to withstand voltages in the 4–7 kV range before breakdown.

A third means of isolation is to use a pair of small (e.g., 1 pF) capacitors to couple a pulse-modulated signal from the isolated input to the output stage. A separate, isolated power supply must be used with the differential capacitor-coupled MIA, too. Table 8.1 lists some of the critical specifications of five types of medical-grade, isolation amplifiers.

The Burr-Brown ISO121 differential capacitor-coupled MIA is used with a separate, isolated clock to run its duty cycle-modulator. The clock frequency can be from 5 to 700 kHz, giving commensurate bandwidths, governed by the Nyquist criterion.

A simplified schematic of an Intronics/Analog Devices Model AD289, magnetically coupled MIA is shown in Figure 8.3. Note that this MIA has a single-ended input. The power oscillator (clock) drives a toroidal core, T1, on which are wound coils for the input and output isolated power supplies, and also for the synchronizing signals for the *double-sideband, suppressed carrier* (DSBSC) modulator and demodulator. A separate toroidal transformer, T2, couples the DSBSCM output signal to the output side of the MIA.

An unmodulated, feedback-type, analog, optical isolation system is used in the Burr-Brown BB3652, differential, optically coupled, linear MIA. This MIA still requires a transformer-isolated power supply for the input headstage and for the driver for the linear optocoupler. A feedback-type linear optocoupler, similar to that used in the BB3652, is shown in Figure 8.4. (In the B3652,

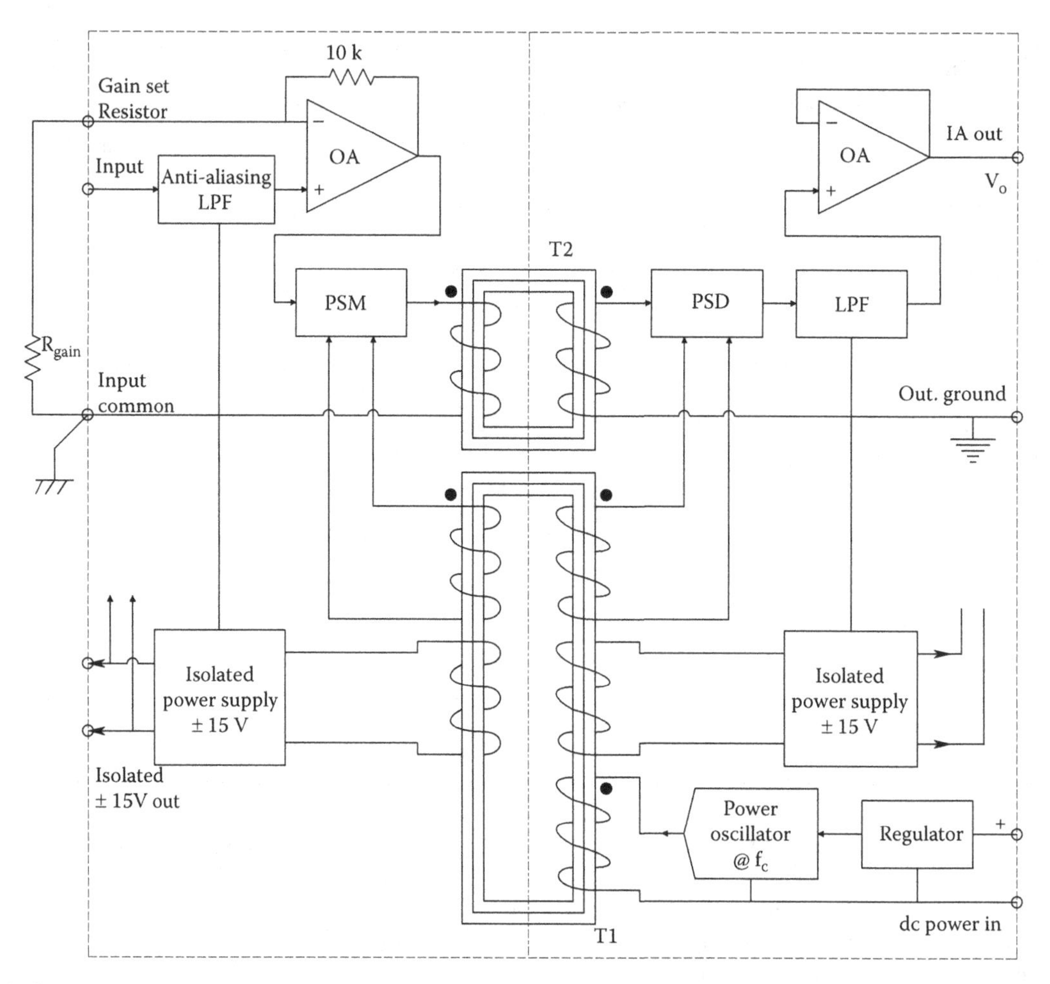

FIGURE 8.3 Simplified schematic of an Analog Devices' AD289, magnetically isolated isolation amplifier (IsoA). An AD620 IA is used as a differential front end for the IsoA; it is powered from the AD289's isolated power supply.

OA1 is replaced with a high input impedance DA headstage.) The circuit works in the following manner: The summing junction of OA2 is at 0 V. DC bias current through R_{B1}, I_{B1}, drives the OA2 output negative, biasing the LED, D2, on at some I_{D20}. D2's light illuminates photodiodes D1 and D3 equally; the reverse photocurrent through D1 drives OA2's output positive, reducing I_{D2}. It thus provides a linearizing, negative feedback around OA2, acting against the current produced by the input voltage, V_{in}/R_1. Because D1 and D3 are matched photodiodes, the reverse photocurrent in D3 equals that in D1, i.e., $I_{D10} = I_{D30}$, and $V_o = R_3 (I_{D30} - I_{B3})$. The bias current I_{B3} makes $V_o \to 0$ when $V_{in} = 0$. Now when $V_{in} > 0$, the input current, V_{in}/R_1, makes the LED D2 brighter, increasing $I_{D1} = I_{D3} > I_{D10} = I_{D30}$, increasing V_o. Thus, $V_o = K_V V_{in}$. Note that analog optoisolation eliminates the need for a high-frequency carrier, modulation and demodulation, while giving a very high degree of Galvanic isolation. Unfortunately, the isolated headstage must still receive its power through a magnetically isolated power supply. It could use batteries, however, which would improve its isolation.

MIAs using capacitor isolation generally use high-frequency, *duty-cycle modulation* to transmit the signal across the isolation barrier using a differential, 1 pF capacitor coupling circuit. This type of MIA also needs an isolated power supply for the input stages, the clock oscillator and

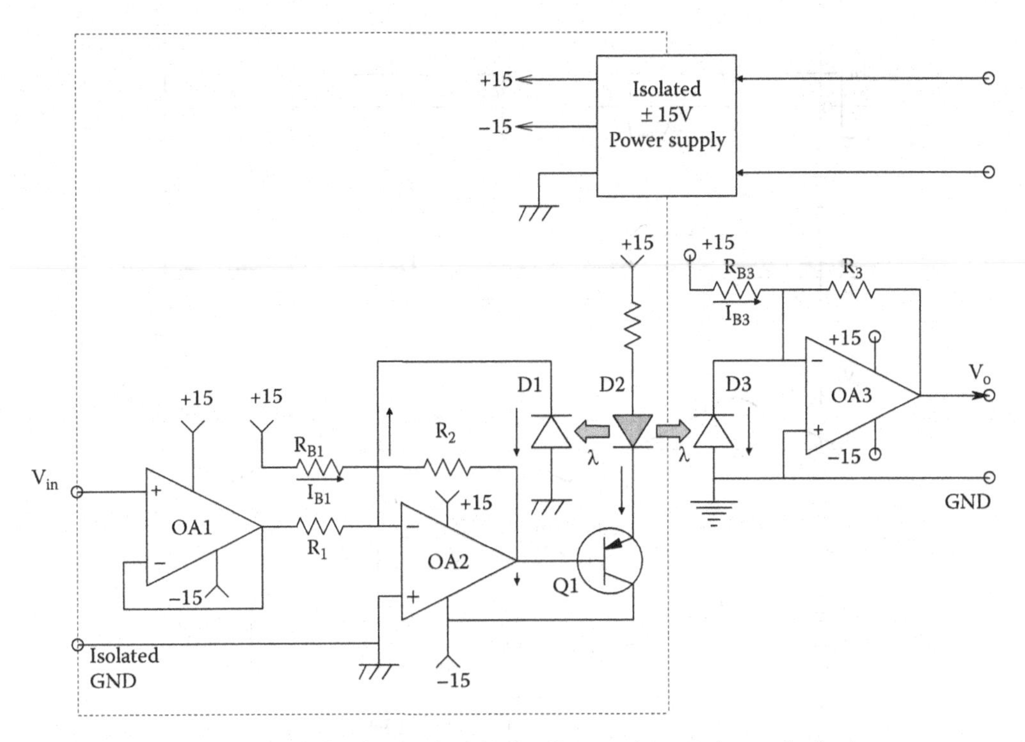

FIGURE 8.4 Simplified schematic of an analog, feedback-type, photo-optic coupler IsoA.

the modulator. Figure 8.5 illustrates schematically a simplified version of how the Burr-Brown ISO121, capacitively isolated, MIA works. The positive signal V_{in} is added to a high-frequency, symmetrical triangle wave, V_T, with peak height, V_{pkT}. The sum of V_T and V_{in} is passed through a comparator which generates a variable-duty-cycle square wave, V_2. Note that the highest frequency in V_{in} is << f_c, the clock frequency, and $|V_{inmax}| < V_{pk}$. The state transitions in V_2 are coupled through the two, 1 pF capacitors as spikes to a flip-flop on the output side of the IA. The flip-flop's transitions are triggered by the spikes. At the flip flop's output, a $\pm V_{3m}$, variable duty-cycle square wave, V_3, is then averaged by low-pass filtering to yield V_o.

The duty cycle of V_2 and V_3 can be shown to be

$$\eta(V_{in}) \equiv T_+ / T = (1/2 + V_{in}/(2V_{pkT})), \quad |V_{in}| < V_{pkT} \tag{8.1}$$

The average of the symmetrical flip-flop output is

$$V_o = \bar{V}_3 = V_{in}(V_{3m}/V_{pkT}) \tag{8.2}$$

Thus, the output signal is proportional to V_{in}. The actual circuitry of the Burr-Brown ISO121 is more complex than that described above, but the basic operating principle has been described.

Certified medical isolation amplifiers *must* be used in surgery and intensive-care hospital environments where cardiac catheters are used. While the scenarios for direct cardiac electroshock do not generally exist for outpatients, MIAs are still used for ECG, EEG, and EMG applications to maximize patient safety and limit liability in the very unlikely event of an electroshock incident.

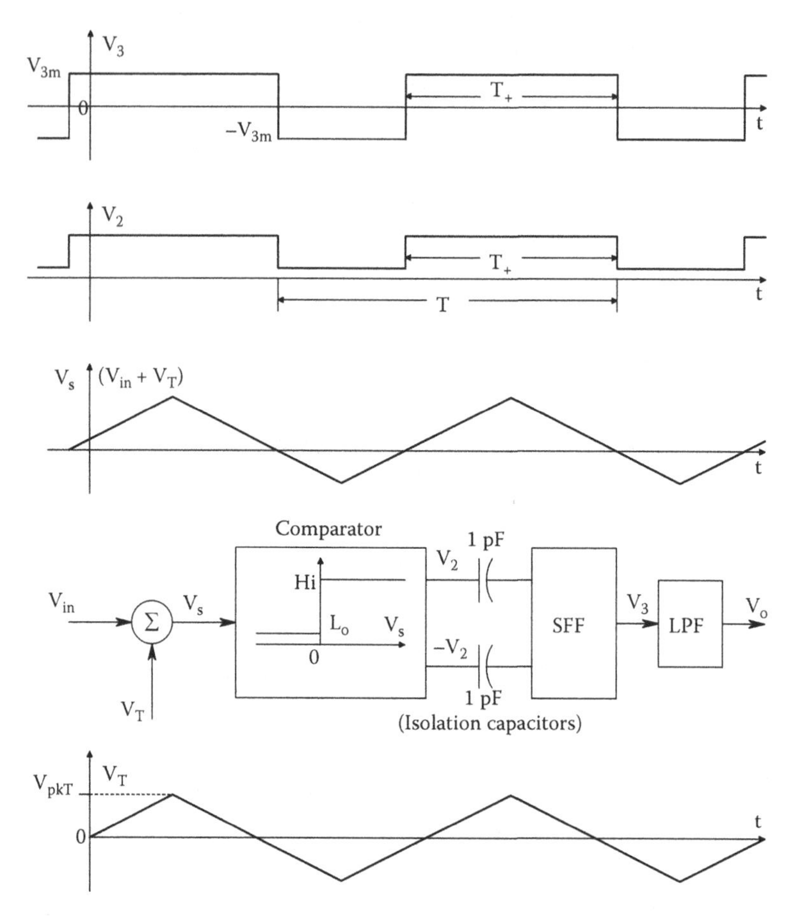

FIGURE 8.5 Waveforms relating to the operation of the Burr-Brown ISO121 capacitively coupled, duty-cycle modulated IsoA system. The low-frequency signal, V_{in}, is added to a symmetrical, 0-mean triangle carrier wave, the sum is passed through a zero-crossing comparator which effectively performs duty-cycle modulation. If $V_{in} > 0$, $T_+ /T > 0.5$; if $V_{in} < 0$, $T_+ /T < 0.5$. The comparator output, V_2, and its compliment, $\overline{V}_2$, are coupled to a flip-flop whose output square wave, V3, has zero mean at 50% duty cycle. It is shown in the text that the time average value of V_3, V_o, is proportional to V_{in}.

8.3.3 A Prototype Magnetic MIA

All of the MIAs we have described earlier use a carrier and can thus face problems of aliasing in the output signal when the input signal's highest frequency approaches ½ the carrier frequency, and also may have carrier-frequency ripple in the output. One way to avoid the problems of carrier-based MIAs is to use a technology that is DC coupled, yet provides the required ohmic isolation. One approach is to use a transduction scheme that uses magnetic fields at signal, rather than carrier frequencies. One such magnetic sensor is the *Hall-effect device* (Yang 1988). Unfortunately, commercial Hall-effect sensors are not particularly sensitive and have low outputs which require amplification. Fortunately, there is another, relatively new technology discovered in the late 1980s by Peter Gruenberg of the KFA Research Institute in Julich, Germany, and independently by Albert Fert at the University of Paris-Sud; this is the *giant magnetoresistive* (GMR) *effect*. Researchers at IBM extended the initial work on GMR devices; they developed sensitive GMR transducers based on sputtered thin film technology. IBM's interest in developing sensitive, miniature GMR devices has been to improve the data density stored on computer floppy and hard drive magnetic disks. IBM also called their GMR sensor the *spin valve read-head*.

GMR sensors have a resistance that is modulated by an imposed magnetic flux density; thus, a Wheatsone bridge can be used to sense the $\Delta R/R_M$, hence the ΔB. Unfortunately, GMRs are not particularly linear, which makes them acceptable for binary applications, but presents problems for linear analog sensing.

A basic GMR sensor is a multiple layer, thin film device. In its simplest form, it has a nonmagnetic, conductive spacing layer sandwiched between two ferromagnetic film layers. Usually, the magnetization in one ferromagnetic layer is fixed or *pinned,* along a set direction. The magnetization of the *free layer* is allowed to rotate in response to an externally applied magnetic field. Low resistance occurs when the pinned and free layer are magnetically oriented in the same direction. This is because electrons in the conductor layer with parallel spin directions move freely in both films. Higher resistance occurs when the magnetic orientations in the two films oppose each other, since movement of electrons in the conductor of either spin direction is hampered by one or the other magnetic films. Depending on the strength and orientation of the applied external **B** field, the pinning direction, the materials used and their thicknesses, the $R_M = f(B, \theta, \varphi)$ curve can have a variety of shapes (Wilson 1996). In many cases, the GMR $R_M = f(B, \theta, \varphi)$ curve exhibits both hysteresis and some dead zone as shown in Figure 8.6. This spin valve has the "crossed easy axis" configuration in which the applied **B** is perpendicular to the free layer easy axis and the pinning direction is parallel to **B**. The response is linear around Q and is relatively hysteresis free (Wilson 1996). Because of its magnetic sensitivity, the GMR must be magnetically shielded from the Earth's (DC) field and stray AC magnetic fields from manmade power wiring and machinery. To use such a sensor as a linear device, it must be magnetically biased around a Q-point.

Research is currently underway to improve the linearity and sensitivity of spin valves or GMR sensors. Attention is being paid to the use of multiple layered thin films of various compositions, including two pinned layers; 6–12 layers are being studied by Fujitsu (Kanai et al. 2001).

GMR sensors are available commercially. *Infineon Technologies* offers a 4-element GMR IC package in which the four GMRs are connected in a bridge (see www.infineon.com/cms/en/products/index.html [accessed 5/5/11]. *Rhopoint Components* of Oxted, Surrey, UK, offers

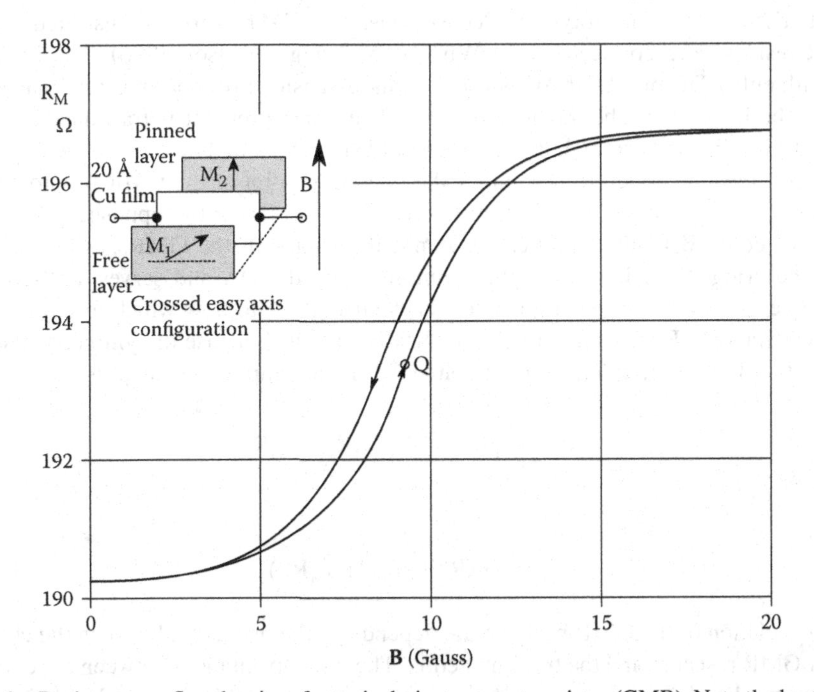

FIGURE 8.6 Resistance vs flux density of a typical giant magnetoresistor (GMR). Note the hysteresis.

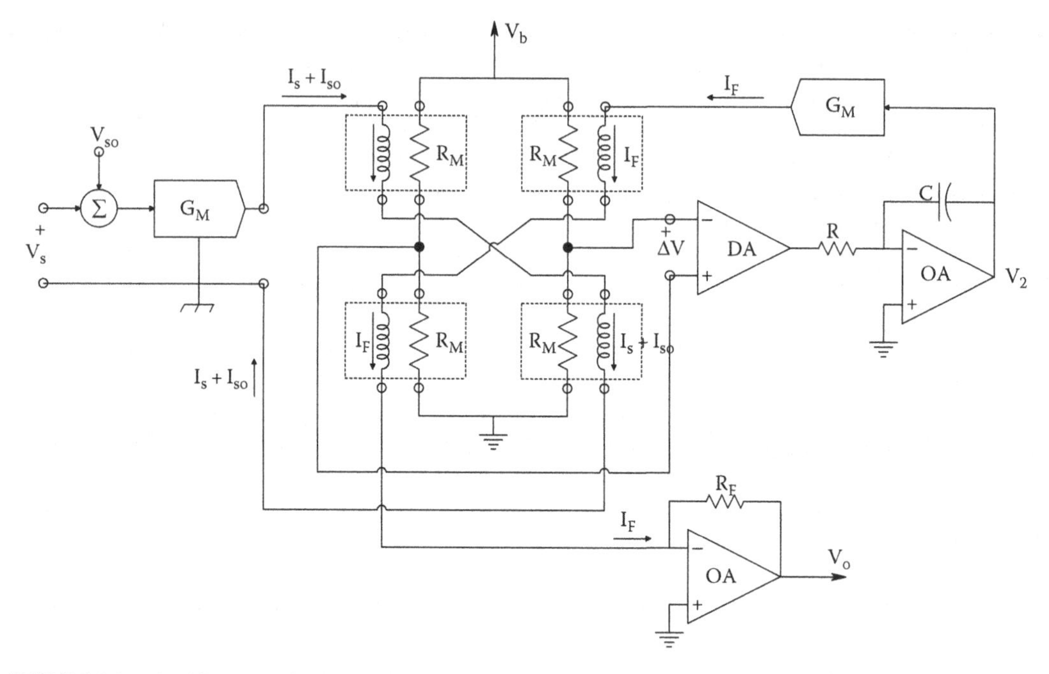

FIGURE 8.7 Architecture of a prototype IsoA designed by the author using four GMR elements in a bridge. A Type 1 feedback loop is used to autonull the bridge. Autonulling insures linear operation of the GMRs. Note that the input circuit ground is separate from the signal conditioning and output ground. V_{so} is a bias voltage that causes the GMRs to operate in their linear ranges.

a 4 sensor GMR device kit (AG003-1) for experimenters and R&D use, and a six-sensor GMR starter engineering kit (AG001-01) (see the Rhopoint website at: www.rhopointcomponents.com/ [Accessed 5/5/11]).

The author's version of a prototype MIA design based on GM resistors is illustrated in Figure 8.7. Four GMR resistors are connected as a Wheatstone bridge (Wilson 1996). The bridge can be powered with either DC or AC; if AC is used, a phase-sensitive rectifier must be placed between the DA and the integrator. The quantity under isolated measurement is transduced to V_s, which is converted to a signal current I_S by a VCCS with transconductance, G_M. A DC bias current component, I_{so}, must be added to I_S to move the operating point of the GMR resistors to a linear region of its $R_M = f(B)$ curve. The current I_S through the coils on the opposite diagonals of the bridge creates equal **B** fields which cause identical changes in the GMRs, ΔR_s, which in turn unbalance the bridge. The bridge output is amplified by the DA and serves as the input to an integrator. The integrator output causes a feedback current, I_F, to flow which forces $\Delta R_f = \Delta R_s$ in the other two diagonal R_Ms, which renulls the bridge output. Because of symmetry, the feedback current $I_F = I_S + I_{so}$ at null, and the output voltage of the op amp transresistor is

$$V_o = -I_F R_F = -V_s G_M R_F + I_{so} R_F \tag{8.3}$$

Thus,

$$V_s = (I_{so} R_F - V_o) / (G_M R_F) \tag{8.4}$$

Galvanic isolation of the GMR bridge MIA depends on the insulation between the chip containing the four GMR resistors and the two input coils. The low capacitances between the coils and R_Ms and the dielectric breakdown of this insulation are important in achieving good isolation.

8.4 SAFETY STANDARDS IN MEDICAL ELECTRONIC AMPLIFIERS

8.4.1 INTRODUCTION

The central rationale for safety standards for medical electronic equipment is based on the need to prevent harm to human patients and health-care workers attached to or using such equipment. Besides user safety, having a biomedical electronic product certified by one or more of the qualified test agencies reduces the litigation risk for those persons who designed it, sold it, and used it in practice should any untoward incident occur. (The United States is legendary for its medical malpractice litigation, and the substantial awards that are made.) Product certification is also necessary in various jurisdictions to be able to sell a biomedical electronic product to hospitals, clinics, physicians, and research labs, etc.

An excellent treatise on electrical safety and the physiological effects of electric currents on the body can be found in Chapter 14 of Webster (1992). A summary of the effects of injuries caused by electric current can also be found in the Online Merk Manual (2010), Section 21, Chapter 316b. An excellent collection of papers on IEC, UL, and ANSI/AAMI safety standards and tests for medical electronic products can be found at the Eisner Safety Consultants website (2010) and in the web paper by Richards (2010). (All Eisner website papers can be downloaded for a fee.) A free, illustrated description on leakage current standards is available in a tutorial paper by Eisner et al. (2004). The book by Geddes (1998) describes case studies of medical device accidents in areas such as anesthesia, electrosurgery, and catheterization.

There are a variety of ways electrical currents can enter the body; probably the most common is through the skin on a hand, the head, or a foot. Note that, for a circuit to exist, the current must also leave the body, also through a hand, the head or feet, or a catheter. Electric shock effects are usually described in terms of the current that flows through the body, and if AC, the frequency. Direct current can also have profound physiological effect, as can transients currents such as from capacitor discharges, static electricity, and lightning. Table 8.2 summarizes typical physiological effects from DC, 60 Hz, and 10 kHz electric currents in a macroshock scenario where the current is applied between the hands. The data are based on several sources, including both human and animal studies.

TABLE 8.2
List of Physiological Effects of Electric Currents in the Body Introduced Through the Hands ("Macroshock")

60 Hz	10 kHz	DC	Effect
0–0.3	0–5	0–0.6	No sensation
2	8	3.5	Slight tingling on hand
1	11	6	"Shock"; Not painful
10	51	58	Painful muscle spasms; May let go
20	60	65	Painful; Muscle tetanus; Cannot let go
>100		>500	Deep burns, edema, cardiac fibrillation, respiratory paralysis
>2000		>2000	All of the above, death

Note that there is a current × time product that determines tissue damage once the power density in tissues reaches the level where temperatures rise to the level where "cooking" occurs. Values are "typical," and can vary widely between individuals due to fat, muscle mass, etc.

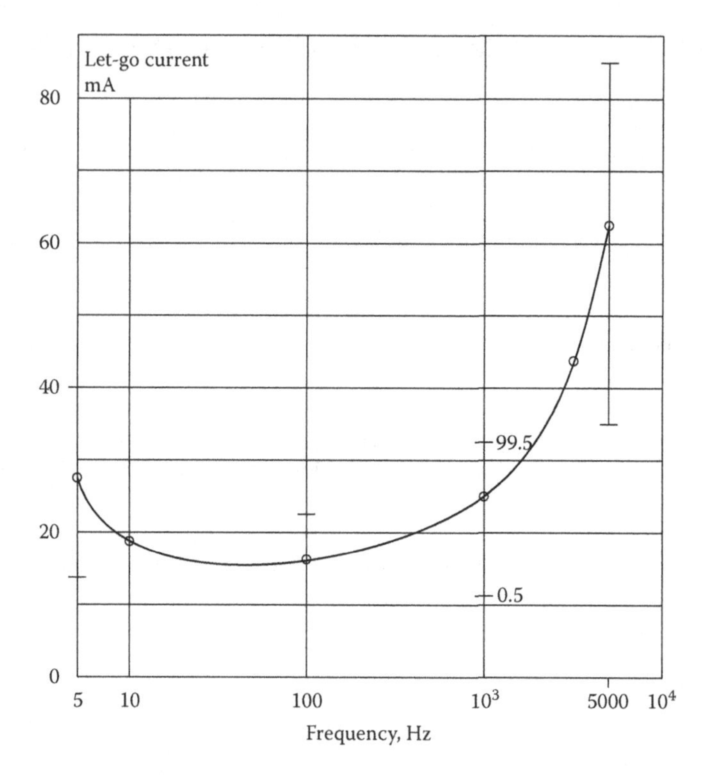

FIGURE 8.8 Let-go current vs frequency for the hand-to-hand current path in humans. Note that the most dangerous frequency is around 50–60 Hz.

Figure 8.8 illustrates let-go current vs frequency for the hand-to-hand current path in humans. Plotted is the current vs frequency for the median of the test population; the bars show the 99.5 and 0.5 percentile limits. What we learn from this curve, and the Table 8.2 is that power line frequency (50 or 60 Hz) is the most physiologically effective in producing electric shock damage to the body and heart. Direct current and AC at 10 kHz is about 1/6th as effective in doing damage. Consequently, impedance pneumographs and plethysmographs typically pass mA-level currents with frequencies ca. 75 kHz through the chest with no untoward effects.

When the heart is stimulated *directly,* as in open-heart surgery or when cardiac pacemaker catheterization is used, the scenario is called *microshock.* The 60 Hz current required to induce ventricular fibrillation can be as low as 20 μA in dogs. In humans, microshock current causing fibrillation is on the order of 80–600 μA (Webster 1990, Chapter 14).

8.4.2 Certification Criteria for Medical Electronic Systems

From the aforementioned data, we see that it is extremely important to prevent harmful currents from flowing into the body under macroshock conditions from any amplifier connected to the body by electrodes, such as in ECG, EEG, EMG, EOG, etc. measurements. In the United States, we have a number of regulatory and certifying agencies that ensure medical electronic devices are safe. These include the following:

- US Food and Drug Administration (FDA)
- National Fire Protection Agency (NFPA) and its National Electrical Code (NEC).
- American National Standards Institute / Assoc. for the Advancement of Medical Instrumentation (ANSI/AAMI ES1-1993)

- Occupational Health & Safety Administration (OSHA)
- Underwriter's Laboratories (UL)

In Europe, there are two major organizations:

- European Committee for Electrotechnical Standardization (CENELEC)
- International Electrotechnical Commission (IEC)

Gradually, the standards in the United States appear to be converging on those established by the IEC. The IEC has developed a set of standards to certify medical instruments called the IEC60601-1 which covers all of the general requirements for all medical based products (St. Onge 2007). (Some papers refer to IEC60601-1 as IEC601-1.) Many of the US standards have been based on IEC requirements set in the past decade, but some such as UL544 were phased out in January, 2003. The new UL2601-1 is largely based on the IEC regulations with some exceptions (Mentelos 2003).

The IEC60601-1 standards are subdivided into several IEC60601-X-YZ parts, which cover specific types of medical equipment. Our interest here, however, is in medical isolation amplifiers used to record potentials from the body surface. There are four classes of basic electrical safety tests defined by the IEC. These include the following:

- Protective Earth Verification
    - Ground Continuity Test
    - Ground Bond Test
- Dielectric Strength
    - AC HiPot Test
    - DC HiPot Test
- High Resistance
    - Insulation Resistance Test
- Leakage Current
    - Earth Leakage, Touch/Chassis (Enclosure),
    - Patient Leakage and Patient Auxiliary Leakage

The *earth* (ground or green wire in the United States) *verification test* passes 25 amps from the line cord plug ground (green) terminal to the chassis to ensure cord-to-chassis ground connection robustness, and measures the voltage between the current source and the chassis or cabinet. The resistance of the grounding system must be $<0.1\ \Omega$ for a detachable line cord, and $<0.2\ \Omega$ for a fixed cord according to IEC60601-1 specifications. Resistance is calculated by Ohm's law.

The *Dielectric Strength Test* applies a high AC or DC voltage to the line power input to ensure no insulation breakdown or flashover (arcing) occurs between ground and the input power line with both terminals tied together. The basic IEC60601-1 standard requires the DUT to with-stand 1250 VRMS at 60 Hz for one minute. Medical isolation amplifiers easily exceed this requirement (see Table 8.1. above). For example, the Intronics IA175 MIA is rated at 3000 V_{pk}, 60 Hz continuous from patient inputs to the outputs/power common. The IA175 runs on +15 VDC, so further isolation can be obtained by using a medical-grade power supply that meets IEC60601-1 standards.

The *insulation resistance test* is a voltmeter–ammeter test of the DUT's insulation using a high-voltage DC source. For example, a high DC potential is applied to the MIA's power input common, say 1000 V, and the steady-state current to ground is measured at the isolated power supply's neutral. Such current would be 1 nA DC if the resistance were $10^{12}\ \Omega$.

Finally *leakage currents are* considered. The four types of leakage current defined by the IEC as described by Eisner et al. (2004):

> Earth Leakage: The most important and most common of the line leakage current tests, earth leakage current is basically the current flowing back through the ground conductor on the power cord [green

TABLE 8.3
Leakage Current Limits for Three Standards

Leakage Type	UL544	UL2601-1	IEC60601-1
Earth leakage	300 μA	300 μA	1 mA
Enclosure leakage	300 μA	300 μA	500 μA
Patient leakage	10 μA Input	50 μA	50 μA
(auxiliary)	20 μA at end of cable		

New units cannot be certified by UL544 after 1/1/03; UL certification expires after 1/1/05. UL2601-1 and IEC60601-1 standards must be used for all new designs of medical electronic equipment

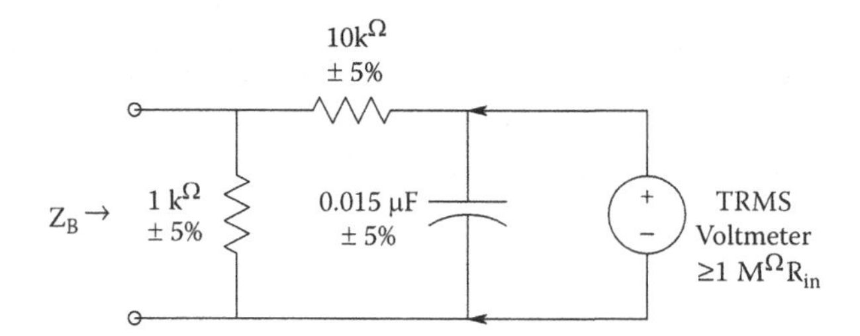

FIGURE 8.9 The IEC body phantom impedance model, defined by the IEC60601-1 standard.

wire]. It is measured by opening the ground conductor, inserting a circuit with the simulated impedance of the human body and measuring the voltage across part of the circuit with a true RMS voltmeter. Patient Leakage: A line leakage current test that measures the current that would flow from or to *applied parts* such as sensor and patient leads.

Patient Auxiliary: line leakage current flowing in the patient in NORMAL use between applied.

Leakage: produce a physiological effect parts of the DUT and not intended to.

Touch/Chassis: A line leakage current test [which] simulates the effect of a person touching exposed

Leakage: metal parts of a product and detects whether or not the leakage current that flows through the person's body remains below a safe level. Line leakage tests are conducted by applying power to the product being tested, then measuring the leakage current from any exposed metal on the chassis of the product under various fault conditions (such as "No Ground"). A special circuit is used to simulate the impedance of the human body.

The circuit that is used to simulate the body's impedance, as defined by IEC60601-1 is shown in Figure 8.9. At 60 Hz, this phantom presents an impedance of $999.7\angle -0.32^\circ$ Ω, basically 1 kΩ. The reactance of the 0.015 μF capacitor is $X_c = -1.768 \times 10^5$ Ω at 60 Hz. (The author finds it curious that leakage currents are measured through this 1 kΩ body phantom, rather than using the short-circuit leakage current; actual human point-to-point body impedances can vary widely.) The Eisner et al. (2004) web paper on leakage current standards illustrates in detail the various circuits used to measure the four types of leakage current; space limitations prevent us from duplicating them here. Below we summarize the leakage current limits from two US standards and IEC60601-1 (Mentelos 2003, 2010):

Modern medical isolation amplifiers such as the Intronics IA175 generally exceed specifications. For example, the maximum leakage currents, inputs to common @ 115 VAC, 60 Hz is only 8 μA max. The actual input impedance of the IA175 is 10^8 Ω||3 pF for DM in and 10^{11} Ω||20 pF for CM inputs. The maximum CM voltage, inputs to outputs/input power common is 3000 Vpk, 60 Hz AC for 1 min. The peak continuous DC CM input voltage is ±5000 V. The CMRR with a balanced differential source is 126 dB at 60 Hz. The small-signal −3 dB frequency is 1 kHz, which is ideal for ECG, EEG, and EOG applications.

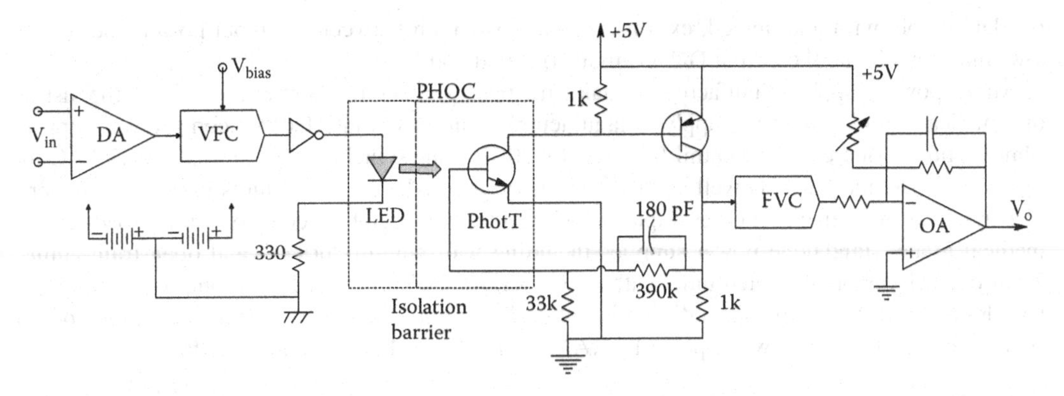

FIGURE 8.10 An IsoA architecture for ECG recording using a digital photo-optic coupler. Pulses from a voltage-to-frequency converter are sent to a frequency-to-voltage converter through the POC to recover a signal proportional to V_{in}.

An inexpensive isolation amplifier to measure the ECG in an experimental setting can be made from a battery-operated AD620 IA connected to a battery-operated, low-current, voltage-to-frequency converter (VFC) such as the AD654. The VFC is given an FM center frequency with a bias voltage (not shown in the figure). The bipolar ECG signal output from the IA frequency-modulates the VFC's digital output. To realize isolation, the VFC drives a photo-optic coupler whose output is the input to a frequency-to-voltage converter (FVC) such as the ADVFC32. The VFC carrier bias at the output of the FVC is subtracted out, and the ECG signal is further amplified and filtered. Figure 8.10 illustrates this system. The photo-optic coupler's phototransistor (PT) is given positive feedback to speed up its switching to a maximum of 500 kHz (Stapleton and O'Grady 2001). Of course, if this design were to be used in a medical or clinical application, it would have to be tested and must meet or exceed IEC60601-1 standards, etc. If the isolation and insulation on the photo-optic coupler were not adequate, one could use a fiberoptic cable to couple the LED to the phototransistor.

Note that radiotelemetry is another means of providing *extreme isolation* between a battery-operated sensor, amplifier, modulator, and RF transmitter and a line-powered receiver, demodulator, and signal conditioner. Wireless patient monitoring (WPM) is an active and growing field in biomedical electronics (see Chapter 13 in this text). Again, extreme isolation is inherent in RF and IR telemetry (see Chapter 14 in this text).

8.5 MEDICAL-GRADE POWER SUPPLIES

The only practical way to achieve extreme galvanic isolation and still couple significant power from the mains to a low-voltage regulated DC supply that powers a medical amplifier is by a toroidal transformer. The transformer can operate at line frequency, but for lighter weight and improved efficiency, should operate at frequencies in the 10–100 kHz range. A power oscillator is used to drive the transformer's primary in the latter case. If a high-frequency oscillator is used, the transformer can be made smaller and lighter (a smaller core and fewer turns on the windings are required), and the output filter capacitor can be smaller and lighter.

A toroidal transformer is used for efficiency in magnetic coupling the primary to secondary windings, and the toroidal core also allows the primary and secondary windings to be physically separate on the core to minimize capacitive coupling between them. By physically separating the windings, and insulating them from the core with special insulation, breakdown voltages between primary and secondary can be made 8 kV or greater, and primary-to-secondary DC resistance can be on the order of 10^{12} Ω and greater. The secondary AC voltage is rectified by the usual means, the raw DC is low-pass filtered by a capacitor, and then regulated by a feedback regulator. The net result is a DC supply with guaranteed, extreme galvanic isolation between the input power lines (high, low, and ground) and the output DC terminals (ground and V_{CC}).

Many power supply manufacturers make medical grade units, for example, see the listing of medical grade power supply manufacturers at www.interfacebus.com/Power_Supply_Manufactures_Medical-Grade.html (Accessed 9/20/10). These include the external "brick" AC-to-low-voltage-DC modules, as well as larger capacity, internal, AC-to-DC units used in computers, displays, and instruments. For example, GlobTek Inc. (www.globtek.com) offers a broad line of medical grade, standalone power supplies including wall plug-in "bricks" and open-frame units. Their class II, double insulated units withstand 4 kV AC or 5.65 kV DC input-output potential and have less than 100 μA leakage. A discussion of design factors used in making medical grade power supplies can be found in a white paper by RAM Technologies LLC (Mentelos 2010).

8.6 CHAPTER SUMMARY

In this chapter, we have described the properties and used of IA ICs, including those we can make from low-noise op amps. We also examined the requirements for and the properties of medical isolation amplifiers. Galvanic isolation is required for patient safety in all settings (surgical, clinical, outpatient). Power supply isolation is achieved by batteries, or special, transformer-coupled power supplies. Isolation amplifier analog output must also be isolated. One way this can be done by DSBSC modulation of a high-frequency ac carrier by the low-frequency physiological signal, and coupling the modulated carrier to the output with a transformer, where the signal is recovered with a demodulator. Another way of coupling the physiological signal to the output with isolation is to use a photo-optic coupler and transmit the signal directly in analog form (cf. Section 6.6.4 of this text). If the isolated physiological signal is sampled and converted by a serial output analog-to-digital converter, the digital output can also be transmitted through a digital photo-optic coupler to the output. Still another way of coupling an isolated signal to the output was shown to be by converting the signal to a pulse-width modulated (PWM) TTL squarewave, and coupling this wave to the output with two, 1 pF capacitors. At the output, this wave is highly differentiated into a spike train. Flip-flops recover the PWM wave at the output, and the signal is demodulated by averaging.

The physiological effects of electroshock were described, including induced cardiac fibrillation, apnea, and burns. Certification agencies for medical electronic devices worldwide were listed and some of their standards compared. The United States was seen to have five major certifying agencies, and Europe, two. There is a trend in the United States to converge on the IEC standards. To meet European marketing standards for medical electronic devices, US manufacturers must meet the IEC and CENELEC standards, which paradoxically in some areas, are less stringent that NFPA and other US standards.

Finally, we discussed medical grade power supplies that run off the mains.

9 Noise and the Design of Low-Noise Signal Conditioning Systems for Biomedical Applications

9.1 INTRODUCTION

Noise and output signal-to-noise ratio provide limitations to the precision of biomedical measurements. Other factors that limit output signal resolution are distortion caused by signal conditioning system nonlinearity and quantization in the analog-to-digital conversion (ADC) of input signals. The degree to which a biomedical signal is resolvable can be determined by the signal-to-noise ratio at the output of the signal conditioning system (SNR_o).

The noise in this chapter is considered to arise in a circuit, measurement system, or electrode from completely random physical and chemical processes. Any measured physical quantity can be "noisy" giving measurement uncertainty; however, in this chapter, consideration will be restricted to completely random noise voltages and currents. These noise voltages and currents are defined as being *stationary* (meaning that the physical process giving rise to the noise does not change with time), and they have *zero means* (meaning that they have zero additive DC components). An unwanted DC component accompanying a noise source, in practice, can be from an electrochemical EMF arising in a recording electrode or from an amplifier's DC offset voltage or bias current. The reduction of unwanted DC components (e.g., from thermally caused drift) will not be treated in this chapter.

Coherent interference (CI) can also be present at the output of biomedical signal conditioning systems. CI, as the name suggests, generally has its origins in periodic, manmade phenomena, such as power line-frequency electric and magnetic fields, radio-frequency sources such as HF and VHF radio and television broadcast antennas, certain poorly shielded computer equipment, spark discharge phenomena such as automotive ignitions and electric motor brushes and commutators, and inductive switching transients generated by SCR motor speed controls, etc. It is well known that minimization of CI is often "arty" and may involve changing the grounding circuits for a system, shielding with magnetic and/or electric conducting materials, filtering, the use of isolation transformers, etc. (see Section 3.10 in Northrop 2005). In this chapter, however, attention will be focused on purely random, stationary, incoherent noise.

As will be seen, minimizing the impact of incoherent noise in a measurement system often involves a prudent choice of low-noise amplifiers and components, certain basic electronic design principles, and band-pass filtering. Below, the commonly used methods for describing stationary random noise are examined.

9.2 DESCRIPTORS OF RANDOM NOISE IN BIOMEDICAL MEASUREMENT SYSTEMS

9.2.1 Introduction

When *stationarity* is assumed for a noise source, averages of noise and functions of noise over time are equivalent to *ensemble averages*. An ensemble average is an average carried out at a given time on data from N separate records, which are generated simultaneously from a *stationary random process* (SRP) (in the limit, $N \rightarrow \infty$). If we can assume that the stationary random process is also *ergodic*, then only one record needs to be examined statistically because it is "typical" of all N records from the SRP.

An example of a *nonstationary noise source* is a resistor, which—at time $t = 0$—begins to dissipate average power such that its temperature slowly rises above ambient, as does its resistance. (As is shown below, the mean-squared noise voltage from a resistor is proportional to its Kelvin temperature.)

Probability and statistics are used to describe random phenomena. Several statistical methods for describing random noise include, but are not limited to: The *mean*, the *root-mean-square* (RMS) value, the *probability density function* (PDF), the *cross*- and *autocorrelation functions* and their Fourier transforms, the *cross*- and *auto-power density spectra* (PDS), and the *root power density spectrum* (RPS, which is simply the square root of the PDS). Both the PDS and root power spectrum (RPS) are, in general, functions of frequency. These descriptors are treated in detail below.

9.2.2 Probability Density Function

The probability density function (PDF) is a mathematical model which describes the probability that any random sample of a noise function, n(t) will lie in a certain range of values. The *univariate* PDF considers only the amplitude statistics of the noise waveform and not how it varies in time. The univariate PDF of the SRV, n(t), is defined as

$$p(x) = \frac{\text{Probability that } [x < n \leq (x + dx)]}{dx} \tag{9.1}$$

where x is a specific value of n taken at some time t, and dx is a differential increment in x. The PDF is the mathematical basis for many formal derivations and proofs in probability theory. The PDF has the following properties:

$$\int_{-\infty}^{v} p(x)\,dx = \text{Prob}[x \leq v] \tag{9.2}$$

$$\int_{v2} p(x)\,dx = \text{Prob}[v_1 < x \leq v_2] \tag{9.3}$$

$$\int_{-\infty}^{\infty} p(x)\,dx = 1 = \text{Prob}[|x| \leq \infty] \text{(a certainty)} \tag{9.4}$$

Several PDFs are widely used as mathematical models to describe the amplitude characteristics of electrical and electronic circuit noises. These include

$$p(x) = \left(\frac{1}{\sigma_x\sqrt{2\pi}}\right)\exp\left[-\frac{(x - <x>)^2}{2\sigma_x^{\,2}}\right] \quad \text{Gaussian or normal PDF ("The bell-shaped curve")} \tag{9.5}$$

$$p(x) = 1/2a, \text{ for } -a < x < a, \text{ and } \quad p(x) = 0, \quad \text{for } x > a \quad \text{Rectangular PDF} \tag{9.6}$$

$$p(x) = \left(\frac{x}{\alpha^2}\right)\exp\left[\frac{-x^2}{2\alpha^2}\right] \quad \text{Rayleigh PDF} \tag{9.7}$$

$$p(x) = \left(\frac{x^2}{\alpha^2}\right)\sqrt{(2/\pi)}\exp\left[\frac{-x^2}{2\alpha^2}\right] \quad \text{Maxwell PDF, } x \geq 0. \tag{9.8}$$

In Equation 9.5 above, $< x >$ is the *true mean or expected value* of the stationary random variable (SRV), x, and $\sigma_x^{\,2}$ is the *variance* of the SRV, x, described below.

The *true mean* of a stationary, ergodic, noisy voltage can be written as a time average over all time:

$$<x> \equiv \lim_{T\to\infty}\frac{1}{T}\int_0^T x(t)dt \tag{9.9}$$

The mean of the SRV, x, can also be written as an expectation, or *probability average* of x:

$$E\{x\} \equiv \int_{-\infty}^{\infty} x\, p(x)\, dx = <x> \tag{9.10}$$

Similarly, the *mean squared value* of x can be expressed by the expectation or *probability average* of x^2:

$$E\{v^2\} \equiv \int_{-\infty}^{\infty} v^2 p(v) dv = <v^2> \tag{9.11}$$

The mean can be *estimated* by a finite average over time. For discrete data, this is called the *sample mean:* The sample mean is a statistical *estimate* of the true mean and as such has uncertainty (noise) itself.

$$\bar{x} = \frac{1}{T}\int_0^T x(t)\, dt, \quad \text{or} \quad \bar{x} = \frac{1}{N}\sum_{k=1}^{N} x_k \text{ (Sample mean)} \tag{9.12}$$

The *variance* of the random noise, $\sigma_x^{\,2}$, is defined by

$$\sigma_x^{\,2} \equiv E\{[x - <x>]^2\} = \int_{-\infty}^{\infty}[x - <x>]^2 p(x) dx = \lim_{T\to\infty}\frac{1}{T}\int_0^T [x(t) - <x>]^2 dt \tag{9.13}$$

It easy to show from Equation 9.13 that $< x^2 > = \sigma_x^2 + < x >^2$, or $E\{x^2\} = \sigma_x^2 + E^2\{x\}$. *Because the random noise considered has zero mean, the mean squared noise is also its variance.*

Under most conditions, we will assume that the random noise arising in a biomedical measurement system has a Gaussian PDF. Many mathematical benefits follow this assumption; for example, the output of a linear system is Gaussian with variance σ_y^2 given its input to be Gaussian with variance σ_x^2. If Gaussian noise passes through a nonlinear system, the output PDF, in general, will not be Gaussian. As you will see, there are ways of describing the transformation of Gaussian input noise by a nonlinear system.

9.2.3 Autocorrelation Function and the Power Density Spectrum

A noise source can be thought of as being the sum of a very large number of sine wave sources with different amplitudes, phases, and frequencies. Very heuristically, an auto power density spectrum (APDS) shows us how the mean squared values of these sine sources are distributed in the frequency domain.

One approach to illustrate the meaning of the APDS of the noise, n(t), uses the *autocorrelation function* (ACF) of that noise. The ACF is defined below by the continuous time integral (Aseltine 1958):

$$R_{nn}(\tau) \equiv \lim_{T\to\infty} \frac{1}{2T}\int_{-T}^{T} n(t)\,n(t+\tau)\,dt = \lim_{T\to\infty} \frac{1}{2T}\int_{-T}^{T} n(t-\tau)\,n(t)\,dt \tag{9.14}$$

The *two-sided PDS* is the continuous Fourier transform (CFT) of the autocorrelation function of the noise:

$$\Phi_{nn}(\omega) \equiv \frac{1}{2\pi}\int_{-\infty}^{\infty} R_{nn}(\tau)e^{-j\omega\tau}\,d\tau \tag{9.15}$$

Because $R_{nn}(\tau)$ is an even function, its Fourier transform, $\Phi_{nn}(\omega)$ is also an even function. Stated mathematically, this means

$$\Phi_{nn}(\omega) = \Phi_{nn}(-\omega) \tag{9.16}$$

In the following discussion, the *one-sided PDS,* $S_n(f)$, will also be considered. $S_n(f)$ is related to the two-sided PDS, $\Phi_{nn}(2\pi f)$, by

$$S_n(f) = 2\Phi_{nn}(2\pi f) \quad \text{for } f \geq 0\text{, and} \tag{9.17}$$

$$S_n(f) = 0 \qquad \text{for } f < 0. \tag{9.18}$$

Note that the radian frequency, ω, is related to the Hz frequency simply by $\omega = 2\pi f$.

To see how one can experimentally find the one-sided PDS, examine the model system shown in Figure 9.1a. Here, a noise voltage is the input to an *ideal* low-pass filter with an adjustable cut-off frequency, f_c.

The output of the ideal low-pass filter is measured with a broadband, true RMS, AC voltmeter. We begin with $f_c = 0$, and systematically increase f_c, each time recording the square of the RMS

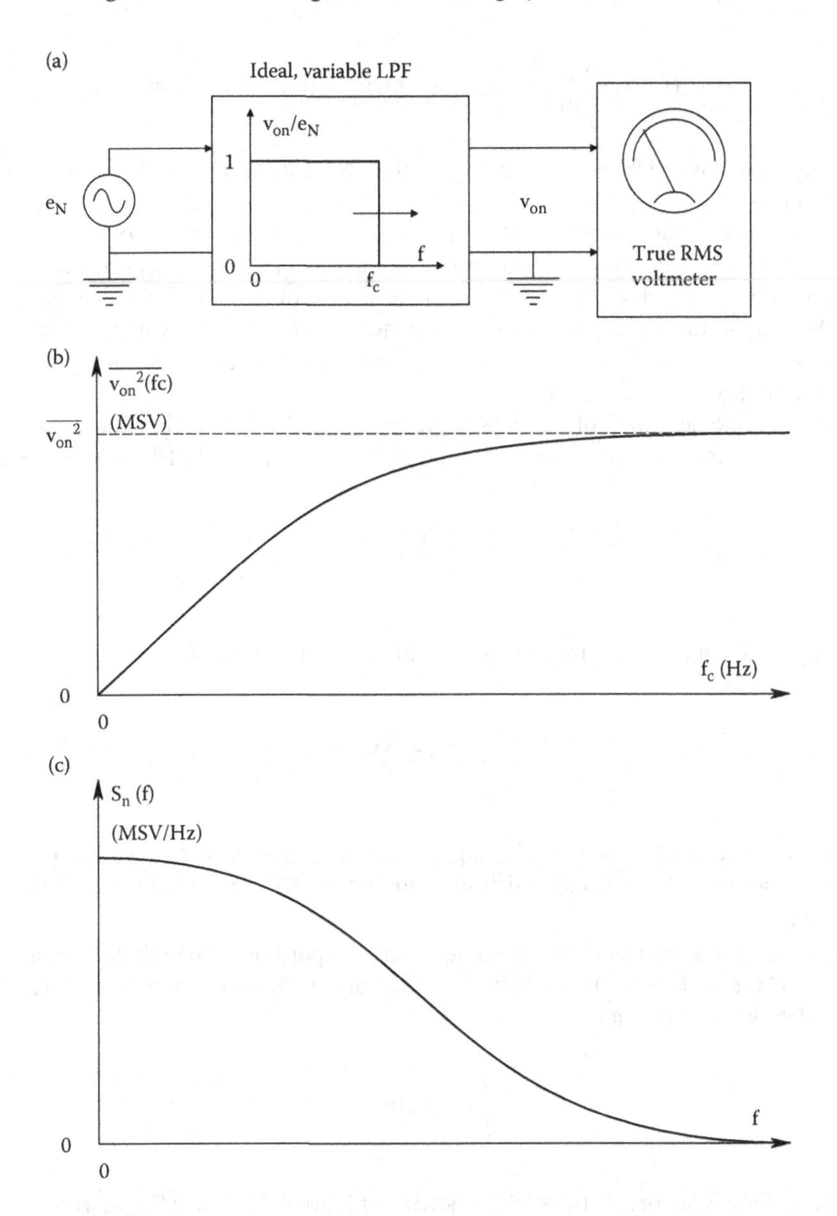

FIGURE 9.1 (a) System for measuring the integral power spectrum (cumulative mean-squared noise characteristic) of a noise voltage source, $e_N(f)$. (b) Plot of a typical integral power spectrum (IPS). (c) Plot of a typical, one-sided, power density spectrum. It is the derivative of the IPS vs. frequency. See Text for description.

meter reading, which is the mean squared output voltage, $\overline{v_{on}^2}$, of the filter. As f_c is increased, $\overline{v_{on}^2}$ increases monotonically, as shown in Figure 9.1b. Because of the finite bandwidth of the noise source, $\overline{v_{on}^2}$ eventually reaches an upper limit which is the total mean-squared noise voltage of the noise source. The plot of $\overline{v_{on}^2}(fc)$ vs. f_c is called the *cumulative, mean-squared noise characteristic* of the noise source. In this example, its units are mean-squared volts.

A simple interpretation of the one-sided, noise power density spectrum, $S_n(f)$, is that it is the derivative, or slope, of the cumulative, mean-squared noise characteristic curve described above. Stated mathematically stated, this is

$$S_n(f) \equiv \frac{d\,\overline{v_{on}^2(f)}}{df}, 0 \leq f \leq \infty \text{ Mean squared volts/Hertz} \tag{9.19}$$

A plot of a typical noise PDS is shown in Figure 9.1c. Note that a practical, one-sided PDS drops off to zero as $f \rightarrow \infty$.

A question which is sometimes asked by those first encountering the PDS concept is why is it called a *power density* spectrum? The power concept has its origin in the consideration of noise in communication systems and has little meaning in the context of noise in biomedical instrumentation systems. One way to rationalize the *power* term is to consider an ideal voltage noise source with a one ohm load. In this case, the average power dissipated in the resistor is simply the total mean-squared noise voltage ($P_{av} = \overline{v_{on}^2} / R$).

From the heuristic definition of the PDS above, it is seen that the total mean-squared voltage in the noise voltage source can be written as the integral of the one-sided PDS from 0 to ∞ Hz:

$$\overline{v_{on}^2} = \int_0^\infty S_n(f)df \tag{9.20}$$

The mean squared voltage in the frequency interval, (f_1, f_2), is found by

$$\overline{v_{on}^2(f_1, f_2)} = \int_{f_1}^{f_2} S_n(f)df \tag{9.21}$$

Often noise is specified or described using *root power density spectra,* which are simply plots of the square root of $S_n(f)$ vs f and which have the units of RMS volts (or other units) per root Hz (RMSV/$\sqrt{Hz}$).

Special (ideal) PDSs are used to model or approximate portions of real PDSs. These include the *White noise PDS,* and the *one-over-f PDS.* A white noise PDS is shown in Figure 9.2a. Note that this PDS is flat; this implies that

$$\int_0^\infty S_{nw}(f)df = \infty \tag{9.22}$$

which is clearly not realistic. A 1/f PDS is shown in Figure 9.2b. The 1/f spectrum is often used to approximate the low-frequency behavior of real PDSs. Physical processes which generate 1/f-like noise include ionic surface phenomena associated with electrochemical electrodes, carbon composition resistors carrying direct current (metallic resistors are substantially free of 1/f noise) and interface imperfections affecting diffusion and recombination phenomena in semiconductor devices. The presence of 1/f noise can present problems in the electronic signal conditioning systems used for low-level, low-frequency, and DC measurements.

9.2.4 Sources of Random Noise in Signal Conditioning Systems

Sources of random noise in signal conditioning systems can be separated into two major categories: noise from passive resistors and noise from semiconductor circuit elements such as bipolar junction transistors, field effect transistors, and diodes. In most cases, the Gaussian assumption for noise amplitude PDFs is valid, and the noise generated can often be assumed to have a white (flat) power over a significant portion of its spectrum.

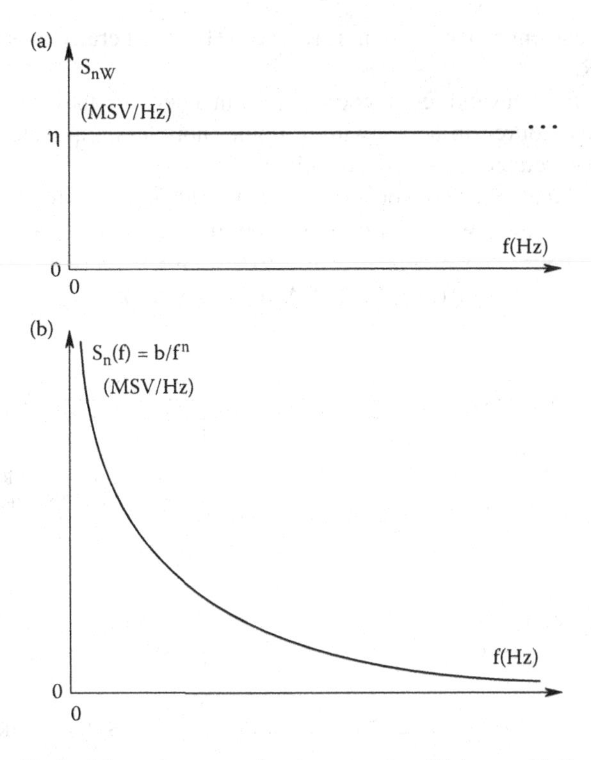

FIGURE 9.2 (a) A one-sided, white-noise power density spectrum. (b) A one-sided, one-over-f power density spectrum. Both of these spectra are idealized, mathematical models. Their integrals are infinite.

9.2.4.1 Noise from Resistors

From statistical mechanics, it can be shown that any pure resistance at some temperature $T > 0°K$ will have a zero mean, broadband noise voltage associated with it. This noise voltage appears in series with the (noiseless) resistor as a Thévènin equivalent noise voltage source. From DC to radio frequencies where the resistor's capacitance to ground and its lead inductance can no longer be neglected, the resistor's noise is well modeled by a Gaussian white noise source. Noise from resistors is called *thermal* or *Johnson noise.* It is described by a one-sided, white, PDS is given by the well-known relation:

$$S_n(f) = 4kTR \text{ mean squared volts / Hz} \tag{9.23}$$

where k is Boltzmann's constant (1.380×10^{-23} J/°K), T is in degrees Kelvin, and R is in ohms.

In a given noise bandwidth $B = f_2 - f_1$, the mean squared thermal white noise from a resistor can be written as

$$\overline{v_{on}^2(B)} = \int_{f_1}^{f_2} S_n(f)df = 4kTR\,(f_2 - f_1) = 4kTRB \text{ MSV} \tag{9.24}$$

A Norton equivalent of the Thévènin Johnson noise source from a resistor can be formed by assuming a MS, white noise, short-circuit current source with PDS:

$$S_{ni}(f) = 4kTG \text{ MS Amps/Hz} \tag{9.25}$$

This Norton noise current root spectrum, i_n RMSA/√Hz, is generally in parallel with a noiseless conductance, G = 1/R.

The Johnson noise from several resistors connected in a network may be combined into a single Thévènin noise voltage source in series with a single, noiseless, equivalent resistor. Figure 9.3 illustrates some of these reductions for two-terminal circuits.

It has been observed that when DC (or an average) current is passed through a resistor, the basic Johnson noise PDS is modified by the addition of a low-frequency, 1/f spectral component. Sic:

$$S_n(f) = 4kTR + A\, I^2 / f \text{ MSV/Hz} \tag{9.26}$$

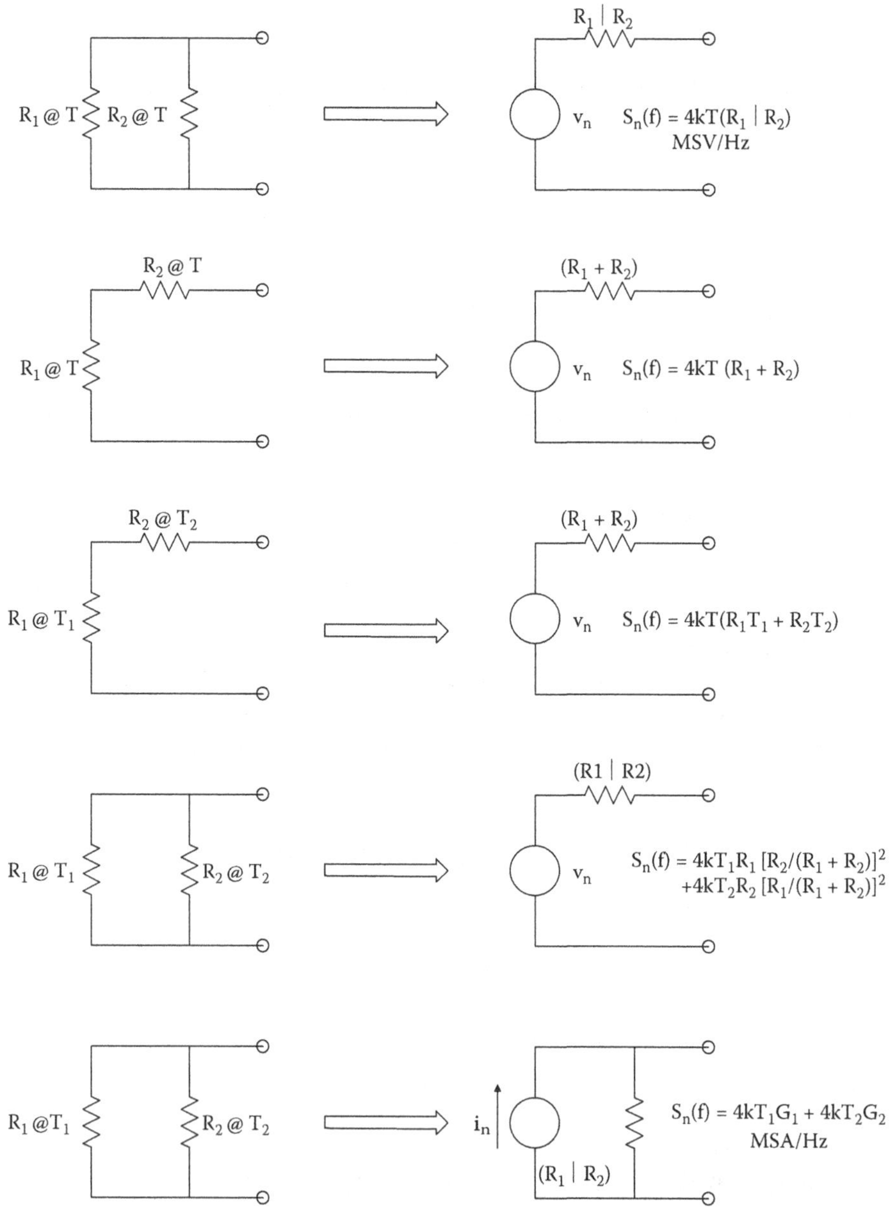

FIGURE 9.3 Examples of combining white, Johnson noise, power density spectra from pairs of resistors. In the resulting Thevenin models, the Thevenin resistors are noiseless.

where I is the average or DC component of current through the resistor, and A is a constant that depends on the material from which the resistor is constructed (e.g., carbon composition, resistance wire, metal film, etc.).

An important parameter for resistors carrying average current is the crossover frequency, f_c, where the MS 1/f PDS equals the MS Johnson noise. f_c is easily shown to be

$$f_c = A I^2/4kTR \text{ Hz} \tag{9.27}$$

It is possible to show that the f_c of a noisy resistor can be reduced by using a resistor of the same type but having a higher wattage or power dissipation rating. As an example of this principle, consider the circuit of Figure 9.4 in which a single resistor of R ohms, carrying a DC current I is replaced by nine resistors of resistance R connected in a series-parallel circuit, which also carries the current I. The 9-resistor circuit has a net resistance, R, which dissipates nine times the power of the single resistor R. The noise PDS in any one of the nine resistors is seen to be

$$S_n'(f) = 4kTR + A\,(I/3)^2/f \text{ MSV/Hz} \tag{9.28}$$

Each of the nine PDSs given by Equation 9.28 above contributes to the net PDS seen at the terminals of the composite 9W resistor. Each resistor's equivalent noise voltage source "sees" a voltage divider formed by the other eight resistors in the composite resistor. The attenuation of *each* of the nine voltage dividers is given by

$$\eta = \frac{3R/2}{3R/2 + 3R} = 1/3 \tag{9.29}$$

The net voltage PDS at the composite resistor's terminals *may only be found by superposition of uncorrelated, MS voltages or PDSs.*

$$S_{n(9)}(f) = \sum_{j=1}^{9} [4kTR + A(I/3)^2 f](\eta)^2 = 4kTR + A\,I^2/9f \text{ MSV/Hz} \tag{9.30}$$

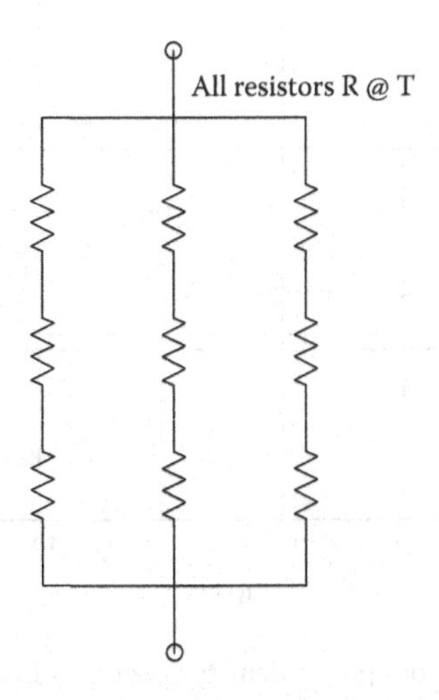

FIGURE 9.4 Nine identical resistors in series-parallel have the same resistance as any one resistor, and nine times the wattage.

Thus, the composite, 9W resistor enjoys a ninefold reduction in the 1/f spectral energy because the DC current density through each element is reduced by 1/3. The Johnson noise PDS remains the same, however. It is safe to generalize that the use of high wattage resistors of a given type and resistance will result in reduced 1/f noise generation when the resistor carries DC (average) current. The cost of this noise reduction is the extra volume required for a high-wattage resistor, and its extra expense.

9.2.4.2 Two-Source Noise Model for Active Devices

Noise arising in JFETs, BJTs, and complicated IC amplifiers is generally described by the *two noise source input model.* The total noise observed at the output of an amplifier, given that its input terminals are short-circuited, is accounted for by defining an equivalent *short-circuited input noise voltage,* e_{na}, which replaces the combined effect of *all* internal noise sources seen at the amplifier's output under short-circuited input conditions. The amplifier, shown in Figure 9.5, is now considered noiseless. e_{na} is specified by manufacturers for many low-noise, discrete transistors and IC amplifiers. e_{na} is in fact a root PDS, i.e., it is the square root of a one-sided PDS and is thus a function of frequency; e_{na} has the units of RMS volts per root Hz. Figure 9.6 illustrates a plot of a typical $e_{na}(f)$ vs. f for a low-noise JFET. Also shown in Figure 9.6 is a plot of the *equivalent input noise current* source, $i_{na}(f)$ vs. f for the same device.

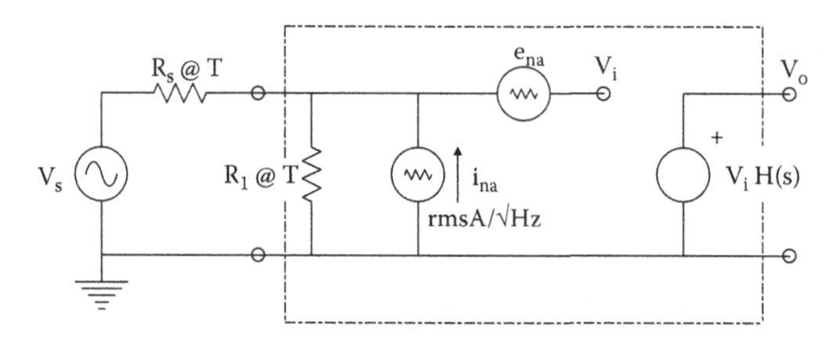

FIGURE 9.5 The two-noise source model for a noisy amplifier. e_{na} and i_{na} are root power density spectra. R_{out} is neglected.

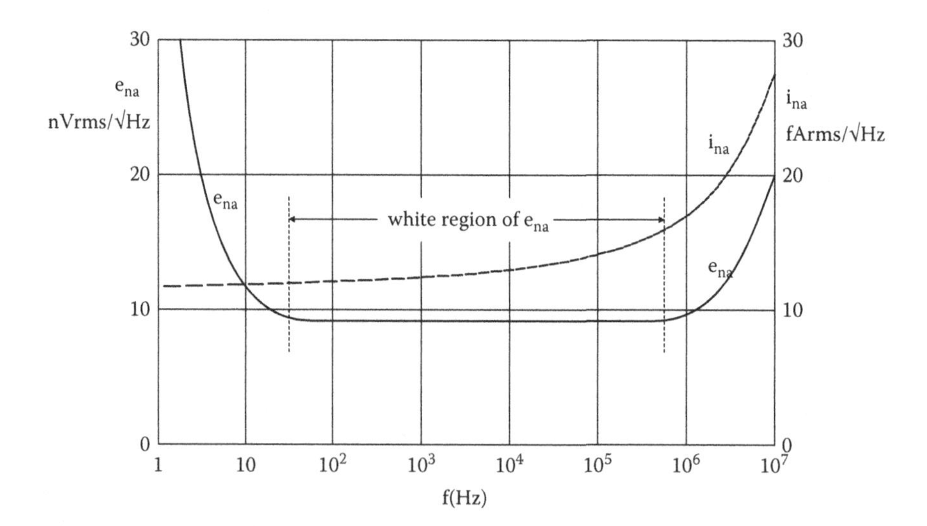

FIGURE 9.6 Plots of the e_{na} and i_{na} root power density spectra vs f for a typical, low-noise FET headstage amplifier. Note that e_{na} has a low frequency $1/\sqrt{f}$ component, and i_{na} does not. Both i_{na} and e_{na} increase at very high frequencies.

In addition to the equivalent short-circuited input noise voltage, the modeling of the net noise characteristics of amplifiers requires the inclusion of current noise, i_{na}, as shown in Figure 9.5. $i_{na}(f)$ is the root PDS of the input equivalent noise current; its units are RMS amps per √Hz. Note that both $e_{na}(f)$ and $i_{na}(f)$ have flat, midfrequency portions, which invite approximation by white noise sources. At high frequencies, both equivalent noise root PDSs slope upward. $e_{na}(f)$ for discrete JFETs and BJTs, and IC amplifiers shows a distinct $1/\sqrt{f}$ region at low frequencies.

9.2.4.3 Noise in JFETs

Certain selected, discrete JFETs are sometimes used in the design of low-noise amplifier headstages for biomedical signal conditioning systems. Some JFETs give good low-noise performance in the audio and subaudio frequency regions of the spectrum, while others excel in the video and radio-frequency end of the spectrum giving them applications for RF oscillators, mixers, and tuned amplifiers used in medical ultrasound applications. Amplifiers using JFET headstages have relatively low input DC bias currents ($I_B \approx 10$ pA) and high input resistances ($> 10^{10}\ \Omega$), both of which are desirable.

Van der Ziel (1974) showed that the theoretical thermal noise generated in the conducting channel of a JFET can be approximated by a white, equivalent short-circuited input voltage noise with PDS given by

$$e_{na}^2 = 4kT/gm = 4kT/g_{m0}\sqrt{\left(\frac{I_{DSS}}{I_{DQ}}\right)} \text{ MSV/Hz} \tag{9.31}$$

where g_{m0} is the JFET's small-signal transconductance measured when $V_{GS} = 0$ and $I_D = I_{DSS}$; I_{DSS} = the DC drain current measured for $V_{GS} = 0$, and $V_{DS} > V_P$, and I_{DQ} = the quiescent DC drain current at the JFET's operating point where $V_{GS} = V_{GSQ}$.

In reality, due to the presence of 1/f noise, the theoretical short-circuited input voltage PDS can be better modeled by

$$e_{na}^2(f) = (4kT/g_m)(1 + f_c/f^n) \text{ MSV/Hz} \tag{9.32}$$

The exponent n has the range $1 < n < 1.5$, and is device and lot determined. n is usually set equal to one for algebraic simplicity. The origin of the $1/f^n$ effect in JFETs is poorly understood. Note that e_{na} given by Equation 9.32 is temperature-dependent. Heatsinking or actively cooling the JFET will reduce e_{na}. The parameter f_c used in Equation 9.32 is the corner frequency of the 1/f noise spectrum. Depending on the device, it can range from below 10 Hz to above 1 kHz. f_c is generally quite high in RF and video frequency JFETs because in this type of transistor, $e_{na}(f)$ dips to around 2 nV/√Hz in the 10^5 to 10^7 Hz region, which is desirable.

JFET gates have a DC leakage or bias current, $I_{GL} = I_B$, which produces broad-band *shot noise*, which is superimposed on the leakage current. This noise component in I_{GL} is primarily due to the random occurrence of charge carriers that have enough energy to cross the reverse-biased gate-channel diode junction. The PDF of the gate current shot noise is generally assumed to be Gaussian, and its PDS is approximated by

$$i_{na}^2 = 2qI_{GL} \text{ MSA/Hz} \tag{9.33}$$

where $q = 1.602 \times 10^{-19}$ coulomb (electron charge) and I_{GL} is the DC gate leakage current in amperes.

I_{GL} is typically about 2 pA; hence, i_{na} is about 1.8 fA RMS/√Hz in the flat midrange of $i_{na}(f)$. $i_{na}(f)$, like $e_{na}(f)$, shows a 1/f characteristic at low frequencies. This can be modeled by:

$$i_{na}^2(f) = 2qI_{GL}(1 + f/f_{ic}) \text{ MSA/Hz} \tag{9.34}$$

where f_{ic} is the current noise corner frequency.

For some transistors, the measured $e_{na}(f)$ and $i_{na}(f)$ have been found to be greater than the predicted, theoretical values; in other cases, they have been found to be less. No doubt the causes for these discrepancies lie in oversimplifications used in their derivations. Note that MOSFETs have no gate-drain diode; hence, generally do not have a significant 1/f component in their i_{na}s.

9.2.4.4 Noise in BJTs

The values of e_{na} and i_{na} associated with bipolar junction transistor amplifiers depend strongly on the device's quiescent, DC operating (Q) point. This is because there are shot noise components superimposed on the quiescent base and collector currents. A midfrequency, small-signal model of a simple, grounded-emitter BJT amplifier is shown in Figure 9.7b. In this circuit, we assume negligible noise from R_L, the voltage-controlled current source, $g_m v_{be}$, and the small-signal base input resistance, r_π. The shot noise PDSs are

$$i_{na}^2 = 2qI_{BQ}\ \text{MSA/Hz} \tag{9.35}$$

$$i_{na}^2 = 2q\beta\ I_{BQ}\ \text{MSA/Hz} \tag{9.36}$$

where $\beta = h_{fe}$ is the BJT's small-signal, forward current gain evaluated at the BJT's quiescent operating (Q) point.

In this example, it is algebraically simpler to not find the equivalent input e_{na} and i_{na}. Rather, one works directly with the two white shot noise sources in the midfrequency, hybrid-pi, small-signal model. It can be shown (Northrop 1990) that the total output white noise voltage PDS is given by

$$S_{NO}(f) = 4kTR_L + 2q(I_{BQ}/\beta)(\beta R_L)^2 + \frac{4kTR_s'(\beta R_L)^2 + 2qI_{BQ}R_s{}^2(\beta R_L)^2}{(V_T/I_{BQ} + r_x)^2}\ \text{MSV/Hz} \tag{9.37}$$

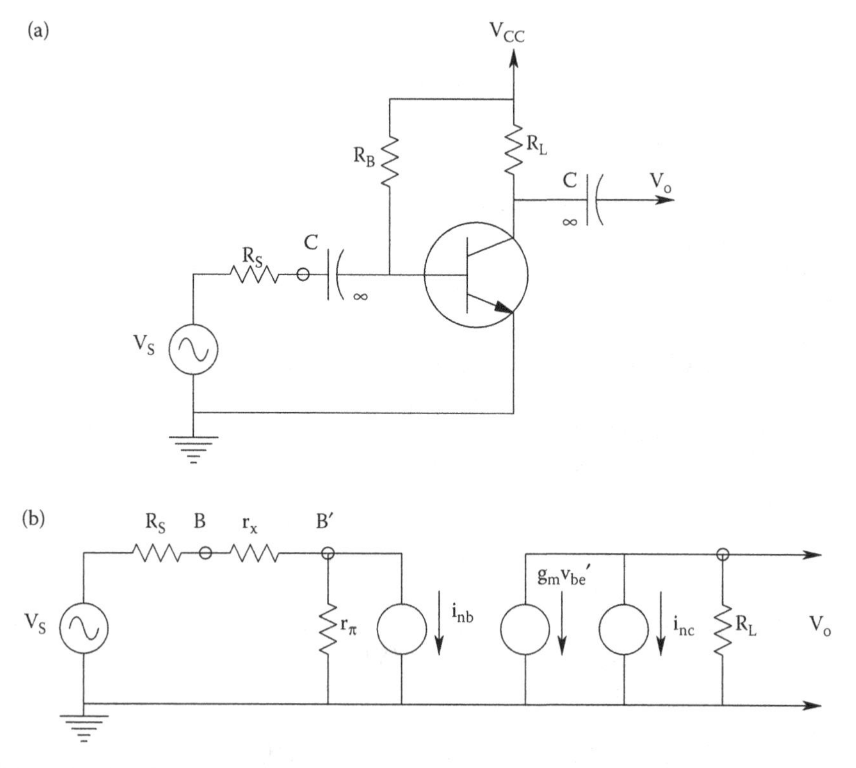

FIGURE 9.7 (a) A simple, grounded emitter BJT amplifier relevant to noise calculations. (b) A noise equivalent circuit for the BJT amplifier.

where it is clear that r_π is approximated by V_T/I_{BQ}, $R_s' = r_x + R_s$, and we will neglect the Johnson noise from R_L because it is numerically small compared to the other terms.

It is easy to show (Northrop 1990) that the mean squared output signal can be written as

$$\overline{v_{os}^2} = \overline{v_s^2}(\beta R_L)^2 B/(V_T/I_{BQ} + r_x)^2 \text{ MSV} \quad (9.38)$$

Thus, the MS signal-to-noise ratio at the amplifier output can be written as

$$SNR_o = \frac{\overline{v_s^2}/B}{4kTR_s' + 2qI_{BQ}R_s'^2 + 2q(I_{BQ}/\beta)(V_T/I_{BQ} + R_s')^2} \quad (9.39)$$

where B is the specified, equivalent (Hz) noise bandwidth for the system. The SNR_O given by Equation 9.39 has a maximum for some non-negative I_{BQMAX}. The I_{BQMAX}, which will give this maximum, can be found by differentiating the denominator of Equation 9.39 with respect to I_{BQ} and setting the derivative equal to zero. This gives

$$I_{BQMAX} = V_T/\left(R_s'\sqrt{\beta+1}\right) \text{ DC amperes} \quad (9.40)$$

What should be remembered from the above exercise is that *the best noise performance for BJT amplifiers is a function of their quiescent biasing conditions (Q-point).* Often these conditions have to be found experimentally when working at high frequencies. While individual BJT amplifiers may best be modeled for noise analysis with the two shot-noise current sources as was done above, it is more customary when describing complex, BJT IC amplifier noise performance to use the more general and more easily used root power spectra, e_{na} and i_{na}, model parameterized for a given BJT Q-point.

9.3 PROPAGATION OF NOISE THROUGH LTI FILTERS

In a formal, rigorous treatment of noise in linear systems, it is possible to show that the PDF of the output of a linear system is Gaussian, given a Gaussian noise input. In addition, it was shown rigorously in the classic text by James et al. (1947) that the one-sided PDS of the system's output noise is given by

$$S_y(f) = S_x(f)\,|\,H(j2\pi f)\,|^2 \quad \text{MS units/Hz} \quad (9.41)$$

This is the scalar product of the positive-real input's one-sided PDS and the magnitude squared of the LTI system's transfer function. This relation can be extended to include two or more cascaded systems, as shown in Figure 9.8:

$$S_y(f) = S_x(f)\,|\,H(j\,2\pi f)^2|\,|\,G(j\,2\pi\,f)^2| \quad \text{MSV/Mz} \quad (9.42)$$

or

$$S_y(f) = S_x(f)\,|\,H(j\,2\pi\,f)\,G(j\,2\pi\,f)\,|^2 \quad \text{MSV/Hz} \quad (9.43)$$

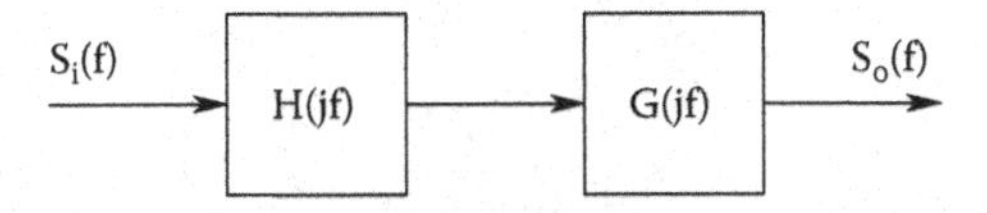

FIGURE 9.8 Two cascaded linear systems through which Gaussian noise is propagating.

If white noise with a PDS, $S_x(f) = \eta$ MSV/Hz is the input to a linear system, then the output PDS is simply

$$S_y(f) = \eta \, |H(j\, 2\pi\, f)|^2 \quad \text{MSV/Hz} \tag{9.44}$$

The total mean-squared output noise of this system is given by

$$\overline{v_{on}^2} = \int_0^\infty S_y(f)df = \eta \int_0^\infty |H(j\, 2\pi\, f)^2|\, df \quad \text{MSV} \tag{9.45}$$

The right-hand integral of Equation 9.45, for transfer functions with one more finite pole than zeros, may be shown to be the product of the transfer function's low-frequency or midband gain squared times the filter's equivalent Hz noise bandwidth. Thus, the filter's *gain squared-bandwidth product* is given by

$$\text{GAIN}^2\text{BW} = \int_0^\infty |H(2\pi\, fj)|^2\, df \tag{9.46}$$

Gain^2-bandwidth integrals have been evaluated for a number of transfer functions using complex variable theory (James et al. 1947). In Table 9.1, we give the gain^2-bandwidth integrals for five common transfer functions. Note that the *equivalent noise bandwidths* (in brackets in each case) *are in* Hz, not radians/s. Also note the absence of any 2π factors in these expressions. Gain^2-bandwidth integrals are used to estimate the total MS output noise from amplifiers having (approximate) white noise input sources, and are thus useful in calculating output signal-to-noise ratios.

TABLE 9.1
Gain^2 Hz Noise Bandwidth Products for Some Common Filter Transfer Functions

Transfer Function, H(s)	Gain^2 {Bandwidth (Hz)}	Filter Type
1. $\frac{K_v}{s\tau + 1}$	$K_v^2 \left\{\frac{1}{4\,\tau}\right\}$	Low-pass, one real-pole
2. $\frac{K_v}{(s\,\tau_1 + 1)(s\,\tau_2 + 1)}$	$K_v^2 \left\{\frac{1}{4(\tau_1 + \tau_2)}\right\}$	Low-pass, 2 real poles
3. $\frac{K_v}{s^2/\omega_n^2 + s2\xi/\omega_n + 1}$	$K_v^2 \left\{\frac{\omega_n}{8\xi}\right\}$ quadratic low-pass	Underdamped
4. $\frac{s\,K_v\,(2\xi/\omega_n)}{s^2/\omega_n^2 + s2\xi/\omega_n + 1}$ bandpass	$K_v^2\{\xi\omega_n\}$	Underdamped quadratic
5. $\frac{s\,\tau_1 K_v}{(s\,\tau_1 + 1)(s\,\tau_2 + 1)}$	$K_v^2 \left\{\frac{1}{4\tau_2(1 + \tau_2/\tau_1)}\right\}$	Overdamped quadratic bandpass

9.4 NOISE FACTOR AND FIGURE OF AMPLIFIERS

9.4.1 Broadband Noise Factor and Noise Figure of Amplifiers

An amplifier's *noise factor,* F, is defined as the ratio of the mean-squared signal-to-noise ratio at the amplifier's input to the MS signal-to-noise ratio at the amplifier's output. Since a real amplifier is noisy and adds noise to the signal as well as amplifying it, the output signal-to-noise ratio (SNR_o) is always less that the input signal-to-noise ratio (SNR_i); hence, the *noise factor* F is always greater than one for a noisy amplifier. F is a figure of merit for an amplifier; the closer to unity the better.

$$F \equiv \frac{SNR_i}{SNR_o} > 1 \tag{9.47}$$

The *noise figure (NF)* is defined as

$$NF \equiv 10 \log_{10}(F) \quad \text{(decibels dB)} \tag{9.48}$$

when the SNRs are in terms of mean squared quantities. The closer NF is to zero, the quieter the amplifier.

Figure 9.9 illustrates a simple, two-noise source model for a noisy amplifier. Here we assume the spectrums of e_{na} and i_{na} are white, and that $R_1 \gg R_s$. The MS input signal is $S_i = \overline{v_s^2}$ so the MS output signal is $S_o = K_V^2 \overline{v_s^2}$, where $K_V{}^2$ is the amplifier's midband gain squared. The *MS input noise* is simply that associated with v_s (here set to zero) plus the Johnson noise from the source resistance, R_s, in a specified Hz noise bandwidth, B. It is

$$N_i = 4kTR_sB \quad \text{MSV} \tag{9.49}$$

The mean-squared noise at the amplifier's output, N_o, is composed of three components: One from the R_s Johnson noise and two from the equivalent noise sources. N_o can be written as the sum of three MS voltages:

$$\begin{aligned} N_o &= (4kTR_s + e_{na}^2 + i_{na}^2R_s^2)\int_0^\infty |H(j\,2\pi\,f)|^2\,df \\ &= (4kTR_s + e_{na}^2 + i_{na}^2R_s^2)\,K_V^2B \quad \text{MSV} \end{aligned} \tag{9.50}$$

Using the definition for F, the noise factor for the simple noisy amplifier model can be written as

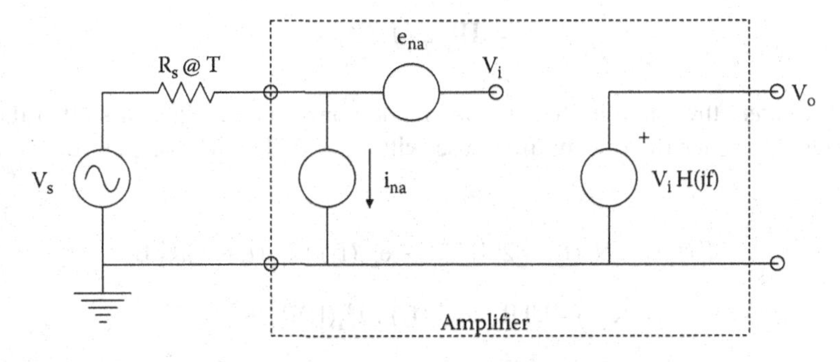

FIGURE 9.9 The simple, two noise source model for a noisy VCVS.

$$F = 1 + \frac{e_{na}^2 + i_{na}^2 R_s^2}{4kTR_s} \tag{9.51}$$

Note that this expression for F contains no bandwidth terms; they cancel out. When the NF is given for an amplifier, R_s must be specified, as well as the Hz bandwidth, B, over which the noise is measured. The temperature should also be specified, although common practice usually sets T at 298°K (25°C).

For practical amplifiers, NF and F are functions of frequency because e_{na} and i_{na} are functions of frequency (see Figure 9.6). For a given R_s, F tends to rise at low frequencies due to the 1/f components in the equivalent input noise sources. F also increases at high frequencies, again, due to the high-frequency increases in e_{na} and i_{na}. Often, we are interested in the noise performance of an amplifier in either low- or high-frequencies where the NF and F are not minimum. To examine the detailed noise performance of an amplifier at low- and high frequencies, the *spot noise figure,* described below, is used.

9.4.2 Spot Noise Factor and Figure

Spot noise measurements are made through a narrow band-pass filter in order to evaluate an amplifier's noise performance in a certain narrow frequency range, particularly where $e_{na}(f)$ and $i_{na}(f)$ are not constant, such as in the 1/f range, and at high frequencies. Figure 9.10 illustrates a set of *spot noise figure* (SNF) contours for a commercial, low-noise preamplifier having applications at audio-frequencies. Note that there is an area in $\{R_s, f\}$ space where the dB spot noise figure is a minimum. For best noise performance, the Thevenin resistance of the source, R_s, should lie in the range of minimum SNF, and the input signal's PDS should contain most of its energy in the range of frequencies where the SNF is minimum.

A system for determining an amplifier's spot noise figure is shown if Figure 9.11. An adjustable white noise voltage source is used at the amplifier's input. Note that the output resistance of the white noise source plus some external resistance must add up to R_s, the specified Thevenin equivalent input resistance. The system is used as follows: *First,* the band-pass filter (BPF) is set to the desired center frequency, f_c, around which we wish to characterize the amplifier's noise performance. Then, the white noise generator is set to $e_N = 0$. Assume that the total mean squared noise at the system output under these conditions can be written as

$$N_o(f_c) = [4kTR_s + e_{na}^2(f_c) + i_{na}^2(f_c)R_s^2]K_V^2 B_F \text{ MSV} \tag{9.52}$$

where $e_{na}(f_c)$ is the value of e_{na} at the center frequency, f_c, B_F is the equivalent noise bandwidth of the BPF, and K_V is the combined midband gain of the amplifier under measurement at f_c, the BPF at f_c, and the postamplifier. K_V can be written as

$$K_V = |\mathbf{H}(j\, 2\pi\, f_c)| K_F K_A \tag{9.53}$$

In the second step, the white noise source is made nonzero and adjusted so that the true RMS voltmeter reads $\sqrt{2}$ higher than in the first case with $e_N = 0$. The MS output voltage can now be written as

$$\begin{aligned} N_o'(f_c) &= 2N_o(f_c) = 2[4kTR_s + e_{na}^2(f_c) + i_{na}^2(f_c)R_s^2]K_V^2 B_F \\ &= [\overline{e_N^2} + 4kTR_s + e_{na}^2(f_c) + i_{na}^2(f_c)R_s^2]K_V^2 B_F \end{aligned} \tag{9.54}$$

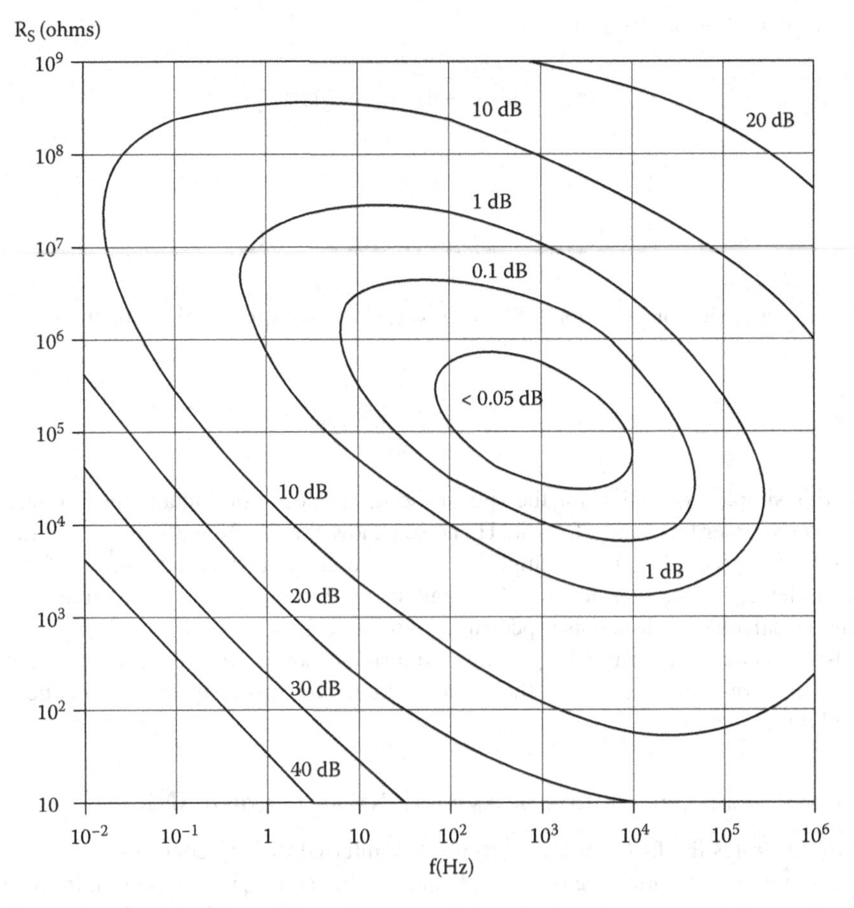

FIGURE 9.10 Curves of constant spot noise figure (SNF) for a typical commercial, low-noise amplifier. Note that there is a region in R_S-f space, where the SNF is minimum (optimum).

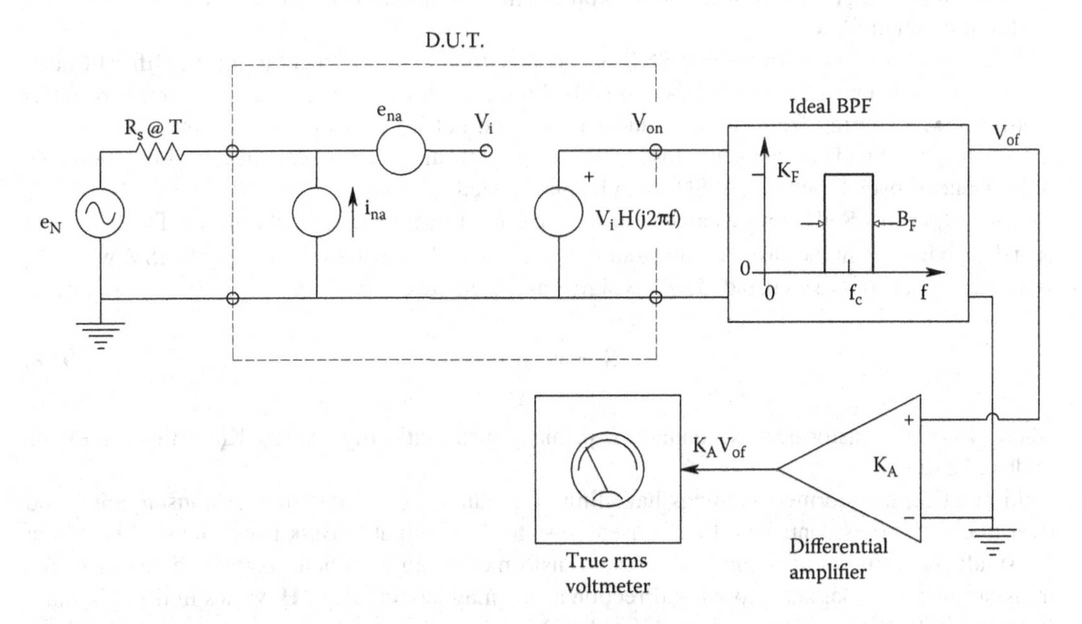

FIGURE 9.11 A test circuit for measuring a noisy amplifier's SNF.

Under this condition, it is evident that

$$\overline{e_N^2} = 4kTR_s + e_{na}^2(f_c) + i_{na}^2(f_c)R_s^2 \quad (9.55)$$

Hence,

$$[e_{na}^2(f_c) + i_{na}^2(f_c)R_s^2] = [\overline{e_N^2} - 4kTR_s] \quad (9.56)$$

When the left-hand side of Equation 9.56 is substituted into Equation 9.51 for the noise factor, F, one finds

$$F_{spot} = \overline{e_N^2}/(4kTR_s) \quad (9.57)$$

Note that this simple expression for the spot noise factor does not contain specific terms for the bandpass filter's center frequency, f_c, or its Hz noise bandwidth, B_F. Note that these parameters must be specified when giving F_{spot} for an amplifier. F_{spot} is actually calculated by setting f_c and R_s, then determining the $\overline{e_N{}^2}$ value that doubles the mean squared output noise. This value of $\overline{e_N{}^2}$ is then divided by the calculated white noise spectrum from the resistor R_s.

It is also possible to measure F_{spot} using a sinusoidal source of frequency f_c, instead of the calibrated white noise source, e_N. See the home problems for this chapter for a detailed treatment of this method.

9.4.3 Transformer Optimization of Amplifier NF and Output SNR

Figure 9.10 illustrates the fact that for a given set of internal biasing conditions, a given amplifier will have an optimum operating region (in R_s, f-space), where NF_{spot} is a minimum. In some practical instances, the input transducer to which the amplifier is connected has an R_s that is *far smaller* than the R_s giving the lowest NF_{spot} on the amplifier's spot NF contours. Consequently, the signal conditioning system (i.e., transducer and amplifier) are not operating to give either the lowest NF or the highest output SNR.

One way of improving the output SNR is to couple the input transducer to the amplifier through a low-noise, low-loss transformer, as shown in Figure 9.12. (Such coupling, of course, presumes that the signal coming from the transducer is AC and not DC, for obvious reasons.) A practical transformer is a bandpass device; it loses efficiency at low and high frequencies, limiting the range of frequencies over which output SNR can be maximized.

The output MS SNR can be calculated for the circuit of Figure 9.12 as follows: The MS input signal is simply $\overline{v_s^2}$. In the case of a sinusoidal input, it is well-known that $\overline{v_s^2} = V_s^2/2$ MSV, where V_s is the peak value of the sinusoid. The MS signal at the output is

$$S_o = \overline{v_s{}^2}\, n^2 K_V{}^2 \quad (9.58)$$

where n is the transformer's secondary-to-primary turns ratio (n_2/n_1), and K_V is the amplifier's midband gain.

In practice, transformer windings have finite resistance; hence, they make Johnson noise, and their magnetic cores contribute Barkhausen noise to their outputs. (Barkhausen noise arises from the small transient voltages induced in the transformer windings when magnetic domains in the transformer's ferromagnetic core flip direction as the magnetizing field, **H**, varies in time. Domain flipping is effectively random at low $|\mathbf{H}|$ values.)

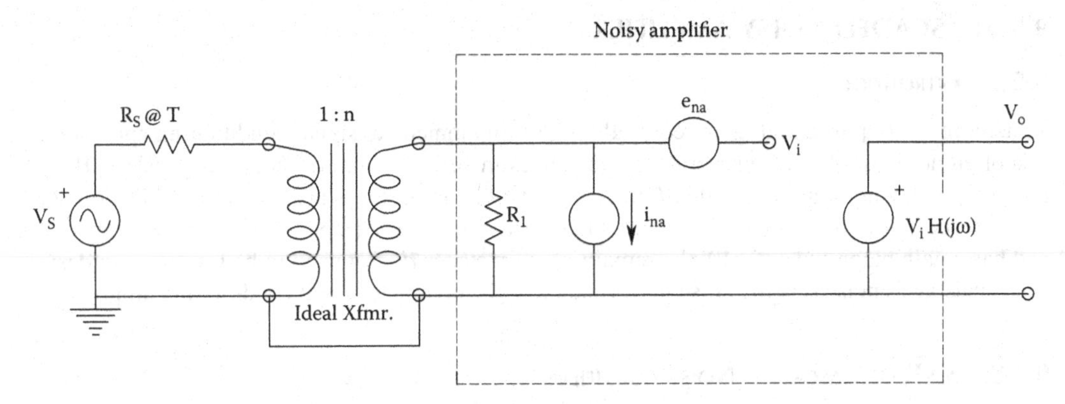

FIGURE 9.12 Use of an ideal transformer in an amplifier's input circuit to both maximize the output MS signal-to-noise ratio, and minimize the SNF, given the optimum turns ratio.

The ideal transformer, besides having infinite frequency response, is also lossless and noiseless. From this latter assumption, it is easy to show that the amplifier "sees" a transformed Thévènin equivalent circuit of the input transducer having an open-circuit voltage of $n\, v_s(t)$, and a Thévènin resistance of $n^2 R_s$ (Northrop 1990). Thus, the mean squared output noise of the transformer-input amplifier can be written as

$$N_o = [n^2 4kTR_s + e_{na}^2 + i_{na}^2 (n^2 R_s)^2] K_V^2 B \text{ MSV} \tag{9.59}$$

And the output SNR is

$$SNR_o = \frac{\overline{v_s^2}/B}{4kTR_s + e_{na}^2/n^2 + i_{na}^2 n^2 R_s^2} \tag{9.60}$$

The SNR_o clearly has a maximum with respect to the turns ratio, n. It can be shown that F is minimum when $n = n_o$ so SNR_o is maximum (Northrop 2005). If the denominator of Equation 9.60 is differentiated with respect to n^2 and set equal to zero, we find that an optimum turns ratio, n_o, exists that will maximize SNR_o. n_o is given by

$$n_o = \sqrt{e_{na}/(i_{na} R_s)} \tag{9.61}$$

If the noiseless (ideal) transformer is given the turns ratio of n_o, then it is easy to show that the maximum output SNR is given by

$$SNR_{Omax} = \frac{\overline{v_s^2}/B}{4kTR_s + 2e_{na} i_{na} R_s} \tag{9.62}$$

The general effect of transformer SNR maximization on the system's noise figure contours is to shift the locus of minimum NF_{spot} vertically to a lower range of R_s; there is no obvious shift of this locus along the f_c axis. Also, the minimum NF_{spot} is higher with a real transformer. This is because a practical transformer is noisy, as discussed above. As a rule of thumb, use of a transformer to improve output SNR and reduce NF_{spot} is justified if $(e_{na}^2 + i_{na}^2 R_s^2) > 20\, e_{na}\, i_{na}\, R_s$ in the range of frequencies of interest (Northrop 1990).

9.5 CASCADED NOISY AMPLIFIERS

9.5.1 Introduction

To achieve the required high gain required for certain biomedical signal conditioning applications, it is often necessary to place several IC gain stages in series. A natural question to ask is: If I am designing a low-noise amplifier, do *all* the component IC gain stages also need to be low-noise? As you will see below, the good news is that as long as the *headstage* (input, or first stage) is low noise, and has a gain magnitude of ≥10, the remaining gain stages *do not* need to be low-noise in design. The headstage's noise sets the noise performance of the complete signal conditioning amplifier.

9.5.2 SNR of Cascaded, Noisy Amplifiers

Figure 9.13 illustrates three, cascaded amplifier stages. The amplifier's overall gain is $K_V = K_{V1}\, K_{V2}\, K_{V3}$. The first stage has a white, short-circuit voltage, root power spectrum of e_{na1} rmsV/$\sqrt{\text{Hz}}$, and an input current noise root power spectrum of i_{na1} rmsV/$\sqrt{\text{Hz}}$. The other two stages have voltage noises of e_{na2} and e_{na3}, respectively, and zero current noises. (We can assume the current noises are zero because the output resistance of the previous stages is assumed to be very low, so that $i_{na2}\, R_{o1} \ll e_{na2}$, and $i_{na3}\, R_{o2} \ll e_{na3}$.) Assume a sinusoidal input signal, $v_s(t) = V_s \sin(2\pi ft)$; thus the MS input voltage is $V_s^2/2$. The MS output voltage is simply: $\overline{v_{os}^2} = (V_s^2/2)(K_{V1}K_{V2}K_{V3})^2$. The total MS noise output voltage is the sum of the MS noise components from the noise sources: $\overline{v_{os}^2} = [e_{na1}^2 + i_{na1}^{2i} R_s^2](K_{v1}K_{v2}K_{v3})^2 + e_{na2}^2(K_{v2}K_{v3})^2 + e_{na3}^2(K_{v3})^2$.

We can now examine the output MS signal-to-noise ratio for the three-stage amplifier:

$$\text{SNR}_o = \frac{(V_s^2/2)(K_{v1}K_{v2}K_{v3})^2}{\{[e_{na1}^2 + i_{na1}^2 R_s^2](K_{v1}K_{v2}K_{v3})^2 + e_{na2}^2(K_{v2}K_{v3})^2 + e_{na3}^2(K_{v3})^2\}B}$$

$$\downarrow \tag{9.63}$$

$$\text{SNR}_o = \frac{(V_s^2/2)/B}{[e_{na1}^2 + i_{an1}R_s^2] + e_{na2}^2/K_{v1}^2 + e_{na3}^2/(K_{v1}K_{v2})^2} \cong \frac{(V_s^2/2)/B}{[e_{na1}^2 + i_{na1}R_s^2]}$$

Thus, the SNR_o of the three-stage, cascaded amplifier is set by the headstage alone, as long as the headstage gain, $|K_{V1}| > 10$.

What if the headstage is of necessity a source- or emitter-follower or other buffer amplifier having near unity gain? If we examine Equation 9.63 above, we see that it reduces to a lower value for $K_{V1} \to 1$, sic:

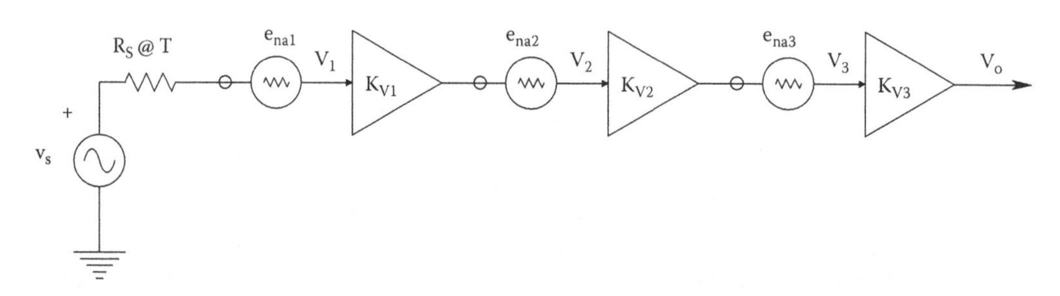

FIGURE 9.13 Three, cascaded noisy amplifiers.

$$\mathrm{SNR_o} \cong \frac{(V_s^2/2)/B}{[e_{na1}^2 + i_{na1}^2 R_s^2] + e_{na2}^2 + e_{na3}^2/(K_{v2})^2} \tag{9.64}$$

Now the second stage's voltage noise, e_{na2}, becomes important, and it is K_{V2} which we wish to be ≥ 10. *Both the first and second stages must now use low-noise amplifiers.*

9.6 NOISE IN DIFFERENTIAL AMPLIFIERS

9.6.1 INTRODUCTION

As we have seen in Chapter 3, the headstage of a differential amplifier contains two active elements (BJTs, JFETs, or MOSFETs), hence two, *independent, uncorrelated* sources of e_{na} and i_{na}. The equivalent input circuit of a DA is shown in Figure 9.14. To simplify analysis, the two amplifier input resistances which appear in parallel with the i_{na}s have been set to infinity (i.e., omitted) because $R_s \ll R_{in}$. All the noise sources are assumed to be white, and $e_{na} = e'_{na}\mathrm{rmsV}/\sqrt{\mathrm{Hz}}$, and $i_{na} = i'_{na}\mathrm{rmsA}/\sqrt{\mathrm{Hz}}$, although certainly $e_{na}(t) \neq e'_{na}(t)$ and $i_{na}(t) \neq i'_{na}(t)$, except very rarely. Recall that for a DA,

$$v_o = A_D v_{id} + A_C v_{ic} \tag{9.65}$$

where A_D is the scalar difference-mode gain, A_C is the scalar common-mode gain, v_{id} is the *difference-mode input signal*, and v_{ic} is the *common-mode input signal*. By definition

$$v_{id} \equiv (v_i - v_i')/2 \tag{9.66a}$$

$$v_{ic} \equiv (v_i + v_i')/2 \tag{9.66b}$$

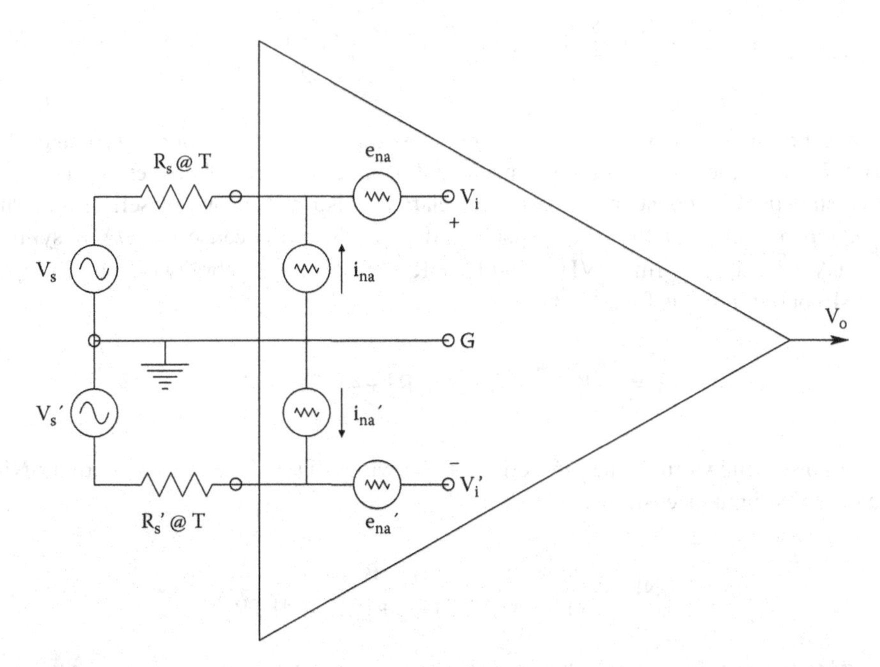

FIGURE 9.14 Equivalent input circuit for a noisy differential amplifier. In this model, both DA input transistors make noise.

Also recall that the common-mode rejection ratio for the simple DA can be expressed as

$$\text{CMRR} \equiv A_D/A_C \tag{9.67}$$

Under normal operating conditions, $|A_D| \gg |A_C|$, and CMRR $\gg 1$.

9.6.2 Calculation of the SNR$_o$ of the DA

Referring to Figure 9.14, we see that the DA noise model circuit has *six*, independent, uncorrelated noise sources. Thus, the total noise PDS at the v_i node can be written as

$$S_{ni} = e_{na}^2 + i_{na}^2 R_s^2 + 4kTR_s \ \text{MSV/Hz} \tag{9.68}$$

The total noise PDS at the v_i' node is similarly

$$S_{ni}' = e_{na}'^2 + i_{na}'^2 R_s'^2 + 4kTR_s' \ \text{MSV/Hz} \tag{9.69}$$

It is of interest to find the MS SNR$_o$ of the noisy DA. Assume that the input signal is pure DM. Thus, $v_{ic} = 0$ and $v_{id} = v_s$, and $\overline{v_{os}^2} = A_D^2 \overline{v_s^2}$ MSV. To find the MS noise output, set $v_s = v_s' = 0$, and consider that the six noise sources add in quadrature (in a MS sense). First, note that in the time domain:

$$v_i(t) = e_{na}(t) + i_{na}(t)R_s + e_{nrs}(t) \ \text{Volts} \tag{9.70}$$

and

$$v_i'(t) = e_{na}'(t) + i_{na}(t)R_s' + e_{nrs}'(t) \ \text{Volts} \tag{9.71}$$

Now let us expand and square Equation 9.65 for the amplifier output:

$$v_{on}^2(t) = A_D^2\left[\frac{v_i^2 - 2v_i v_i' + v_i'^2}{4}\right] + 2A_D A_C\left[\frac{v_i - v_i'}{2}\right]\left[\frac{v_i + v_i'}{2}\right] + A_C^2\left[\frac{v_i^2 + 2v_i v_i' + v_i'^2}{4}\right] \tag{9.72}$$

When the expressions for $v_i(t)$ and $v_i'(t)$ are substituted from Equations 9.70 and 9.71 into Equation 9.72, and the expectation or mean is taken, cross-terms between v_i and v_i' vanish because of statistical independence and no correlation. Also, the means of self cross-terms such as $e_{na}'(i_{na}'R_s')$ also vanish for the same reasons. Also recall that because the DA is symmetrical, $e_{na} = e_{na}'$ rmsV/$\sqrt{\text{Hz}}$, $i_{na} = i_{na}'$ rmsA/$\sqrt{\text{Hz}}$, and $R_s = R_s'$. After some algebra (which is not reproduced here), the MS output noise is found to be

$$\overline{v_{on}^2} = \frac{(A_D^2 + A_C^2)}{2}(e_{na}^2 + i_{na}R_s^2 + 4kTR)B \ \text{MSV} \tag{9.73}$$

B is the Hz noise bandwidth of the DA acting on the white PDSs. Now the MS output SNR of the DA for a pure DM input is easily written as

$$\text{SNR}_o = \frac{2\overline{v_{sd}^2}/B}{(1 + \text{CMRR}^{-2})(e_{na}^2 + i_{na}R_s^2 + 4kTR_s)} \tag{9.74}$$

Note that CMRR$^{-2} \ll 1$, and is negligible. The 2 in the numerator is real, however, and illustrates the advantage of using a DA with pure DM signals.

9.7 EFFECT OF FEEDBACK ON NOISE

9.7.1 Introduction

Chapters 4 and 5 have shown that negative voltage feedback (NVFB), correctly applied, has many important beneficial effects in signal conditioning. These include but are not limited to: *reduction of harmonic distortion, extension of bandwidth, and reduction of output impedance.* There is a common misconception that negative voltage feedback also acts to improve output SNR and reduce the NF. It is shown below that NVFB has quite the opposite effect; it *reduces* the output SNR and *increases* the NF.

9.7.2 Calculation of SNR_o of an Amplifier with NVFB

Figure 9.15 illustrates a noisy differential amplifier with NVFB applied through a voltage divider to the inverting input. To simplify calculations, assume that the DA has a finite difference-mode gain, A_D, and an infinite CMRR, that is, $A_C \to 0$. Also, neglect the input voltages produced by the current noise sources. The DA's output is given by

$$v_o = A'_D(v_i - v'_i) \tag{9.75}$$

The noninverting input node signal voltage is $v_i = v_s$. The inverting input node voltage is

$$v'_i = v_o\left(\frac{R_1}{R_1 + R_F}\right) = v_o\,\beta \tag{9.76}$$

The expressions for v_i and v'_i above are substituted into Equation 9.75 above, and v_o is found to be

$$v_o = \frac{v_s A'_D}{1 + \beta A'_D} \tag{9.77}$$

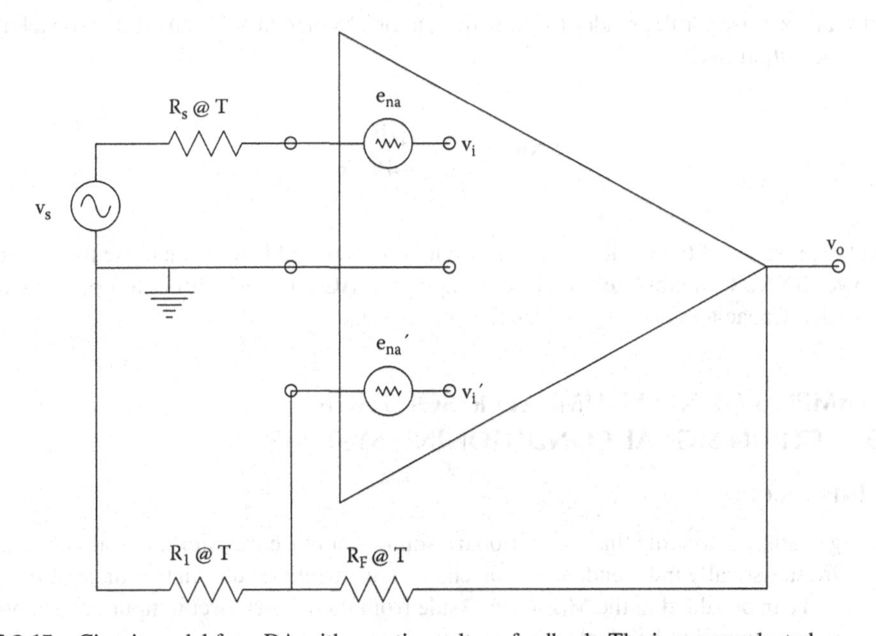

FIGURE 9.15 Circuit model for a DA with negative voltage feedback. The i_{na}s are neglected.

The mean-squared output signal voltage is thus

$$\overline{v_{os}^2} = \overline{v_s^2}\frac{A_D'^2}{(1+\beta\, A_D')^2} \tag{9.78}$$

When considering the noises, v_s is set to zero and the time signals can be written as

$$v_o = A_D'[e_{na} + e_{ns} - \{e_{na}' + \beta v_o + \beta e_{nf} + (1-\beta)e_{n1}\}] \tag{9.79}$$

Equation 9.79 is solved for $v_o(t)$:

$$v_o(1+\beta A_D') = A_D'[e_{na} + e_{ns} - e_{na}' - \beta e_{nf} - (1-\beta)e_{n1}\}] \tag{9.80}$$

Note that $\beta \equiv R_1/(R_1 + R_F)$ and $e_{na} = e_{na}'$ statistically (but not necessarily in the time domain), e_{ns}, e_{n1}, and e_{nf} equals the thermal noise voltages from R_s, R_1, and R_F, respectively, all at Kelvin temperature T. One can now write the expression for the mean-squared v_o over a Hz noise bandwidth B; this can be shown to be

$$\overline{v_{on}^2} = \frac{A_D^2}{(1+\beta A_D')^2}[2e_{na}^2 + 4kTR_s + \beta^2 4kTR_F + (1-\beta)^2 4kTR_1]B \tag{9.81}$$

The MS signal-to-noise ratio of the feedback amplifier is found by taking the ratio of Equation 9.78 to Equation 9.81:

$$SNR_o = \frac{\overline{v_s^2}/B}{2e_{na}^2 + 4kT[R_s + \beta^2 R_F + (1-\beta)^2 R_1]} \tag{9.82}$$

It is left for an exercise for the reader to show that in the absence of feedback (no feedback resistors at all) that the output SNR is

$$SNR_o = \frac{\overline{v_s^2}/B}{2e_{na}^2 + 4kTR_F} \tag{9.83}$$

Note that the presence of the feedback voltage divider resistors adds Johnson noise to the output and gives a lower SNR_o. Contemplate the effect of applying AC feedback through a purely capacitive voltage divider. Capacitors do not generate thermal noise.

9.8 EXAMPLES OF NOISE-LIMITED RESOLUTION OF CERTAIN SIGNAL CONDITIONING SYSTEMS

9.8.1 Introduction

In following examples, assume that the stationary sources of noise (resistor thermal noise, amplifier e_{na} and i_{na}) are statistically independent, uncorrelated, have white spectra in the range of frequencies of interest, and can be added in the MS sense. Aside from their short-circuit input voltage noise, e_{na}, the op amps are assumed to be ideal.

9.8.2 Calculation of the Minimum Resolvable AC Input Voltage to a Noisy Op Amp

Figure 9.16 illustrates a simple, inverting op amp circuit with a sinusoidal input. Assume that $i_{na} R_F \ll e_{na}$; hence, i_{na} produces negligible noise at the amplifier output and thus is deleted from the model. Only amplifier e_{na} and resistor Johnson noise contribute to the amplifier's noise output. The mean-squared *signal* output is given by

$$\overline{v_{os}^2} = (V_S^2/2)(-R_F/R_1)^2 \tag{9.84}$$

The noise voltages in this circuit are all conditioned by different gains: e_{n1} is the thermal noise from R_1; it is conditioned by the same gain as v_s, i.e., $(-R_F/R_1)$. Because the summing junction is at zero volts due to the ideal op amp assumption, the thermal noise in R_F, e_{nf}, is seen at the output as simply e_{nf} (a gain of unity). Again, the gain for e_{na} is found by assuming $v_i' = 0$. The voltage at the R_1–R_F node thus must be e_{na}; hence, the voltage divider ratio gives us $v_o = e_{na}(1 + R_F/R_1)$. Note that these three gains are derived assuming e_{na}, e_{nf}, and e_{n1} are voltages varying in time. When we examine the MS noise at the output, the gains must be squared. Using the principles described above, we find that the total MS noise at the op amp output is

$$\overline{v_{on}^2} = \{4kTR_1(-R_F/R_1)^2 + 4kTR_F + e_{na}^2(1 + R_F/R_1)_2\}B \tag{9.85}$$

Note that the equivalent noise bandwidth, B, must be used to effectively integrate the white output PDS, giving MSV. The MS SNR_o of the amplifier is thus

$$SNR_o = \frac{(V_S^2/2)(-R_F/R_1)^2}{\{4kTR_1(-R_F/R_1)^2 + 4kTR_F + e_{na}^2[1 + 2R_F/R_1 + (R_F/R_1)^2]\}B} \tag{9.86}$$

$$\downarrow$$

$$SNR_o = \frac{(V_S^2/2)/B}{\{4kTR_1 + 4kTR_F(R_1/R_F)^2 + e_{na}^2[1 + 2R_F/R_1 + (R_F/R_1)^2](R_1/R_F)^2\}} \tag{9.87}$$

$$\downarrow$$

$$SNR_o = \frac{(V_S^2/2)/B}{\{4kTR_1 + 4kT(R_1^2/R_F) + e_{na}^2[(R_1 + R_F)^2 + 2R_1/R_F + 1)^2]\}} \tag{9.88}$$

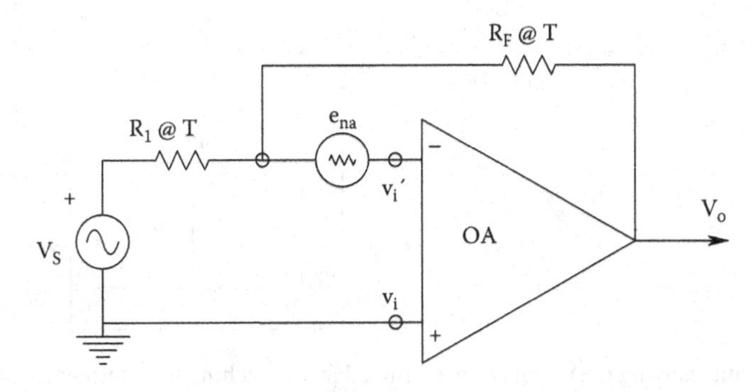

FIGURE 9.16 A simple inverting op amp circuit with a sinusoidal voltage input. White thermal noise is assumed to come from the two resistors and also from the op amp's e_{na}.

↓

$$SNR_o = \frac{(V_S^2/2)/B}{\{4kTR_1(1+R_1/R_F)+e_{na}^2[1+(R_1/R_F)]^2\}} \tag{9.89}$$

To maximize Equation 9.89 for SNR_o, it is clear that R_1/R_F must be small, or equivalently, the amplifier's signal gain magnitude, R_F/R_1, must be large. This is an unusual result because it says that in this case, the SNR_o is gain-dependent. Most SNR_os calculated are independent of gain. Equation 9.89 can be solved for the minimum V_S to give a specified SNR_o. *For example,* let the required MS SNR_o be set to 3; $4kT \equiv 1.656 \times 10^{-20}$; $R_1 = 1k$, $R_F = 10k$; $e_{na} = 10\,nVrms/\sqrt{Hz}$; B = 1000 Hz. The source frequency is 10 kHz and lies in the center of B. The minimum peak sinusoidal input voltage, V_S, is found to be 0.914 microvolts for the output $SNR_o \geq 3$.

9.8.3 Calculation of the Minimum Resolvable AC Input Signal to Obtain a Specified SNR_O in a Transformer-Coupled Amplifier

Figure 9.17 illustrates an op amp circuit used to condition an extremely small AC signal from a low impedance source. An impedance-matching transformer is used because R_S is much less than $R_{Sopt} = (e_{na}/i_{na})$ ohms. Assume that the op amp is ideal except for e_{na} and i_{na}. The summing junction of the op amp, looking into the transformer's secondary winding, can be shown to "see" an input Thevenin equivalent circuit with an open-circuit voltage of $n\,v_s$, and a Thevenin resistance of $n^2 R_S$ (Northrop 1990). Thus the output voltage due to the signal is $v_{os} = n\,v_s\,[-R_F/n^2 R_S]$, and the MS signal is

$$\overline{v_{os}^2} = \overline{v_s^2}[R_F/n\,R_S]^2 \text{ MSV} \tag{9.90}$$

The op amp's output is filtered by an (ideal) bandpass filter with peak gain = 1, and noise bandwidth, B Hz centered at f_s, the signal frequency. The filter is used to restrict the noise power at the output, while passing the signal.

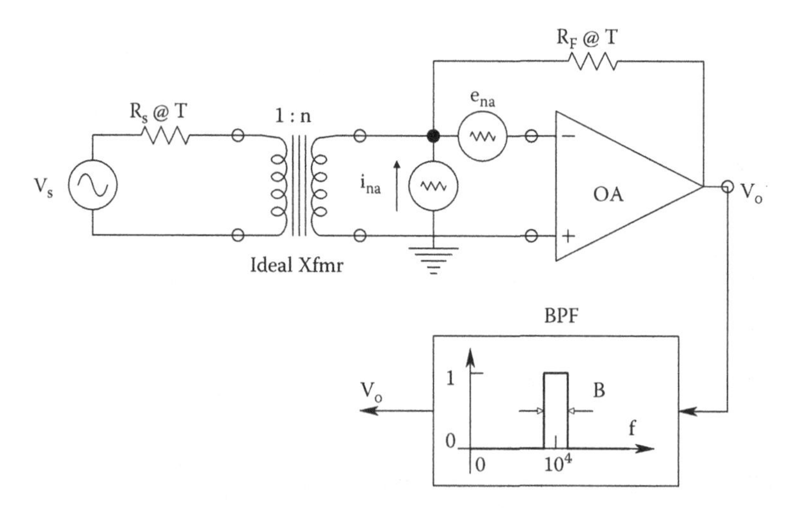

FIGURE 9.17 Circuit showing the use of an ideal, impedance-matching transformer to maximize the output SNR. R_s and R_F are assumed to make thermal white noise; e_{na} and i_{na} are assumed to have white spectra. An ideal, unity gain BPF is used to limit output noise MSV.

Finding the output noise is more complicated. The gain for e_{ns}, the thermal noise from R_S, is the same as for v_s; i.e., $[R_F/n^2R_S]$. The gain for i_{nf}, the thermal noise from R_F, is 1. The gain (transresistance) for i_{na} is R_F. The gain for e_{na} can be shown to be $[1 + R_F/(n^2R_S)]$ (Northrop 1990). By using the superposition of mean-squared voltages, we can write the total noise MS output voltage:

$$\overline{v_{on}^2} = \{e_{na}^2[1+R_F/(n^2R_S)]^2 + i_{na}^2R_F^2 + 4kTR_F + 4kTR_S[R_F/nR_S]^2\}B \text{ MSV} \tag{9.91}$$

The output SNR is easily written as

$$SNR_o = \frac{\overline{v_s^2}/B}{4kTR_S + e_{na}^2[nR_S/R_F + 1/n]^2 + i_{na}^2R_S^2n^2 + 4kTR_F[nR_S/R_F]^2} \tag{9.92}$$

The denominator of Equation 9.92 has a *minimum* for some non-negative, transformer turns ratio, n_o; thus, SNR_o is *maximum* for $n = n_o$. To find n_o, we differentiate the denominator with respect to n^2, and set the derivative equal to zero, then solve for n_o:

$$0 = \frac{d}{dn^2}\{4kTR_S + e_{na}^2[nR_S/R_F + 1/n]^2 + i_{na}^2R_S^2n^2 + 4kTR_F[nR_S/R_F]^2\} \tag{9.93}$$

$$\downarrow$$

$$0 = e_{na}^2[R_S/R_F]^2 + e_{na}^2[-1/n_o^{\,4}] + i_{na}^2R_S^2 + 4kTR_F[R_S/R_F]^2 \tag{9.94}$$

$$\downarrow$$

$$n_o = \frac{\sqrt{e_{na}/R_S}}{\{(e_{na}^2/R_F)^2 + 4kTR_F + i_{na}^2\}^{1/4}} \tag{9.95}$$

Let us now calculate the numerical turns ratio, n_o, that will maximize SNR_o. Define the parameters: $e_{na} = 3$ nVrms/$\sqrt{\text{Hz}}$ (white), $i_{na} = 0.4$ pArms/$\sqrt{\text{Hz}}$ (white), $R_F = 10^4$ ohms, $R_S = 10$ ohms, $4kT = 1.656 \times 10^{-20}$, and $B = 10^3$ Hz. Using Equation 9.95, one finds that $n_o = 14.73$ (note that the secondary-to-primary ratio does not need to be an integer).

Using $n_o = 14.73$, we define the desirable MS $SNR_o = 3$, and substitute the numerical values above into Equation 9.92, and solve for the RMS v_s required; $v_s = 28.3$ nVrms. If no transformer is used (equivalent to $n = 1$ in Equation 9.92), we find we need $v_s = 166$ nVrms for the same MS $SNR_o = 3$.

9.8.4 Effect of Capacitance Neutralization on the SNR_o of an Electrometer Amplifier Used for Glass Micropipette, Intracellular, Transmembrane Voltage Recording

Measurement of the transmembrane potential of neurons, muscle cells, and other cells is generally done with hollow, glass, micropipettes filled with a conductive electrolyte solution, such as 3M KCl (La Vallee et al. 1969). In order for the glass micropipette electrode to penetrate the cell membrane, the tips are drawn down to diameters of the order of −0.5 μm. It is the small diameter tips that give micropipettes their high series resistance, R_μ. Figure 9.18 illustrates a simplified, lumped-parameter model for a glass microelectrode with its tip in a cell. R_μ is on the order of 50–500 MΩ,

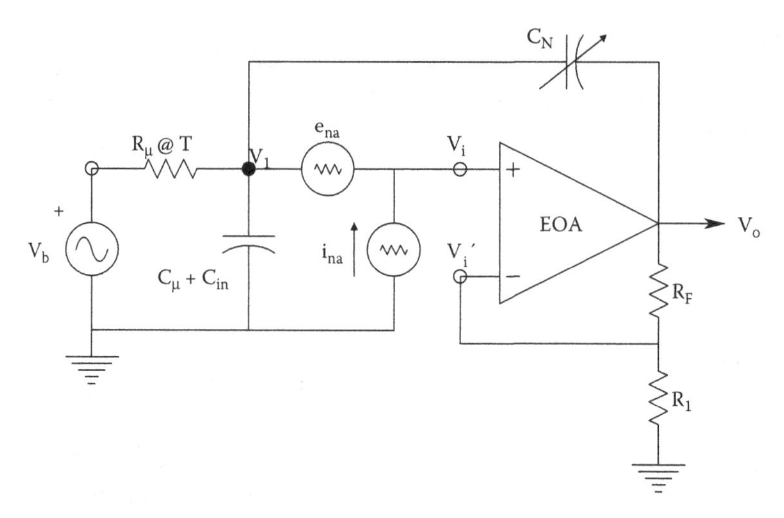

FIGURE 9.18 Circuit used to model noise in a capacity-neutralized electrometer amplifier supplied by a glass micropipette electrode. Only white thermal noise from the microelectrode's internal resistance is considered along with the white noises, e_{na} and i_{na}.

depending on the filling electrolyte and tip diameter. C_T is the sum of the equivalent, lumped, shunt capacitance across the electrode's glass tip (C_μ), plus the capacitance looking into the EOA's summing junction, C_{in}. C_T is on the order of single pFs. An electrometer op amp (EOA) is used to condition signals recorded intracellularly with a glass micropipette microelectrode is direct-coupled, has a low, noninverting gain between 2 and 5, and is characterized by its extremely high input impedance (ca. 10^{15} Ω), very low DC bias current (ca. 100 fA) and high e_{na}. The first two properties are necessary because the Thevenin source resistance of the microelectrode is so high, and for practical reasons, negligible DC bias current should flow through it to prevent ion drift at the tip. For all practical purposes, we can treat the EA as a noisy but otherwise ideal voltage amplifier. Capacitive neutralization is used to extend the high frequency bandwidth of the glass micropipette electrode-EOA system. Capacitance neutralization is accomplished by positive feedback applied though the variable capacitor, C_N.

The transfer functions for the bio-signal, V_b, and the amplifier noises, e_{na} and i_{na} will now be found.

Assume the EOA's DC gain is made to be +3. First, write the node equation for the noninverting v_1 node in terms of the Laplace variable, s:

$$V_1[G_\mu + sC_T + sC_N] - 3V_1 sC_N = V_b G_\mu \tag{9.96}$$

Equation 9.96 can be solved for V_1:

$$V_1 = \frac{V_b}{1 + sR_\mu(C_T - 2C_N)} \tag{9.97}$$

Hence,

$$V_o = \frac{+3V_b}{1 + sR_\mu(C_T - 2C_N)} \tag{9.98}$$

Note that in this simple case, when C_N is made $C_T/2$, the amplifier's time constant → 0, hence the break frequency $f_b = 1/2\pi\tau \to \infty$, and $V_o = 3V_b$.

Now consider the transfer function for the EOA's current noise, i_{na}:

$$V_1[G_\mu + s(C_T + C_N)] - 3V_1C_N = i_{na} \tag{9.99}$$

This node equation leads to the transfer impedance:

$$\frac{V_o}{i_{na}} = \frac{3R_\mu}{1 + sR_\mu(C_T - 2C_N)} \text{ Ohms} \tag{9.100}$$

Now find the transfer function for e_{na}. Again, one writes a node equation:

$$V_1'[G_\mu + s\,(C_T + C_N)] - 3V_1C_N = 0 \tag{9.101}$$

Note that when $V_i' = V_1 - e_{na}$ is substituted into Equation 9.101, one can solve for the transfer function:

$$\frac{V_o}{e_{na}} = \frac{3[1 + sR_\mu(C_T + C_N)]}{1 + sR_\mu(C_T - 2C_N)} \tag{9.102}$$

In summary, when $C_N = C_T/2$, the amplifier is neutralized, and the noise gains are

$$V_o = 3e_{n\mu}\ (e_{n\mu} \text{ is the thermal noise from } R_\mu)\text{RMSV}/\sqrt{\text{Hz}} \tag{9.103a}$$

$$V_o = 3R_\mu i_{na} \qquad \text{RMSV}/\sqrt{\text{Hz}} \tag{9.103b}$$

$$V_o = 3[1 + sR_\mu(3C_T/2)]e_{na} \qquad \text{RMSV}/\sqrt{\text{Hz}} \tag{9.103c}$$

The total MS noise output of the C-neut. amp is found by superposition of the three mean-squared noise components:

$$N_o = \{9(4kTR_\mu) + 9R_\mu^2 i_{na}^2\}B + \int_0^B 9e_{na}^2\,|1 + j2\pi fR_\mu(3C_T/2)|^2\,df \text{ MSV} \tag{9.104a}$$

$$\downarrow$$

$$N_o = \{(4kTRm) + R_\mu^2\, in_a^2 + e_{na}^2\}9B + 9\,e_{na}^2(B^3/3)\,[2\pi\,R_\mu(3C_T/2)^2] \text{ MSV} \tag{9.104b}$$

The fourth term in Equation 9.104B represents excess noise introduced by the positive feedback through the neutralizing capacitor. B is the Hz noise bandwidth of the unity-gain, ideal lowpass filter used to limit the output noise. For example, calculate the RMS output noise of the neutralized amplifier. The parameters are as follows: Amplifier gain = 3, e_{na} = 35 nV rms/√Hz (white), $i_{na} = 1.1 \times 10^{-16}$ A rms/√Hz (white), $R_\mu = 10^8\ \Omega$, C_T = 5 pF, $4kT = 1.656 \times 10^{-20}$, B = 5E3 Hz. When substituted into Equation 9.104b, one finds that $v_{on} = 2.915 \times 10^{-4}$ V rms, or about 0.3 mV RMS. The corner frequency for the output noise due to e_{na} under conditions of neutralization is

$$f_c = 1/[2\pi R_\mu(3C_T/2)] \quad \text{Hz} \tag{9.105}$$

Numerically, this is 212 Hz. Finally, the SNR_o of the neutralized amplifier can be written as

$$SNR_o = \frac{\overline{V_b^2}}{\{(4kTR_\mu) + R_\mu^2 i_{na}^2 + e_{na}^2\}B + e_{na}^2(B^3/3)[2\pi R_\mu(3C_T/2)]^2} \tag{9.106}$$

As a final example, find the RMS V_b required to give a MS $SNR_o = 9$. Substituting the numerical values from above, one finds $V_b = 8.75 \times 10^{-4}$ V rms.

9.8.5 Calculation of the Smallest Resolvable ΔR/R in a Wheatstone Bridge Determined by Noise

9.8.5.1 Introduction

One typically associates the Wheatstone bridge with the precision measurement of resistance. However, this simple, ubiquitous circuit is used as a output transducer in many biomedical measurement systems in which the quantity under measurement (QUM) causes a sensor to change resistance. Some examples of variable resistance sensors include: thermistors, platinum resistance thermometers (RTDs), photoconductors, strain gauges, hot-wire anemometers, and direct resistance change by mechanical motion (potentiometers). Bridges used with ΔR sensors generally have AC sources for increased sensitivity. The output of a balanced Wheatstone bridge under AC excitation can be shown to be double-sideband, suppressed-carrier (DSBSC) modulated AC (Northrop 1997). DSBSC operation allows enhanced detection sensitivity and noise reduction by bandpass filtering.

9.8.5.2 Bridge Sensitivity Calculations

Figure 9.19 illustrates a Wheatstone bridge whose output is conditioned by a noisy but otherwise ideal DA. The AC output of the bridge is then passed through a simple, quadratic bandpass filter to reduce noise, and then is demodulated by a phase-sensitive rectifier/low-pass filter to give an analog voltage proportional to the QUM causing the sensor's ΔR. The system appears complicated but, in reality, is exquisitely sensitive.

In the bridge, two arms are fixed with resistance R, and two vary with the QUM; one increasing (R + ΔR) and the other decreasing (R − ΔR), a situation often found in strain gauge systems used in blood pressure sensors. In the circuit, there are five sources of white noise; the amplifier's e_{na}, and the thermal noise from the four bridge resistors. Assume that the DA has ∞ CMRR. The voltage at the left-hand corner of the bridge is: $v_i' = v_s/2$. The voltage at the right-hand corner is: $v_l = (v_s/2)(1 + \Delta R/R)$. The voltage at the DA output is thus

$$v_o' = K_d(v_l - v_l') = K_d(v_s/2)(\Delta R/R) \tag{9.107}$$

$$v_s(t) = V_s \sin(2\pi f_s t) \tag{9.108}$$

v_o' passes through the BPF with unity gain, so the MS output due to ΔR/R is

$$\overline{v_{os}^2} = (v_s^2/2)(1/4)[K_d(\Delta R/R)]^2 \quad \text{MSV} \tag{9.109}$$

9.8.5.3 Bridge SNR_o

The noise power density spectrum at the DA output is found by superposition of PDSs:

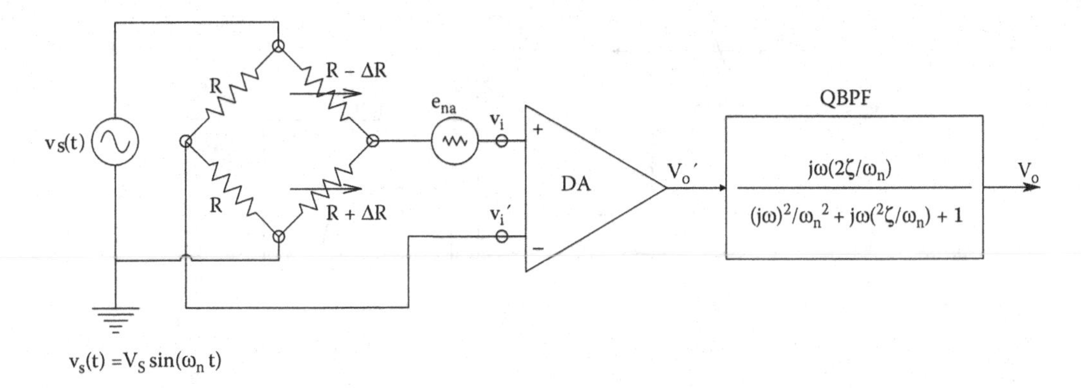

FIGURE 9.19 Schematic of a DA and BPF used to condition the AC output of a two-active arm Wheatstone bridge. The thermal noise from the bridge resistors is assumed white as is the DA's e_{na}. The quadratic BPF is used to limit the output noise far from ω_n.

$$S'_{no}(f) = [4kTR/2 + 4kTR/2 + e_{na}^2]\, K_d^2 \quad \text{MSV/Hz (white)} \tag{9.110}$$

The gain²-bandwith integral for the unity-gain, quadratic BPF with $Q = 1/2\xi$ has been shown to be $(2\pi fs/2Q)$ Hz. Thus, the MS noise at the filter output is

$$\overline{v_{on}^2} = [4kTR + e_{na}^2]\, K_d^2 (2\pi fs/2Q) \quad \text{MSV} \tag{9.111}$$

And the SNR_o is thus

$$SNR_o = \frac{(V_s^2/2)(1/4)[K_d(\Delta R/R)]^2}{[4kTR + e_{na}^2]\, K_d^2 (2\pi fs/2Q)} \tag{9.112}$$

Equation 9.112 can be used to find the numerical $\Delta R/R$ required to give a $SNR_o = 1$. Let $f_s = 1$ kHz, $4kT = 1.656 \times 10^{-20}$, $Q = 2$, $e_{na} = 10\ \text{nVrms}/\sqrt{\text{Hz}}$, $R = 400\ \Omega$, $K_d = 10^3$, and $V_s = 5$ Vpk. From these values, the minimum $\Delta R/R$ is found to be 2.315×10^{-7}, and $\Delta R = 0.2315$ mΩ. Also, the DA output is 0.579 mVpk.

For a blood pressure sensor, if the sensor's sensitivity and how many mmHg causes a given $\Delta R/R$ are known, it is easy to find the noise-limited ΔP from Equation 9.112.

9.8.6 Calculation of SNR Improvement Using a Lock-In Amplifier

A lock-in amplifier (LIA) is used to measure coherent signals, generally at audio frequencies, that are "buried in noise." More precisely, the input RMS signal-to-noise ratio is very low, often as low as −60 dB. There are two, basic architectures used for LIAs. One uses an analog multiplier for signal detection followed by a low-pass filter; this system is shown in Figure 9.20a. A second LIA architecture, shown in Figure 9.20b, uses a synchronous rectifier followed by a low-pass filter to measure the amplitude of a coherent signal of constant frequency, which is present in an overwhelming amount of noise. Assume the input to the LIA is

$$x(t) = n_i(t) + V_s \cos(\omega_o t) \tag{9.113}$$

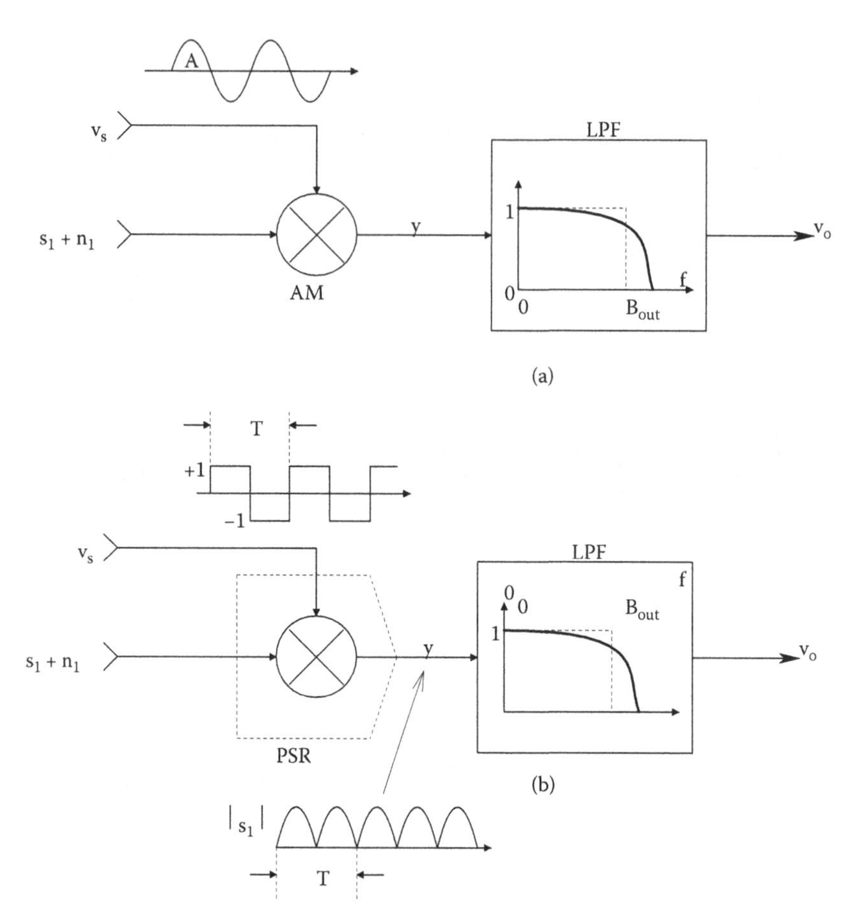

FIGURE 9.20 (a) Basic model for synchronous detection by a lock-in amplifier. A sinusoidal sync. signal is used with an ideal analog multiplier and a low-pass filter. (b) Lock-in operation when the sinusoidal signal to be detected, s_1, is effectively multiplied by a ± 1 sync signal with the same frequency and phase as s_1. Note that s_1 is effectively full-wave rectified by the multiplication, but n_1 is not.

Assume the noise is zero-mean, Gaussian white noise with one-sided power density spectrum, $S_n(f) = \eta$ ms V/Hz. The input MS SNR is

$$SNR_{in} = \frac{V_s^2/2}{\eta\, B_{in}} \tag{9.114}$$

where B_{in} is the Hz bandwidth over which the input noise is measured.

In the analog multiplier form of the LIA, x(t) is multiplied by an in-phase sync signal, $v_s(t) = A\cos(\omega_o t)$.

The multiplier output is thus

$$\begin{aligned} y &= v_s(n_i + s_i) = A\cos(\omega_o t)[n_i(t) + V_s\cos(\omega_o t)] = A\, n_i(t)\cos(\omega_o t) + A\, V_s\cos^2(\omega_o t) \\ y(t) &= A\, n_i(t)\cos(\omega_o t) + (AV_s/2)[1 + \cos(2\omega_o t)] \end{aligned} \tag{9.115}$$

Note that the one-sided power spectrum of the first term in Equation 9.115 is the noise PDS shifted up to be centered at $\omega = \omega_o$. Because $S_n(f)$ is white, shifting the center of $S_n(f)$ from 0 to $f_o = \omega_o/2\pi$

does not change the noise output of the LIA's output bandpass filter Thus the MS output noise voltage from the LIA is $v_{on}^2 = A^2 \eta(1/4\tau)$ msV, where $(1/4\tau)$ can be shown to be the equivalent Hz noise bandwidth of the simple output R-C low-pass filter, and τ is the output LPF's time constant. The output LPF removes the $2\omega_o$ frequency term in the right-hand term of Equation 9.115, *leaving a DC output proportional to the peak value of the sinusoidal signal.* Clearly, $v_{os} = AV_s/2$. Thus, the MS SNR at the LIA output is

$$SNR_{out} = \frac{A^2 V_s^2/4}{A^2\eta(1/4\tau)} = V_s^2(\tau/\eta) \tag{9.116}$$

The noise figure, F, is defined as the ratio of SNR_{in} to SNR_{out}. For an amplifier, F is desired to be as small as possible. In a noise-free amplifier (the limiting case), F = 1. It is easy to show that F for this kind of LIA is

$$F_{LIA} = B_{out}/B_{in} \tag{9.117}$$

where $B_{out} = 1/4\tau$ is the Hz noise bandwidth of the LIA's output LPF, and B_{in} is the Hz noise bandwidth over which the input noise is measured.

Since the LIA's desired output is a DC signal proportional to the peak sinusoidal input signal, B_{out} can often be made on the order of single Hz, and F_{LIA} can be $\ll 1$.

In the second model for LIA noise, consider the synchronous rectifier LIA architecture of Figure 9.20b. Now the sinusoidal signal is full-wave rectified by passing it through an absolute value function which models the synchronous rectifier. The full-wave rectified, sinusoidal input signal can be shown to have the Fourier series (Aseltine 1958):

$$y(t) = |v_s(t)| = V_s(2/\pi)[1 - (2/3)\cos(2\omega_o t) - (2/15)\cos(4\omega_o t) - \ldots] \tag{9.118}$$

Clearly, the average (or DC) value of y is $V_s(2/\pi)$.

Curiously, the zero-mean white noise *is not* conditioned by the absolute value function of the synchronous rectifier. This is because the synchronous rectifier is really created by effectively multiplying $x(t) = n_i(t) + V_s\cos(\omega_o t)$ by an even ± 1 square wave having the same frequency as, and in-phase with $V_s\cos(\omega_o t)$. This square wave can be represented by the Fourier series:

$$SQWV(t) = \sum_{n=1}^{\infty} a_n \cos(n\omega_o t) \tag{9.119}$$

where $\omega_o = 2\pi/T$, and

$$a_n = (2/T)\int_{-T/2}^{T/2} f(t)\cos(n\omega_o t)\,dt = (4/n\pi)\sin(n\pi/2) \quad \text{[nonzero for n odd]} \tag{9.120}$$

For a unit cosine (even) square wave can be written in expanded form:

$$SQWV(t) = (4/\pi)[\cos(\omega_o t) - (1/3)\cos(3\omega_o t) + (1/5)\cos(5\omega_o t) - (1/7)\cos(7\omega_o t) + \ldots] \tag{9.121}$$

The input Gaussian noise is multiplied by SQWV(t):

$$y_n(t) = n(t) \times (4/\pi)[\cos(\omega_o t) - (1/3)\cos(3\omega_o t) + (1/5)\cos(5\omega_o t) - (1/7)\cos(7\omega_o t) + \ldots] \tag{9.122}$$

The white, one-sided noise power density spectrum before passing through the LIA's output LPF can be shown to be

$$S_n(f) = \eta(4/\pi)^2[1-(1/3)+(1/5)-(1/7)+(1/9)-(1/11)+(1/13)-\ldots]^2 = \eta \text{ msV/Hz} \quad (9.123)$$

This white noise is conditioned by the output LPF, so the output MS SNR is

$$SNR_{out} = \frac{V_s^2(2/\pi)^2}{\eta\, B_{out}} \quad (9.124)$$

The MS SNR at the input to the LIA is

$$SNR_{in} = \frac{V_s^2/2}{\eta\, B_{in}} \quad (9.125)$$

Thus, the noise factor (F) for this LIA architecture is found to be

$$F = \frac{SNR_{in}}{SNR_{out}} = \frac{\pi}{2^3}\frac{B_{out}}{B_{in}} = 1.23\frac{B_{out}}{B_{in}} \quad (9.126)$$

which can be made quite small by adjusting the ratio of B_{out} to B_{in}.

As an example of signal recovery by an LIA, consider an LIA using the analog multiplier architecture. Let the signal to be measured be: $v_s(t) = 20 \times 10^{-9} \cos(2\pi\, 50 \times 10^3\, t)$. The Gaussian white noise present with the signal has a root power spectrum of $\sqrt{\eta} = 4$ nVrms/$\sqrt{\text{Hz}}$. The input amplifier has a voltage gain of $K_v = 10^4$ with a 100 kHz noise and signal bandwidth. Thus, the raw input MS SNR is

$$SNR_{inl} = \frac{(20\times10^{-9})^2/2}{(4\times10^{-9})^2\times10^5} = \frac{2\times10^{-16}\text{msV}}{1.6\times10^{-12}\text{msV}} = 1.25\times10^{-4}, \text{ or } -39 \text{ dB} \quad (9.127)$$

If the sinusoidal signal is conditioned by an (ideal) unity-gain LPF with a Q = 50 = center freq./bandwidth, the noise bandwidth B = 50 × 10³/50 = 1 kHz. The MS SNR at the output of the ideal BPF is still poor:

$$SNR_{filt} = \frac{2\times10^{-16}\text{msV}}{(4\times10^{-9})^2\times10^3} = 1.25\times10^{-2}, \text{ or } -19 \text{ dB} \quad (9.128)$$

Now the signal plus noise are amplified and passed directly into the LIA, and the LIA's output LPF has a noise bandwidth of 0.125 Hz. The output DC component of the signal is $K_vV_s/2$ V. Thus, the MS DC output signal is $\overline{v_{so}^2} = K_v^2V_s^2/4 = K_v^2\times1\times10^{-16}$ MSV. The MS noise output is $\overline{v_{no}^2} = K_v^2(4\times10^{-9})^2\times0.125$ msV. Thus, the MS $SNR_{out} = 50$, or + 17 dB.

The costs paid for using a LIA are that the AC signal is reduced to a proportional DC level, and the output LPF means that the LIA does not reach a new steady-state output, given a step change in V_s, until about three time constants of the LPF (about 3 s in the example above). The benefit of using a LIA is that coherent signals buried in up to 60 dB of noise generally can be measured.

9.8.7 Signal-to-Noise Ratio Improvement by Signal Averaging of Evoked Transient Signals

9.8.7.1 Introduction

The SNR of a periodic signal recorded with additive noise is an important figure of merit, which characterizes the expected resolution of the signal. SNRs are typically given at the input to a signal conditioning system and also at its output. A SNR can be expressed as a positive, real number, or in decibels (dB). The SNR can be calculated from the MS, the RMS, or peak signal voltage divided by the MS or RMS noise voltage in a defined noise bandwidth. If the MS SNR is computed, the $SNR_{(dB)} = 10\log_{10}(\text{MS SNR})$; otherwise, it is $SNR_{(dB)} = 20\log_{10}(\text{RMS SNR})$.

Signal averaging is widely used in both experimental and clinical electrophysiology in order to extract a repetitive, quasi-deterministic, electrophysiological transient response buried in broadband noise. One example of the type of signal being extracted is the evoked cortical response recorded directly from the surface of the brain (or from the scalp) by an electrode pair while the subject is given a repetitive, periodic, sensory stimulus, such as a tone burst, a flash of light, or a tachistoscopically presented picture. Every time the stimulus is given, a "hard-wired," electrophysiological transient voltage, $s_j(t)$, lasting several hundred milliseconds is produced in the brain by the massed activity of cortical (and deeper) neurons. When viewed directly on an oscilloscope or recorder, each evoked cortical response is generally invisible to the eye because of the accompanying noise from electrodes, amplifiers, and neural activity in the CNS.

Signal averaging is used to extract the small evoked potential, s(t), from the noise accompanying it. Signal averaging is also used to extract evoked cortical magnetic field transients recorded with SQUID sensors (Northrop 2002), and to extract *multifocal electroretinogram* (ERG) *signals* obtained when testing the competence of macular cones in the retina of the eye. A small spot of light illuminating only a few cones is repetitively flashed on the macular retina. ERG averaging is done over N flashes for a given spot position in order to extract the local ERG flash response, then the spot is moved to a new, known, position on the macula, and the process is repeated until a 2-D, macular, ERG response for one eye is mapped (Northrop 2002).

Signal averaging is *ensemble averaging*. Following each identical, periodic stimulus, the response can be written for the jth stimulus:

$$x_j(t) = s_j(t) + n_j(t), \quad 1 \le j \le N \tag{9.129}$$

where $s_j(t)$ is the jth evoked transient response, and $n_j(t)$ is the jth noise following the stimulus. t is the local time origin taken as 0 when the jth stimulus is given. The noise is assumed to be, in general, *nonstationary*, i.e., its statistics are affected by the stimulus. We assume that the noise has zero mean, however, regardless of time following any stimulus. That is, $E\{n(t)\} = 0$, $0 \le t < T_i$. T_i is the interstimulus interval, and $E\{n(t)\}$ denotes the probability operation of taking the expected value of the noise. Also, to be general, we assume that the evoked response varies from stimulus to stimulus. That is, $s_j(t)$ is not exactly the same as $s_{j+1}(t)$, etc.

We assume that each $x_j(t)$ is sampled and digitized beginning with each stimulus; the sampling period is T_s, and M samples are taken following each stimulus. Thus there are N sets of sampled $x_j(k)$, $0 \le k \le (M - 1)$, also, $(M - 1)T_s = T_D < T_i$. T_D is the total length of analog $x_j(t)$ digitized following each input stimulus (epoch length).

When the jth stimulus is given, the x(k)th value is summed in the kth data register with the preceding x(k) values. At the end of an experimental run, we have $[x_1(k) + x_2(k) + x_3(k) + \ldots + x_N(k)]$ in the kth data register. Figure 9.21 illustrates the organization of a signal averager. Early signal averagers were standalone, dedicated instruments. Modern signal averagers typically use a PC or laptop computer with a dual-channel, A/D interface to handle the trigger event that initiates sampling

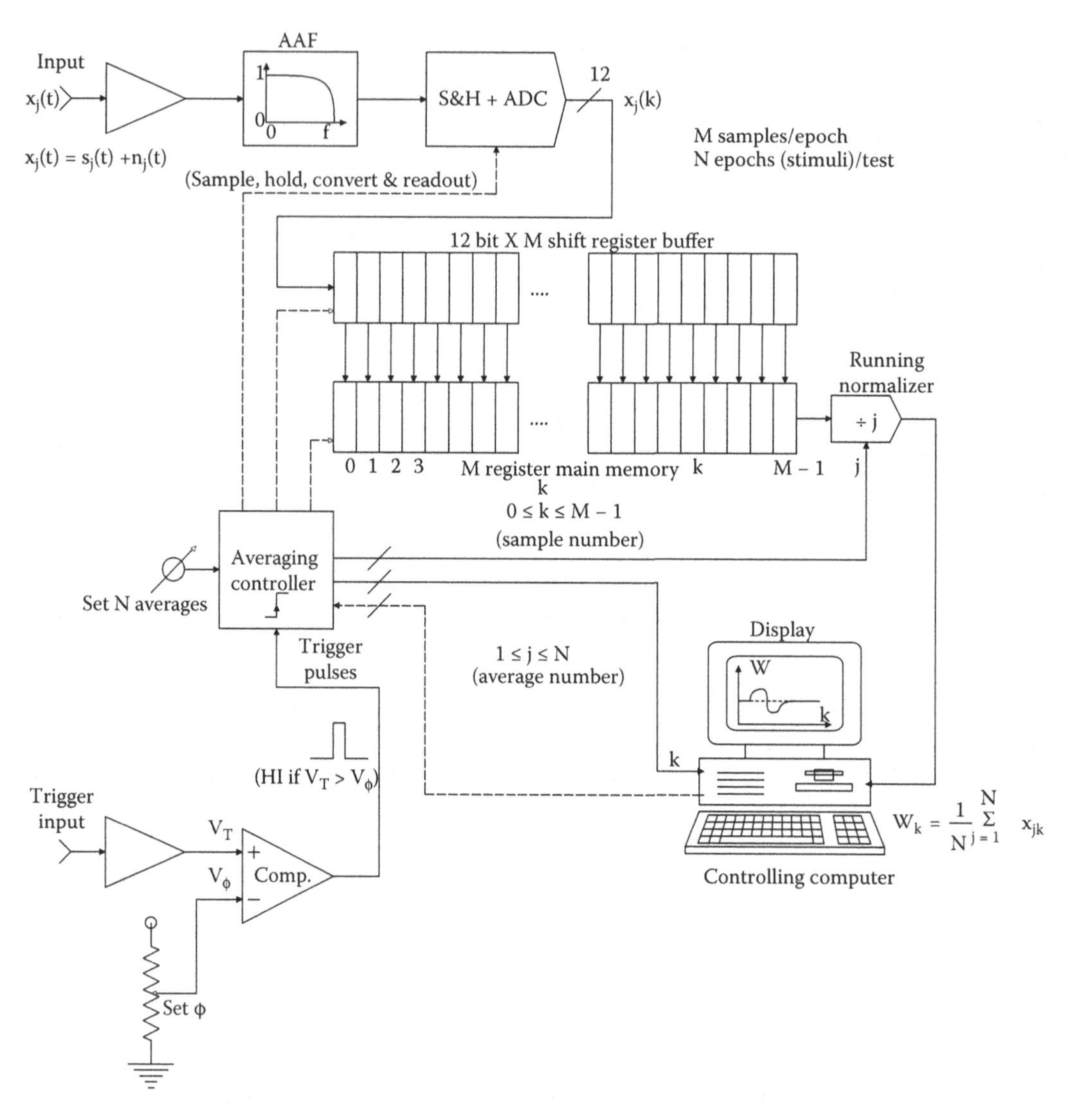

FIGURE 9.21 Block diagram of a signal averager. The memory and averaging controller are actually in the computer, and are drawn outside for clarity.

the evoked transient plus noise, $x_j(t) = s_j(t) + n_j(t)$. Modern averagers give a running display in which the main register contents are continually divided by the running j value as j goes from 1 to N.

9.8.7.2 Analysis of SNR Improvement by Averaging

The average contents of the kth register after N epochs are sampled can be written formally:

$$\overline{x(k)_N} = \frac{1}{N}\sum_{j=1}^{N} s_j(k) + \frac{1}{N}\sum_{j=1}^{N} n_j(k), \quad 0 \leq k \leq (M-1) \tag{9.130}$$

where the left-hand summation is the *signal sample mean* at $t = kT_s$ after N stimuli, and the right-hand summation is the *noise sample mean* at $t = kT_s$ after N stimuli. The *variance of the sample mean* was shown above to be a statistical measure of its noisiness. In general, the larger N is, the smaller the noise variance will be. The variance of the sample mean of x(k) is written as

$$\mathrm{Var}\{\bar{x}(k)_N\} = E\left\{\left[\frac{1}{N}\sum_{j=1}^{N} x_j(k)\right]^2\right\} - \langle x(k)\rangle^2$$

$$\downarrow$$

$$\mathrm{Var}\{\bar{x}(k)_N\} = E\left\{\frac{1}{N}\sum_{j=1}^{N} x_j(k)]\left[\frac{1}{N}\sum_{i=1}^{N} x_i(k)\right]\right\} - \langle x(k)\rangle^2$$

$$\downarrow$$

$$\mathrm{Var}\{\bar{x}(k)_N\} = \frac{1}{N^2}\sum_{j=1}^{N}\sum_{i=1}^{N} E\ \{x_j(k)\, x_i(k)\} - \langle x(k)\rangle^2$$

$$\downarrow$$

$$\mathrm{Var}\{\bar{x}(k)_N\} = \underset{(N\text{ terms, } j=i)}{\frac{1}{N^2}\sum_{j=1}^{N}} E\ \{x_j{}^2(k)\} + \underset{(N^2-N\text{ terms})}{\frac{1}{N^2}\sum_{j=1}^{N}\sum_{\substack{i=1\\ j\neq 1}}^{N}} E\{x_j(k)\, x_i(k)\} - \langle x(k)\rangle^2 \quad (9.131)$$

Now for the N squared terms,

$$\begin{aligned} E\{x_j^2(k)\} &= E\{[s_j(k) + n_j(k)]^2\} = E\{s_j^2(k)\} + 2E\{s_j(k)\}\ E\{n_j(k)\} + E\{n_j^2(k)\} \\ &= \sigma_s^2(k) + \langle s(k)\rangle^2 + \sigma_n^2(k) \end{aligned} \quad (9.132)$$

For the $(N^2 - N)$ terms with unlike indices,

$$\begin{aligned} E\{x_j(k)\, x_i(k)\} = E\{[s_j(k) + n_j(k)][s_i(k) + n_i(k)]\} = E\{s_j(k)\, s_i(k)\} \\ + E\{n_j(k)\ ni(k)\} + E\{s_j(k)\, n_i(k) + s_i(k) n_j(k)\} \end{aligned} \quad (9.133)$$

Several important assumptions are generally applied to Equation 9.133: First, noise and signal are uncorrelated and statistically independent. This means that $E\{s\, n\} = E\{s\}E\{n\} = E\{s\}\, 0 = 0$. Also, assume that noise samples taken at or more than $t = T$ seconds apart are uncorrelated; these assumptions lead to $E\{n_j(k)\ n_i(k)\} = E\{n_j(k)\}\ E\{n_i(k)\} \to 0$. So $E\{x_j(k)\, x_i(k)\} = E\{[s_j(k)\ s_i(k)\}$. Also assume that $s_j(k)$ and $s_i(k)$ taken at or more than T seconds apart are independent. Finally, the expected signal + noise squared is

$$E\{x_j(k)\, x_i(k)\} = E\{[s_j(k)\, s_i(k) = E\{s_j(k)\}\ E\{s_i(k)\} = \overline{s(k)}^2 \quad (9.134)$$

Putting all the terms together,

$$\text{Var}\{\overline{x}(k)_N\} = \frac{1}{N^2}\{N[\sigma_s^2(k) + \overline{s}(k)^2 + \sigma_n^2(k)] + (N^2 - N)\overline{s}(k)^2\} - \overline{s}(k)^2 \quad (9.135)$$

$$\downarrow$$

$$\text{Var}\{\overline{x}(k)_N\} = \frac{\sigma_s^2(k) + \sigma_n^2(k)}{N} \quad (9.135)$$

The variance of the sample mean for the kth sample following a stimulus is a measure of the noisiness of the averaging process. The variance of the averaged signal, x, is seen to decrease as 1/N, where N is the total number of stimuli given and of responses averaged.

Another measure of the effectiveness of signal averaging is the averager's *noise factor,*

$$F \equiv \frac{S_{in}/N_{in}}{S_o/N_o}$$

where S_{in} is the *mean-squared input signal* to the averaging process, N_{in} is the MS input noise, S_o is the *MS output signal*, and N_o is the MS output noise.

The noise factor is normally used as a figure of merit for amplifiers; amplifiers generally add noise to the input signal and noise, so the output signal-to-noise ratio is less than the input SNR, so for a nonideal amplifier, $F > 1$. For an ideal, noiseless amplifier, $F = 1$. The exception to this behavior is in signal averaging, where the averaging process generally produces an output SNR > the input SNR, making $F < 1$. Note that the MS *noise figure* of a signal conditioning system is defined as 10 × the logarithm of the MS noise factor:

$$NF \equiv 10 \log_{10}(F) \text{ dB} \quad (9.136)$$

From the calculations above on the averaging process,

$$S_{in}(k) = E\{s_j^2(k)\} = \sigma_s^2(k) + \overline{s}(k)^2 \quad (9.137)$$

$$N_{in}(k) = E\{n_j^2(k)\} = \sigma_n^2(k) \quad (9.138)$$

$$S_o(k) = E\{s_o^2(k)\} = \frac{\sigma_s^2(k)}{N} + \overline{s}(k)^2 \quad (9.139)$$

$$N_o(k) = \frac{\sigma_n^2(k) + \sigma_s^2(k)}{N} \quad (9.140)$$

These terms can be put together to calculate the noise factor of the averaging process:

$$F_K = \frac{[\sigma_s^2(k) + s(k)^2]\left[1 + \overline{\sigma_s^2(k)}/\sigma_n^2(k)\right]}{[\sigma_s^2(k) + N\,\overline{s}(k)^2]} \quad (9.141)$$

Note that if the evoked transient is exactly the same for each stimulus, $\sigma_s^2(k) \to 0$, and $F = 1/N$.

The reader should appreciate that this is an idealized situation; in practice, a constant level of noise, σ_a^2, is present on the output of the signal averager. This noise comes from the signal conditioning amplifiers, the quantization accompanying analog-to-digital conversion, and arithmetic round-off. The averager's MS output noise can thus be written as

$$N_o = \frac{\sigma_n^2(k) + \sigma_s^2(k)}{N} + \sigma_a^2 \text{ mean-squared volts} \quad (9.142)$$

And as before, the MS signal is

$$S_o(k) = \frac{\sigma_s^2(k)}{N} + \overline{s(k)}^2 \quad (9.143)$$

The averager's output MS SNR is just

$$SNR_o = \frac{\sigma_s^2(k) + N\,\overline{s(k)}^2}{\sigma_s^2(k) + \sigma_n^2(k) + N\,\sigma_a^2} \quad (9.144)$$

And if the evoked response is deterministic, $\sigma_s^2(k) \rightarrow 0$, and we have

$$SNR_o = \frac{N\,\overline{s(k)}^2}{\sigma_n^2(k) + N\,\sigma_a^2} \quad (9.145)$$

Note that if the number of stimuli and responses averaged, N becomes very large, then

$$SNR_o \rightarrow \frac{\overline{s(k)}^2}{\sigma_a^2} \quad (9.146)$$

and also in the limit,

$$F \rightarrow \frac{\sigma_a^2}{\sigma_n^2(k)} \quad (9.147)$$

Thus, signal averaging can recover a good estimate of s(k) even when $\sigma_n(k)$ is 60 dB larger than s(k).

From Equation 9.145, we can find the N required to give a specified SNR_o, given $\sigma_n^2(k)$, σ_a^2, and $\overline{s(k)}^2$.

9.8.7.3 Discussion

Signal averaging is widely used in biomedical research and diagnosis. A periodic stimulus (e.g., a noise, a flash, an electric shock, a pin prick, etc.) is given to a subject. The response is generally electrophysiological, i.e., an evoked cortical potential (ECP), an electrocochleogram (ECoG), or an electroretinogram (ERG), all richly contaminated with noise. By averaging, the noise is reduced (its sample mean tends to zero) as the number of averaging cycles, N, increases, while the signal remains the same. Hence, signal averaging increases the SNR in the averaged signal. However, it was shown that there are practical limits to the extent of SNR improvement.

9.9 SOME LOW-NOISE AMPLIFIERS

In Table 9.2, TYPE refers to whether the amplifier is an op amp (OA) or an instrumentation amplifier (IA), and whether it has a BJT or FET headstage. e_{na} is given in nV RMS/√Hz measured at 1 kHz, i_{na} is given either in picoamps (pA) or femtoamps (fA)RMS/√Hz measured at 1 kHz. Low Freq. V_n is the equivalent, peak-to-peak, short-circuit input noise measured over a standard 0.1 Hz to 10 Hz bandwidth. R_{in} is the input resistance, f_T is the unity gain bandwidth in MHz, unless followed by (–3), in which case it is the high frequency –3 dB frequency. A_{V0} for op amps is their open-loop, DC gain; the useful gain range is given for IAs. (Manufacturers: AD = Analog Devices, BB = Burr-Brown, MAX = Maxim, PMI = Precision Monolithics, LT = Linear Technologies).

9.10 ART OF LOW-NOISE SIGNAL CONDITIONING SYSTEM DESIGN

Consider the scenario where a physiological signal such as nerve action potentials (spikes) are to be recorded extracellularly from the brain with a metal micro-electrode embedded in the cortex. The signal has a peak amplitude, v_{spk}, generally in the 10s of μV. Assume that the input signal is accompanied by additive white noise and must be resolved above the total broadband noise at the preamplifier's input. It was shown previously that the MS input noise is

$$N_i = [e_{na}^2 + i_{na}^2 R_s^2 + 4kTR_s + e_{ns}^2]\, B \quad \text{MSV} \tag{9.148}$$

where e_{na} and i_{na} are white root noise spectra that are properties of the amplifier used, and e_{ns} is a white noise root power spectrum added to the recorded signal in the brain. We also assume that the thermal noise in the source resistance, R_s, is white, and B is the Hz bandwidth over which the signal and input noises are considered.

The first step in designing a low-noise signal conditioning system is to choose a low-noise headstage amplifier that also meets other design criteria for parameters such as bandwidth, slew rate, input DC offset voltage (V_{OS}) and bias current (I_B), and V_{OS} and I_B tempcos. Modern low-noise, IC amplifiers typically have e_{na}s < 6 nV/$\sqrt{\text{Hz}}$ in the white (flat spectral) region. Such amplifiers may use super-beta BJT headstages which unlike FET headstages have higher values of I_B and i_{na}, and a relatively lower R_{in}.

Because the noise performance of a multistage amplifier used for signal conditioning is set by the noise characteristics of the (input) headstage, we must give the low-noise headstage at least a gain of 5, preferably 10. Having done this, following amplifier stages need not be expensive low-noise types. Any resistance used in an input high-pass filter coupling the electrode to the headstage should be a low-noise, metal film type, not carbon composition.

Finally, a bandpass filter with noise bandwidth B should follow the amplifier stages. The filter's corner frequencies to pass nerve spikes and to exclude high- and low-frequency noise should be at 30 Hz and 3 kHz. The noise Hz BW, B, is generally close to but greater than the signal passband. For a simple, two-real-pole BPF with low break frequency at $f_{lo} = 1/(2\pi\tau_1)$ Hz and a high break frequency at $f_{hi} = 1/(2\pi\tau_2)$ Hz, the noise BW from Table 9.1 is

$$B = \frac{1}{4\tau_2(1 + \tau_2/\tau_1)}\ \text{Hz} \tag{9.149}$$

The *signal's* –3 dB Hz bandwidth is easily seen to be

$$\text{SBW} = \frac{(\tau_1 - \tau_2)}{2\pi\, \tau_1\, \tau_2}\ \text{Hz} \tag{9.150}$$

TABLE 9.2
A Partial Listing of Some Commercially Available, Low-Noise Op Amps and Instrumentation Amplifiers Having Low Noise Characteristics Suitable for Biomedical Signal Conditioning Applications

Amp. Model	Type	e_{na}	i_{na}	Low Freq V_n	R_{in}	f_T(MHz)	A_{V0}
AD8597	OA/BJT	1.1	2.4 pA/√Hz	76 nVppk	—	10	116 dB
AD743	OA/FET	3.2	6.9 fA/√Hz	0.38 μVppk	10^{10} Ω (DM) 3×10^{11} Ω (CM)	4.5	4×10^3
OP27 (PMI)	OA/BJT	3	0.4 pA/√Hz	0.08 μVppk	6 M	5	10^6
OP61AP (PMI)	OA/BJT	3.4	0.8 pA/√Hz	—	—	200	4×10^5
NE5532	OA/BJT	5.0	0.7 pA/√Hz	—	300kΩ	10	2.2×10^3
OPA111 (BB)	OA/FET	6	0.4 fA/√Hz	1.6 μVppk	10^{13} (DM) 10^{14} (CM)	2	125 dB
MAX410	OA/BJT	1.5	1.2 pA/√Hz	—	20kΩ (DM)	28	122 dB
LT1028	OA/BJT	0.85	1 pA/√Hz	35 nVppk	20M (DM) 300M (CM)	75	7×10^6
INA163 (BB)	IA/BJT	1.0	0.8 pA/√Hz	—	60 MΩ (DM) 60 MΩ (CM)	3.4 kHz	$1-10^3$
INA103 (BB)	IA/BJT	1.0	2.0 pA/√Hz	—	60 MΩ (DM) 60 MΩ (CM)	6	$1-10^2$
AD624	IA/BJT	4	60 pAppk (0.1 – 10 Hz)	—	1G‖10 pF (DM,CM)	25 MHz	$1-10^3$
MAX2641	UHF Amp	NF = 1.5 dB @ 2.45 GHz	—	50 Ω,	Rev. isol. = −24 dB,	—	13.5 dB @ 2.45 GHz
MAX2656	UHF Amp	NF = 1.9 dB @ 1.96 GHz	—	50 Ω,	Rev. isol, = −28 dB,	—	13.5 dB @ 1.96 GHz

For example, if $\tau_2 = 10^{-4}$ s and $\tau_1 = 10^{-2}$ s, then B = 2.475 × 10³ Hz for noise, and the signal BW is SBW = 1.576 × 10³ Hz.

In Section 9.4.3, the use of an input transformer to maximize the SNR at the output of the analog signal conditioning system was described. It may be worthwhile to consider transformer coupling of the source to the headstage if the Thevenin source resistance of the electrode, R_s, is less than 1/10th of $R_{sopt} = e_{na}/i_{na}$ Ω. Transformer coupling carries a price tag, however. Special, expensive, low-loss, low-noise transformers are used, generally having extensive magnetic shielding to prevent the pickup of unwanted, time-varying magnetic fields, such as from power lines, etc. The author has never heard of SNR_o-maximizing coupling transformers being used with metal microelectrodes. The R_s of a typical metal microelectrode with its tip platinized is on the order of 15 kΩ @ 1 kHz (Northrop and Guignon 1970). If an instrumentation amplifier such as the AD624 is used as the headstage, its $e_{na} = 4\ \text{nV}/\sqrt{\text{Hz}}$, its $i_{na} = 0.4\ \text{pA}/\sqrt{\text{Hz}}$, so its $R_{sopt} = e_{na}/i_{na} = 10^5$ Ω. If a transformer were to be used, its turns ratio to maximize SNR_o would be 2.58. Experience tells us that while SNR_o improvement would occur, it would be too small to justify the expense of the transformer. (It would be only 1.08 times the SNR of the amplifier with no transformer.) On the other hand, if the same amplifier were to be used with a transducer having R_s = 10 Ω, the transformer turns ration would be n_o = 100, and the improvement in SNR_o over an amplifier with no transformer would be

$$\begin{aligned}\rho &= \frac{4kTR_s + e_{na}^2 + i_{na}^2 R_s^2}{4kTR_s + 2e_{na} i_{na} R_s} \\ &= \frac{1.656\times10^{-19} + 16\times10^{-18} + 16\times10^{-26}\times100}{1.656\times10^{-19} + 2\times4\times10^{-9}\times4\times10^{-13}\times10} = 81.81\end{aligned} \tag{9.151}$$

Thus, the use of the transformer under the conditions above would lead to a significant improvement in the output MS SNR.

In Sections 9.7 and 9.8.2 above the effect on output noise of negative feedback applied around an amplifier through a resistive voltage divider was examined. A surprising result was found for a sinusoidal voltage source connected to a standard inverting, ideal op amp circuit with short-circuit equivalent input noise root power spectrum, e_{na} (i_{na} = 0 in this case), and noisy resistors. Namely, the amplifier's SNR_o increases monotonically with amplifier gain magnitude, R_F/R_1, to a best, asymptotic value of

$$SNR_{outmax} \cong \frac{(V_s^2/2)/B}{4kTR_1 + e_{na}^2} \tag{9.152}$$

Thus, the output MS SNR depends on both the absolute value of the input resistor and the amplifier's overall, closed-loop gain.

As a design example, examine the SNR_o for an op amp used in the noninverting mode. Although both op amp inputs are properly characterized with their own e_{na} and i_{na}, it is common practice to assume infinite CMRR and combine the noises as one net e_{na} and i_{na} at the amplifier's summing junction (inverting input node), as shown in Figure 9.22. Assume that the three resistors make thermal white noise. The signal is assumed to be sinusoidal. The MS output signal is

$$S_o = (V_s^2/2)(1 + R_F/R_1)^2 \text{ MSV} \tag{9.153}$$

The MS output noise has five independent components:

$$N_o = \left\{(4kTR_s + e_{na}^2)(1 + R_F/R_1)^2 + (i_{na}^2 + 4kTG_1 + 4kTG_F)G_F^2\right\} B \text{ MSV} \tag{9.154}$$

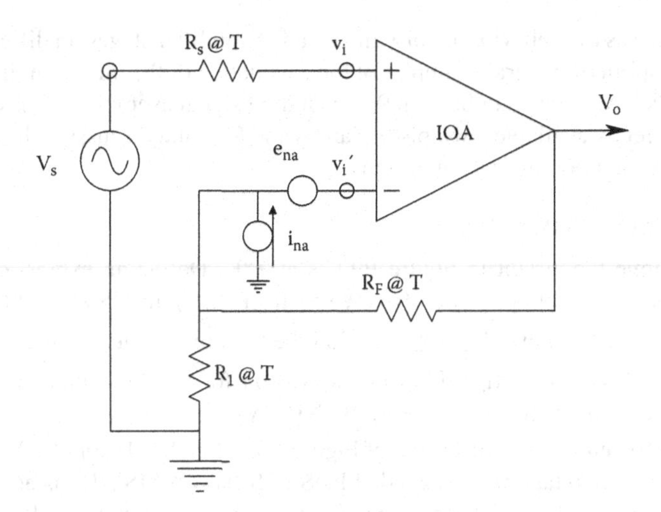

FIGURE 9.22 Noisy, noninverting op amp amplifier relevant to the design example in Section 9.10.

Now, the output MS SNR can be written as

$$SNR_o = \frac{(V_s^2/2)/B}{4kTR_s + e_{na}^2 + i_{na}^2(R_F \| R_1)^2 + 4kT(R_F \| R_1)} \tag{9.155}$$

where $(R_F||R_1) = R_F R_1/(R_F + R_1)$.

SNR_{out} is maximized by (1) choosing an op amp with low i_{na} and e_{na}, and (2) making $(R_F||R_1)$ small. The latter condition says nothing about the amplifier's voltage gain $(1 + R_F/R_1)$, only that $R_F R_1/(R_F + R_1)$ must be small. For example, for small-signal operation, let $R_1 = 100\ \Omega$, and $R_F = 99.9$ kΩ, for a gain of 10^3. R_F and R_1 should be low excess noise types, i.e., wire-wound or metal film.

Low-noise amplifier design also includes strategies to minimize the pickup of coherent interference. These strategies are not covered here; the interested reader can find descriptions of shielding, guarding, and ground loop elimination in Section 3.9 in Northrop (1990), Barnes (1987), and Ott (1976).

9.11 CHAPTER SUMMARY

In this chapter, the key mathematical ways of describing the random noise accompanying recorded signals, and also originating in resistors and amplifier, have been introduced. The concepts, properties, and significance of the probability density function, the auto- and cross-correlation functions, and their Fourier transforms, the auto- and cross-power density spectrums were examined.

Random noise was shown to arise in all resistors, the real parts of impedances or admittances, diodes, and active devices including BJTs, FETs, and IC amplifiers. It was stressed that to find the total noise from a circuit, one must add the mean squared noise voltages rather than the RMS noises; then the square root is taken to find the total RMS noise. The same superposition of mean squared noises can also be applied to noise power density spectra (PDS).

After showing that the output noise PDS from a linear system can be expressed as the product of the input power density spectrum and the magnitude squared of the system's frequency response function as shown in Equation 9.41 above, the concepts of noise factor (F), noise figure (NF), and signal-to-noise ratio (SNR) were introduced as figures of merit for low-noise amplifiers and signal conditioning systems. Clearly, it is desired to maximize the amplifier's output SNR, and minimize F and NF. Both broadband and spot noise factor were treated, as well as the use of an input transformer to minimize F and maximize the output SNR when the Thévènin source resistance is significantly lower than e_{na}/i_{na}.

Also considered was the behavior of noise in cascaded amplifier stages, in differential amplifiers, and in feedback amplifiers. Several examples of the calculation of the minimum input signal to get a specified output SNR were given in Section 9.8, including signal averaging. This chapter concluded by listing some currently available low-noise op amps and IAs, and discussing the general principles of low-noise signal conditioning system design.

CHAPTER 9 HOME PROBLEMS

9.1 (A) Assume the circuit in Figure P9.1 is at T°K. Derive an expression for the one-sided, noise voltage power density spectrum, $S_n(f)$, in MSV/Hz at the v_o node.

(B) Integrate $S_n(f)$ over $0 \leq f \leq \infty$ to find the total mean-squared noise voltage at v_o.

(C) Let $i_s(t) = I_s \sin(2\pi f_o t)$. Find an expression for the MS output voltage signal to noise ratio. Sketch and dimension SNR_{out} vs. C.

9.2 Repeat Problem 9.1 for the circuit of Figure P9.2. Let $f_o = 1/(2\pi\sqrt{LC})$

9.3 A white noise voltage with one-sided PDS of $S_n(f) = \eta$ MSV/Hz is added to the sinusoidal signal, $v_s(t) = V_s \sin(2\pi f_o t)$. Signal plus noise are conditioned by a simple low-pass filter with transfer function: $H(s) = 1/(\tau s + 1)$. See Figure P9.3.

(A) Find an expression for the mean-squared output signal voltage, $\overline{v_{os}^2}$.

(B) Find an expression for the mean-squared output noise voltage, $\overline{v_{on}^2}$.

(C) Find an expression for the optimum filter break frequency, $f_{opt} = 1/(2\pi\tau_{opt})$, that will maximize the mean-squared output signal-to-noise ratio. Give an expression for the MS optimum output SNR.

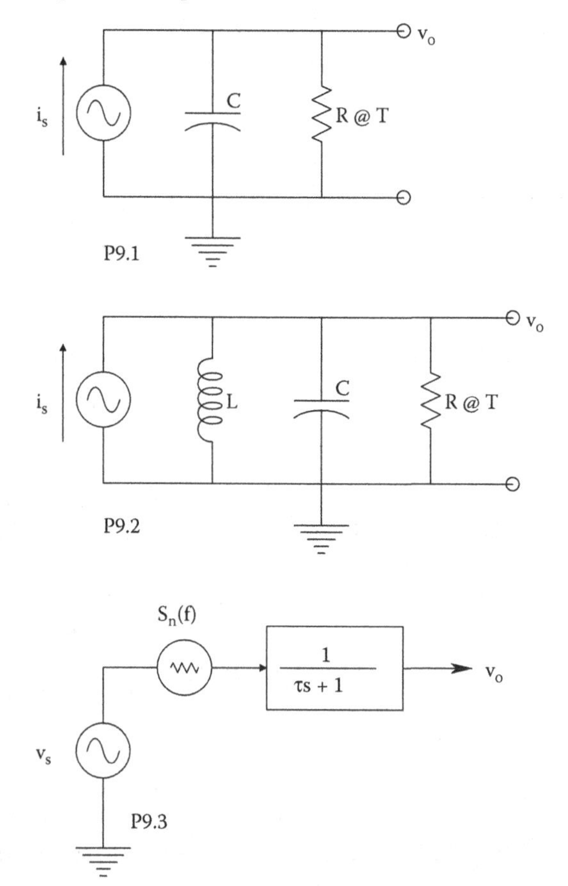

9.4 See Figure P9.4. A noisy but otherwise ideal op amp is used to condition a small AC current, $i_s(t) = I_s \sin(2\pi f_o t)$. It is followed by a noiseless, ideal bandpass filter with center frequency, f_o and Hz bandwidth B. Let $I_s = 10^{-11}$ A, $f_o = 10^4$ Hz, $4kT = 1.66 \times 10^{-20}$, $e_{na} = 100\ \text{nVrms}/\sqrt{\text{Hz}}$, $i_{na} = 1\ \text{pArms}/\sqrt{\text{Hz}}$. Assume all noise sources are white.

(A) Find an expression for and the numerical value of the ms output signal voltage.

(B) Find an expression for and the numerical value of the ms output noise voltage.

(C) Find B in Hz required to give an ms output SNR = 10.

9.5 A tuned (bandpass) video amplifier, shown in Figure P9.5, is used to condition a 900 kHz Doppler ultrasound signal to which various uncorrelated noise signals are added. The amplifier's peak gain is 10^4, and its noise bandwidth B is 10 kHz centered on 900 kHz. Let $e_{na} = 10$ nVRMS/$\sqrt{\text{Hz}}$ (white), $e_{ns} = 25$ nVRMS/$\sqrt{\text{Hz}}$ (white), $R_s = 1200\ \Omega$, $4kT = 1.66 \times 10^{-20}$, $v_s(t) = V_s \sin(2\pi 9.01 \times 10^5 t)$.

(A) Find the RMS output noise voltage.

(B) Find the peak signal voltage, Vs, to give an RMS SNRout = 10.

9.6 A noisy but otherwise ideal op amp is used to condition the signal from a silicon photoconductor (PC) light sensor as shown in Figure P9.6. Resistor R_c is used to compensate for the PC's dark current so that $V_{os} = 0$ in the dark. $i_{na} = 0.4$ pA RMS/$\sqrt{\text{Hz}}$ (white), $e_{na} = 3$ nV RMS/$\sqrt{\text{Hz}}$ (white), $R_c = 2.3 \times 10^5\ \Omega$, $R_F = 10^6\ \Omega$, & $4kT = 1.66 \times 10^{-20}$. The photoconductor can be modeled by a fixed, dark conductance, $G_D = 1/R_D$, in parallel with a light-sensitive conductance given by $G_P = I_P/V_C = P_L \times 742.27$ Siemens. P_L is the incident optical power in Watts, and the photoconductance parameter is computed from various physical constants (cf. Section 2.6.5). The amplifier is followed by a noiseless LPF with $\tau = 0.01$ s.

(A) Derive an expression for and calculate the numerical value of the RMS output noise voltage, v_{on}, in the dark. Assume all the resistors make thermal white noise and are at the same temperature. (Note that there are five uncorrelated noise sources in the dark.)

(B) Give an expression for the DC V_{os} as a function of I_P. What is the PC's dark current, I_D?

(C) What photon power in Watts, P_L, must be absorbed by the PC in order that the DC V_{os} be equal to three times the RMS noise voltage, v_{on}, found in part A).

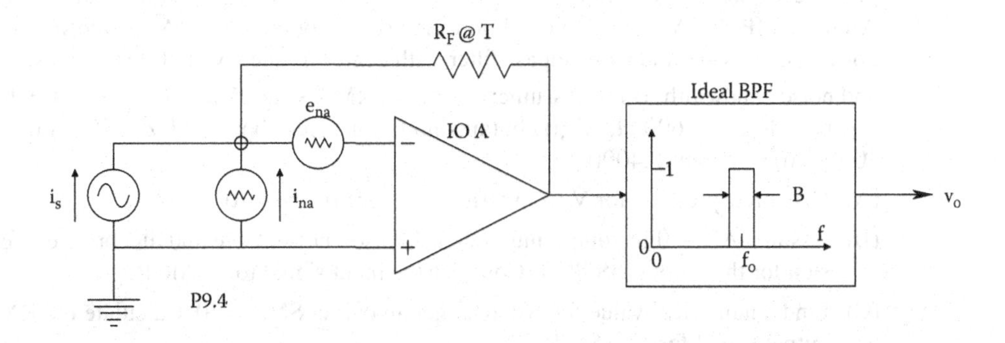

P9.4

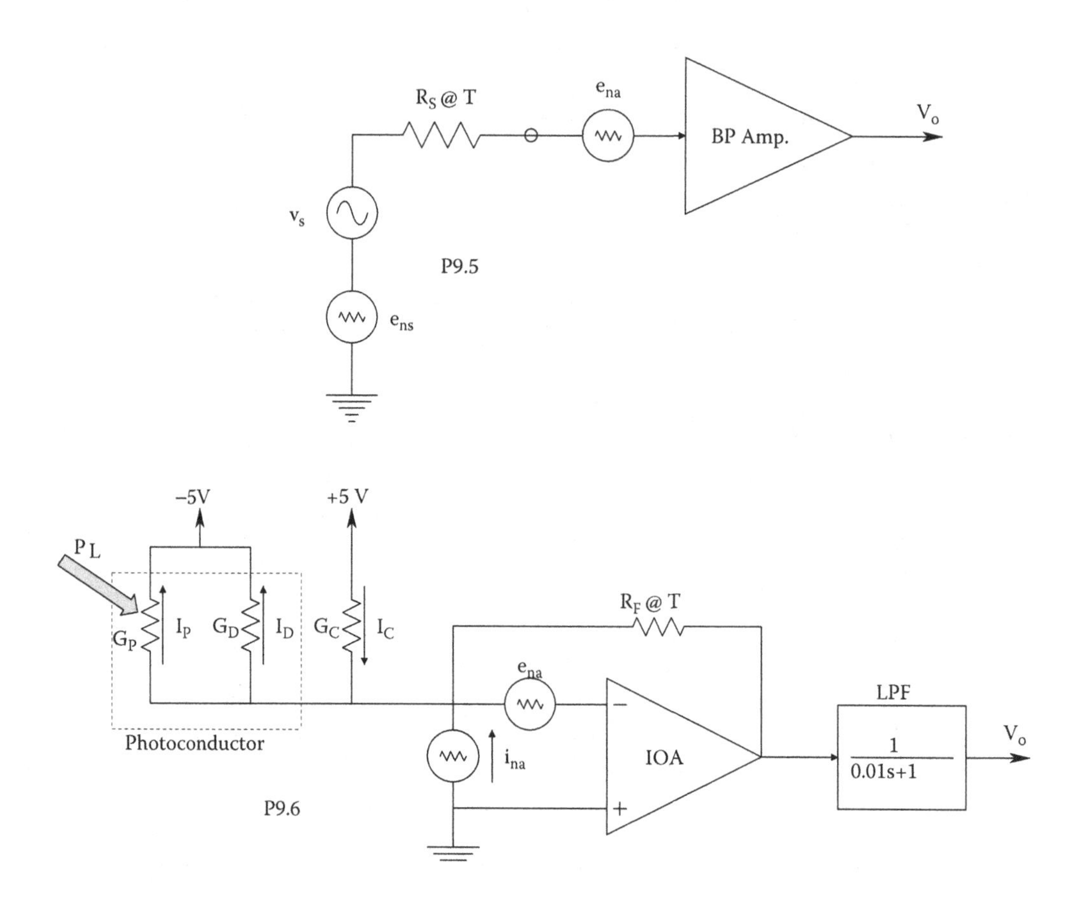

9.7 In an attempt to increase the output SNR of a signal conditioning system, the circuit architecture of Figure P9.7 is proposed. N low-noise preamplifiers, each with the same value of short-circuit input voltage noise, e_{na}, are connected as shown. The ideal op amp and resistors R and R/N are assumed to be noiseless. R_S, however, is at temperature T°K and makes Johnson noise. *Find* an expression for the MS output SNR.

9.8 A four-arm, unbonded strain gauge (Wheatstone) bridge is used in a physiological pressure sensor, shown in Figure P9.8. The bridge is excited by a 400 Hz AC signal. A PMI AMP-01 IA is used to condition the bridge's output. The IA is followed by a noiseless, unity-gain ideal bandpass filter with center frequency at 400 Hz, and signal and noise bandwidth, B Hz. Assume: $e_{na} = 5\ \text{nVRMS}/\sqrt{\text{Hz}}$, $V_B = 5$ V peak, B = 100 Hz, $K_v = 10^3$, R = 600 Ω, ΔR(t) contains no frequencies above 50 Hz. $4kT = 1.656 \times 10^{-20}$. $v_b(t) = V_B \sin(2\pi 400t)$.

(A) Give an expression for $V_u(t)$ in terms of R, ΔR(t), and $v_b(t)$.

(B) Assume ΔR ≡ 0 in computing system Johnson noise. Give and algebraic expression for the output MS SNR. Consider the input signal to be ΔR/R.

(C) Find a numerical value for ΔR/R to get an output SNR = 10. Calculate the RMS output signal for this ΔR/R.

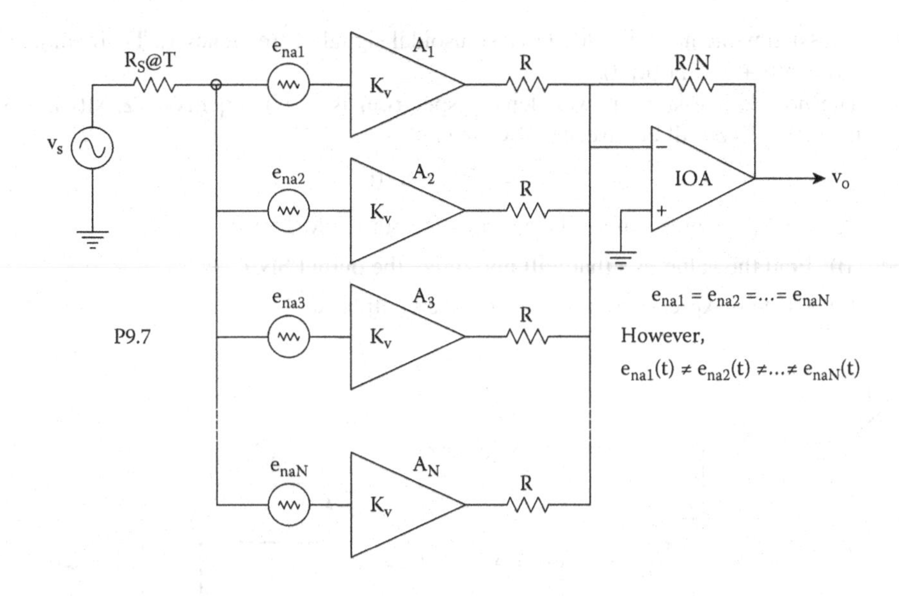

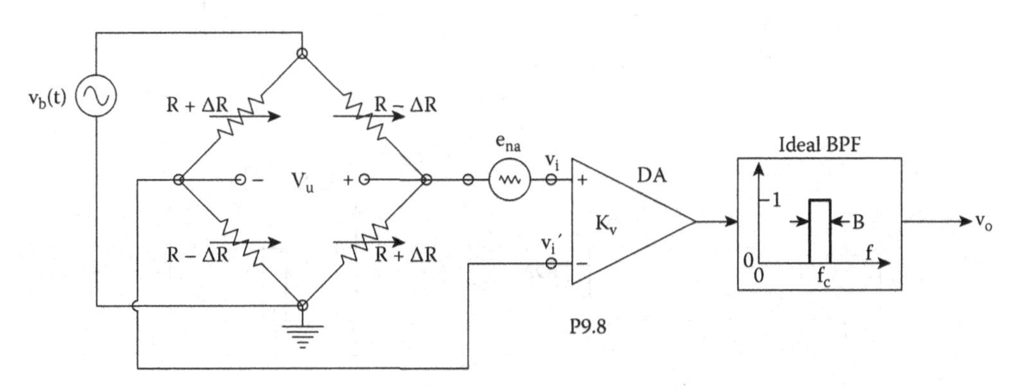

9.9 A PIN photodiode is used in the biased (fast) mode, as shown in Figure P9.9. The op amp used has $e_{na} = 3\ \text{nV}/\sqrt{\text{Hz}}$, $i_{na} = 0.4\ \text{pA}/\sqrt{\text{Hz}}$, $R_F = 1\ \text{M}\Omega$, $4kT = 1.656 \times 10^{-20}$. The PD is biased so that its dc dark current is $I_{DK} = 10$ nA, $[\eta q/(h\nu)] = 0.34210$ A/W @ 850 nm. Assume that the PD makes only shot noise MS current given by $i_{sh}^2 = 2q(I_{DK} + I_P)B$ mean square amperes. Let $B = 10^6$ Hz, $T = 300$ °K, and $I_{rs} = 0.1$ nA, and assume the biased PD presents an infinite dynamic resistance to e_{na}. Also, assume that all noises are white, and that the feedback resistor makes thermal noise.

(A) Derive an algebraic expression for the ms voltage SNR at the output of the amplifier.

(B) Find the input photon power, P_i, that will give a ms output voltage exactly equal to the total ms noise output voltage.

(C) Examine $\overline{v_{on}^2}$ numerically. Use the P_i value above. Which noise source in the circuit contributes the most to $\overline{v_{on}^2}$? The least ?

9.10 Gaussian white noise is added to a sinusoidal signal of frequency f_o. Their sum, x(t), is $x(t) = n(t) + V_s \sin(2\pi f_o t)$.
The noise's one-sided power density spectrum is: $S_n(f) = \eta$ msV/Hz. x(t) is passed through a linear filter described by the ODE:

$$\dot{v}_o = -av_o + Kx(t)$$

(A) Find an expression for the steady-state output, MS SNR.
(B) Find the value of a that will maximize the output SNR.
(C) Give an expression for the maximized output SNR.

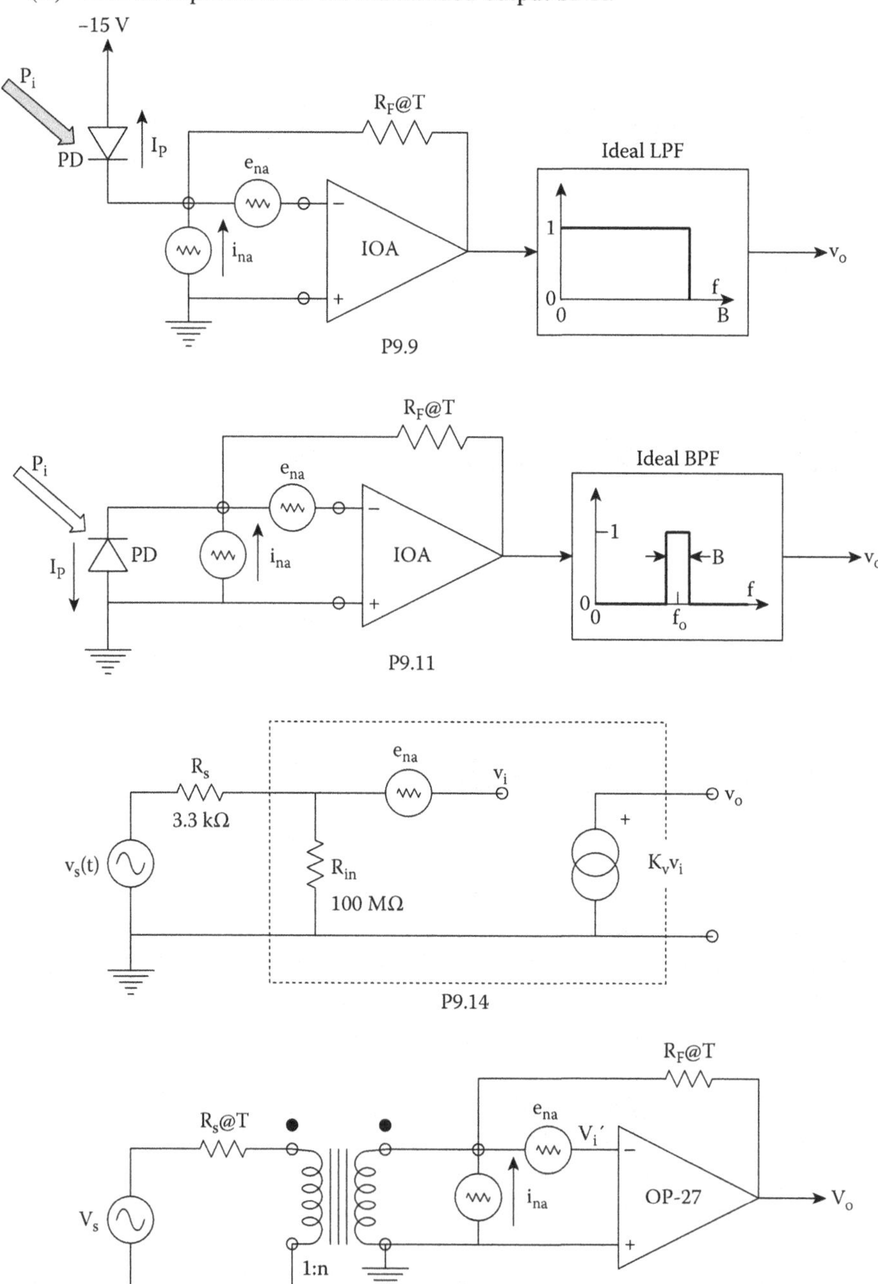

9.11 The current output of a PIN photodiode operating in the zero voltage mode is conditioned by an OP37 op amp (see Figure P9.11). The input signal is sinusoidally modulated light power at 640 nm wavelength: $P_i(t) = 0.5\ P_{pk}\ [1 + \sin(\omega_o t)]$. *Assume:* The PD's $I_{rs} = 0.1$ nA, $V_T = 0.0259$ V, the photocurrent $I_P = [\eta q/(h\nu)]\ P_i$ A, and the PD makes shot noise *and* white thermal noise currents with the one-sided power density spectrum: $S_{Dn}(f) = [2q\ I_{Pave} + 4kTg_d]$ MSA/Hz. g_d is the PD's small-signal conductance at zero bias, easily shown to be: $g_d = I_{rs}/V_T$, where $V_T \equiv kT/q$; q is the electron charge magnitude, T is the Kelvin temperature, and k is Boltzmann's constant (1.38×10^{-23} J/°K). The op amp has $e_{na} = 3\ \text{nV}/\sqrt{\text{Hz}}$ (white) and $i_{na} = 0.4\ \text{pA}/\sqrt{\text{Hz}}$. R_F makes thermal white noise. Use $4kT = 1.656 \times 10^{-20}$. The noise bandwidth is B = 1 kHz around $f_o = \omega_o/2\pi = 10$ kHz.

(A) Write an expression for the ms output voltage SNR.

(B) Find a numerical value for P_{pk} that will make the output MS SNR = 1.0.

(C) What P_{pk} will saturate v_o at 12.5 V?

9.12 Calculate the RMS thermal noise voltage from a 0.1 MΩ resistor at 300°K in a 100 to 10 kHz bandwidth. Boltzmann's constant is 1.38×10^{-23}.

9.13 A certain amplifier has an equivalent, short-circuit, white input noise root power spectrum, $e_{na} = 10\ \text{nVRMS}/\sqrt{\text{Hz}}$. What value equivalent series input resistor at 300°K will give the same noise spectrum?

9.14 An amplifier shown in Figure P9.14, has a 100 MΩ input resistance, $e_{na} = 12\ \text{nVRMS}/\sqrt{\text{Hz}}$, and a sinusoidal (Thevenin) source $v_s(t)$ in series with a 3.3 kΩ resistor. Both resistors are at 300°K. Amplifier bandwidth is 100 Hz to 20 kHz. Assume the resistors make white noise, and e_{na} is white. The sinusoidal source's frequency is 1 kHz, and the amplifier's gain is 10^3. Find the RMS value of $v_s(t)$ so that the output mean-squared SNR = 1.

9.15 An OP-27 low-noise op amp is connected to a Thevenin source [v_s, R_s @ T] through an *ideal, noiseless transformer* to maximize the ms output SNR. Consider the op amp ideal except for its noises. R_F makes thermal noise. See Figure P9.15.

(A) Give an expression for the mean-squared output signal voltage, $\overline{v_{os}^2}$. *Hint:* What is the Thevenin equivalent circuit looking back from the summing junction toward the transformer?

(B) Give an expression for the MS output noise, $\overline{v_{on}^2}$.

(C) Find a numerical value for the transformer's turns ratio, n_o, will maximize SNR_{out}. Let $4kT = 1.66 \times 10^{-20}$, $R_F = 10^5\ \Omega$, $e_{na} = 3\ \text{nVRMS}/\sqrt{\text{Hz}}$ (white), $i_{na} = 0.4\ \text{pARMS}/\sqrt{\text{Hz}}$ (white), $R_s = 50\ \Omega$, the noise bandwidth $B = 10^4$ Hz.

9.16 Signal averaging: A periodically evoked transient signal, which can be modeled by $s(t) = (V_{so}/2)[1 + \sin(2\pi t/T)]$ for $3T/4 \le t \le 7T/4$, 0 elsewhere, is added to Gaussian broad-band noise having zero mean and variance, σ_n^2. *Assume:* The averager is noiseless ($\sigma_a^2 = 0$), and the signal is deterministic, and so its variance, $\sigma_s^2 = 0$.

(A) Find an algebraic expression for the number of averages, N, required to get a specified MS $SNR_{out} > 1$ at the peak of the signal.

(B) Evaluate N numerically so that when $(V_{so}/2) = 1\ \mu$V, and $\sigma_n = 10\ \mu$Vrms, the MS SNR_{out} at peak s(t) will equal 10.

10 Digital Interfaces

10.1 INTRODUCTION

Digital interfaces enable the conversion of analog signals to a digital format that can be an input to a computer or a digital data storage system and, conversely, take digital data from a computer or digital storage system and convert it to an analog signal (voltage or current, thence to sound, light intensity, etc.). An *analog-to-digital converter* (ADC) performs the former task, whereas a *digital-to-analog converter* (DAC) does the latter operation. As will be seen, there are many types of ADCs and DACs.

The majority of ADC and DAC operations involve *sampling,* i.e., the periodic conversion of signals to digital or analog format. Because sampling occurs in the time domain, it can also be described in the frequency domain by an appropriate transformation. It will be shown that there are *two major sources of error in periodic data conversion:* The first involves a phenomenon known as *aliasing,* where an analog signal is effectively sampled at too low a rate for its bandwidth. The second has to do with the finite number of binary digits used to characterize an analog signal; the finite-size binary words produce *quantization error,* effectively introducing noise into the sampled signal. In Section 10.2, the problem of aliasing in sampled data is considered.

10.2 ALIASING AND THE SAMPLING THEOREM

10.2.1 Introduction

As illustrated in Figure 10.1, a modern biomedical instrumentation system generally includes a digital computer, which is used to supervise, coordinate, and control the measurements, and which often is used to condition data, store data (data logging), and to display it in a meaningful summary form on a monitor.

In describing signal conversion interfaces, it is expedient to first consider DACs because these systems are also used in the designs of several designs of ADCs. Data conversion from analog-to-digital form or digital-to-analog form is generally done periodically. Periodic data conversion has a great effect on the information content of the converted data, as is shown in Section 10.2.2.

10.2.2 Sampling Theorem

The *sampling theorem* describes the analog filter required to recover an analog signal, x(t), from its sampled (impulse-modulated) form, x*(t). The theorem states that if the highest frequency present in the continuous Fourier transform (CFT) of y(t) is f_{max}, then when x(t) is sampled at a rate $f_s = 2 f_{max}$, x(t) can be exactly recovered from x*(t) by passing x*(t) through an *ideal low-pass filter (LPF),* $\mathbf{H}_{IL}(j2\pi f)$. The weighting function (impulse response) of $\mathbf{H}_{IL}(j2\pi f)$ is (Proakis and Manolakis 1989):

$$h_{IL}(t) = \frac{\sin(2\pi f_{max} t)}{(2\pi f_{max} t)}, \quad -\infty \le t \le \infty \tag{10.1}$$

Thus, in the time domain, x(t) is given by the real convolution operation:

$$x(t) = x^*(t) \otimes h_{IL}(t) \tag{10.2}$$

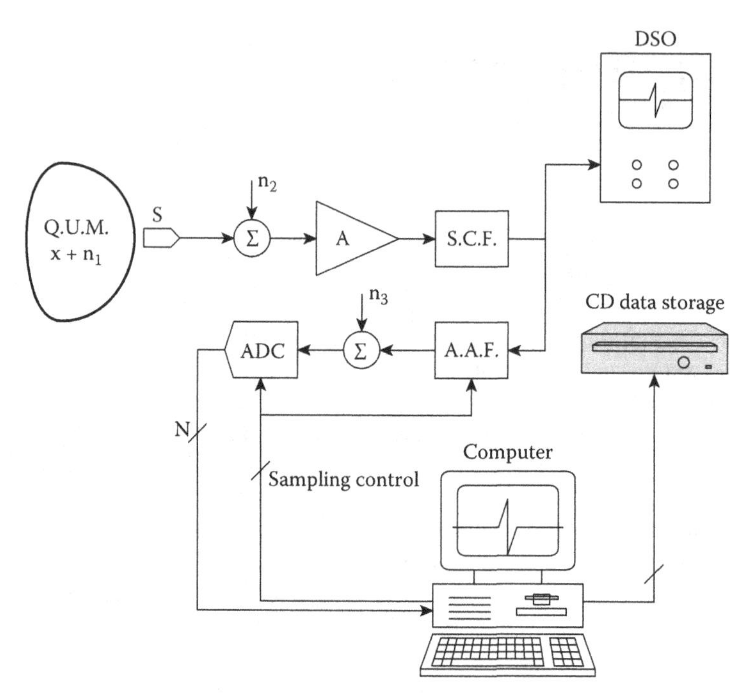

FIGURE 10.1 A typical instrumentation system. DSO = digital storage oscilloscope. ATR = analog tape recorder, SCF = signal conditioning filter (analog), AAF = antialiasing low-pass filter (analog), ADC = N-bit, analog-to-digital converter under computer control, QUM = noisy quantity under measurement.

The sampling rate, $f_s = 2 f_{max}$, *must be at least twice the highest frequency of the signal,* x(t). Note that many practical x(t)s can have spectra in which their RMS values approach zero asymptotically as $f \to \infty$. In this case, the Nyquist frequency can be chosen to be the value at which the RMS value of x(t) is some fraction of its max value, e.g., say $1/10^3$, or −60 dB.

Note that $\mathbf{H}_{IL}(j2\pi f)$ is an *ideal* LPF and is not physically realizable because $h_{IL}(t)$ exists for negative time. In practice, the sampling rate is made 3 to 5 times f_{max} to compensate for the finite attenuation characteristics of the real antialiasing, LPF, and for any "long tail" on the spectrum of x(t). Even so, some small degree of aliasing is often present in $\mathbf{X}^*(j2\pi f)$.

The *sampling theorem* is important because it establishes a criterion for the minimum sampling rate, which must be used to digitize a signal with a given low-pass, power density spectrum. The relation between the highest significant frequency component in the signal's power density spectrum and the sampling frequency is called the *Nyquist criterion*; the implications of the Nyquist criterion and aliasing are discussed later.

Because analog-to-digital data conversion is generally a periodic process, we will first analyze what happens when an analog signal, x(t), is periodically and ideally sampled. The ideal sampling process generates a data sequence from x(t) defined only and exactly at the sampling instants, when $t = nT_S$, where n is an integer ranging from $-\infty$ to $+\infty$, and T_S is the *sampling period.* It is easy to show that an ideal sampling process is mathematically equivalent to *impulse modulation,* as shown in Figure 10.2. Here, the continuous analog time signal x(t) is multiplied by an infinite train of unit impulses or delta functions that occur only at the sampling instants. This time-domain multiplication process produces a periodic number sequence, x*(t), at the sampler output. The numbers in the number sequence exist only at sampling times, $t = nT_s$. In the frequency domain, $\mathbf{X}^*(j\omega)$ is given by the *complex convolution* of $\mathbf{X}(j\omega)$ with the Fourier transform of the pulse train, $\mathbf{P}_T(j\omega)$. In the time domain, the pulse train can be written as

$$P_T(t) = \sum_{n=-\infty}^{\infty} \delta\,(t - nT_s) \tag{10.3}$$

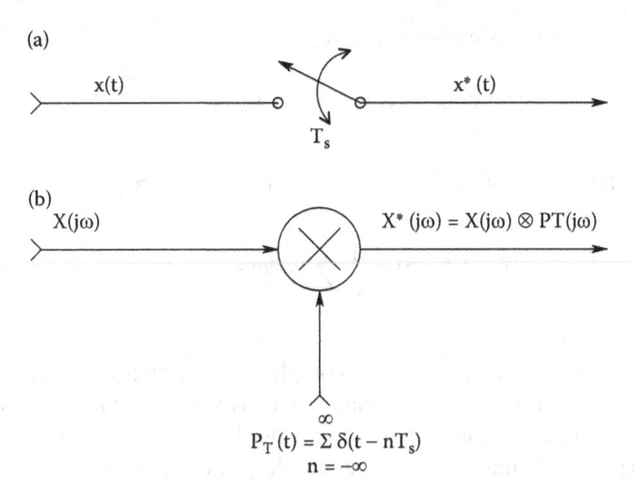

FIGURE 10.2 (a) A sampler equivalent of periodic analog-to-digital conversion. (b) An impulse modulator equivalent to a sampler.

The periodic impulse function, $P_T(t)$, can be represented in the time domain by a *Fourier Series* in a complex form:

$$P_T(t) = \sum_{n=-\infty}^{\infty} C_n \exp(+j\omega_s t) \tag{10.4}$$

where

$$\omega_s = \frac{2\pi}{T_s} \text{ r/s} \tag{10.5}$$

and the complex-form Fourier series coefficients are given by the well-known integral:

$$C_n = \frac{1}{T_s} \int_{-T_s/2}^{Ts/2} P_T(t) \exp(-j\omega_s t)\, dt = \frac{1}{T_s} \tag{10.6}$$

Thus, the complex Fourier series for the pulse train is found to be

$$P_T(t) = \frac{1}{T_S} \sum_{n=-\infty}^{\infty} \exp(+jn\omega_s t) \tag{10.7}$$

The sampler output in the time-domain is the product of $P_T(t)$ and x(t) (this is impulse modulation):

$$x^*(t) = x(t) \times \frac{1}{T_S} \sum_{n=-\infty}^{\infty} \exp(+jn\omega_s t)$$

$$= \frac{1}{T_S} \sum_{n=-\infty}^{\infty} x(t) \exp(+jn\omega_s t) \tag{10.8}$$

The Fourier theorem for complex exponentiation is

$$F\{y(t)\exp(+jat)\} \equiv Y(j\omega - ja) \tag{10.9}$$

Using this theorem, the Fourier transform for the sampler output, x*(t), can be simply written as

$$X^*(j\omega) = \frac{1}{T_S}\sum_{n=-\infty}^{\infty} x(j\omega - jn\omega_s) \tag{10.10}$$

Equation 10.10 for **X***(jω) is the result of the complex convolution of **X**(jω) and $\mathbf{P_T}$(jω); it is in the *Poisson sum form*, which helps us to visualize the effects of (ideal) sampling in the frequency domain and to understand the phenomenon of aliasing. In Figure 10.3a, we plot the magnitude of **X**(jω); note that **X**(jω) is assumed to have negligible power above the Nyquist frequency, $\omega_s/2$. When x(t) is sampled, we see a periodic spectrum for **X***(jω).

Note that x(t) can be recovered from the sampler output by passing x*(t) through an ideal LPF, as shown in Figure 10.3a. In Figure 10.3b, it was assumed that the base-band spectrum of x(t) extends beyond $\omega_s/2$. When such an x(t) is sampled, the resultant **X***(jω) is also periodic, but the high-frequency corners of the component spectra overlap. An ideal LPF thus cannot uniquely recover the base-band spectrum, hence x(t). This condition of overlapping spectral components in **X***(jω) illustrates *aliasing*, which can lead to serious errors in subsequent digital signal processing.

Because of the problem of aliasing, all properly designed analog-to-digital conversion systems used in FFT spectrum analyzers, time-frequency analyzers, and related equipment must operate on input signals that obey the *Nyquist criterion,* i.e., the power density spectrum of x(t), $S_{xx}(f)$, must have no significant power at frequencies above one-half the sampling frequency. One way to ensure that this criterion is met is to use a properly designed, analog low-pass, *antialiasing filter* immediately preceding the sampler.

Antialiasing filters are generally high-order, linear phase, LPFs that attenuate the input signal at least by 40 dB at the Nyquist frequency. Many designs are possible for high-order antialiasing filters. For example, Chebychev filters maximize the attenuation cutoff rate at the cost of some pass-band ripple. Chebychev filters can achieve a given attenuation cutoff slope with a lower order (fewer poles) than other filter designs. It should be noted that in the limit as passband ripple approaches zero, the Chebychev design approaches the Butterworth form of the same order, which has no ripple

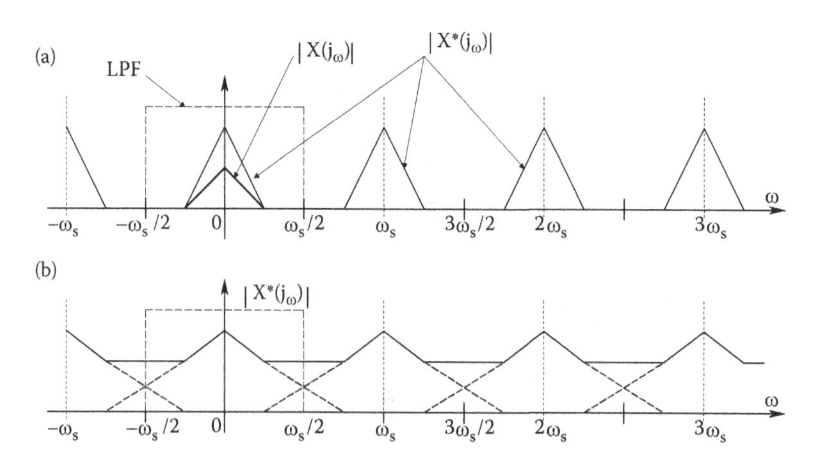

FIGURE 10.3 (a) The spectrum of a signal, and spectrum of an ideally-sampled signal which is not aliased. (b) Spectrum of an aliased, sampled signal.

in the passband. Chebychev filters are designed in terms of their order, n, their cutoff frequency, and the maximum allowable peak-to-peak ripple (in decibels) of their passband.

If ripples in the frequency response stopband of antialiasing filter are permissible, then elliptical or Cauer filter designs may be considered. With stopband ripple allowed, even sharper attenuation in the transition band than obtainable with Chebychev filters of a given order can be obtained. Elliptic LPFs are specified in terms of their order, their cutoff frequency, the maximum peak-to-peak passband ripple, and their minimum stopband attenuation.

Bessel or Thomson filters are designed to have linear phase in the passband. They generally have a "cleaner" transient response, i.e., less ringing and overshoot at their outputs, given transient inputs.

One problem in the design of analog antialiasing filters to be used with instruments having several different sampling rates is adjusting the filters to several different Nyquist frequencies. One way of handling this problem is to have a fixed filter for each separate sampling frequency. Another way is to make the filters easily tunable, either by digital or analog voltage means. Some approaches to the tunable filter problem are discussed in Section 7.3 of this text and in Chapter 10 of the text by Northrop (1990).

Antialiasing LPFs are generally not used at the inputs of digital oscilloscopes, because one can generally see directly on the display if the sampled waveform is sampled too slowly for resolution. An optional analog LPF is often used to cut high-frequency interference on digital oscilloscope inputs; this, however, is not an antialiasing filter.

10.3 DIGITAL-TO-ANALOG CONVERTERS

10.3.1 Introduction

A *digital-to-analog converter* accepts as inputs an N-bit digital word (0s and 1s) representing a numerical value of an analog output signal and a convert enable (CE) command. A DAC's output is a voltage or current determined by the digital word input. The output is *held* until the next word is presented (either as parallel or serial data) and the next CE command is given.

DACs (voltage or current output) are used in many applications, which include but are not limited to high-fidelity sound systems; analog CRT display systems used in computers and TV; generation of analog signals used in test and measurement systems, motion control systems, waveform synthesis, etc.

10.3.2 DAC Designs

DACs can be classified by whether they use bipolar junction transistor switches, or MOS transistor technology. The following DAC architectures are found with MOS technology:

- Binary-weighted resistor DAC
- R-2R ladder
- Inverted R-2R ladder
- Inherent monolithic ladder
- Switched-capacitor DAC.

The following DAC designs use BJT technology:

- Binary-weighted current sources
- R-2R Ladder using current sources.

Figure 10.4 illustrates four common DAC architectures. Figure 10.4a shows the *binary weighted resistor DAC.* This is an impractical design for IC fabrication; one needs accurate resistor ratios over a wide range of resistor values. Also, the op amp is presented with varying input impedances,

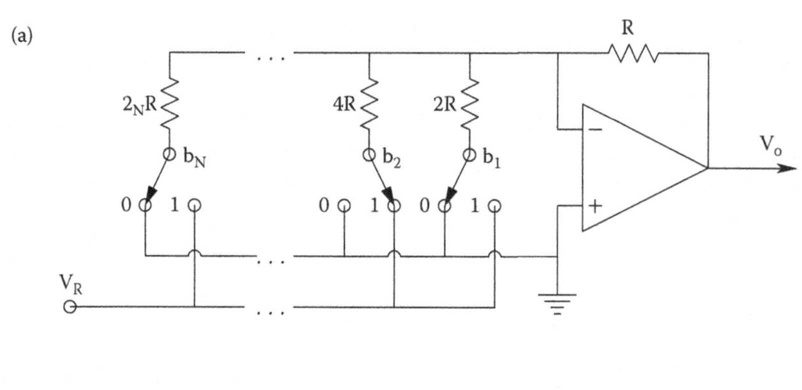

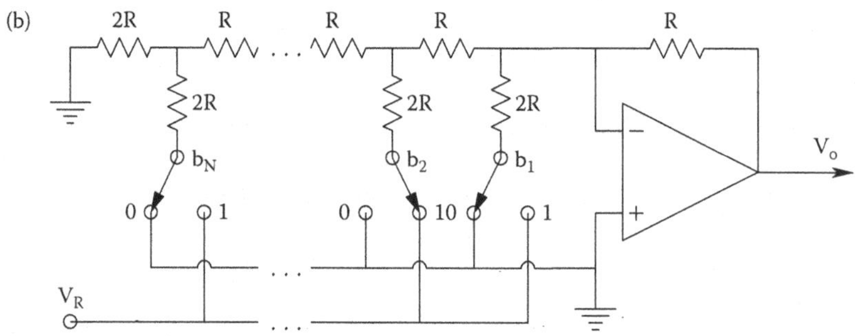

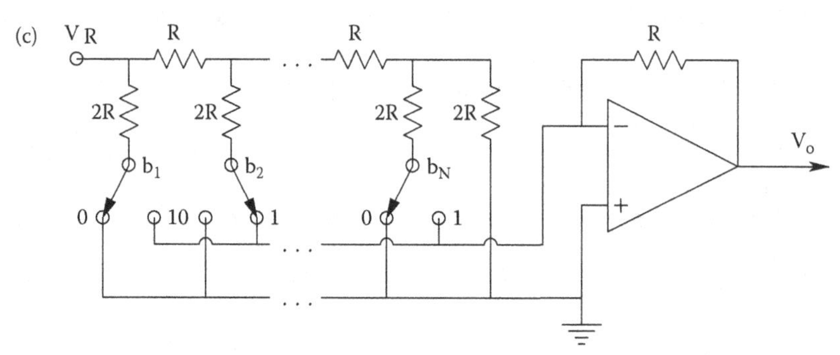

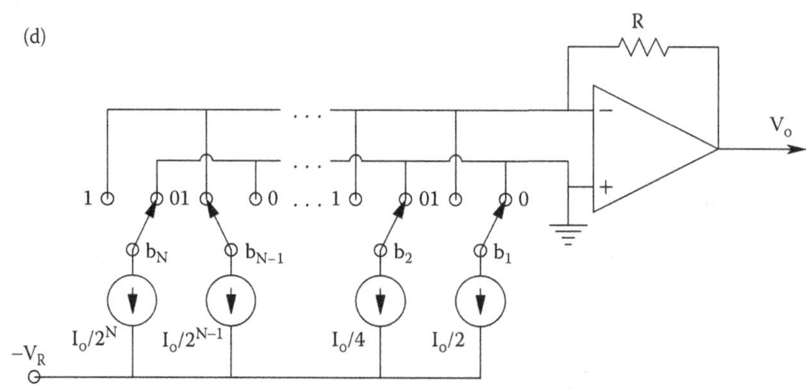

FIGURE 10.4 Four kinds of DAC circuits using op amps: (a) A binary-weighted resistor DAC (not practical for $N > 8$). (b) The R-2R ladder DAC. (c) The inverted R-2R ladder DAC. (d) A binary-weighted current source DAC (not practical for $N > 8$).

depending on the input word, making the DAC subject to op amp DC bias current errors. The SPDT switches used in this design are generally MOS transistors which are designed to have very low ON resistance, and high OFF resistance. The output voltage of this DAC is given by

$$V_o = \frac{-V_R}{2^N} \sum_{k=1}^{N} b_k 2^k \tag{10.11}$$

where N is the bit length of the binary "word" being converted, and b_k is either "0" or "1," depending on the word.

The circuit design of the popular R-2R ladder DAC is illustrated in Figure 10.4b. Here, only two resistor values are used; their exact values are not critical; however, the ratio must be *exactly* 2 between *all* 2R and R valued resistors. Switches with low ON resistance and zero offset voltage are required. The output can be shown to be

$$V_o = \frac{-V_R}{2^{N+1}} \sum_{k=1}^{N} b_k 2^k \tag{10.12}$$

Full-scale output voltage occurs when all the switches are set to V_R. This is

$$V_{oFS} = -V_R(1 - 2^{-N}) \tag{10.13}$$

The inverted R-2R DAC architecture is shown in Figure 10.4c. This is a relatively switching glitch-free DAC, well suited for CMOS switches. Note that the ladder resistors' currents are constant, independent of the switch positions because the op amp's summing junction is at virtual ground. Bit b_1 is the most significant bit (MSB). With $b_1 = 1$ and all others = 0, $V_o = -V_R/2$.

Figure 10.4d illustrates the overall architecture of the *binary-weighted current source DAC*. This circuit is easily implemented with BJT current sources and switches. There are a number of approaches of realizing the switches and current sources for this type of DAC (Franco 1988). The output voltage of this DAC is given by

$$V_o = (I_o R) \sum_{k=1}^{N} b_k 2^{-k} \tag{10.14}$$

When the MSB is HI ($b_1 = 1$), and all other $b_k = 0$, $V_o = I_o R/2$, and when the LSB is HI ($b_N = 1$) and all other $b_k = 0$, then $V_o = I_o R/2^N$.

Figure 10.5 illustrates a simplified schematic of a low-power DAC using *switched, weighted capacitors* (SWC). The MSB output of the SWC DAC can be found by observing that when $b_1 \rightarrow 1$, all other $b_k = 0$, the charge in C_1 is also the charge in C_F. Also, the summing junction is assumed to be at virtual ground. Thus, the charge in C_1 can be written as

$$Q_1 = 2^{N-1} C V_R = Q_F = V_o 2^N C \tag{10.15}$$

$$\downarrow$$

$$V_o = V_R/2 \tag{10.16}$$

The LSB output of the SWC DAC is found the same way by assuming $b_N \rightarrow 1$, all other $b_k = 0$.

$$Q_N = V_R 2^0 C = Q_F = V_o 2^N C \tag{10.17}$$

$$\downarrow$$

$$V_o = \frac{V_R}{2^{N-1}} \tag{10.18}$$

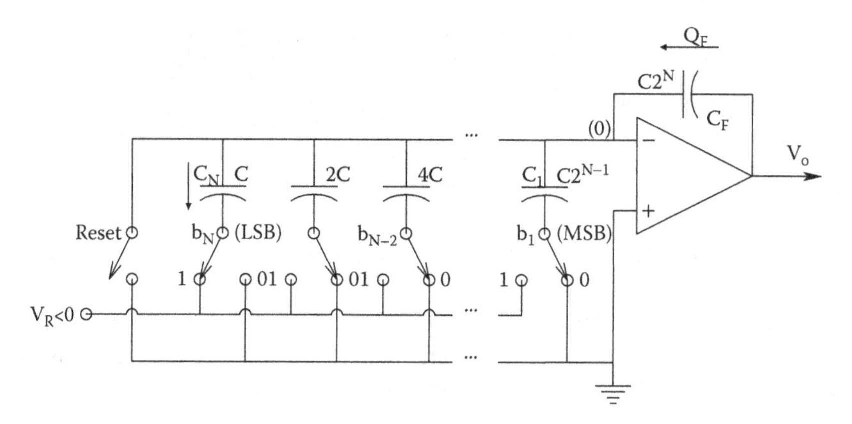

FIGURE 10.5 A switched, weighted capacitor DAC (not practical for N > 8).

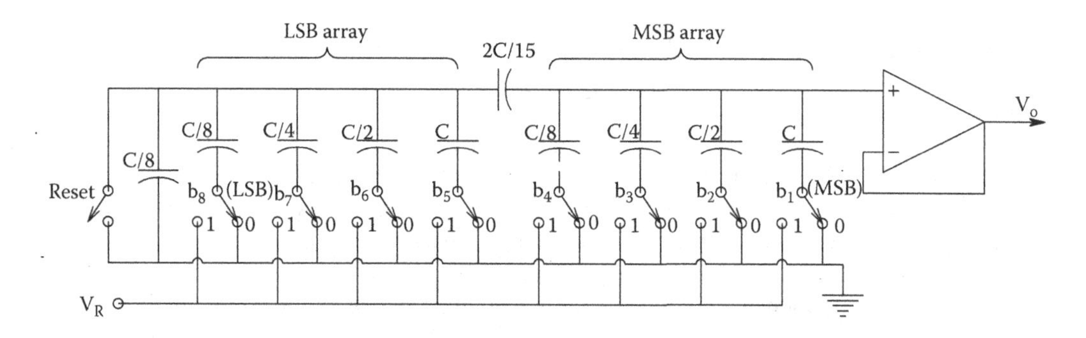

FIGURE 10.6 A charge scaling, switched-capacitor DAC.

Thus, the general output can be written as

$$V_o = \frac{V_R C}{2^N} \sum_{k=1}^{N} b_k 2^{k-1} \tag{10.19}$$

Two practical problems emerge in considering the SWC DAC: (1) C_1 must have 2^{N-1} times the area of C_N on the substrate. This limits N practically to 8. (2) The op amp must have a MOS transistor front end to obtain ultralow bias current so V_o will not significantly drift over a sampling period.

Figure 10.6 illustrates a design strategy that enables the use of a 1:8 capacitor area ratio, rather than a 1:128 area ratio required for the 8-bit DAC shown in Figure 10.5. The MSB output is found from the capacitive voltage divider made from the input array. The input capacitor is $C_1 = C$. It can be shown that the series-parallel combination of the rest of the capacitors having $b_k = 0$ so they are grounded is C. Thus, $V_{o\,(MSB)}$ is simply $V_R/2$. The LSB output is found the same way by considering the capacitor voltage divider and can be shown to be $V_{o\,(LSB)} = V_R/256$. The complete charge-scaling DAC output is given by

$$V_o = V_R \sum_{k=1}^{N} b_k 2^{-k} \tag{10.20}$$

Multiplying DACs (MDACs) are a special class of DAC in which the reference signal is made variable and the DAC output is the product of the analog value of $v_R(t)$ and the digital scaling input. Thus, 2-quadrant multiplication can be realized for a *straight unipolar binary* input:

$$v_o(t) = v_R(t)\left[2^{-N}\sum_{k=1}^{N} 2^k\right] \tag{10.21}$$

If the DAC is set up for *bipolar offset binary* (BOB) operation, one has true, 4-quadrant multiplication. The output of a DAC configured for BOB, such as the AD7845, 12-bit MDAC, is given by

$$v_o(t) = v_R(t)\left[-1 + \frac{1}{2^{N-1}}\sum_{k=1}^{N} b_k 2^{k-1}\right] \tag{10.22}$$

For N = 12,

$$\{b_k\} = 1111\ 1111\ 1111,\ V_o = +v_R(t)\frac{2047}{2048} \tag{10.23a}$$

$$\{b_k\} = 1000\ 0000\ 0001,\ V_o = +v_R(t)\frac{1}{2048} \tag{10.23b}$$

$$\{b_k\} = 1000\ 0000\ 0000,\ V_o = v_R(t)\frac{0}{2048} = 0 \tag{10.23c}$$

$$\{b_k\} = 0111\ 1111\ 1111,\ V_o = -v_R(t)\frac{1}{2048} \tag{10.23d}$$

$$\{b_k\} = 0000\ 0000\ 0000,\ V_o = -v_R(t)\frac{2048}{2048} = -v_R(t) \tag{10.23}$$

MDACs find application in waveform generation, digitally controlled attenuators, digitally controlled filters, programmable power supplies, programmable gain amplifiers, and self-nulling systems. The unity gain, small-signal bandwidth (f_T) of the AD7845 is 600 kHz, and its full-power bandwidth is 250 kHz.

10.3.3 Static and Dynamic Characteristics of DACs

Figure 10.7 illustrates the input/output characteristic of an ideal, binary, N = 3-bit DAC (in practice the smallest N you will find is typically 8 bits). Note that the analog output has ½ LSB of output added to it to minimize conversion error. In general, the LSB and full-scale output of the 3-bit binary input DAC is given by

$$\text{LSB} = V_R/2^N \tag{10.24}$$

$$V_{oFS} = V_R - \text{LSB}/2 = V_R[1 - 2^{-(N+1)}] \tag{10.25}$$

For the N = 3 DAC, $V_{oFS} = V_R \times 0.9375$.

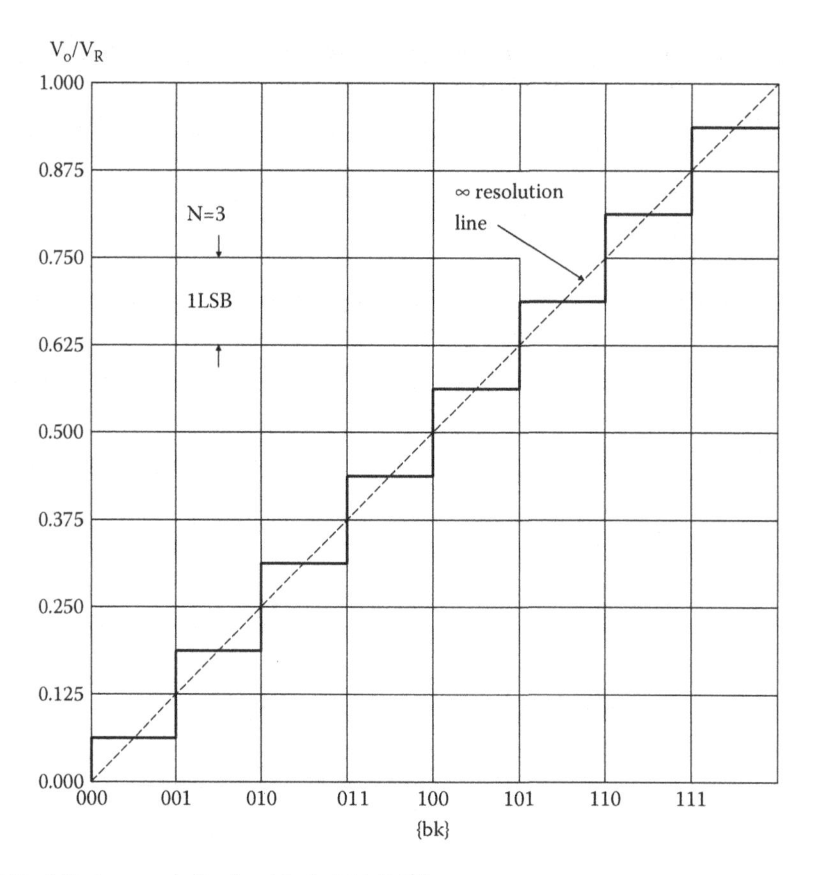

FIGURE 10.7 I/O characteristic of an ideal, 3-bit DAC.

DAC static errors can be described by the *integral nonlinearity* (INL) and the *differential nonlinearity* (DNL). Allen and Holberg (2002) stated

> [The] *INL* is the maximum difference between the actual finite resolution characteristics and the ideal finite resolution characteristic measured vertically. Integral nonlinearity can be expressed as a percentage of the full scale range or in terms of the least significant bit. Integral nonlinearity has several subcategories, which include absolute, best-straight-line, and end-point nonlinearity. The *INL* of a 3-bit [DAC] characteristic is illustrated in Figure 10.8. The *INL* of an N-bit DAC can be expressed as a positive *INL* and a negative *INL*. The positive *INL* is the maximum positive *INL*. The negative *INL* is the maximum negative *INL*. In Figure 10.8, the maximum +*INL* is 1.0LSB and the maximum −*INL* is −1.5LSB.

The differential nonlinearity (DNL) is a measure of the separation between adjacent levels measured at each vertical discontinuity in quantization. The DNL measures bit-to-bit deviations from ideal output steps, rather than along the entire output range. If V_{cx} is the actual voltage change on a bit-to-bit basis and V_s is the ideal change, then the differential nonlinearity can be written as

$$\text{DNL} = \frac{V_{cx} - V_s}{V_s} \times 100\% = (V_{cx}/V_s - 1)\ \text{LSBs} \tag{10.26}$$

For an N-bit DAC and a full-scale voltage range of VFSR,

$$V_s = V_{FSR}/2^N \tag{10.27}$$

Figure 10.8 also illustrates *differential nonlinearity*. Note that DNL is a measure of the step size and is totally independent of how far the actual step change may be away from the infinite resolution characteristic at the jump. The change from 101 to 110 results in a maximum +DNL of 2.5LSBs (V_{cx}/V_s = 2.5LSBs). The maximum negative DNL is found when the digital input code changes from 011 to 100. The change is −0.5 LSB (V_{cx}/V_s = −0.5LSB), which gives a DNL of −0.5LSB. It is of interest to note that as the digital input code changes from 100 to 101, no change occurs (point ***P***). Because we know that a change should have occurred, one can say that the DNL at point ***P*** is −0.5LSB.

Dynamic DAC characteristics limit the speed at which they can convert digital words to analog signals. If a DAC IC has an on-chip op-amp for current-to-voltage conversion, the op amp's f_T and slew rate, h, provide one factor that limits conversion speed. Another factor comes from on-chip parasitic capacitances that shunt all resistors and transistors to substrate ground. Conversion speed is also limited by the rate at which MOS and/or BJT switches can turn on and off.

Glitches are another problem with high-speed DACs. Glitches are unwanted (artifactual) transients on the DAC output immediately following a digital word input. Franco (1988) described their origin and a cure:

> ... these are due to the internal circuitry's non-uniform response to input bit changes and to poor synchronization of the bit changes themselves. For instance, if during the center-scale transition from 011...1 to 100...0 the MSB is perceived as going on before (after) all other bits go off, the output will momentarily [try to] swing to full-scale (to zero), thus causing an output glitch.
>
> Glitches can be minimized either by synchronizing the input bit changes with a high-speed parallel latch register, or by processing the DAC output with a S/H [sample and hold] deglitcher circuit. The circuit is switched to hold mode just prior to the input code change and is returned to the track mode only after the DAC gas settled to its new level, thus preventing any glitches from reaching the output.

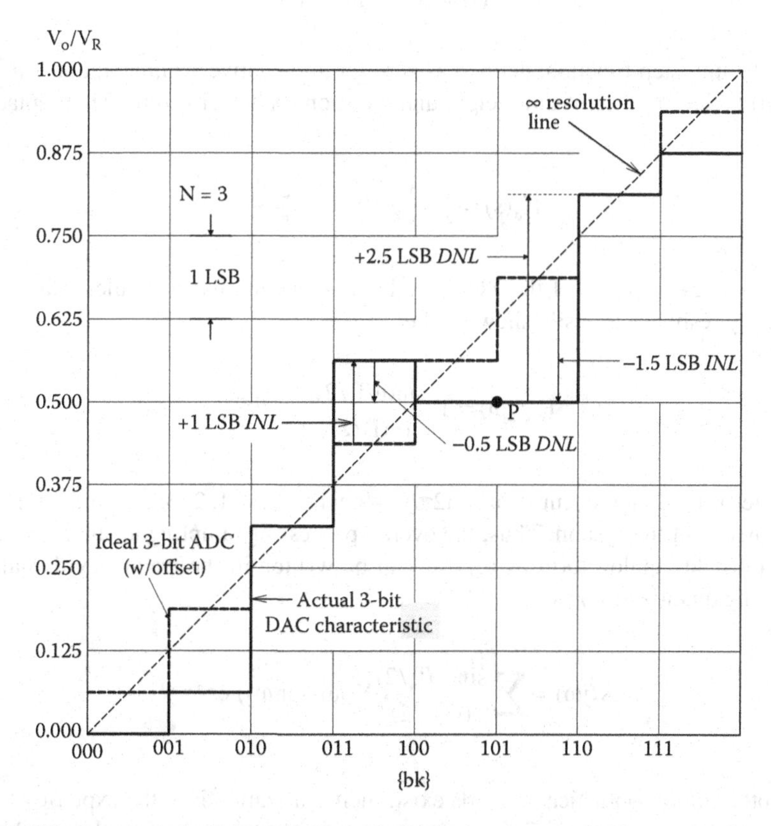

FIGURE 10.8 I/O characteristic of a nonideal, 3-bit DAC, showing types of errors. (Adapted from Allen, P.E. and Holberg, D.R., CMOS *Analog Circuit Design*, Oxford University Press, New York, 2002.)

The very fast, video, voltage-output DACs now available (2011) can convert at above 200 MSPS. For example, the 10-bit, Analog Devices AD9732 DAC are rated at 200 MSPS, and take 5 ns to settle to ½ LSB.

The Maxim MAX5891 is a 16-dit DAC that can update at 600 Msps. The Texas Instruments DAC3283 is a 16-bit DAC that has an 800 Msps update rate. The Faraday 8-bit, DAC8001, is rated at 200 MSPS and claims a 4 ns analog settling time. The AD9122 is a two-channel, 16-bit, current output DAC that is rated at 1.23 Gsps. The MAX5581 is a 12-bit, current-steering, 4.3-Gsps cable downstream, direct RF synthesis DAC.

Many high-speed DACs exist; the faster ones generally have current outputs, and the slower tend to have voltage outputs. Some have two parallel channels on a chip. For further insight into the design and application of ultra-high speed DACs, see the 2010 Analog Devices App. Note, AN928, *Understanding High Speed DAC Testing and Evaluation.*

10.4 SAMPLE-AND-HOLD CIRCUITS

Just as the sampling process can be interpreted in the frequency domain, so can the process of sample (or track) and hold of analog signals from a DAC. Note that the digital input to a DAC is generally periodic with period T_s. The DAC's analog output from the nth digital input is generally held constant until the (n + 1)th input updates it. This process generates a stepwise output waveform if $\{b_k\}$ is changing. This process can be viewed as linear filtering operation. The impulse response of the *zero-order hold* (ZOH) filter to a unit input word at t = 0, and zero inputs at sampling instants thereafter is

$$h_o(t) = U(t) - U(t - T_s) \tag{10.28}$$

where U(t) is the unit step function, defined as zero for all negative argument, and 1 for all positive argument. $h_o(t)$ is thus a pulse of unit height and duration (0, T_s), else zero. The Laplace transform of $h_o(t)$ is

$$H_o(s) = \frac{1}{s} - \frac{1}{s}e^{-sTs} = \frac{1 - e^{-sTs}}{s} \tag{10.29}$$

To find the frequency response of the ZOH, we let s → jω, and use the Euler relation for $e^{j\theta}$. The ZOH's frequency response is easily shown to be

$$H_o(j\omega) = T_s \frac{\sin(\omega T_s/2)}{(\omega T_s/2)} e^{-j\omega Ts/2} \tag{10.30}$$

Note that the zeros in $\mathbf{H}_o(j\omega)$ occur at $\omega = n2\pi/T_s$ r/s, where n = 1, 2, 3, … , and $2\pi/T_s$ is the radian sampling frequency of the system. Thus, the overall process of sampling an analog signal, x(t), and reconverting to (held) analog form by a DAC can be written in the frequency domain (Northrop 1990) (neglecting quantization) as

$$X(j\omega) = \sum_{n=0}^{\infty} \frac{\sin(\omega T_s/2)}{(\omega T_s/2)} X(j\omega - jn\omega_s)\, e^{-j\omega Ts/2} \tag{10.31}$$

Note that other more sophisticated holds exist; their realization is at the expense of some circuit or software complexity, however. For example, the first-difference extrapolator-hold which generates linear slope transitions between sampling instants (instead of steps) can be realized with three DACs, a resetable analog integrator, and an analog adder (Northrop 1990). From its impulse response, its transfer function can be shown to be

$$H_{1D}(s) = \frac{1-e^{-sT}}{s} + \frac{1-2\,e^{-sT}+e^{-2sT}}{s^2} - \frac{(1-e^{-sT})\,e^{-sT}}{s} = \frac{(1+e^{-sT})^2+(1-e^{-sT})^2}{s^2} \quad (10.32)$$

10.5 ANALOG-TO-DIGITAL CONVERTERS

10.5.1 Introduction

While the technology for DACs is relatively simple, there are many diverse kinds of ADCs and ADC algorithms. There are five major categories of ADC: (1) *Tracking (servo)* converters; (2) *Successive approximation* converters; (3) *Integrating* converters; (4) *Flash (parallel)* converters; (5) *Oversampled (sigma–delta)* converters. Each category will be examined below and how it works will be described.

Figure 10.9 shows the transfer characteristic of a 3-bit, binary-output ADC. Note that an infinite-resolution analog signal, x(t), is *quantized* into 8, 3-bit binary words, depending on its value. Figure 10.10 illustrates the *normalized quantization error* (NQE) ° v_e/LSB of this converter; the quantization error voltage is given by

$$V_e = V_x - V_{FS}\sum_{k=1}^{N} b_k 2^{-k} = v_x - V_{FS}(b_1 2^{-1} + b_2 2^{-2} + b_3 2^{-3}),\quad \text{for } N = 3 \quad (10.33)$$

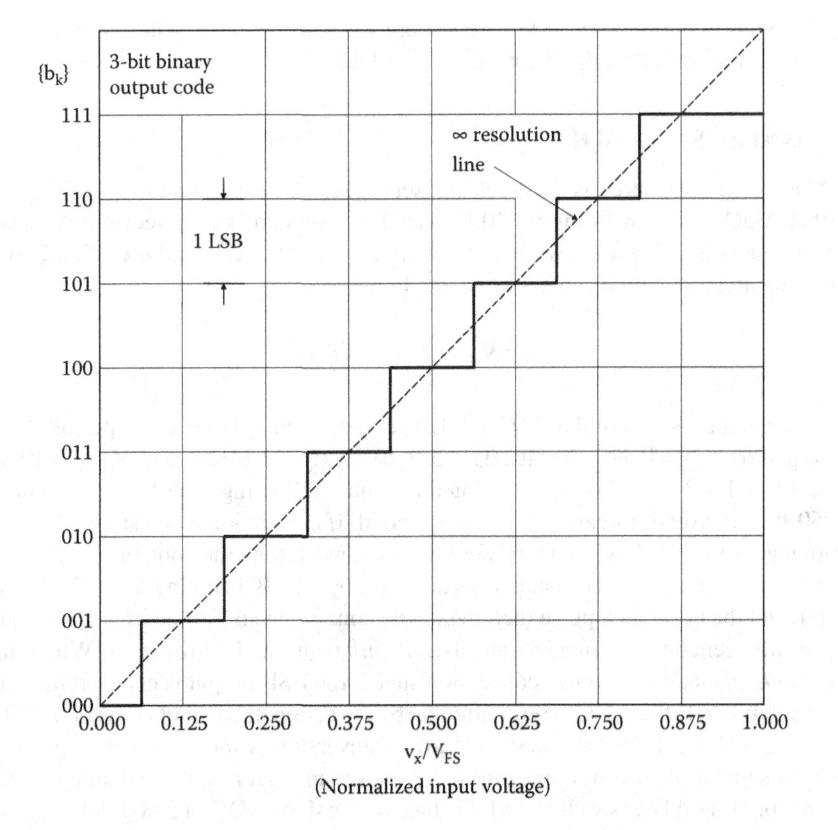

FIGURE 10.9 Transfer characteristic of an ideal, 3-bit, binary-output ADC.

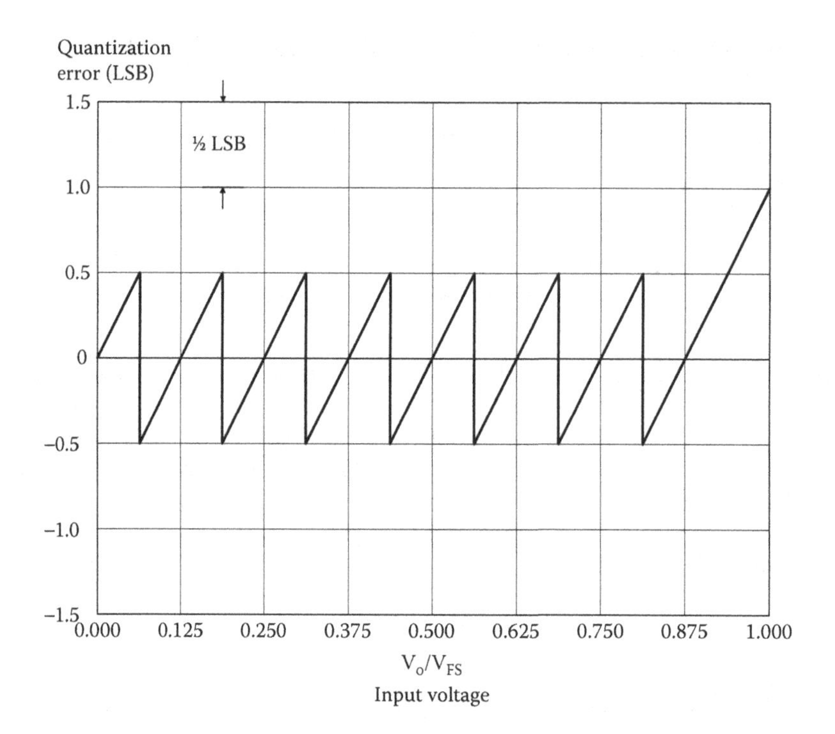

FIGURE 10.10 Normalized quantization error vs input voltage for an ideal, 3-bit, binary ADC.

Note that the NQE is bounded by ± ½ LSB except for $v_x/V_{FS} \geq 7/8$, where it reaches +1LSB at $v_x/V_{FS} = 1$. 1 LSB = $V_{FS}/2^3 = V_{FS}/8$ for this 3-bit ADC.

10.5.2 Tracking (Servo) ADC

The first ADC to be considered is the tracking (servo) ADC, aka the counting ADC. A block diagram for this ADC is shown in Figure 10.11. When conversion is initiated, the up/down counter is reset, then counts up. The up/down counter's digital output goes to a DAC. The DAC's voltage output ramps up at a rate which can easily shown to be

$$\eta = V_{oFS}/(2^N T_c) \quad \text{V/Sec.} \tag{10.34}$$

where N is the number of bits of the DAC and U/D counter and T_c is the clock period. V_{oFS} is generally made equal to V_{xmax}. If N = 10 bits, $T_c = 5 \times 10^{-7}$ s, (f_c = 2 MHz), and V_{omax} = 10 V, then the V_o slew rate is h = 1.953×10^4 V/s. By resetting the counter following each 10 V conversion, one sees that ca. 1950 10 V conversions can be made per second. If conversion is not stopped when the comparator output goes LO ($V_o > V_x$), and the counter is not reset, then the counter will increment down by 1 LSB at the next clock cycle, causing V_o to decrease by 1 LSB, bringing $V_o < V_x$; the comparator then goes HI, and the next clock pulse increments the counter up so V_o then exceeds V_x. The process repeats cyclically, generating a steady-state, 1-LSB *dither* in the digital output. When this ADC is used in the *tracking mode* to improve conversion speed, the LSB output is not used in order to avoid the steady-state dither. If the ADC is reset after each conversion, the end of conversion (EOC) signal occurs when $V_o > V_x$ by 1 LSB the first time after conversion is initiated. Although this mode of operation avoids dither, it is slower, and still has a conversion error between 0 and +1 LSB.

The servo counting ADC is well suited for data conversion of DC or low-frequency AC signals. It is also easy to implement in hardware (ICs). One disadvantage is that conversion time depends on

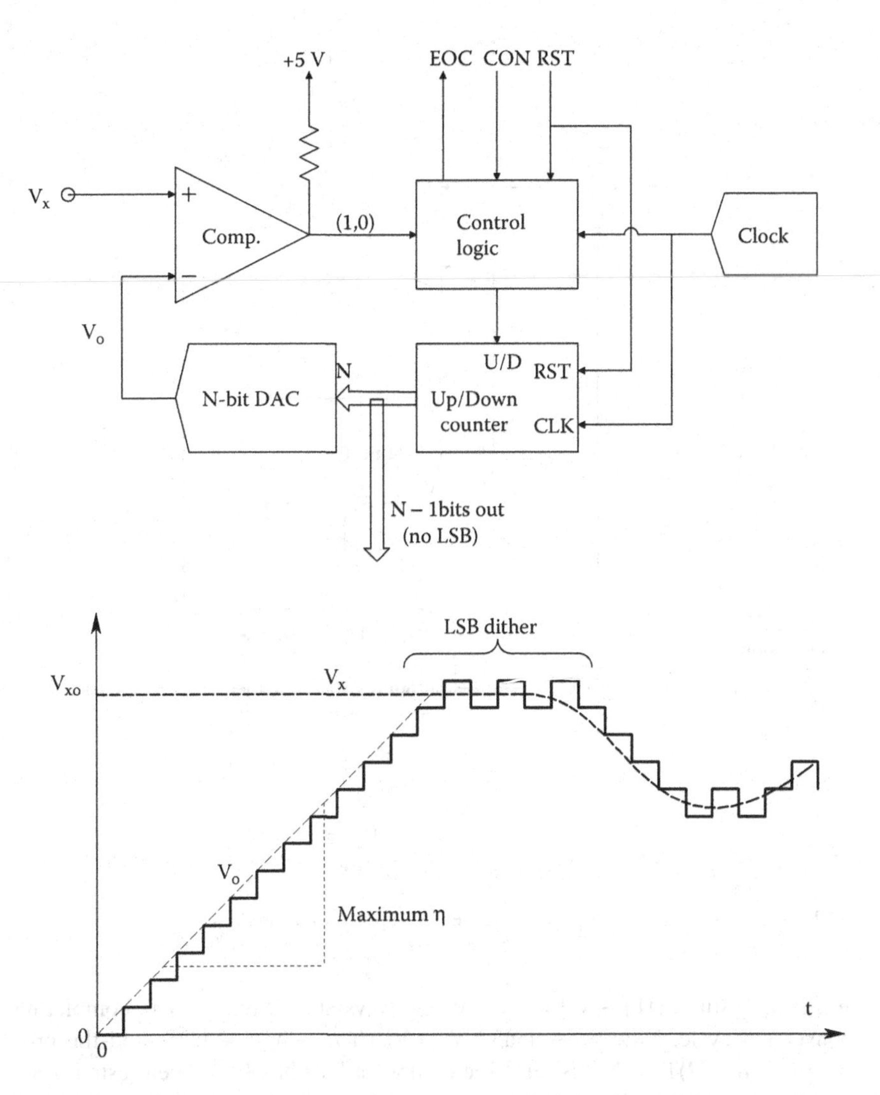

FIGURE 10.11 *Top:* Block diagram of a tracking or servo ADC. *Bottom:* DAC output of the servo ADC showing numerical slew-rate limiting and dither.

the value of v_x/V_{xmax}, i.e., it is variable. Another disadvantage is the LSB dither seen in the steady-state tracking mode.

10.5.3 Successive Approximation ADC

Like the servo counting ADC, the *successive approximation ADC* (SAADC) also uses a comparator and a DAC in a closed-loop architecture, as shown in Figure 10.12. The conversion cycle for a 10-bit SAADC begins with a *start* signal from the controlling computer's I/O interface at t = nT. *Start* causes the analog input signal, V_x, to be held at $[V_x(nT)]$, and the counter's output register is cleared (all $b_k \rightarrow 0$ except for $b_1 = 0$ (MSB)). This action causes the DAC output, V_o, to go to $512V_R/1024 = V_R/2$. The comparator subtracts this V_o from $[V_x(nT)]$ and performs the operation:

$$Q = \text{sgn}\ \{[V_x(nT)] - V_R/2\} \tag{10.35}$$

If Q = 1, then b_1 is kept 1 (HI); if Q = −1, then b_1 is set to 0 (LO). Next, b_2 is set to 1 (b_1 retains the value determined in the first cycle). Now the DAC output is $V_o = V_R(b_1/2 + 1/2^2)$. The comparator

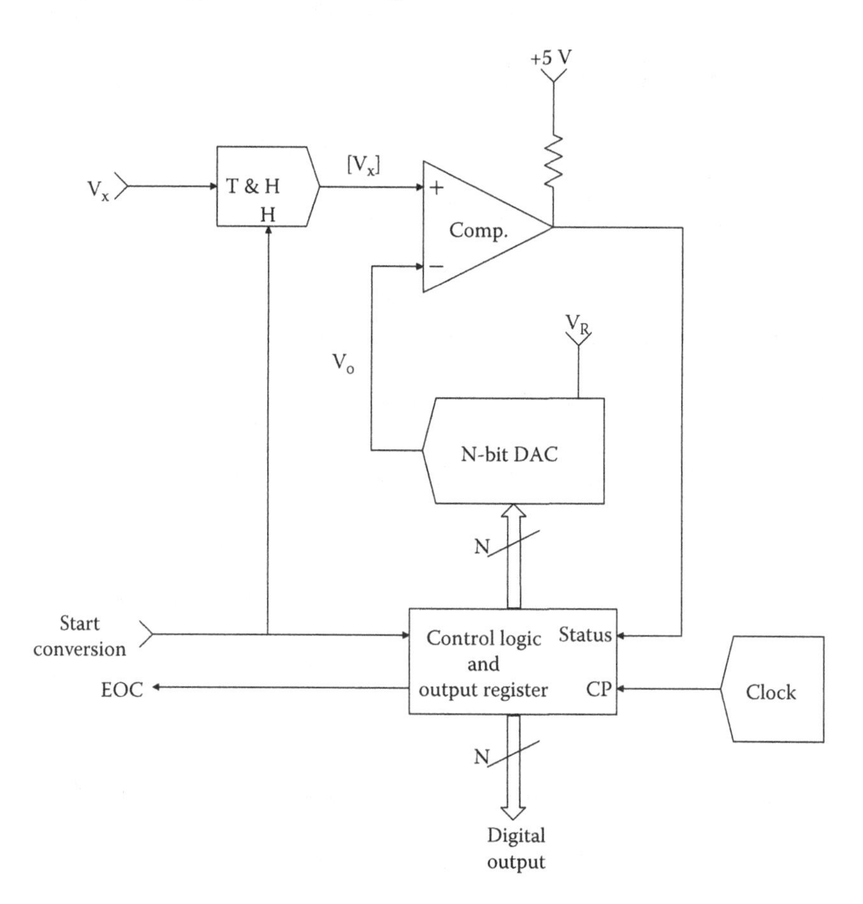

FIGURE 10.12 Block diagram of the popular successive-approximation ADC.

tests to see if $\text{sgn}\{[V_x((n + 1)T] - V_o\} = 1$. If *yes*, b_2 stays at 1, if no, $b_2 \rightarrow 0$, completing the second bit's conversion cycle. Now $b_3 \rightarrow 1$ and $V_o = V_R (b_1 /2 + b_2 /4 + 1/2^3)$, and the process continues. $Q = \text{sgn}\{V_x((n + 2)T] - V_o\}$ is tested, etc., until all 10 bits have been tested. Figure 10.13, adapted from Northrop 1990, illustrates a logical flowchart for the operation of a 10-bit SAADC; note b_1 = MSB and b_{10} = LSB.

The conversion time of a SAADC is $T_c = NT$, i.e., about N clock periods. For example, the Texas Instruments TLC1225 12-bit SAADC can convert in 12 ms, given a 2 MHz clock input. The TI TLC1550I 10-bit SAADC can convert in 6 ms given a 7.8 MHz clock, which is about 166 kSa/s.

10.5.4 Integrating Converters

Integrating converters are also called serial analog DACs. There are two basic architectures that we will consider in this section: the *single-slope* and the *dual-slope integrating DAC* (IDAC). Figure 10.14 illustrates the block diagram of one version of a single-slope IDAC (SSIDAC). A resetable op amp integrator is used as a ramp generator; it integrates the DC $V_R < 0$ to produce a positive ramp with slope V_R/RC. The ramp, V_2, is the negative input to a comparator, the positive input to which is the held signal being converted, $[V_x] > 0$. At the start of conversion, $[V_x] > V_2$, so the comparator output, Q, is HI, enabling the AND gate to pass clock pulses to the binary counter. When $V_2 > [V_x]$, Q goes LO. This event stops the counting, and through the control logic, causes the integrator to be reset to $V_2 \rightarrow 0$, and the track and hold circuit to again track $v_x(t)$. $Q \rightarrow 0$ also causes the counter to present the total count at its parallel output, and the control logic to signal *end of conversion* (EOC).

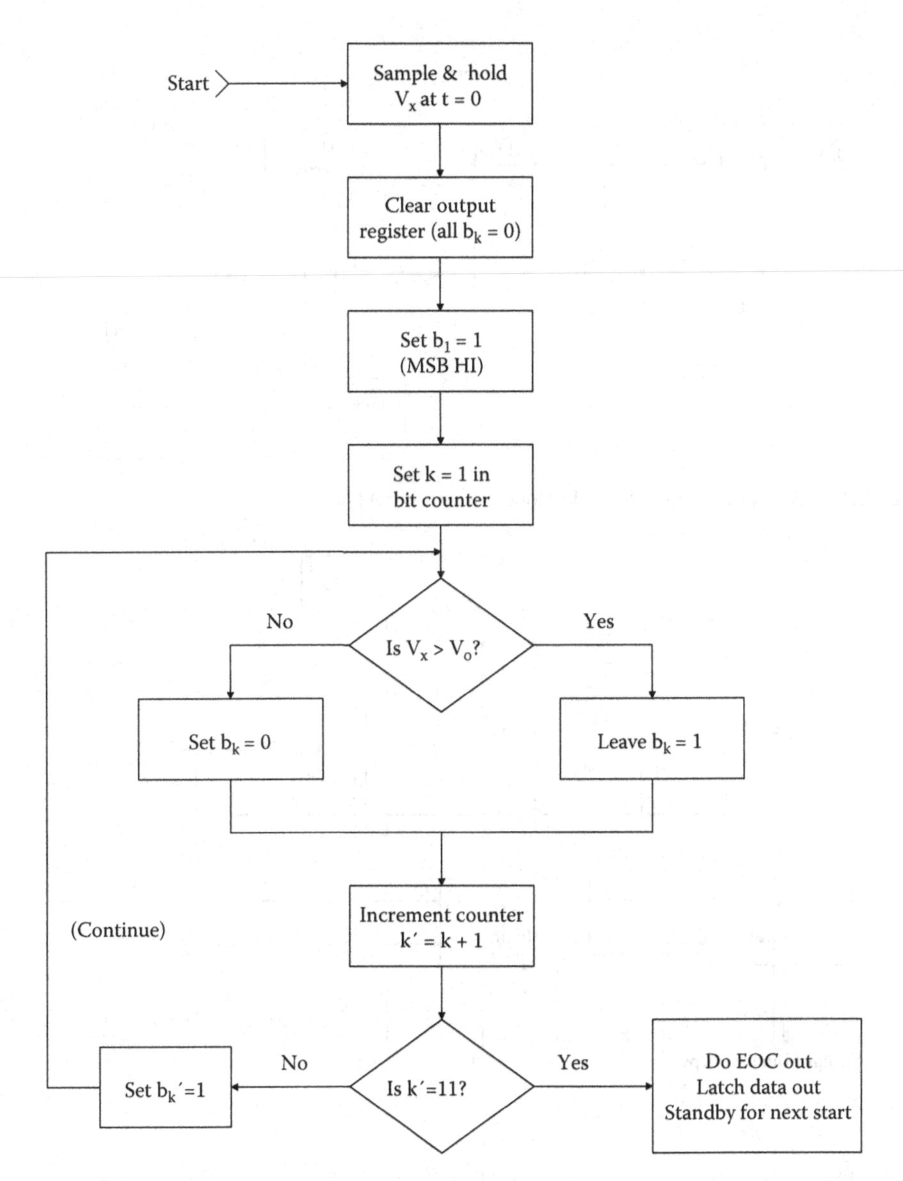

FIGURE 10.13 Logical flowchart illustrating the steps in one conversion cycle of a successive-approximation ADC.

The SSIDAC is now in standby mode waiting for the next convert (CONV) command. The leading edge of the CONV command causes the counter to be reset, $v_x(t)$ to be held, the integrator to begin integrating V_R, and the counter to begin counting. Each completed conversion count, M, is proportional to that $[V_x]$. From the SSIDAC architecture, one can write for the jth conversion:

$$\frac{1}{RC}\int_0^{M_jT} V_R\, dt = [V_x]_j \tag{10.36}$$

$$M_j = \frac{[V_x]_j RC}{V_R T} \tag{10.37}$$

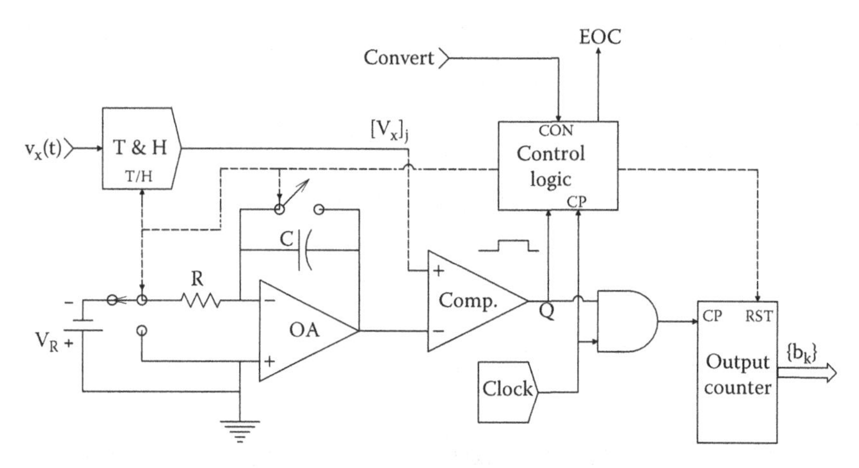

FIGURE 10.14 Block diagram of a single-slope, integrating ADC.

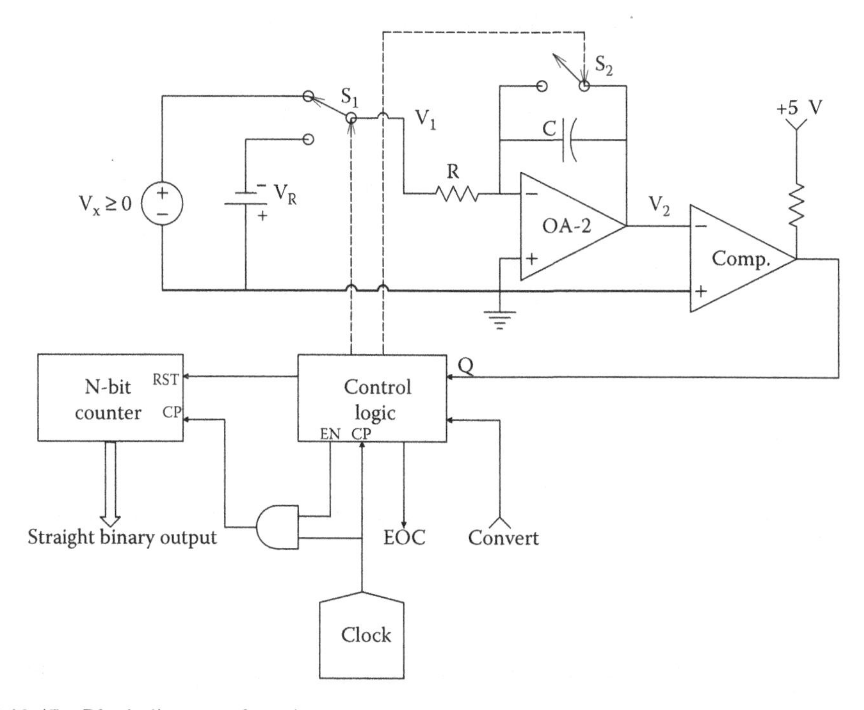

FIGURE 10.15 Block diagram of a unipolar input, dual-slope, integrating ADC.

Suppose a 10 bit converter is desired, where V_x ranges fro 0 to 10 V. Let $V_R = 1.00$ V, and $T = 10^{-6}$s. Then, from Equation 10.37, one finds that $RC = 1.023 \times 10^{-4}$ s, so if $C = 10^{-8}$ F, then $R = 1.023 \times 10^4\ \Omega$. With these parameters, the SSIADC will output $M_j = 2^{10} - 1$ when $[V_x]_j = 10.0$V. Note that SSIADC conversion time is variable; the larger $[V_x]_j$, the longer it takes. When $[V_x]_j = 10$ V, conversion takes 1.023 ms. Thus, integrating ADCs (IADCs) are relatively slow, suitable for ECG and DC applications. Also, accuracy of the SSIADC depends on the stability of the R-C product and clock period over time and temperature changes. To overcome these problems, the clever design of the dual-slope, integrating ADC was developed.

Figure 10.15 illustrates the circuit of a unipolar, dual-slope, integrating ADC. Note that this ADC does not require a DAC. On receiving the *convert* command, this ADC first resets its integrator output to $V_2 = 0$, and clears its counter to zero. S_1 connects the integrator to $V_x > 0$. V_x is integrated for 2^N clock cycles, or $2^N T_c$ seconds, causing V_2 to go negative. At the end of this integration time, the counter is again cleared and S_1 switches to $-V_R$ which is integrated, causing V_2 to ramp positively toward zero. During this interval, the counter counts up from zero because Q is high. When V_2 reaches zero, the comparator output Q goes from HI to LO, stopping the counter and signaling the end of the conversion cycle. Mathematically, the integrator output when the counter reaches $T_1 = 2^N T_c$ is

$$V_2(2^N T_c) = -\frac{1}{RC}\{\int_0^{T_1} v_x(t)/(T_1)\, dt\}\ T_1 = \frac{-2^N T_c}{RC}\ \{\overline{V_x(T_1)}\} \quad (10.38)$$

In the second part of the conversion cycle, the integrator integrates until V_2 reaches zero. This takes M clock cycles. M is given by

$$\underset{\downarrow}{V_2} = 0 = \frac{-2^N T_c}{RC}\{\overline{V_x(T_1)}\} + \frac{M T_c V_R}{RC} \quad (10.39)$$

$$M = \frac{\{\overline{V_x(T_1)}\}\ 2^N}{V_R} \quad (10.40)$$

Thus, the count down time, hence M, is proportional to the average of the input signal over $T_1 = 2^N T_c$ seconds. Note that this ADC is independent of RC and T_c; these parameters are determined from practical considerations. Often T_1 is made 1/60 s to make the ADC reject 60 Hz hum on $v_x(t)$ (Northrop 1990). Figure 10.16 illustrates the block diagram of a *dual-slope, integrating ADC* (DSIADC).

This ADC gives an *offset binary output code* for bipolar DC input signals. When the convert command is given, the input is held, the counter is cleared (reset to zero) and V_2 is set to zero with S_2. Next, S_2 is opened and S_1 is set to integrate the output of OA-1, V_2, for a time equal to 2^N clock

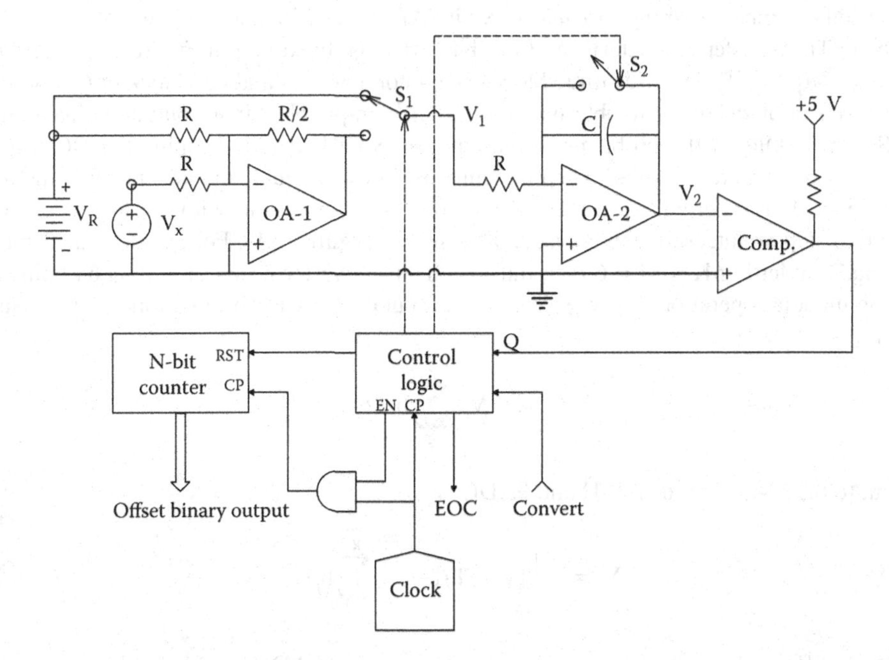

FIGURE 10.16 Block diagram of a bipolar input, dual-slope, integrating ADC. The output is in offset binary code.

cycles ($T_1 = 2^N T_c$). V_2 goes positive, so Q = LO, disabling the output counter. When $T_1 = 2^N T_c$, the counter is enabled and counts clock pulses, and S_1 is set to integrate $+V_R$. V_2 now ramps down to zero, which is sensed by the comparator output Q going HI. The number of clock cycles required for V_2 to go to 0 is M. The peak V_2 is found by

$$V_2(2^N T_c) = \frac{1}{2RC} \int_0^{2^N T_c} (V_R + [V_x])\, dt = \frac{V_R 2^N T_c}{2RC} + \frac{[V_x] 2^N T_c}{2RC} \tag{10.41}$$

The number of clock cycles required to integrate $V_2(2^N T_c)$ to zero is M:

$$\frac{V_R 2^N T_c}{2RC} + \frac{[V_x] 2^N T_c}{2RC} - \frac{V_R M T_c}{RC} = 0 \tag{10.42}$$

Solving for M:

$$M = 2^{N-1}(1 + [V_x]/V_R) \tag{10.43}$$

Note that when $[V_x] = -V_R$, M = 0; when $[V_x] = 0$, $M = 2^{N-1}$ (1 MSB), and when $[V_x] = + V_R$, $M = 2^N$, giving a *true offset binary output code.* Note that this dual-slope, integrating ADC also has accuracy independent of RC and T_c.

10.5.5 Flash Converters

The fastest ADCs are *flash converters.* Flash converters (FADCs) enable signal sampling in the ns range and thus are widely used in medical ultrasound systems, sonar and radar data conversion, and certain communications applications (Kester 2008; Sexton et al. 2008; Kulkarni et al. 2010). Data conversion rates into the hundreds of MSa/s are typical. Figure 10.17 illustrates an N = 3-bit flash ADC with straight binary output. $2^N - 1 = 7$ voltage comparators are used for conversion; comparator C_1 is used to signal over-range. (Thus, an 8-bit FADC uses 255 analog comparators, plus one for over-range.) The transfer characteristic of a 3-bit FADC is illustrated in Figure 10.18. The Analog Devices AD770 8-bit FADC uses three blocks of 64 comparators and one block of 65 comparators and two levels of bit decoding to obtain an 8-bit, ECL-compatible, binary output with a guaranteed 200 MSa/s rate. One of the problems in realizing an 8-bit FADC is keeping the DC offset voltages of the 256 comparators small, keeping tempcos, low and equal, and also keeping the resistors matched in the 2^N-resistor voltage divider. To realize flash conversions with resolutions greater than 8 bits, a two-step architecture can be used, as shown in Figure 10.19. For example, a 12-bit FADC can be made by letting K = M = 6 bits; thus, each subconverter needs only $2^6 = 64$ comparators. Assuming unipolar operation, $0 \le v_x \le V_{FS}$. The output of the K-MSB DAC following a conversion of $[v_x(nT)]$ is

$$V_1 = V_{FS} \sum_{i=1}^{K} b_i / 2^i \tag{10.44}$$

The input to the M-lesser bits T & H and FADC is

$$V_2 = 2^K \left([v_x(nT)] - V_{FS} \sum_{i=1}^{K} b_i / 2^i \right) \tag{10.45}$$

The voltage difference in parentheses is V_e. Thus, the second FADC generates a binary code on the quantized remnant, V_e, to give a net N = (K + M)-bit output. Because the K- and M-bit FADCs use

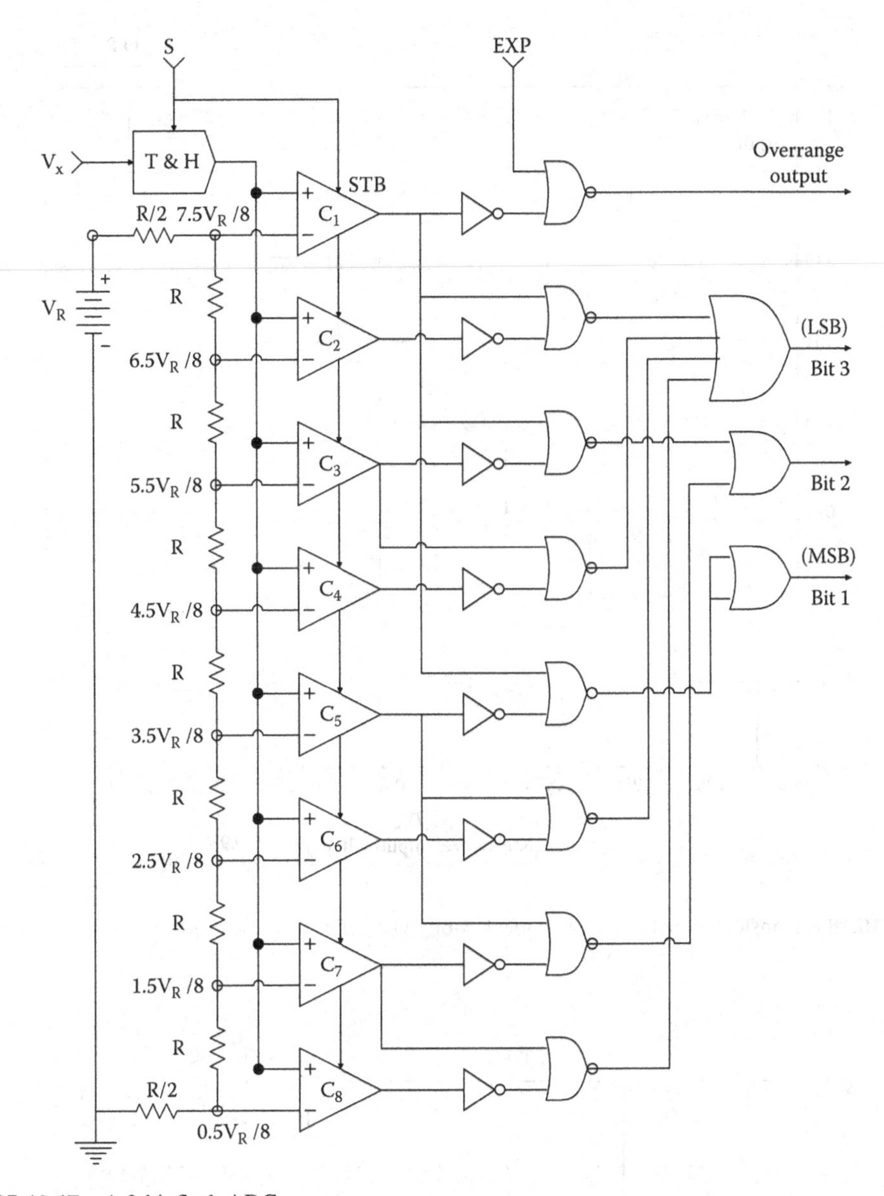

FIGURE 10.17 A 3-bit flash ADC.

$(2^K - 1)$ and $(2^M - 1)$ comparators, respectively, the system is generally less expensive and easier to build than a single N-bit FADC. The total coded output of the system is

$$[V_x(nT)] = V_{FS}\left\{\sum_{i=1}^{K} b_i / 2^i + \sum_{j=1}^{M} b_j / 2^j\right\} = V_{FS}\sum_{k=1}^{N} b_k / 2^k \tag{10.46}$$

The growth of digital, GHz communications has pushed the demand for very fast ADCs (Ali et al. 2006). Sandner et al. (2005) described the design of a 6-bit FADC that converted at a rate of 1.2 GSps, which provided an effective resolution bandwidth (ERBW) of 700 MHz. This FADC had an input capacitance of only 400 fF. The Maxim MAX5881 12-bit FADC converts at 4.3 GSps; such speed is not without cost, this ADC consumes 1.4 W at 4 GSps. Four digital input channels

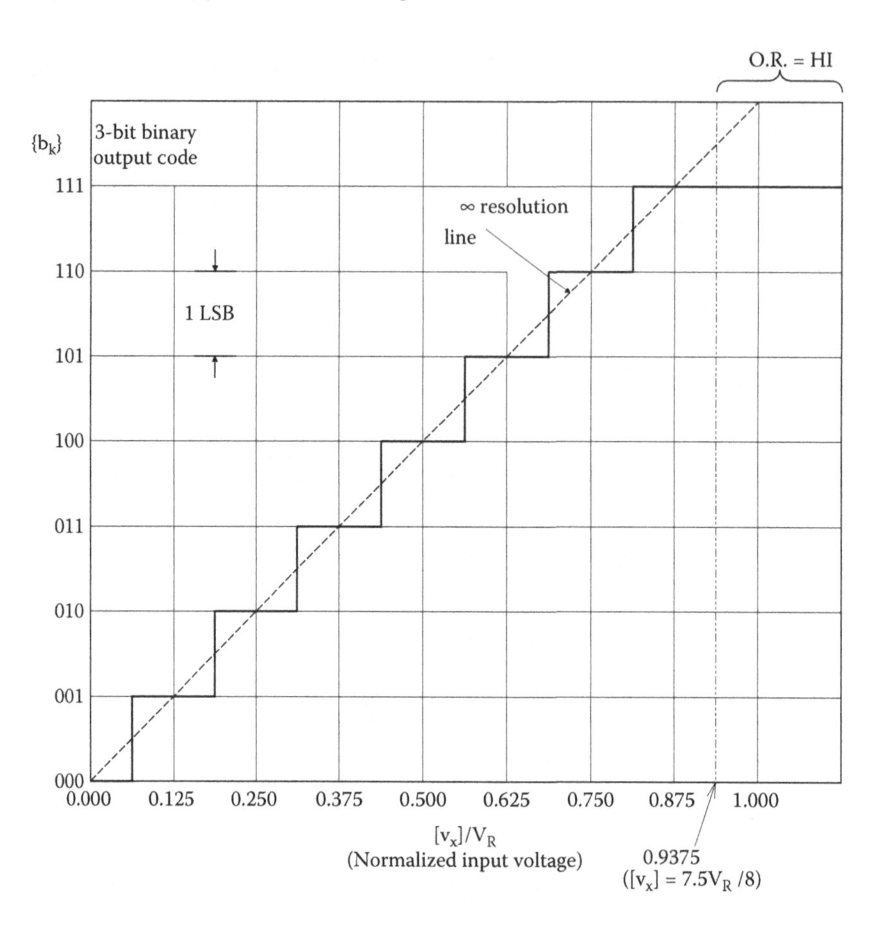

FIGURE 10.18 Transfer characteristic of an ideal, 3-bit, flash ADC.

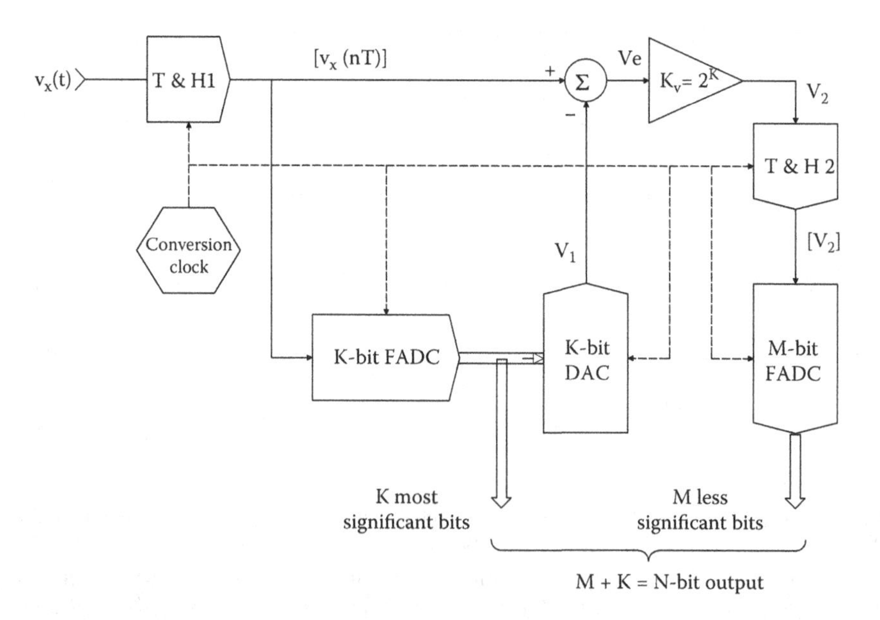

FIGURE 10.19 Architecture of a two-step flash ADC. This design is more efficient when $N \geqslant 8$ is desired.

can be multiplexed.When flash converters are used that sample at over 100 MSa/s, special attention must be paid to how the digital data is handled. High-speed logic (e.g., ECL) must be used, and data must be stored temporarily in shift registers and high-speed RAM before permanent recording can take place on a magnetic hard disk or optical disk. FADCs also are greedy for die size and operating power. For every bit increase in FADC resolution, the ADC core circuitry size (comparators, resistors, decoding logic) essentially doubles, as does the chip's power dissipation. Conversion time, however, is independent of the bit resolution, N, and is fast, the state of the art for 2 and 4 bit FADCs is a sample rate of about 1 GSa/s.

10.5.6 Delta–Sigma ADCs

Delta-sigma ADCs are also called sigma–delta ADCs and *oversampled* or *noise-shaping converters.* Oversampling ADCs are based on the principle of being able to trade-off accuracy in time for accuracy in amplitude. Figure 10.20 illustrates the circuit of a *first-order, Δ-Σ ADC.* The circuit in the box is a first-order Δ-Σ modulator. The digital filter and decimator produces the N-bit, digital output.

How the Δ-Σ modulator operates in the time domain will be analyzed first. Set $V_x \to 0$. Let the MOS switch apply $-V_R$ to the integrator (the Q output of the DFF is LO) so that the integrator output, V_1, goes positive. The comparator output, V_2, applied to the D input of the D flip-flop (DFF) now will be HI. At the rising edge of the next clock pulse, HI is seen at the Q output of the DFF. This HI causes the MOS switch to switch the integrator input, V_s, to $+V_R$, so that now the integrator output V_1 begins to ramp down. When V_1 goes negative, the comparator output V_2 goes LO. Again when the clock pulse goes HI, the LO at D is sent to the DFF Q output. This LO again sets the MOS switch to $-V_R$, causing V_2 to ramp positively until it goes positive, setting V_2 HI, etc. Figure 10.21 shows the Δ-Σ modulator's waveforms for $V_x = 0$. Q is the DFF output which is the comparator

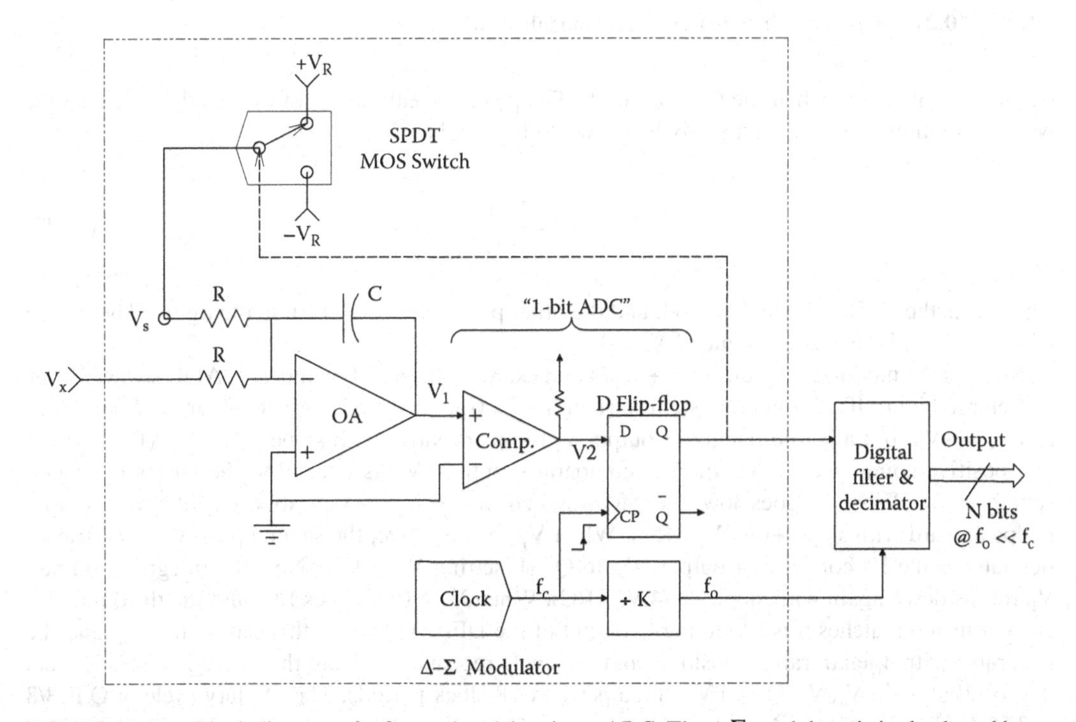

FIGURE 10.20 Block diagram of a first-order, delta-sigma ADC. The Δ-Σ modulator is in the dotted box.

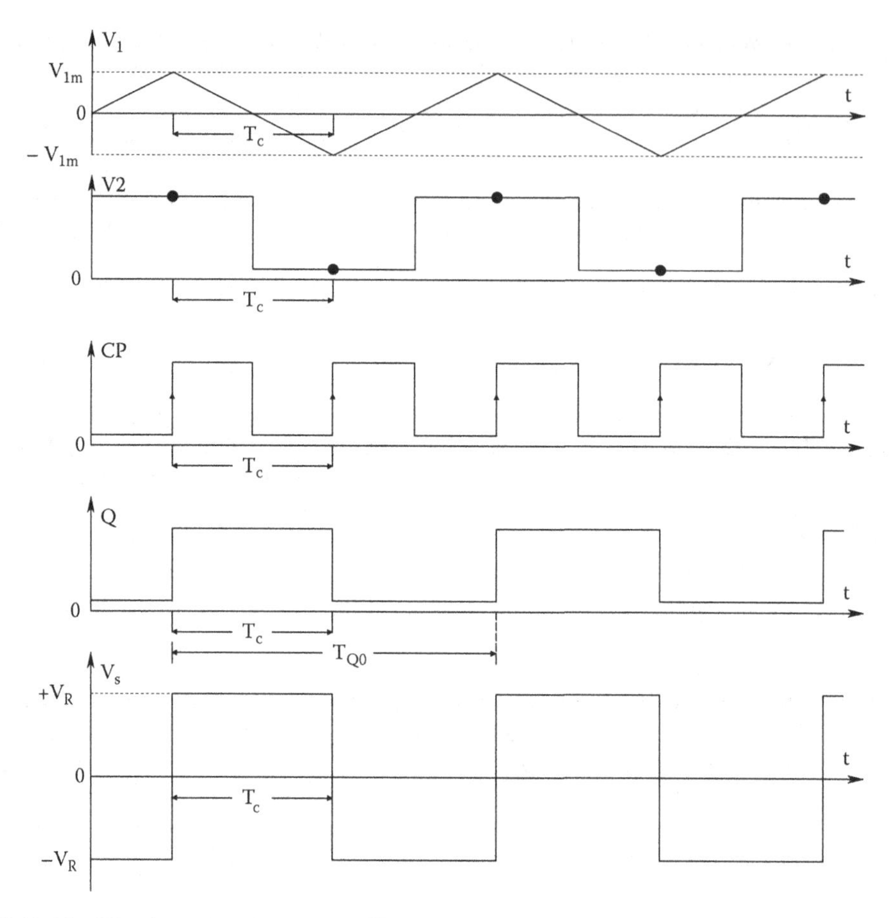

FIGURE 10.21 Waveforms in a first-order Δ-Σ modulator when $V_x = 0$.

output, V_2, latched in when the CP goes high. The peak-to-peak height of the steady-state triangle wave oscillation seen at V_1 can easily be shown to be equal to

$$2V_{1m} = \frac{V_R T_c}{RC} \tag{10.47}$$

where T_c is the DSDAC's clock period, and the other parameters are given in the figure. The period of V_1 is $2T_c$, and the average value of $V_s = 0$.

Now set the modulator input, $V_x = +\ V_R/4$ and examine the steady-state, Δ-Σ ADC's waveforms.

Refer to Figure 10.22. Let the system start with $V_1 = 0$ at $t = 0$, and begin to integrate $V_x = +V_R/4$ and $V_s = +V_R$. Initially, the integrator output V_1 ramps negative with slope $-(5/4)\ V_R/(RC)$. At the first positive-going clock wave, the LO comparator output, V_2, is latched to the DFF's Q output, setting it low. When Q goes low, the MOS switch makes $V_s = -V_R$. Now the integrator output ramps upward with slope $+(3/4)V_R/(RC)$. When V_1 goes positive, the second positive clock transition latches the HI comparator output, V_2, to Q HI, setting V_s to $+V_R$. Now the integrator output, V_1, ramps down again with slope $-(5/4)V_R/(RC)$. When $V_1 < 0$, V_2 goes LO, and the third positive clock transition latches this LO to the Q output of the DFF. As before, this sets V_s to $-V_R$, and the integrator output again ramps positive, and the cycle repeats, etc. Note that there is a steady-state (SS) oscillation in V_1, V_2, Q and V_s with a period of 8 clock periods. The SS duty cycle of Q is 3/8 or 37.5% when $V_x = +V_R/4$.

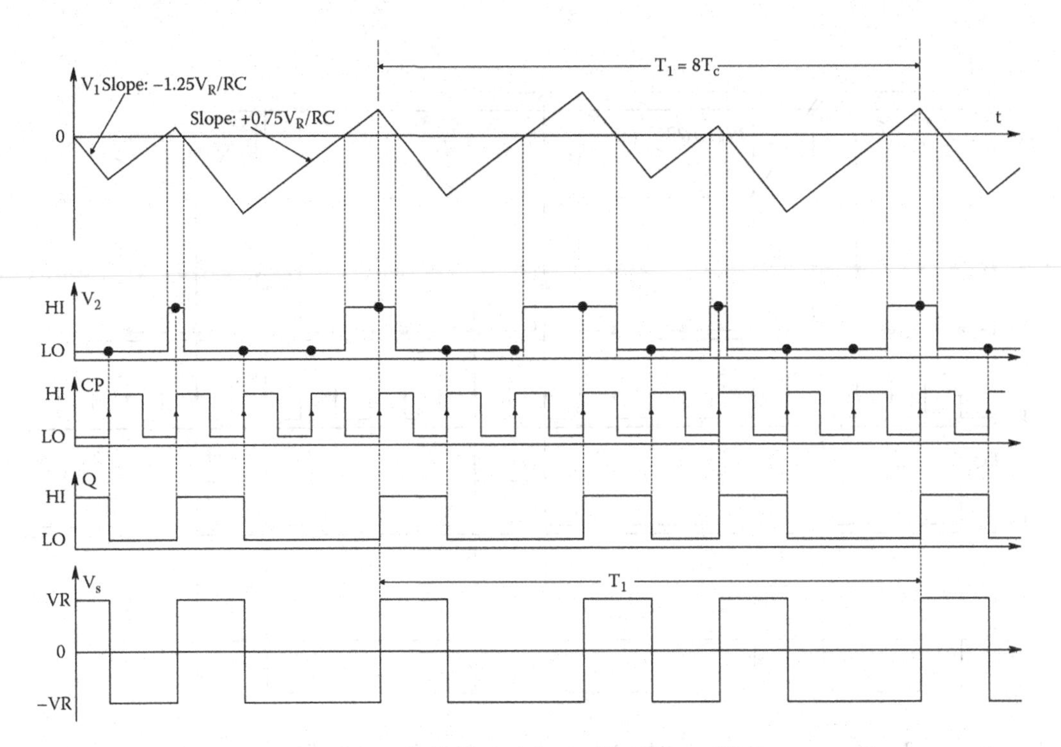

FIGURE 10.22 Waveforms in a first-order Δ-Σ modulator when $V_x = +V_R/4$.

It is also of interest to examine the Δ-Σ ADC's steady-state waveforms when $V_x = +V_R/2$. Let the system start with $V_1 = 0$ at $t = 0$, and begin to integrate $V_x = V_R/2$ with $V_s = +V_R$. Assuming V_x is constant, V_1 ramps negative with slope $-(3/2)V_R/(RC)$, causing the comparator output, V_2, to be LO. At the first positive-going clock pulse, the DFF latches the low D input to Q, causing the MOS switch to make $V_s = -V_R$. Now the net input to the integrator is $-V_R/2$, and the integrator output begins to go positive with slope $+ (1/2)V_R/(RC)$, as shown in Figure 10.23. When V_1 first goes positive, V_2 goes HI. At the third clock HI transition, the DFF output goes HI, setting the MOS switch to $-V_R$. Now the net input to the integrator is $+3V_R/2$, and V_1 begins to ramp down again with slope $-(3/2)V_R/(RC)$, and the ADC process repeats itself indefinitely until V_x changes. From the waveforms in this figure where $V_x = V_R/2$, we see that the duty cycle of Q is ¼ (25%), and the average $V_s = -½$. From the three sets of V_s waveforms, we see that, in general, $V_x = -V_R V_{s(Ave)}$.

Now consider the operation of first-order, Δ-Σ ADC. If the number of ones in the output data stream (i.e., the DFF's Q output) is counted over a sufficient number of samples (clock cycles), the counter's digital output will represent the digital value of the analog input, V_x. Obviously, this method of averaging will only work for DC or low-frequency V_x. In addition, at least 2^N clock cycles must be counted in order to obtain N-bit effective resolution. In the Δ-Σ ADC, the modulator's DFF's Q output is the input to the block labeled "digital filter & decimator." The digital LPF precedes the decimator. The digital LPF serves two functions: (1) It acts as an antialiasing filter for the final sampling rate, f_o. (2) It filters out the higher frequency noise produced by the Δ-Σ modulator.

Quoting Analog Devices' AN-283 on *Sigma–Delta ADCs and DACs:*

> The final data rate reduction is performed by digitally resampling the filtered output using a process called decimation. The decimation of a discrete-time signal is shown in Fig. 6.12, where the sampling rate of the input signal x(n) is at a rate which is to be reduced by a factor of 4. The signal is resampled at the lower rate (the decimation rate), s(n) [f_o]. Decimation can also be viewed as the method by which the redundant signal information introduced by the oversampling process is removed.

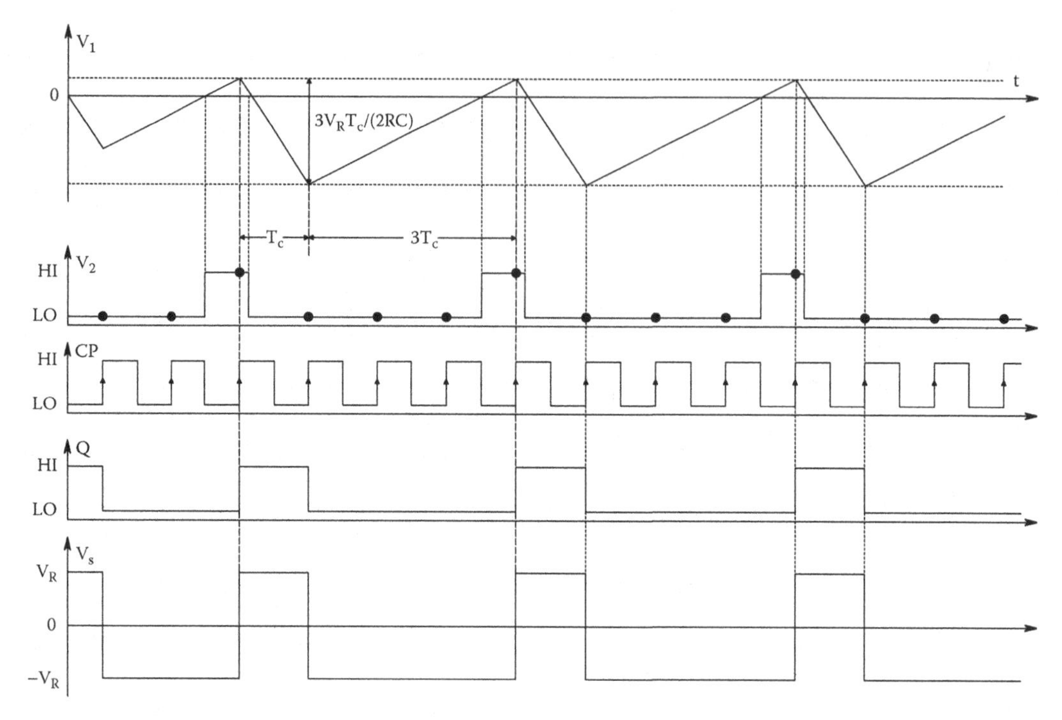

FIGURE 10.23 Waveforms in a first-order Δ-Σ modulator when $V_x = + V_R/2$.

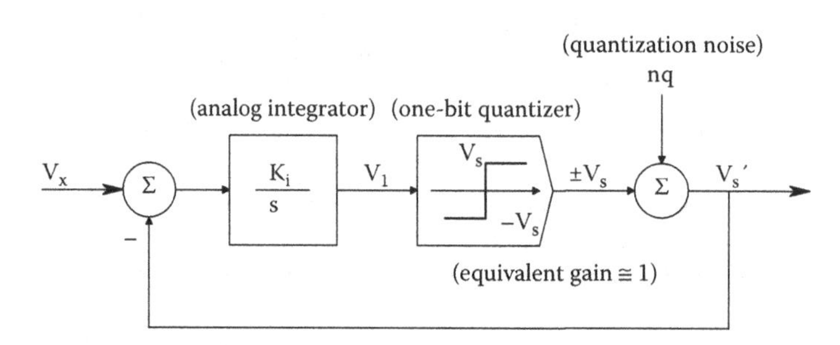

FIGURE 10.24 A heuristic, frequency domain block diagram of a first-order, Δ-Σ modulator.

In sigma–delta ADC designs, it is common to combine the decimation function with the digital filtering function. If done correctly, this can lead to an increase in computational efficiency.

Figure 10.24 illustrates a frequency-domain block diagram approximation for a first-order Δ-Σ ADC. To appreciate what happens in the system in the frequency domain, we can find the transfer function for the analog input, V_x, and the internal quantization noise, n_q (see the following section). Assuming a linear system, we find

$$V_s' = \frac{V_x K_i}{j\omega + K_i} + \frac{j\omega\, n_q}{j\omega + K_i} \tag{10.48}$$

Thus, the 1-bit quantization noise in the output is boosted at high frequencies so $V_s' \cong j\omega\, n_q/K_i$. The signal component in V_s' rolls off at −6 dB/octave above $\omega = K_i$ r/s. At low frequencies, the noise in V_s' is negligible and $V_s' \cong V_x$. Because the Δ-Σ modulator is really a sampled system at frequency f_c, the noise in V_s and Q has the root power density spectrum shown in Figure 10.25: Note that the

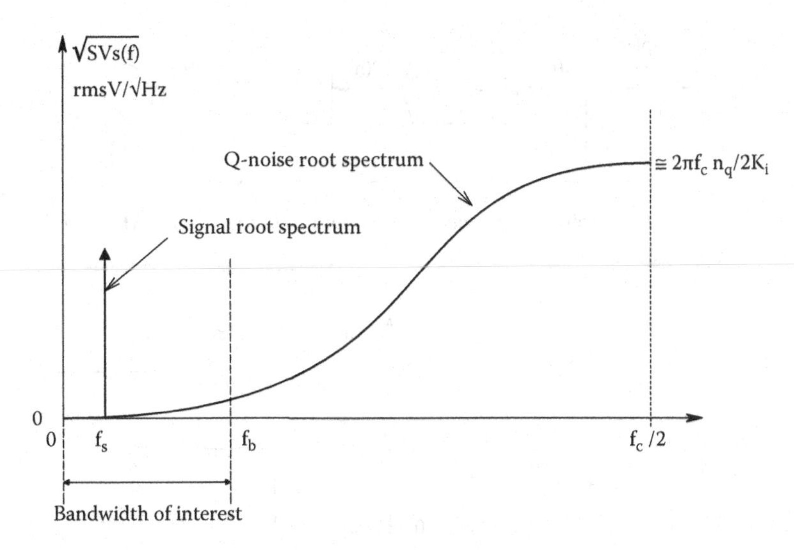

FIGURE 10.25 A typical, one-sided, root power density spectrum of signal and quantization noise in a first-order, Δ-Σ modulator.

broadband quantization noise is concentrated at the upper end of the root spectrum. The range from $0 \leq f \leq f_b$ is relatively noise-free. Operation in this range is achieved by first having the FIR LPF operate on the data stream from Q at clock rate f_c, then decimation so $f_b = f_o/2$, the Nyquist frequency of the decimation frequency. Lastly, the counter counts the decimated data for $2^N f_o$ clock periods.

More on the sigma-delta ADC can be found in Maxim's *Application Note 1870 Demystifying Sigma–Delta ADCs,* 31 Jan. 2003 (go to: www.maxim-ic.com/an1870). Intersil's App. Note AN9504 (May, 1995), *A Brief Introduction to Sigma Delta Conversion,* also gives a clear detailed description of sigma-delta conversion. See also Beis (2008) for another good tutorial on sigma-delta conversion.

10.6 QUANTIZATION NOISE

In this section, an important source of noise in signals that are periodically sampled and converted to numerical form by an ADC is described. These numerical samples can then be digitally-filtered or processed, and then returned to analog form, $v_y(t)$, by a digital-to-analog converter. Such signals include modern digital audio, video, and static images. The noise created by converting from analog to digital form is called *quantization noise* (QN), and it is associated with the fact that when a noise-free analog signal, $v_x(t)$, having almost infinite resolution, is sampled and digitized, each $v_x^*(nT)$ is described by a binary number of finite length, introducing an uncertainty between the original $v_x(nT)$ and $v_x^*(nT)$. This uncertainty gives rise to the quantization noise which can be considered to be added to either $v_y(t)$ or $v_x(t)$. (A paper by Kollár, 1986, has a comprehensive review of quantization noise. Also, Chapter 14 in the text by Phillips and Nagle (1984) has a rigorous mathematical treatment of QN.)

When a Nyquist band-limited analog signal is sampled and then converted by an N bit ADC to digital form, a statistical uncertainty in the digital signal amplitude exists which can be considered to be equivalent to a broad-band, *quantization noise* added to the analog signal input *before sampling.* In the quantization error-generating model of Figure 10.26, a noise-free, Nyquist-limited, analog signal, $v_x(t)$, is sampled and digitized by an N-bit ADC of the *round-off type.* The ADC's numerical output, $v_x^*(nT)$, is the input to an N-bit DAC. The *quantization error,* e(n), is defined *at sampling instants* as the difference between the sampled analog input signal, $v_x(nT)$ and the analog

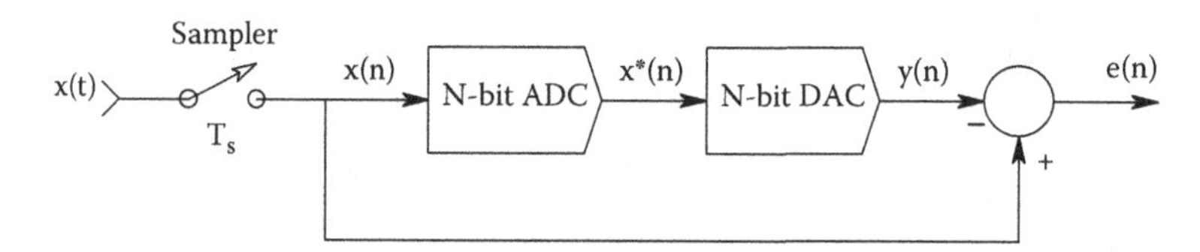

FIGURE 10.26 A quantization noise error-generating model for an ideal N-bit ADC driving an N-bit ideal DAC.

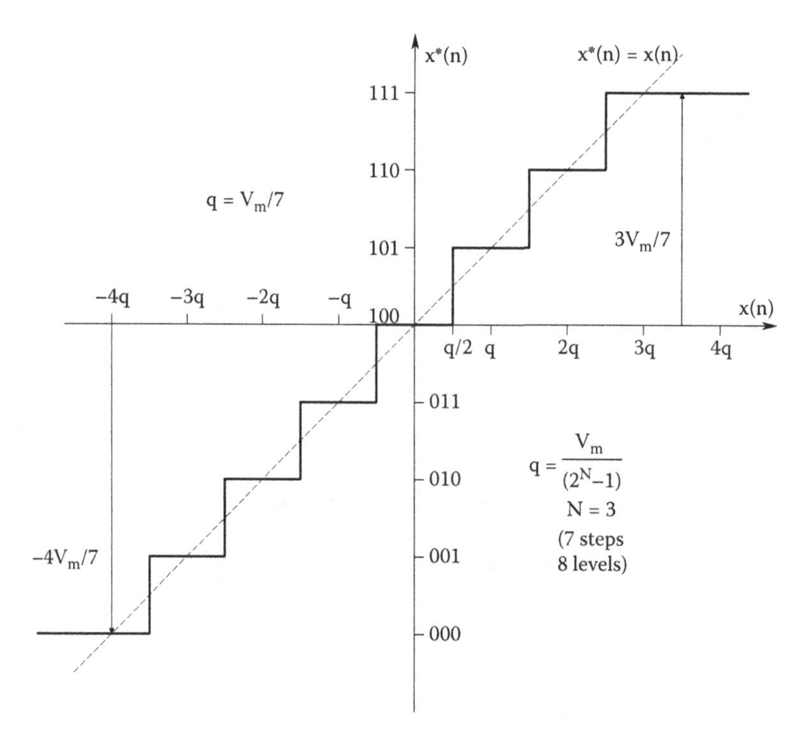

FIGURE 10.27 A 3-bit, rounding quantizer I/O function.

DAC output, $v_y(nT)$. (Henceforth the shorter notation, x(n), y(n), etc., will be used) The ADC/DAC channel has unity gain. Thus, the quantization error is simply

$$e_q(n) = x(n) - y(n) \tag{10.49}$$

Figure 10.27 illustrates a bipolar, rounding quantizer function relating analog sampler output, x(n), to the binary DAC output, x*(n). In this example, N = 3. (This uniform rounding quantizer has 2^N levels and $(2^N - 1)$ steps.) When y(n) is compared to the direct path, the error, $e_q(n)$, can range over ±q/2 in the center of the range, where q is the voltage step size of the ADC/DAC. It is easy to see that for full dynamic range, q should be

$$q = \frac{V_{xMax}}{(2^N - 1)} \text{ volts} \tag{10.50}$$

where V_{xMAX} is the maximum (peak-to-peak) value of the input, $v_x(t)$, to the ADC/DAC system. For example, if a 10-bit ADC is used to convert a signal ranging from −5 to + 5 V, then by Equation 10.50, q = 9.775 mV. If x(t) has *zero mean,* and its probability density function (PDF) has a standard

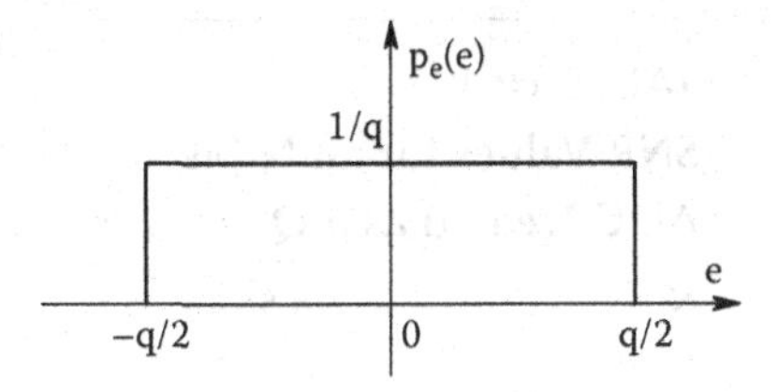

FIGURE 10.28 The rectangular probability density function generally assumed for quantization noise.

deviation $\sigma_x > q$, then it can be shown that the PDF of $e_q(n)$ is well-modeled by a uniform (rectangular) density, $f_e(e)$ over $e = \pm q/2$. This rectangular PDF is shown in Figure 10.28; it has a peak height of 1/q. The mean-squared error voltage is found from the expectation

$$E\{e^2\} = \overline{e^2} = \int_{-\infty}^{\infty} e^2 f_e(e)\, de = \int_{-q/2}^{q/2} e^2 (1/q)\, de = \left.\frac{(1/q)e^3}{3}\right|_{-q/2}^{q/2} = \frac{q^2}{12} = \sigma_q^{\,2} \text{ MSV} \quad (10.51)$$

Thus, it is possible to treat quantization error noise as a zero-mean, broad-band noise with a standard deviation of $\sigma_q = q/\sqrt{12}$ RMSV, added to the ADC/DAC input signal, x(t). We assume the QN spectral bandwidth to be flat over $\pm f_s/2$, where f_s is the sampling frequency, i.e., the Nyquist range.

To minimize the effects of quantization noise for an N-bit ADC, it is important that the analog input signal, $v_x(t)$, use nearly the full dynamic range of the ADC. In the case of a zero-mean, time-varying signal which is Nyquist band-limited, gains and sensitivities should be chosen so that the peak expected x(t) does not exceed the maximum voltage limits of the ADC.

If x(t) is a SRV and has a Gaussian PDF with zero mean, the dynamic range of the ADC should be about ±3 standard deviations of the signal. Under this particular condition, it is possible to derive an expression for the mean-squared signal-to-noise ratio of the ADC and its quantization noise. Let the signal have an RMS value σ_x volts. From Equation 10.50, the quantization step size can be written as

$$q \approx \frac{6\,\sigma_x}{(2^N - 1)} \text{ volts} \quad (10.52)$$

or

$$\sigma_x = q(2^N - 1)/6 \quad (10.53)$$

From which note that $\sigma_x > q$ for $N \geq 3$. Relation 10.52 for q can be substituted into Equation 10.51 for the variance of the quantization noise. Thus, the mean-squared output noise is

$$N_o = \frac{q^2}{12} = \frac{36\sigma_x^2}{12\,(2^N - 1)} = \frac{3\sigma_x^2}{(2^N - 1)} = \sigma_q^2 \text{ MSV} \quad (10.54)$$

Hence, the mean-squared signal-to-noise ratio of the N-bit, rounding quantizer is

$$SNR_q = (2^N - 1)/3 \text{ MSV/MSV} \quad (10.55)$$

Note that the quantizer SNR is independent of σ_x as long as σ_x is held constant under the dynamic range constraint described above. In dB, $SNRq = 10 \log[(2^N - 1)/3]$. Table 10.1 summarizes the SNR_q of the quantizer for different bit values.

TABLE 10.1
SNR Values for an N-bit ADC Treated as a Quantizer

N	dB SNRq
6	31.2
8	43.4
10	55.4
12	67.5
14	79.5
16	91.6

Note: Total input range is assumed to be 6 σ_x volts. Note that about 6 dB of SNR improvement occurs for every bit added to the ADC word length.

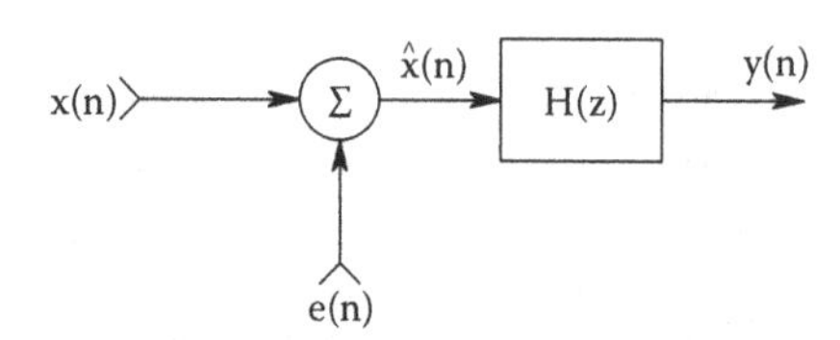

FIGURE 10.29 Block diagram of a model where quantization noise is added to a noise-free sampled signal at the input to a digital filter.

16- to 24-bit ADCs are routinely used in modern, precision digital audio systems because of their low quantization noise. Other classes of input signals to uniform quantizers, such as sine waves, triangle waves, and narrow-band Gaussian noise were discussed by Kollár (1986).

Figure 10.29 illustrates a model whereby the equivalent QN is added to the ideal, sampled signal at the input to some digital filter, H(z). Note that the quantization error sequence, $e_q(n)$, is assumed to be from a wide-sense stationary, white noise process, where each sample, $e_q(n)$, is uniformly distributed over the quantization error. The error sequence is also assumed to be uncorrelated with the corresponding input sequence, x(n). Furthermore, the input sequence is assumed to be a sample sequence of a stationary random process, {**x**}. Note that $e_q(n)$ is treated as *white sampled noise* (as opposed to sampled white noise). The auto-power density spectrum of $\mathbf{e}_q(n)$ is assumed to be flat (constant) over the *Nyquist range:* $-\pi/T \leq \omega \leq \pi/T$ r/s. (T is the sampling period.) $\mathbf{e}_q(n)$ propagates through the digital filter; in the time domain this can be written as a real, discrete convolution:

$$y(n) = \sum_{m=-\infty}^{\infty} e_q(m)h(n-m) \tag{10.56}$$

σ_q^2 is the variance of the white quantization noise, and the variance of the filter's output noise can be shown (Northrop 2010) to be expressed as

$$\sigma_y^2 = \sigma_q^2 \sum_{k=0}^{\infty} h^2(k) \tag{10.57}$$

10.7 CHAPTER SUMMARY

Digital interfaces generate sampled data when they periodically convert an analog signal to numerical form, or numerical data to an analog voltage or current. Sampled data are subject to the sampling theorem, which describes the conditions under which unwanted aliasing can take place. Sampling as impulse modulation was described in this chapter and also shown was how sampled data can be described in the frequency domain by a repeated spectrum Poisson sum. In the frequency domain, aliasing was shown to exist when the edges of the repeated spectra in the Poisson sum overlapped. This overlapping occurred when the power density spectrum of the sampled analog signal contained significant power above one-half the sampling frequency, also known as the Nyquist frequency.

DACs were next covered; their circuit architecture and factors affecting the speed of conversion were described. Hold circuits were next described. The transfer function of the zero-order hold, and a simple extrapolator-hold were derived.

Many types of ADCs were described, including the tracking or servo ADC, the successive approximation ADC, integrating ADCs, and flash ADCs. Flash ADCs were seen to be the fastest because they convert in parallel.

Finally, quantization noise was described and an expression for ADC SNR due to quantization noise was derived as a function of the number of binary bits in the converted signal. The more bits, the higher the ADC's SNR.

CHAPTER 10 HOME PROBLEMS

10.1 A 16-bit ADC is used to convert an audio signal ranging over ± 1 V.

(A) Find the size of the quantization step, q, required.

(B) Find the RMS quantization noise associated with full-scale operation of this ADC.

(C) Let $v_{in}(t) = 1 \sin(\omega_o t)$. Find the RMS SNR at the ADC output in dB.

10.2 Consider the 4-bit, resistive ladder DAC shown in Figure P10.2.

(A) Use superposition to find an expression for $V_o = f(I_o, I_1, I_2, I_3)$. Let R = 1 kΩ, I_o = 1 mA dc.

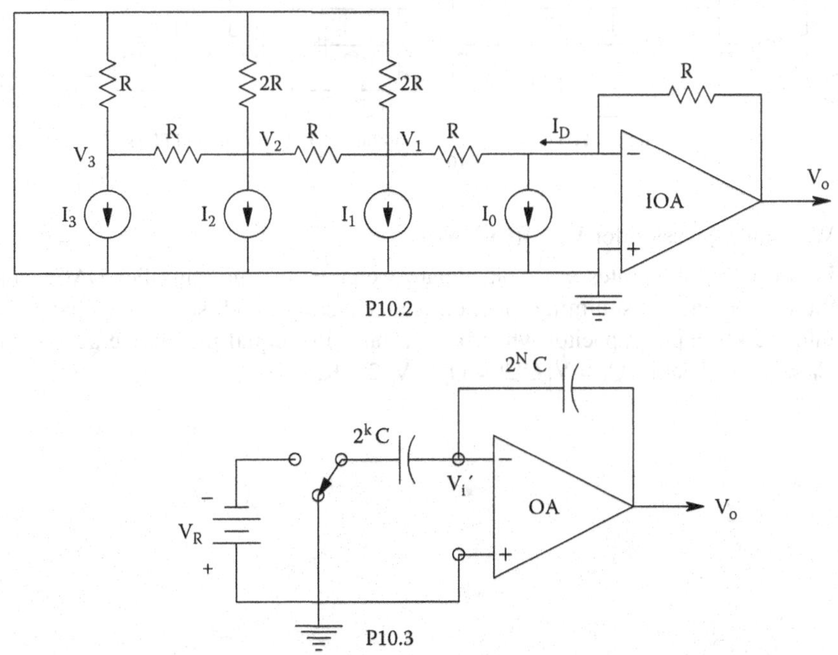

(B) What values should I_1, I_2, and I_3 have to make a binary DAC? What is the max. V_o?

10.3 Refer to Text Figure 10.5 for the switched weighted capacitor DAC. In this problem you will examine the dynamics of this system. A simplified circuit is shown in Figure P10.3. In this circuit, k = 0, 1, 2, . . ., N − 1. The op amp is characterized by: $R_{in} = \infty$, $I_B = V_{os} = R_{out} = 0$ and $V_o = (-K_{vo}\,\omega_b)/(s + \omega_b)$.

(A) Find an algebraic expression for $\frac{V_o}{V_R}(s)$.

(B) Assume $V_R(s) = V_{Ro}/s$ (step input). Give an expression for $V_o(s)$. Plot and dimension a general $v_o(t)$.

(C) Let k = 0, N = 8; sketch and dimension $v_o(t)$.

(D) Let k = N − 1 = 7; sketch and dimension $v_o(t)$.

(E) Find a general expression for the maximum slope of $v_o(t)$ in terms of k and other system parameters.

(F) Let $V_{Ro} = 1$ V, The op amp's GBWP = $K_{vo}\,\omega_b = 3 \times 10^8$. Find V_{omax} for k = 0 and k = 7.

What must the op amp's slew rate be to avoid slew-rate limiting of $V_o(t)$?

10.4 Figure P10.4 illustrates an N = 8 bit MOSFET current-scaling DAC. The feedback action of the left-hand op amp forces the Q_1 drain current to be $I_D = V_R/(2^N R)$. The left-hand op amp also puts all the connected FET gates at virtual ground (0). The right-hand op amp forces the FET drains connected to it to also be at virtual ground (0). Because all of the MOSFETs are matched, and they all have the same drain, gate and source voltage, they all have the same drain current, I_D.

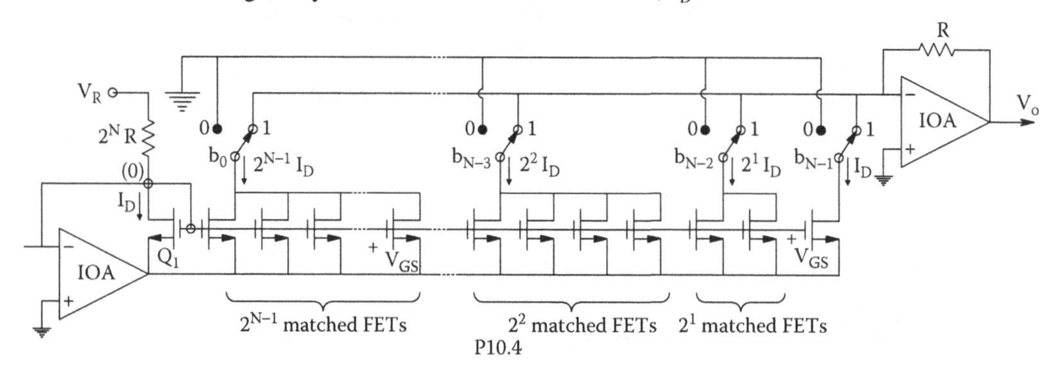

P10.4

Write an expression for $V_o = f(\{b_k\}, V_R)$.

10.5 Figure P10.5 illustrates an N-bit, binary-weighted charge amplifier DAC. Note that the ideal op amp's summing junction is at virtual ground, so the net charge flowing into the kth input capacitor when $b_k = 1$, must also equal the charge accumulated in $C_F = 2C/K$. That is, $Q_k = V_R C/2^k = Q_F = V_o\,2C/K$.

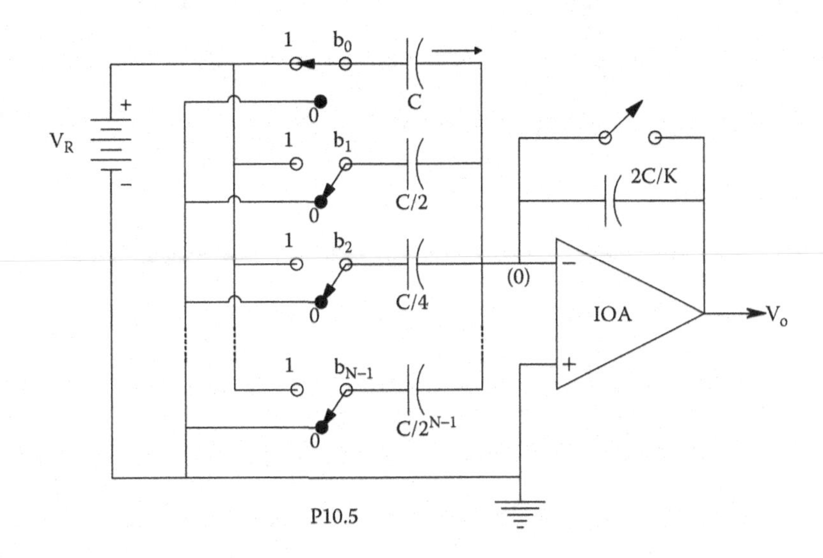

P10.5

Write an expression for $Vo = f(\{b_k\}, V_R, K)$; use superposition.

10.6 An 8-bit, successive approximation ADC has a reference voltage, V_R, set to 10.0 V at 25°C. Find the maximum allowable temperature coefficient of VR in μV/°C that will allow an error of no more than ± ½ LSB over an operating temperature range of 0 to 50°C.

10.7 A 100 mV peak-to-peak sinusoidal signal is the input to a 12 bit ADC which has a bipolar offset binary output and a full-scale input range of ±2.5 V.

(A) Find the output RMS SNR in dB when the input is a 2.5 V peak sinewave.

(B) Find the output RMS SNR in dB when the input is the 50 mV peak sinewave.

10.8 A unipolar, 3-bit successive-approximation ADC has $V_R = 8.0$ V, and a ½ LSB offset as shown in Text Figure 10.27. $V_{in} = 2.832$ V. Find the LSB voltage, and the intermediate and final DAC output voltages during conversion.

10.9 Explain the differences between *Nyquist-Rate data converters and oversampling data converters.*

10.10 Find the maximum magnitude of quantization error for a 10-bit ADC with $V_R = 10$ V, and ½ LSB absolute accuracy.

10.11 Draw to-scale the impulse response of the First-Difference Extrapolator-Hold system whose transfer function is given by Text Equation 10.32.

11 Modulation and Demodulation of Biomedical Signals

11.1 INTRODUCTION

In general, modulation is a process whereby a DC or low-frequency signal of interest is combined nonlinearly with a high-frequency carrier wave to form a *modulated carrier* suitable for transmission to a receiver/demodulator where the signal is recovered. Modulators and demodulators form essential components of most wire and wireless communication and other data transmission systems (e.g., fiber optic, ultrasound, light beam). Some modulation schemes involve multiplication of the carrier with a function of the modulating signal.

In biomedical engineering, recorded physiological signals are modulated because modulation permits robust transmission by wire (twisted pair), coaxial cable, fiber optic cable, or radio telemetry from the recording site to the site where the signal is demodulated, processed, and stored. As an example, in *biotelemetry,* physiological signals such as the ECG and blood pressure modulate a carrier, which is sent as an FM radio signal from an ambulance to a remote receiver (e.g., in a hospital ER) where the signals are demodulated, filtered, displayed, interpreted, digitized, and stored.

Five major forms of modulation involve altering a high-frequency, *sinusoidal carrier wave.* These modulation schemes include (1) *amplitude modulation* (AM); (2) *single-sideband AM* (SSBAM); (3) *frequency modulation* (FM), including *narrow-band FM* (NBFM); (4) *phase modulation* (PhM); and (5) *double-sideband, suppressed-carrier modulation* (DSBSCM).

Modulation can also be done using a square wave (or TTL) carrier, and can involve FM, NBFM, and PhM. Digital carriers at constant frequency are used with delta–sigma modulation, pulse-position modulation (PPM), and pulse-width modulation (PWM). They are also used in class D audio systems.

AM, FM, and DSBSCM are expressed mathematically below for a sinusoidal carrier. Let $v_m(t)$ be the actual physiological signal. The highest frequency in $v_m(t)$'s power spectrum must be $<< \omega_c$, the carrier frequency. The *normalized modulating signal,* m(t), is defined by Equation 11.1a:

$$m(t) = \frac{v_m(t)}{V_{mmax}}, 0 \leq |m(t)| \leq 1 \quad \text{Normalized modulating signal} \tag{11.1a}$$

$$y_m(t) = A[1 + m(t)]\cos(\omega_c t) \quad \text{AM} \tag{11.1b}$$

$$y_m(t) = Am(t)\cos(\omega_c t) \quad \text{DSBSCM} \tag{11.1c}$$

$$y_m(t) = A\cos[\omega_c t + K_f \int^t m(t)\,dt] \quad \text{FM} \tag{11.1d}$$

$$y_m(t) = A\cos[\omega_c t + K_p m(t)] \quad \text{phM} \tag{11.1e}$$

11.2 MODULATION OF A SINUSOIDAL CARRIER VIEWED IN THE FREQUENCY DOMAIN

It is interesting to examine the frequency spectrums of the modulated signals. For illustrative purposes, let the modulating signal be a pure cosine wave, $m(t) = m_o \cos(\omega_m t)$, $0 < m_o \leq 1$. Thus, by using Equation 11.1B and a trig identity, the amplitude-modulated (AM) signal can be rewritten as

$$y_m(t) = A\cos(\omega_c t) + (A\,m_o/2)\{\cos[(\omega_c + \omega_m)t] + \cos[(\omega_c - \omega_m)t]\} \tag{11.2}$$

Thus, the AM signal has a carrier component and two *sidebands,* each spaced by the amount of the modulating frequency above or below the carrier frequency. In SSBAM, a sharp cutoff filter is used to eliminate either the upper or lower sideband; the information in both sidebands is redundant, so removing one means less bandwidth is required to transmit the SSBAM signal. SSBAM signals are more noise resistant than conventional AM because they require less bandwidth to transmit the same m(t).

FM and PhM are subsets of *angle modulation.* FM can be further classified as *broadband* (BBFM) or *narrowband FM* (NBFM). In BBFM, $K_f \equiv 2\pi f_d$, where f_d is called the frequency deviation constant. In NBFM, $f_d/f_{mmax} << 1$ (f_{mmax} is the highest expected frequency in $v_m(t)$, which is bandwidth-limited). Unlike AM, the frequency spectrum of an FM carrier is tedious to derive. Using $m(t) = m_o \cos(\omega_m t)$, we can write the FM carrier as

$$y_m(t) = A\cos[\overset{\alpha}{\omega_c t} + (K_f/\omega_m)\overset{\beta}{\omega_o \sin(\omega_m t)}] \tag{11.3}$$

Using the trig identity, $\cos(\alpha + \beta) = \cos(\alpha)\cos(\beta) - \sin(\alpha)\sin(\beta)$, Equation 11.3 can be written as

$$y_m(t) = A\cos(\omega_c t)\cos[K_f/\omega_m)m_o\sin(\omega_m t)] - A\sin(\omega_c t)\sin[K_f/\omega_m)m_o\sin(\omega_m t) \tag{11.4}$$

Now the $\cos[(K_f/\omega_m)m_o \sin(\omega_m t)]$ and $\sin[(K_f/\omega_m)m_o \sin(\omega_m t)]$ terms can be expressed as two Fourier series whose coefficients are *ordinary Bessel functions of the first kind* and argument β (Clarke and Hess 1971); note that $\beta \equiv m_o 2\pi f_d/\omega_m$:

$$\cos[\beta \sin(\omega_m t)] = J_0(\beta) + 2\sum_{n=1}^{\infty} J_{2n}(\beta)\cos(2b\omega_m t) \tag{11.5a}$$

$$\sin[\beta \sin(\omega_m t)] = 2\sum_{n=0}^{\infty} J_{2n+1}(\beta)\sin[2(n+1)\omega_m t] \tag{11.5b}$$

The two Bessel sum relations for $\cos[\beta \sin(\omega_m t)]$ and $\sin[\beta \sin(\omega_m t)]$ can be recombined with Equation 11.4 using the trig identities, $\cos(x)\cos(y) = ½[\cos(x + y) + \cos(x - y)]$, and $\sin(x)\sin(y) = ½[\cos(x - y) - \cos(x + y)]$, and we can finally write for the FM carrier spectrum, letting $m_o = 1$:

$$\begin{aligned} y_m(t) = A\{&J_0(\beta)\cos(\omega_c t) + J_1(\beta)[\cos((\omega_c + \omega_m)t) - \cos((\omega_c - \omega_m)t)]\} \\ &+ J_2(\beta)[\cos((\omega_c + 2\omega_m)t) + \cos((\omega_c - 2\omega_m)t)] \\ &+ J_3(\beta)[\cos((\omega_c + 3\omega_m)t) + \cos((\omega_c - 3\omega_m)t)] \\ &+ J_4(\beta)[\cos((\omega_c + 4\omega_m)t) + \cos((\omega_c - 4\omega_m)t)] \\ &+ J_5(\beta)[\cos((\omega_c + 5\omega_m)t) + \cos((\omega_c - 5\omega_m)t)] \end{aligned} \tag{11.6}$$

At first inspection, this result appears quite complicated. However, it is evident that the numerical values of the Bessel terms tend to zero as n becomes large. For example, let $\beta = 2\pi f_d/\omega_m = 1$, then $J_0(1) = 0.7852$, $J_1(1) = 0.4401$, $J_2(1) = 0.1149$, $J_3(1) = 0.01956$, $J_4(1) = 0.002477$, $J_5(1) = 0.0002498$,

$J_6(1) = 0.00002094$, etc. All the Bessel constants $J_n(1)$ for $n \geq 4$ contribute less than 1% together to the $y_m(t)$ spectrum, so we can neglect them. Thus, the practical bandwidth of the FM carrier, $y_m(t)$, for $\beta = 1$ is $\pm 3\omega_m$ around the carrier frequency, ω_c. In general, as β increases, so does the effective bandwidth of the FM $y_m(t)$. For example, when $\beta = 5$, the bandwidth becomes $\pm 8\omega_m$ around ω_c, and when $\beta = 10$, the bandwidth required is $\pm 14\omega_m$ around ω_c (Clarke and Hess 1971).

In the case of NBFM, $\beta << 1$. Thus, the modulated carrier can be written as

$$y_m(t) = A\cos[\overset{\alpha}{\omega_c t} + (K_f/\omega_m)\sin(\overset{\beta}{\omega_m t})] \tag{11.7a}$$

$$\downarrow$$

$$\begin{aligned} y_m(t) &= A\{\cos(\omega_c t)\cos[\beta\sin(\omega_m t)] - \sin(\omega_c t)\sin[\beta\sin(\omega_m t)]\} \\ &\cong A\{\cos(\omega_c t)(1) - \sin(\omega_c t)\sin[\beta\sin(\omega_m t)]\} \\ &= A\{\cos(\omega_c t) - (\beta/2)[\cos((\omega_c - \omega_m)t) - \cos((\omega_c + \omega_m)t)]\} \end{aligned} \tag{11.7b}$$

With the exception of signs of the sideband terms, the NBFM spectrum is very similar to the spectrum of an AM carrier (Zeimer and Tranter 1990); sum and difference frequency sidebands are produced around a central carrier.

The spectrum of a *double-sideband suppressed carrier* (DSBSCM) signal is given by

$$y_m(t) = A\,m_o\cos(\omega_m t)\cos(\omega_c t) = (A\,m_o/2)[\cos((\omega_c + \omega_m)t) + \cos((\omega_c - \omega_m)t)] \tag{11.8}$$

That is, ideally the information is contained in the two sidebands, and *there is no carrier.* DSBSCM is widely used in instrumentation and measurement systems. For example, it is the natural result when a light beam is chopped in a photonic instrument such as a spectrophotometer and also results when a Wheatstone bridge is given AC (carrier) excitation and nulled, then one (or more) arm resistances is slowly varied in time around its null value (see Figure 11.1a). DSBSCM is also present

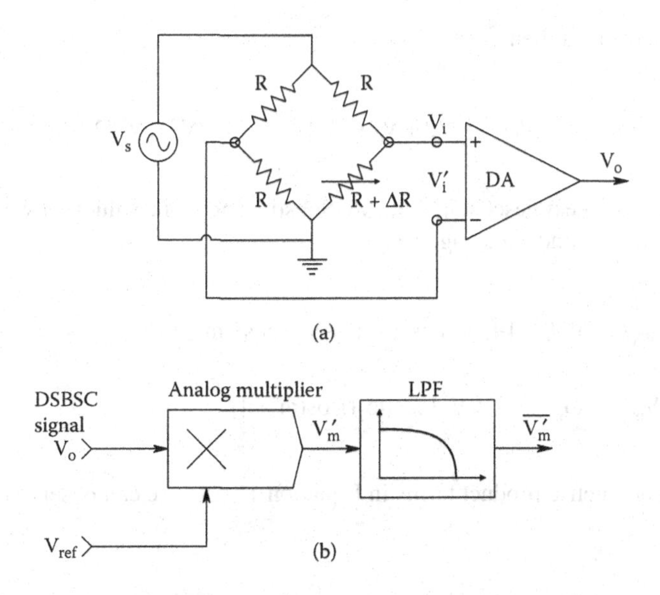

FIGURE 11.1 (a) A one active-arm Wheatstone bridge. When AC excitation is used, the output is a double-sideband, suppressed-carrier modulated (DSBSCM) carrier. (b) An analog multiplier and a low-pass filter are used to demodulate the DSBSCM signal.

at the output of an LVDT (linear variable differential transformer) length sensor as the core is moved in and out (Northrop 2005). Figure 11.1b illustrates a simple system used to demodulate DSBSCM signals.

11.3 IMPLEMENTATION OF AM

11.3.1 INTRODUCTION

Equation 11.1b indicates that *multiplication* is inherent in the AM process. In practice, an actual analog multiplier can be used, or effective multiplication can be realized by passing $v_c(t)$ and $[1 + m(t)]$ through a square-law nonlinearity, such as a field-effect transistor. Note that in Equation 11.1b, $|m(t)| \leq 1$ so $[1 + m(t)] \geq 0$. If $[1 + m(t)]$ were to go < 0, there would be an 180° phase-shift in the AM output, which is an undesirable condition called *overmodulation*. Overmodulation also occurs when the modulator output stage is driven so hard that the output transistor stage is cutoff, giving zero output for several carrier cycles. Hard cutoff also distorts the AM carrier and produces unwanted harmonics in the demodulated signal.

There are many types of circuits which have been devised to do AM. Clearly, we cannot examine all of them here; several representative circuits are described in the next section.

11.3.2 SOME AMPLITUDE MODULATION CIRCUITS

Figure 11.2a illustrates the use of a tuned, grounded source JFET amplifier as a square-law, amplitude modulator. Figure 11.2b illustrates the power-law, i_D vs v_{GS} curve for the JFET. The gate-source voltage (v_{GS}) is the sum of a DC bias voltage that places the quiescent operating point of the JFET at the center of its saturated channel region, plus the carrier signal and the modulating signal. In this and the other examples below, $\omega_m << \omega_c$ is asserted. Let the JFET gate-source voltage be

$$v_{GS} = V_p/2 + V_c \cos(\omega_c t) + V_m \cos(\omega_m t), \quad V_p = -4V. \tag{11.9}$$

The JFET's drain current is then

$$i_D = (I_{DSS}/V_P^2)\{V_P - [V_P/2 + V_c + V_m]\}^2 = (I_{DSS}/V_P^2)\{V_P/2 + V_c + V_m\}^2 \tag{11.10a}$$

Note that if $v_c = v_m = 0$, the quiescent $i_D = I_{DSS}/4$. Substituting in the values for v_c and v_m in Equation 11.9 into Equation 11.10A and squaring, we get

$$i_D = (I_{DSS}/V_p^2)\{V_p^2/4 + V_c^2 \cos^2(\omega_c t) + V_m^2 \cos^2(\omega_m t) - V_p[\overset{v_c}{V_c \cos(\omega_c t)}$$

$$+ \overset{v_m}{V_m \cos(\omega_m t)}] + 2V_c V_m[\cos(\omega_c t)\cos(\omega_m t)]\} \tag{11.10b}$$

Expanding the trigonometric product terms in Equation 11.10B, we can observe the harmonics and sideband products:

$$i_D = (I_{DSS}/V_p^2)\{V_p^2/4 + V_c^2 \tfrac{1}{2}[1 + \cos(2\omega_c t)] + V_m^2 \tfrac{1}{2}[1 + \cos(2\omega_m t]$$

$$- V_p[V_c \cos(\omega_c t) + V_m \cos(\omega_m t)] + V_c V_m[\cos((\omega_c + \omega_m)t) + \cos((\omega_c - \omega_m)t)]\} \tag{11.10c}$$

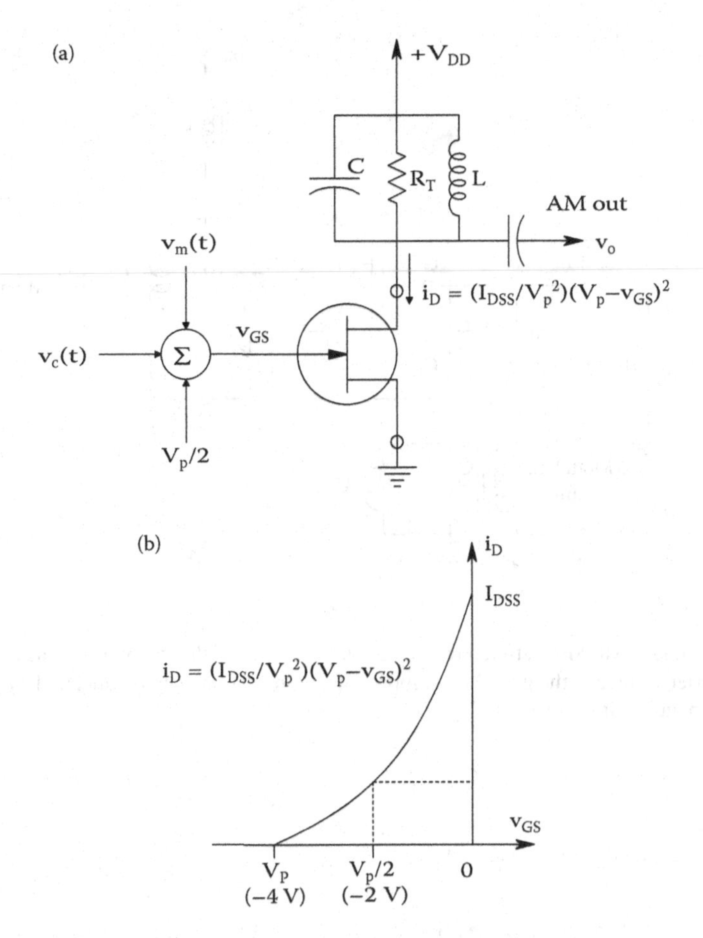

FIGURE 11.2 (a) Schematic of a tuned-output JFET square-law amplitude modulator. (b) Square-law drain current versus gate-source voltage curve for a JFET operated under saturated drain conditions $[v_{DS} > |v_{GS} + V_P|]$.

Equation 11.10c shows that the drain current has three DC terms, terms at ω_m and $2\omega_m$, terms at ω_c and $2\omega_c$, and the sideband terms at $(\omega_c + \omega_m)$ and $(\omega_c - \omega_m)$. The DC terms are eliminated by the output coupling capacitor. The parallel RLC "tank" circuit is resonant around ω_c, and so selects the ω_c and sideband terms. The AM output voltage is approximately

$$v_o \cong -R_T(I_{DSS}/V_p^2)\{-V_pV_c\cos(\omega_c t) + V_cV_m[\cos((\omega_c + \omega_m)t) + \cos((\omega_c - \omega_m)t)]\} \quad (11.11)$$

That is, the resonant circuit attenuates all frequencies not immediately around ω_c.

Figure 11.3 illustrates the architecture of a class C, MOSFET RF power amplifier with a high Q output resonant circuit. The modulating signal, $v_m(t)$, is added to a DC gate bias and the RF carrier source. The radio-frequency chokes (RFC) are inductors with very high reactance around ω_c; they pass currents from DC to ω_{mmax}. The principle of sideband generation is very similar to the JFET example above. Both JFETs and MOSFETs have square-law i_D vs v_{GS} curves.

The BJT circuit of Figure 11.4 illustrates yet another amplitude modulator architecture. Q3 and Q4 modulate the collector currents in Q1 and Q1 by changing the g_m of these transistors, for example, $g_{m1} = I_{CQ1} / V_T$. The operating points of Q1 and Q2 are identical; they are affected by $I_{C4} = I_{E1} + I_{E2}$, which is in turn a function of the modulating signal, $v_m(t)$. Clarke and Hesse (1971) gave a detailed analysis of this transconductance modulator.

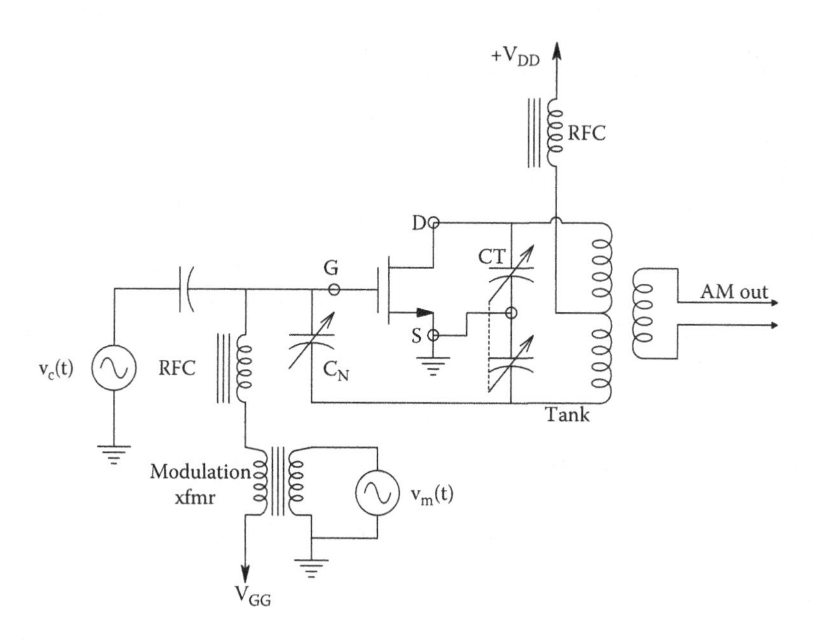

FIGURE 11.3 A class C MOSFET, tuned RF power amplifier in which the low-frequency modulating signal is added to the carrier voltage at the gate. Miller input capacitance at the gate is cancelled by positive feedback through the small neutralizing capacitor, C_N.

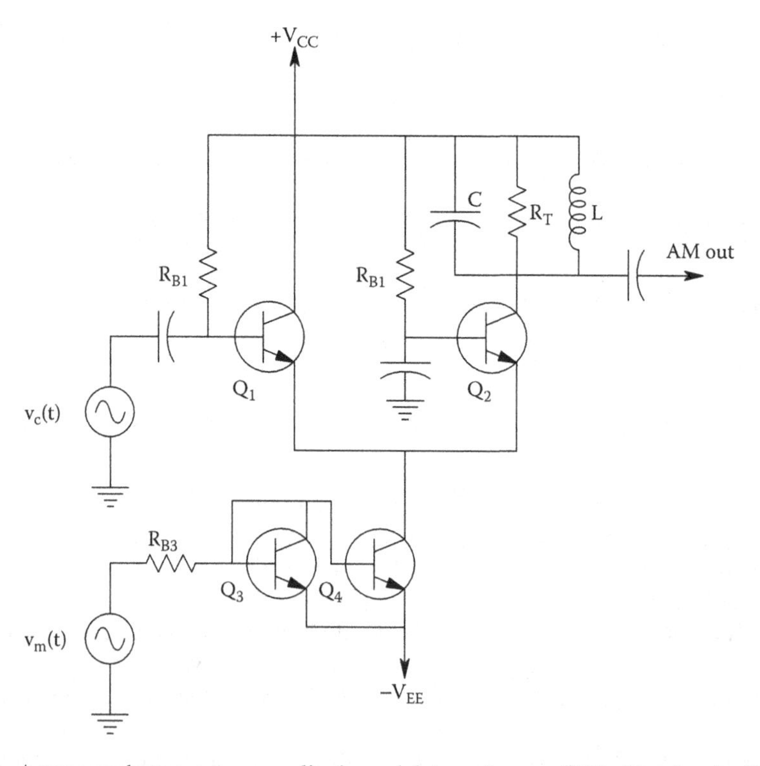

FIGURE 11.4 A transconductance-type amplitude modulator using *npn* BJTs. The circuit effectively multiplies the carrier by the modulating signal, producing an AM output.

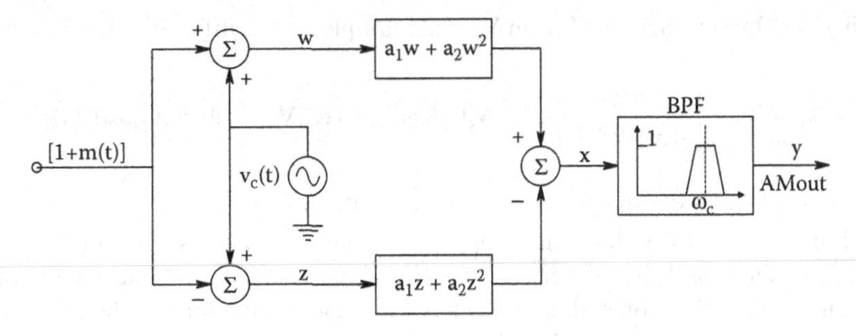

FIGURE 11.5 Block diagram of a quarter-square multiplier used for amplitude modulation.

Still another approach to AM generation is illustrated in the block diagram of Figure 11.5. This system is basically a *quarter square multiplier,* except the nonlinearities contain a linear (a_1) term as well as the square-law (a_2) term. The signals are as follows:

$$w(t) = V_c \cos(\omega_c t) + [1 + m(t)], \ |m_{max}| \leq 1 \tag{11.12a}$$

$$z(t) = V_c \cos(\omega_c t) - [1 + m(t)] \tag{11.12b}$$

$$u(t) = a_1 V_c \cos(\omega_c t) + a_1[1 + m(t)] + a_2\{V_c^2 \cos^2(\omega_c t) + 2V_c[1 + m(t)]\cos(\omega_c t) + [1 + 2m(t) + m^2(t)]\} \tag{11.12c}$$

$$v(t) = a_1 V_c \cos(\omega_c t) + a_1[1 + m(t)] + a_2\{V_c^2 \cos^2(\omega_c t) - 2V_c[1 + m(t)]\cos(\omega_c t) + [1 + 2m(t) + m^2(t)]\} \tag{11.12d}$$

$$x = u - v \tag{11.12e}$$

$$x(t) = 2a_1 + 2a_1 m_c \cos(\omega_m t) + [(4a_2 V_c)\cos(\omega_c t) + (4a_2 V_c)1/2\{\cos[(\omega_c + \omega_m)t] + \cos[(\omega_c - \omega_m)t]\} \tag{11.12}$$

The bandpass filter around ($\omega_c - \omega_m$) to ($\omega_c + \omega_m$) selects the AM output and blocks DC and the ω_m signal. Many other AM circuits exist; some are practical for high-power RF output, and others assume the AM output will be amplified by a linear RF amplifier.

Double-sideband, suppressed carrier modulation (DSBSCM) is another form of AM in which there is little or no carrier frequency power in the output spectrum. Ideally, DSBSCM follows Equation 11.1c. That is, DSBSCM results as the product of a low-frequency modulating signal multiplying a high-frequency carrier voltage.

Many processes are inherent generators of DSBSCM. For example, see Figure 11.1a for a Wheatstone bridge initially nulled, whose output depends on $\Delta R/R$. The bridge is given AC excitation so that its sensitivity is enhanced. Let us develop an expression for V_o using voltage-divider relations:

$$V_i = V_s \frac{R + \Delta R}{2R + \Delta R} \tag{11.13}$$

$$V_i' = V_s \frac{R}{2R} \tag{11.14}$$

The output is found by subtracting V_i' from V_i, and multiplying the difference by the DA's gain, K_D.

$$V_o = K_D V_s \left[\frac{\Delta R}{4R + 2\Delta R} \right] \cong K_D V_s [\Delta R/4R] = (K_D V_s/4R)[\Delta R(t)\cos(\omega_c t)] \qquad (11.15)$$

The quantity in the brackets is the DSBSCM product. $\Delta R(t)$ varies at ω_m.

DSBSCM also occurs for light-beam chopping in photonic systems, and for the output of the linear, variable differential transformer (LVDT) linear position sensor. A schematic of an LVDT is shown in Figure 11.6. Seen on end, an LVDT is a cylinder with a tube in the center running the length of the cylinder. In the center of the tube slides a cylindrical, high-permeability, magnetic core that couples magnetic flux from the excitation coil to the two secondary coils, which are wound in opposite directions with the same number of turns. When the core is centered (x = 0), equal flux intercepts the winding of both secondary coils, and the net output EMF is zero. If the core position is up ($x = +x_m$), most of the flux is coupled to the upper secondary coil, and $|V_o|$ is maximum,

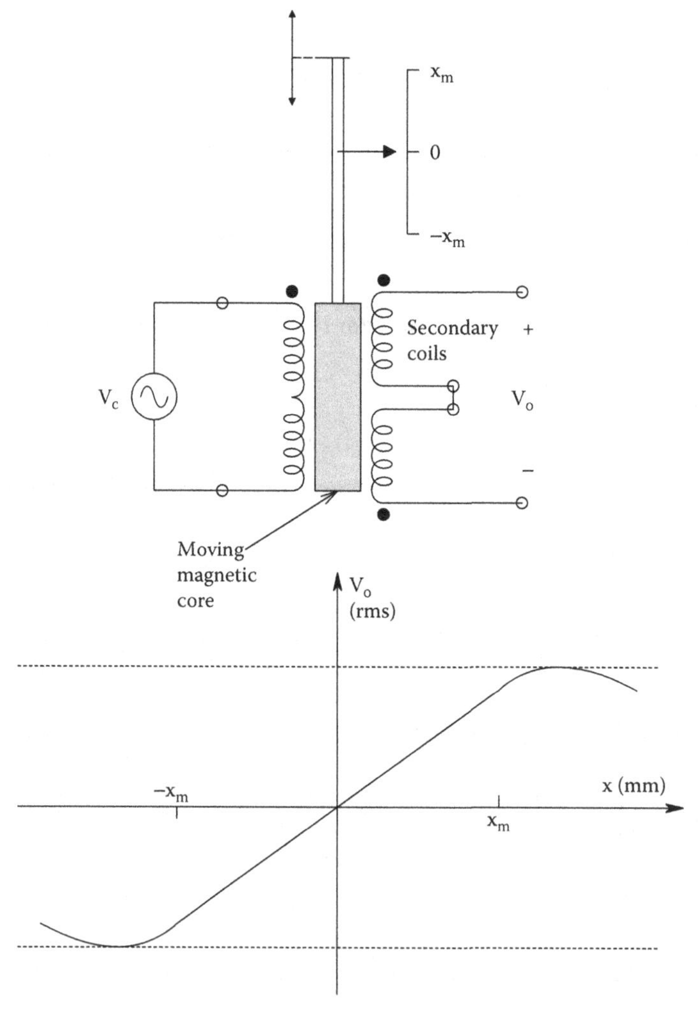

FIGURE 11.6 *Top:* Cross sectional schematic of a linear variable differential transformer (LVDT). The output is a DSBSC modulated carrier. *Bottom:* Transfer curve of the peak voltage output of the LVDT vs. core position. A 180° phase shift in the output is signified by $V_o(x) < 0$.

having the same phase as V_c. If $x = -x_m$, $|V_o|$ is maximum and the phase is 180° from V_o with $x = +x_m$. In general, the linear part of the output can be written as

$$V_o = N(\dot{\varphi}_u - \dot{\varphi}_l) = Kx(t)V_c \cos(\omega_c t) \quad (11.16)$$

where $\dot{\varphi}_u$ is the time rate of change of the AC flux intercepting the N turns of the upper secondary coil, and K is the slope of the linear V_o vs x curve.

Refer to Figure 11.5. If one replaces [1 + m(t)] by simply $v_m(t)$, it is easy to see that the output x(t) is given by

$$\begin{aligned} x(t) &= u(t) - v(t) = 2a_1 v_m(t) + 4a_2 v_c(t) v_m(t) \\ &= 2a_1 V_m \cos(\omega_m t) + 2a_2 V_c V_m [\cos((\omega_c + \omega_m)t) + \cos((\omega_c - \omega_m)t)] \end{aligned} \quad (11.17)$$

The BPF centered on ω_c removes the $2a_1 V_m \cos(\omega_m t)$ term, leaving the DSBSCM output, so

$$y(t) = 2a_2 V_c V_m [\cos((\omega_c + \omega_m)t) + \cos((\omega_c - \omega_m)t)] \quad (11.18)$$

In summary, DSBSCM is widely encountered in all phases of instrumentation and measurement systems; it is simply the direct result of multiplying the carrier times the modulating signal.

11.4 GENERATION OF PHASE AND FREQUENCY MODULATION

11.4.1 Introduction

Phase- and *frequency-modulation* are subsets of *angle modulation,* which has the general form

$$y_m(t) = A \cos[\omega_c t + \Phi(t)] \quad (11.19)$$

The phase argument of the modulated carrier is $[\omega_c t + \Phi(t)]$ radians, and the frequency of the modulated carrier is $[\omega_c + \dot{\Phi}]$r/s. When $\Phi(t) = K_f \int^t m(t)\, dt$, we have FM, when $\Phi(t) = K_p\, m(t)$, PhM is the result. Many practical angle modulation and demodulation circuits have been developed since Edwin H. Armstrong invented frequency modulation in 1933. Like many innovations in technology, FM radio did not really "catch on" at once; it did not become widely used commercially until after World War II (Stark et al. 1988). A useful, practical source of PhM and FM circuits can be found in the ARRL's *Radio Amateur's Handbook*.

11.4.2 NBFM Generation by Phase-Lock Loop

Figure 11.7 illustrates at the systems level the processes of generating NBFM using a *phase-lock loop* (PLL) IC. From a system's viewpoint, a PLL is a type 1, negative feedback system that continually tries to match the phase of the periodic output of a voltage-controlled oscillator (VCO) to the phase of its input signal (Northrop 1990). A basic PLL consists of a phase detector, a loop filter, and a VCO. The VCO output may be sinusoidal or digital. (PLLs are covered in detail in Chapter 12.) The frequency output of the VCO is given by: $\omega_o = K_v V_c$. However, it is the VCO's *phase* that is compared with the carrier's input phase by the *phase detector* (PhD) module having output, $V_p = K_P(\theta_i - \theta_o)$. Note that phase is the integral of frequency: $\theta_o = V_c(K_v/s)$. When a PLL is *locked,* both the frequency and phase of the VCO equal the frequency and phase of the input signal.

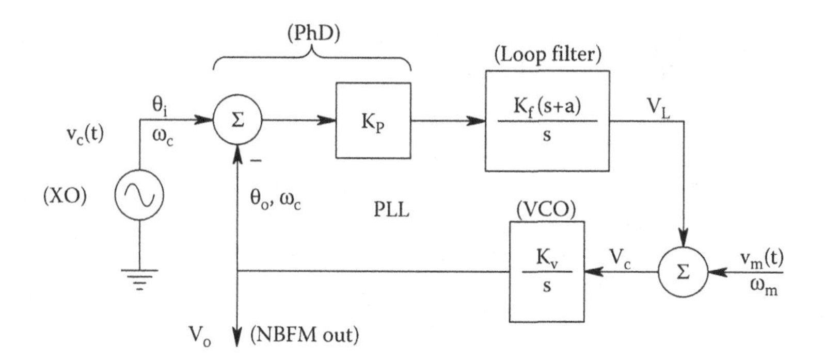

FIGURE 11.7 Block diagram of a phase-lock loop used to generate narrow-band FM (NBFM).

Let us examine the transfer function between the VCO's output phase and the modulating signal, $v_m(t)$:

$$\frac{\theta_o}{V_m}(s) = \frac{K_v/s}{1+K_pK_fK_v(s+a)/s^2} \tag{11.20}$$

To optimize the dynamics of the closed-loop PLL, it is prudent to make $K_P K_f K_v = 2a$ (Northrop 1990). Thus, the frequency response of the output phase can be written as

$$\frac{\boldsymbol{\theta}_o}{\mathbf{V}_m}(j\omega) = \frac{j\omega K_v/2a^2}{(j\omega)^2/2a^2+(j\omega)/a+1} \tag{11.21}$$

Note that ω in the frequency response function above is the radian frequency of the modulating signal. Now for $\omega_m > 2a\sqrt{2}$, the VCO's output phase is approximately

$$\frac{\boldsymbol{\theta}_o}{\mathbf{V}_m}(j\omega_m) \cong \frac{K_v}{j\omega_m} \tag{11.22}$$

Equation 11.22 implies that the phase of the constant-amplitude VCO output is proportional to the integral of $v_m(t)$, which is the condition present in FM. The VCO frequency when $v_m(t) = 0$ is simply that of the carrier input oscillator (XO), ω_c. The PLL is a compact, useful way of generating NBFM for a variety of communications applications. The NBFM output of the PLL can be conditioned by a linear RF amplifier to boost its power level, or can be amplified by a frequency multiplier to convert it to wide-band FM (Stark et al. 1988). Note that if the modulation input signal to the PLL is the *derivative* of $v_m(t)$, PhM results for $\omega_m > 2a\sqrt{2}$ r/s.

Figure 11.8 illustrates another PLL angle modulator system. Inspection of the figure gives us the transfer function for the phase, θ_o, of the VCO output as a function of V_m:

$$\frac{\boldsymbol{\theta}_o}{\mathbf{V}_m}(s) = \frac{K_v/s}{1+K_pK_fK_v/[s(s+b)]} = \frac{K_v(s+b)}{s^2+sb+K_pK_fK_v} \tag{11.23}$$

To make the closed loop system have a damping factor of $\xi = 0.707$, it can be shown that the gain product, $K_P K_f K_v$, must equal $b^2/2$. Thus, the frequency response function of the PLL angle modulator can be written as

$$\frac{\boldsymbol{\theta}_o}{\mathbf{V}_m}(j\omega) = \frac{(2Kv/b)(j\omega/b+1)}{(j\omega)^2/(b^2/2)+j\omega 2/b+1} \tag{11.24}$$

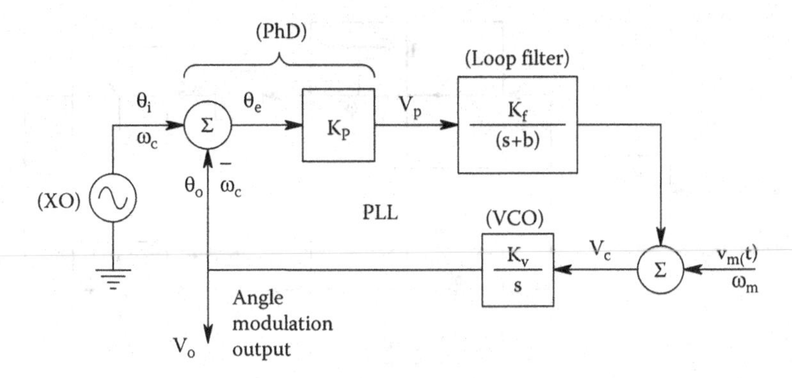

FIGURE 11.8 A PLL used for a frequency-dependent angle modulator.

In the modulating signal frequency range from $0 \leq \omega_m \leq b/2$ r/s, $\theta_o/V_m \cong 2K_v/b$. That is, θ_o is proportional to V_m, and we have *phase modulation*. In the frequency range, $2b/\sqrt{2} \leq \omega_m \leq \infty$, the VCO output phase is given by

$$\frac{\boldsymbol{\theta}_o}{\mathbf{V}_m} = K_v/(j\omega_m) \quad (11.25)$$

Because the phase is proportional to the integral of $v_m(t)$, we have FM again taking place in this frequency range.

While the PLL method of generating PhM and NBFM can produce a modulated sinusoidal carrier, it is often desired to generate an angle-modulated TTL wave or pulse train. Such TTL FM can drive a fiber optic, pulsed laser data transmission system.

11.4.3 Integral Pulse Frequency Modulation as a Means of FM

Consider *integral pulse frequency modulation* (IPFM). A systems model for a *two-sided IPFM system* is shown in Figure 11.9. A positive modulating signal, v_m, is integrated; the integrator output, v, is sent to two threshold nonlinearities. When v reaches the positive threshold, φ_+, the nonlinearity's output, w^+, jumps to +1. This step is differentiated to make a positive unit impulse at time t_k, $\delta(t - t_k)$. This impulse is fed back, given a weight of φ/K_i, and subtracted from the input to form $e(t_k) = v_m(t_k) - (\varphi/K_i)\delta(t - t_k)$. When integrated, this $e(t_k)$ resets the integrator output to zero, and the process repeats. If $v_m < 0$, v approaches the negative threshold, φ^-. When φ^- is reached, the output from the two-sided IPFM system is a negative unit impulse which is also fed-back to reset the integrator. The net output from the two-sided IPFM system can be written as a superposition of the positive and negative impulse outputs:

$$y(t) = \sum_{k=1}^{\infty} \delta(t - t_k) - \sum_{j=1}^{\infty} \delta(t - t_j) \quad (11.26)$$

where $\{t_k\}$ are the times that + pulses are emitted and $\{t_j\}$ are the times that negative pulses occur. A simpler way of dealing with negative $v_m(t)$ is to add a DC bias V_B to $v_m(t)$ so $[V_B + v_m(t)]$ is always > 0. Now the negative pulse generation and integrator reset channel can be eliminated. Many low-frequency physiological signals such as body temperature and blood pressure are always positive, so the negative pulse channel on the IPFM system can be deleted, and V_B set to 0 in a one-sided system.

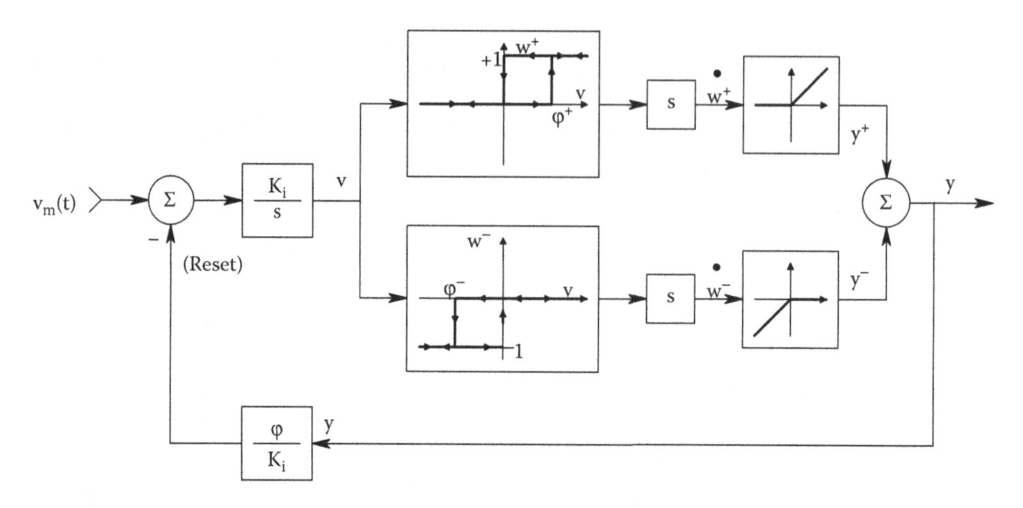

FIGURE 11.9 Block diagram of a two-sided, integral pulse frequency modulation (IPFM) system.

Note that a one-sided IPFM system behaves like a classical pulse FM system, given a non-negative modulating signal input and *zero carrier frequency.* If the modulating signal is small, the output pulse rate will be low, and the IPFM system will be poor at following high-frequency components of $v_m(t)$. By establishing a carrier frequency with input bias voltage, V_B, one has a classic pulse FM system with a carrier frequency, r_c pps. A carrier FM system is better able to follow high-frequency changes in small v_m.

One-sided IPFM can be described mathematically by a set of integral equations:

$$v = \int K_i e(t)dt \tag{11.27}$$

$$\varphi = \int_{t_{k-1}}^{t_k} K_i\ e(t)dt,\ K = 2, 3, \ldots, \infty \tag{11.28}$$

where K_i is the integrator gain; e(t) is its input; $e(t) = [v_m(t) + V_B]$ for $t_{k-1} < t < t_k$. t_k is the time the kth output pulse occurs. $v(t_{k-1}) = 0$, due to the feedback pulse resetting the integrator. Thus, Equation 11.28 can be rewritten as

$$r_k = \frac{1}{t_k - t - 1} = (K_i/\varphi)\frac{1}{t_k - t_{k-1}}\int_{t_{k-1}}^{t_k} e(t)\ dt,\ k = 2, 3 \ldots \tag{11.29}$$

Here r_k is the kth *element of instantaneous frequency,* defined as the reciprocal of the interval between the kth and (k − 1)th output pulses, $\tau_k \equiv (t_k - t_{k-1})$. So the kth element of instantaneous (pulse) frequency is given by

$$r_k \equiv 1/\tau_k = (K_i/\varphi)\{\bar{e}\}_{\tau k} \tag{11.30}$$

If v_m is zero and the input to the IPFM system is a constant $V_B \geq 0$, $r_c = (K_i/\varphi)\ V_B$ pps. That is, the IPFM output carrier center frequency, r_c, is proportional to the bias, V_B.

As an example of finding the pulse emission times for a one-sided IPFM system, consider the input, $v_m(t) = (4e^{-7t})\,U(t)$, the threshold $\varphi = 0.025$ V, $K_i = 1$ and $V_B = 0$. The first pulse is emitted at t_1, which is found from the definite integral:

$$\varphi = \int_0^{t1} v_m(t)dt \rightarrow 0.025 = \int_0^{t1} \frac{4(e^{-7t})(-7)dt}{(-7)} \rightarrow \frac{0.025(-7)}{4} = (e^{-7t1} - 1) \rightarrow \tag{11.31}$$

$$e^{-7t1} = 1 - \frac{7 \times 0.025}{4} = 0.95625 \xrightarrow{\ln(*)} -7t_1 = -4.47359 \times 10^{-2} \tag{11.32}$$

The time the first pulse is emitted, t_1, is found to be at 6.391×10^{-3} s.

The general pulse emission time, t_k, is found by recursion. For example, once t_1 is known, t_2 is found by solving

$$\varphi = \int_{t1}^{t2} v_m(t)dt \tag{11.33}$$

In this simple case, it is found that $t_2 = 13.081$ E–3 seconds. A general formula for t_k is found for this problem by logical induction:

$$t_k = (-1/7)\ln\left[1 - \frac{k \times 7 \times 0.025}{4}\right] \tag{11.34}$$

From Equation 11.34, one sees that t_k is only defined for a positive ln [*] argument. That is, for

$$k \le \frac{4}{7 \times 0.025} = 22.875 \tag{11.35}$$

Thus, $k_{max} = 22$; only 22 pulses are emitted.

Demodulation of IPFM positive pulse trains can be done by passing the pulses through a low-pass filter, or actually calculating the pulse train's instantaneous frequency by taking the reciprocal of the time interval between any two pulses and holding that value until the next pulse [(k + 1)th] occurs in the sequence, then repeating the operation. Stated mathematically, instantaneous pulse frequency demodulation (IPFD) can be written as

$$\hat{v}_m(t) = \sum_{k=2}^{\infty} r_k\{U(t - t_k) - U(t - t_{k+1})\} \tag{11.36}$$

where

$$r_k \equiv 1/\tau_k = \frac{1}{t_k - t_{k-1}}, \quad k = 2, 3, \ldots$$

is the kth element of instantaneous frequency, and $\hat{v}_m(t)$ is analog output of the IPFM demodulator.

Note that two pulses (k = 2) are required to define the first pulse *interval.* $\hat{v}_m(t)$ is a series of steps, the height of each being the (previous) r_k. Note that the IPFD system is not limited to the demodulation of IPFM, it has been experimentally applied as a descriptor to actual neural spike signals (Northrop 2001).

11.5 DEMODULATION OF MODULATED SINUSOIDAL CARRIERS

11.5.1 Introduction

Of equal importance in the discussion of modulation is the process of *demodulation* or *detection*, in which the modulating signal, $v_m(t)$, is recovered from the modulated carrier, $y_m(t)$. There are generally several circuit architectures that can be used to modulate a given type of modulated signal, and several ways to demodulate it. In the case of AM (or single-sideband AM), the signal recovery process is called *detection.*

11.5.2 Detection of AM Signals

There are several practical means of *AM detection* (Clarke and Hess 1971, Chapter 10). One simple form of AM detection is to rectify and low-pass filter $y_m(t)$. Because rectification is difficult at high radio frequencies, *heterodyning* or mixing the incoming high-frequency AM signal with a local oscillator (in the receiver) whose frequency is separated by a fixed interval, Δf, from that of the incoming signal produces mixing frequencies of $(f_c - f_{lo}) = \Delta f$. Δf is called the intermediate frequency of the receiver and is typically 50–455 kHz, or 10.7 MHz in commercial FM receivers. High-frequency selectivity IF transformers are used that have tuned primary and secondary windings. Very high-IF frequency selectivity can be obtained with piezoelectric crystal filters or *surface acoustic wave* (SAW) tuned IF filters.

Another form of AM detection passes $y_m(t)$ through a square-law nonlinearity followed by a low-pass filter. However, the square-law detector suffers from the disadvantage that it generates a second harmonic component of the recovered modulating signal.

A third way to demodulate an AM carrier, of the form given by Equation 11.1b, is to mix it (multiply it) by a sinusoidal signal of the same frequency and phase as the carrier component of the $y_m(t)$. A phase-lock loop system architecture can be used for this purpose; see Figure 11.10 (Northrop 1990). This PLL system uses three multiplicative mixers. The AM input after RF amplification is

$$x_1 = A[1 + m(t)]\sin(\omega_c t + \theta_c) \quad (11.38)$$

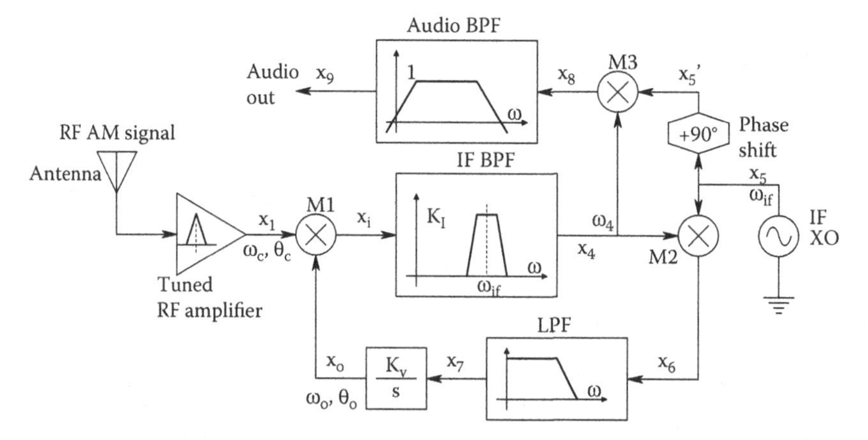

FIGURE 11.10 Block diagram of a PLL system used to demodulate AM audio signals. Note that three mixers (multipliers) are used; M_1 is the quadrature phase detector of the PLL.

Mixer M1 effectively multiplies $x_1 \times x_o$. (x_o is the output of the PLL's VCO.) Thus,

$$x_1 = A[1+m(t)]\sin(\omega_c t+\theta_c)\times X_o\cos(\omega_o+\theta_o)$$
$$=[AX_o[1+m(t)/2]\{\sin[\omega_c+\omega_o)t+\theta_c+\theta_o]+\sin[\omega_c-\omega_o)t+\theta_c-\theta_o]\} \quad (11.39)$$

The IF bandpass filter selects the second term which has frequency close to ω_{if} when the PLL is near lock. This means that x_4 is

$$x_4 = \{K_i AX_o[1+m(t)]/2\}\ \sin[\omega_c-\omega_o)t+\theta_c-\theta_o] \quad (11.40)$$

Also, the output of the crystal-controlled oscillator (XO) is

$$x_5 = X_5\cos(\omega_{if}t) \quad (11.41)$$

Mathematically, one forms the product, $x_6 = x_4 \times x_5$:

$$x_6 = [K_i AX_o[1+m(t)]/2]\ \sin[\omega_c-\omega_o)t+\theta_c-\theta_o]\times X_5\cos(\omega_{if}t) \quad (11.42a)$$

$$x_6 = [K_5\{K_i AX_o[1+m(t)]/4\}\{\sin[(\omega_c-\omega_o+\omega_{if})t+\theta_c-\theta_o]$$
$$+\sin[(\omega_c-\omega_o-\omega_{if})t+\theta_c-\theta_o]\} \quad (11.42b)$$

At lock, $(\omega_c - \omega_o) = \omega_{if}$ r/s, and $(\theta_c - \theta_o) \to 0$. The low-pass filter acts on x_6; its output x_7 is the low-frequency component of x_6. Thus,

$$x_7 = X_5\{K_i AX_o[1+m(t)]/4\}\ \sin[(\omega_c-\omega_o+\omega_{if})t+\theta_c-\theta_o] \quad (11.43)$$

Note that from the conditions above, $x_7 \to 0$ at lock. Now, $x_5' = X_5\sin(\omega_{if}t)$, so x_8 can be written as

$$x_8 = x_4\times x_5' = [K_i AX_o[1+m(t)]/2]\ \sin[(\omega_c-\omega_o)t+\theta_c-\theta_o]\times X_5\sin(\omega_{if}t) \quad (11.44a)$$

$$x_8 = \{X_5K_i AX_o[1+m(t)]/4\}\{\cos[(\theta_c-\theta_o-\omega_{if})t+\theta_c-\theta_o]$$
$$-\cos[(\theta_c-\theta_o]-\cos[(\theta_c-\theta_o+\omega_{if})t+\theta_c-\theta_o]\} \quad (11.44b)$$

Again, at lock,

$$x_8 = [X_5K_i AX_o[1+m(t)]/4]\{\cos(0)-\cos[(2\ \omega_{if})t+\theta_c-\theta_o]\} \quad (11.44c)$$

The bandpass filter cuts the DC term in x_8 given by Equation 11.44C and also the $2\omega_{if}$ term. Thus, the output of the BPF is proportional to the low-frequency modulating signal:

$$x_9 = X_5K_i AX_o m(t)/4 \quad (11.45)$$

Thus, we recover the normalized modulating signal, $[m_o\cos(\omega_m t)]$, times a scaling constant.

A fourth kind of AM demodulation can be done by finding the magnitude of the modulated signal's *analytical signal* (Northrop 2003).

A fifth kind of AM demodulation uses the widely used, rectifier + low-pass filter (average envelope) AM detection system. Figure 11.11a illustrates a low-frequency modulating signal, m(t). Figure 11.11b shows the amplitude-modulated carrier (the sinusoidal carrier is drawn with straight lines for simplicity). Figure 11.11c illustrates the block diagram of a simple, half-wave rectifier circuit followed by a bandpass filter to exclude DC and terms of carrier frequency and higher. The half-wave rectification process can be thought of as multiplying the AM $y_m(t)$ by a 0,1 switching function, SQ(t), in phase with the carrier. Mathematically, this can be stated as

$$y_{mr}(t) = A[1 + m \cos(\omega_c t) \times SQ(t) = A \cos(\omega_c t)\ SQ(t) + A\ m_o \cos(\omega_m t) \cos(\omega_m t) \cos(\omega_c t)\ SQ(t) \tag{11.46}$$

Sq(t) can be written as a *Fourier series* (Northrop 2003):

$$SQ(t) = 1/2 + (2/\pi) \sum_{n=1}^{\infty} (-1)^{n+1} \frac{\cos[(2n-1)\omega_c t]}{(2n-1)} \tag{11.47a}$$

$$\downarrow$$

$$SQ_q(t) = 1/2 + (2/\pi)\ \{\cos(\omega_c t) - (1/3)\cos(3\omega_c t) + (1/5)\cos(5\omega_c t) - \ ...\ \} \tag{11.47b}$$

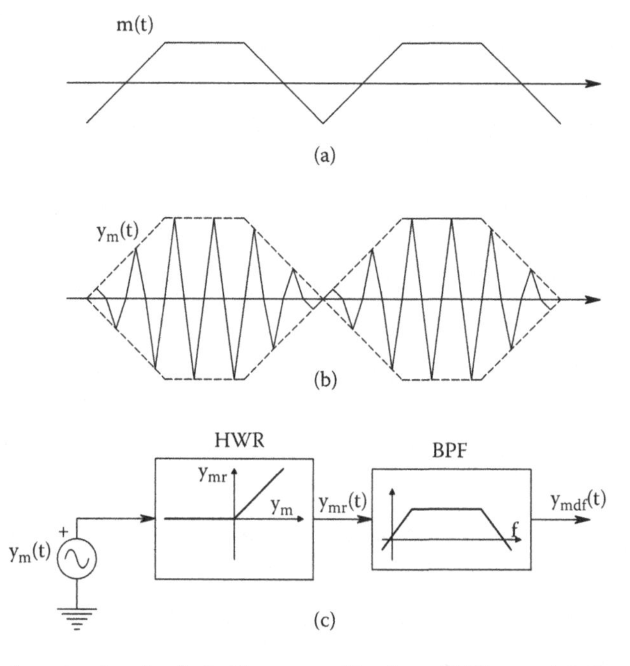

FIGURE 11.11 AM detection by simple half-wave rectification: (a) The modulating signal. (b) The AM carrier (drawn as a triangle wave instead of a sinusoid). (c) An ideal half-wave rectifier followed by an audio bandpass filter.

Now multiply the Fourier series by the terms of Equation 11.46 and examine what happens when we pass the terms of Equation 11.48 through a bandpass filter that attenuates to zero DC and all terms at above $(\omega_c - \omega_m)$.

$$\begin{aligned} y_d(t) = {} & 1/2A\cos(\omega_c t) + (2\pi)A\{\cos^2(\omega_c t) - (1/3)\cos(3\omega_c t)\cos(3\omega_c t) \\ & + (1/5)\cos(\omega_c t)\cos(5\omega_c t) - \ldots\} + (1/2A\, m_o)\cos(\omega_m t)\cos(\omega_c t) \\ & + (2A\, m_o/\pi)\cos(\omega_m t)\cos^2(\omega_c t) - (2A\, m_o/3\pi)\cos(\omega_m t)\cos(\omega_c t)\cos(3\omega_c t) \\ & + (2A\, m_o/5\pi)\cos(\omega_m t)\cos(\omega_c t)\cos(5\omega_c t) \\ & - (2A\, m_o/7\pi)\cos(\omega_m t)\cos(\omega_c t)\cos(7\omega_c t) + \ldots \end{aligned} \quad (11.48)$$

Trigonometric expansions of the form cos(x) cos(y) = (1/2)[cos(x + y) + cos(x − y)] are used. The BPF's output can be shown to be $y_{mdf}(t)$:

$$y_{mdf}(t) = (A/\pi)[m_o \cos(\omega_m t)] \quad (11.49)$$

The BPF output contains a term proportional to the desired $m_o \cos(\omega_m t)$. Since AM radio is usually used to transmit audio signals, which do not extend to zero frequency, the *bandpass filter* blocks the DC but passes modulating signal frequencies. It cuts all frequencies that are harmonics of the carrier frequency ω_c, as well as mixing terms of the form $(n\omega_c \pm \omega_m)$. Thus, $y_{mdf}(t)$ µ m_o $\cos(\omega_m t)$.

Several other AM detection schemes exist, including *peak envelope detection and synchronous detection,* described below in the detection of DSBSCM signals; the interested reader can find a good description of these modes of AM detection in the communications text by Clarke and Hess (1971).

11.5.3 Detection of FM Signals

When it is desired to modulate and transmit signals with a DC component, FM is the desired modulation scheme because a DC signal, V_m, produces a fixed frequency deviation from the carrier at ω_c given by

$$\Delta\omega = K_f V_m \quad (11.50)$$

As in the case of AM, *FM demodulation* can done by several means: The first step in any FM demodulation scheme is to *limit the received signal.* Mathematically, limiting can be represented as passing the sinusoidal FM $y_m(t)$ through a signum function (symmetrical clipper). Mathematically, the clipper output is a square wave of peak height, $y_{mcl}(t) = B\,\mathrm{sgn}[y_m(t)]$. (The $\mathrm{sgn}(y_m)$ function is 1 for $y_m \geq 0$, and −1 for $y_m < 0$.) Clipping removes most unwanted amplitude modulation including noise on the received $y_m(t)$, one reason FM radio is relatively noise free compared to AM. The frequency argument of $y_{mcl}(t)$ is the same as for the FM sinusoidal carrier, i.e., $\omega_{FM} = \omega_c + K_f v_m(t)$. Once limited, there are several means of FM demodulation, including the *phase-shift discriminator,* the *Foster–Seely discriminator,* the *ratio detector, pulse averaging,* and certain *phase-lock loop* circuits (Chirlian 1981; Northrop 1990). It is beyond the scope of this text to describe all of these FM demodulation circuits in detail, so we will first examine the simple *pulse averaging discriminator.* In this FM demodulation means, the limited signal is fed into a one-shot multivibrator that triggers on the rising edge of each cycle of $y_{mcl}(t)$, producing a train of standard TTL pulses, each of fixed width $\delta = \pi/\omega_c$ sec. For simplicity, assume the peak height of each pulse is 5 V, and low is 0 V. Now the average pulse voltage is $v_{av}(t)$:

$$v_{av}(t) = \frac{1}{T}\int_0^{\delta} 5\, dt = \frac{\omega_c + K_f v_m}{\pi}\int_0^{\pi/\omega c} 5\, dt = (5/2)(1 + K_f v_m/\omega_c) \tag{11.51}$$

Thus, recovery of $v_m(t)$, even a DC v_m, requires the linear operation:

$$v_m(t) = [(2/5)v_{av}(t) - 1](\omega_c/K_f) \tag{11.52}$$

In practice, the averaging is done by a low-pass filter with break frequency $\omega_{mmax} << \omega_f << \omega_c$. In *phase modulation,* the modulated carrier is given by

$$y_m(t) = A\cos[\omega_c t + K_p v_m(t)] \tag{11.53}$$

Because the frequency of the PhM carrier is the derivative of its phase, we have

$$\omega_{PhM} = \omega_c + K_p \dot{v}_m(t) \tag{11.54}$$

PhM carriers can be both generated and demodulated using phase-locked loops (Northrop 1990).

Figure 11.12 illustrates an example of a PLL used to recover the modulating signal, $v_m(t)$, in a NBFM carrier. Note that the PLL input is the *phase* of the NBFM signal, θ_i, which is proportional to the integral of $v_m(t)$. The PLL tries to track $\theta_i(t)$, and in doing so generates the VCO control signal, $v_c(t)$, which is of interest. The frequency in the transfer function of the PLL is the frequency of $v_m(t)$, not ω_c. The loop gain of the PLL is

$$A_L(s) = -\frac{K_p K_f K_v}{s(s+b)} \tag{11.55}$$

To give the closed loop PLL a damping of $\xi = 0.707$, it is easy to show using root locus that $K_P K_f K_v = b^2/2$, and the undamped natural frequency of the PLL is $\omega_n = b\sqrt{2}/2$ r/s. The frequency response function for the PLL demodulator can be shown to be

$$\frac{\mathbf{V_c}}{\mathbf{V_m}}(j\omega) = \frac{(K_m/j\omega)\,K_P K_f/(j\omega + b)}{1 + K_P K_f K_v/[j\omega(j\omega + b)]} = \frac{K_m/K_v}{(j\omega)^2/(b^2/2) + j\omega(2/b) + 1} \tag{11.56}$$

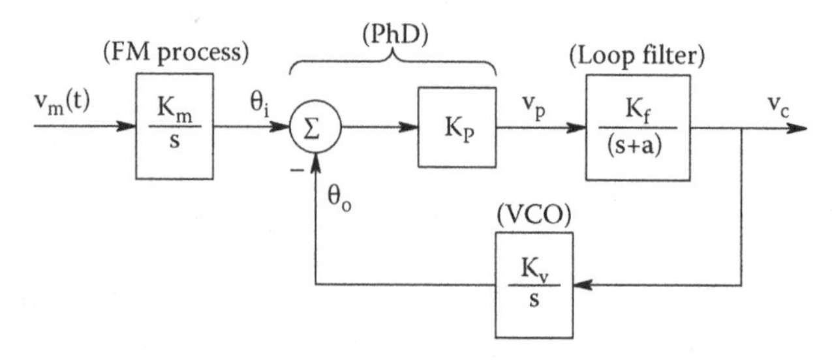

FIGURE 11.12 A PLL used to demodulate a NBFM carrier.

So, at signal frequencies below the loop's $\omega_n = b\sqrt{2}/2$ r/s, the PLL demodulates the NBFM input; the output is proportional to $v_m(t)$. That is,

$$v_c(t) \cong (K_m/K_v)v_m(t) \tag{11.57}$$

Thus, the loop filter output is proportional to $v_m(t)$ for v_m frequencies between zero and about $\omega_n/2$.

11.5.4 Demodulation of DSBSCM Signals

The demodulation of DSBSCM carriers is generally done by a phase-sensitive rectifier (PSR) (also known as a synchronous rectifier) followed by a low-pass filter. One version of this system is shown in Figure 11.13. In this op amp version of a PSR, an analog MOS switch is made to close for the positive half-cycles of the reference signal which has the same frequency and phase as the unmodulated carrier. Figure 11.14 illustrates a low-frequency modulating signal, $v_m(t)$, thence the DSBSCM signal, and finally $V_z(t)$, the unfiltered output of the PSR. Note that "**c**" means the MOS switch is closed, "**o**" means it is open in the circuit of Figure 11.13. The simple op amp low-pass filter also inverts, so its output $\overline{V}_z$ is proportional to $-v_m(t)$.

Another means of demodulating a DSBSC signal is by an *analog multiplier* followed by a LPF. In the latter means, the multiplier output voltage, $V_o'(t)$, is the product of a *reference carrier* and the DSBSCM signal:

$$V_o'(t) = (0.1)B\ \cos(\omega_c t) \times (A\ m_o 2)[\cos((\omega_c + \omega_m)t) + \cos((\omega_c - \omega_m)t)] \tag{11.58}$$

The constant 0.1 is inherent to all IC analog multipliers. By trig identity, noting that $\cos\theta$ is an even function, and the multiplier output can be written as

$$V_o'(t) = (0.1)(A\ m_o B/4)[\cos((2\omega_c + \omega_m)t) + \cos(\omega_m t)] \tag{11.59}$$

After unity-gain low-pass filtering, we have

$$\overline{V}_o'(t) = (0.1)(A\ B/4)m_o \cos(\omega_m t) \tag{11.60}$$

which is certainly proportional to $v_m(t)$.

Still another way to demodulate DSBSC signals is by a special PLL architecture called the Costas loop shown in Figure 11.15 (Northrop 1990). Its successful operation requires that the

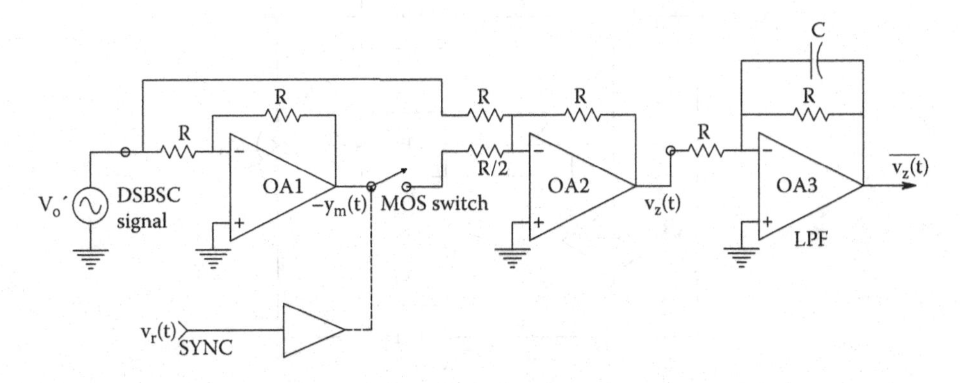

FIGURE 11.13 Schematic of a 3-op amp synchronous (phase-sensitive) rectifier used to demodulate a DSBSC-modulated carrier.

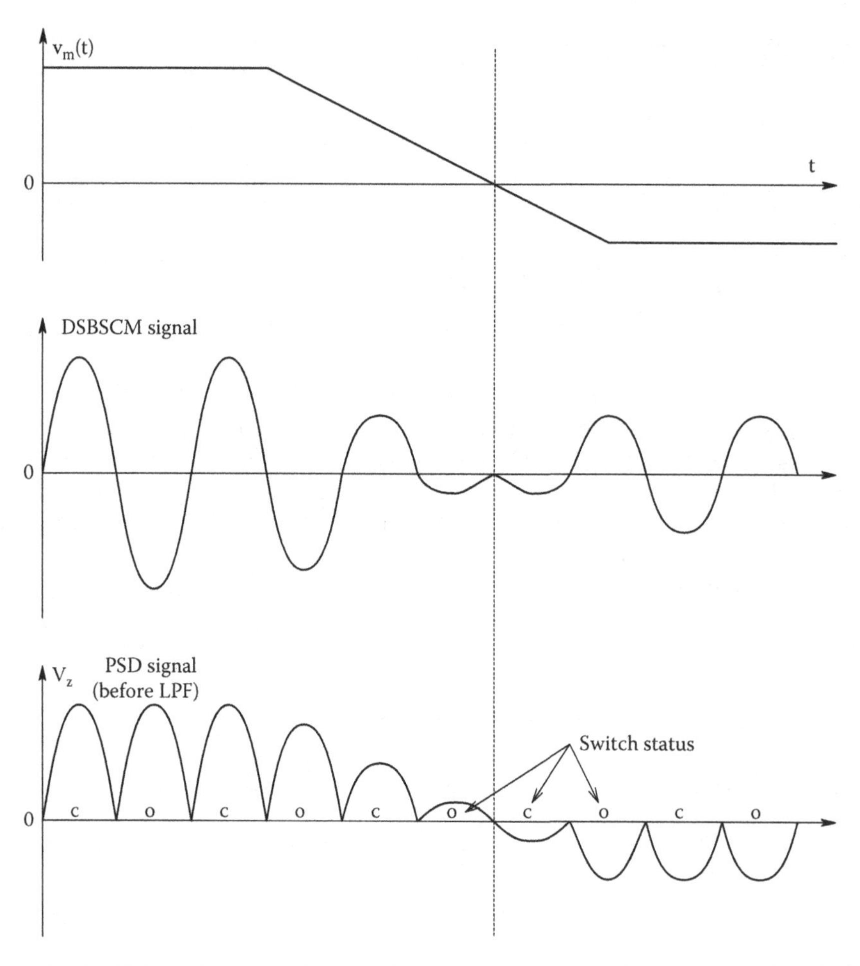

FIGURE 11.14 DSBSC modulation and demodulation by a phase-sensitive detector (PSD). *Top:* The low frequency modulating signal. *Middle:* The DSBSCM AC carrier. *Bottom:* The raw (not low-pass filtered) output of a PSD.

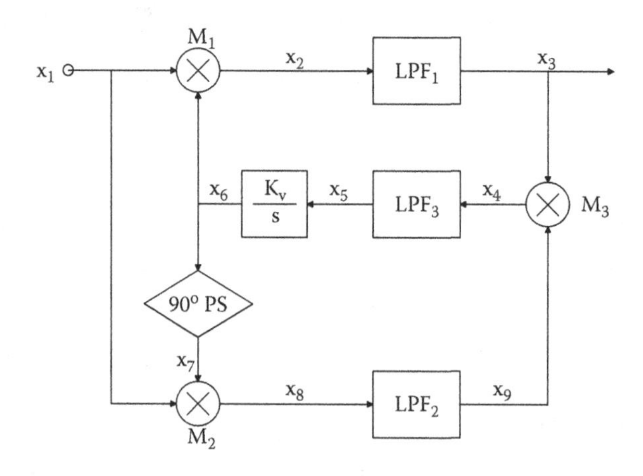

FIGURE 11.15 The Costas phase-lock loop. See text for analysis.

modulating signal, $v_m(t)$, be zero only for short intervals so that the PLL does not loose lock. The input DSBSCM signal can be written as

$$x_1 = v_m(t)\, V_c \cos(\omega_c t + \theta_c) \tag{11.61}$$

The output of the PLL's VCO is

$$x_6 = X_6 \cos(\omega_o t + \theta_o) \tag{11.62}$$

The output of mixer M1 is

$$\begin{aligned} x_2 = x_1 \times x_6 &= v_m(t) V_c X_6 \cos(\omega_c t + \theta_c)\cos(\omega_o t + \theta_o) \\ &= [v_m(t) V_c X_6/2]\{\cos[(\omega_c + \omega_o)t + \theta_c + \theta_o] + \cos[(\omega_c - \omega_o)t + \theta_c - \theta_o]\} \end{aligned} \tag{11.63}$$

At lock, $\omega_o \rightarrow \omega_c$ and $\theta_o \rightarrow \theta_c$, and LPF1 passes only the low-frequency components of x_2. Thus,

$$x_3 = v_m(t) V_c X_6/2 \tag{11.64}$$

which is the desired output. Now examine how the other signals in the Costas loop contribute to its operation. By trigonometric identity, the output of the quadrature phase shifter is

$$x_7 = -X_6 \sin(\omega_o t + \theta_o) \tag{11.65}$$

The output of the second mixer is thus

$$x_8 = -X_6 v_m(t) V_c \sin(\omega_o t + \theta_o)\, \cos(\omega_c t + \theta_c) \tag{11.66a}$$

$$x_8 = [-X_6 v_m(t) V_c/2]\{\sin[(\omega_o + \omega_c)t + \theta_o + \theta_c] + \sin[(\omega_o - \omega_c)t + \theta_o - \theta_c]\} \tag{11.66b}$$

Near lock, at the output of LPF2, we have

$$x_9 \cong [-X_6 v_m(t) V_c/2][(\omega_o - \omega_c)t + \theta_o - \theta_c] \tag{11.67}$$

Thus, the output of mixer M3 is

$$\begin{aligned} x_4 = x_9 \times x_3 &= [-X_6 v_m(t) V_c/2][v_m(t) V_c X_6/2][\omega_o - \omega_c)t + \theta_o - \theta_c] \\ &= -[v_m(t) V_c X_6/2]^2[(\omega_o - \omega_c)t + (\theta_o - \theta_c)] \end{aligned} \tag{11.68}$$

x_4 tends to zero when the loop locks, leaving the VCO with phase $\theta_o = \theta_c$, and $\omega_o = \omega_c$.

11.6 MODULATION AND DEMODULATION OF DIGITAL CARRIERS

11.6.1 Introduction

TTL NBFM carriers can be modulated using *voltage-to-frequency converter* or voltage-controlled oscillator (VCO) integrated circuits. The frequency output of such an IC is given by

$$f_o = k_1 + K_v v_m(t) \text{ Hz.} \tag{11.69}$$

Obviously, $k_1 = f_c$, the unmodulated carrier frequency. Many VCO ICs will give simultaneous TTL, triangle, and sinusoidal wave outputs over a millihertz to over 10 MHz range.

In one design to produce a TTL wave whose *duty cycle is modulated* by $v_m(t)$, we begin with a constant frequency, zero mean, symmetrical triangle wave, $v_T(t)$, as shown in Figure 11.16. $v_T(t)$ is one input to an analog comparator with a TTL output. The other input is $v_m(t)$. As $v_m(t)$ approaches the peak voltage of the triangle wave, V_p, the duty cycle, η, of the TTL wave approaches unity; similarly, as $v_m(t) \rightarrow -V_p$, $\eta \rightarrow 0$. Mathematically, the duty cycle is defined as the positive pulse width, δ, divided by the triangle wave period, T. In other words, the comparator TTL output is HI for $v_m(t) > v_T(t)$. From the foregoing, it is easy to derive the TTL wave's duty cycle:

$$\eta = \delta/T = 1/2[1 + v_m(t)/V_p] \tag{11.70}$$

Here assume $v_m(t)$ is changing slowly enough to be considered to be constant over T/2. Demodulation of a pulse-width-modulated TTL carrier is done by averaging the TTL pulse train and subtracting out the DC component present when $v_m = 0$.

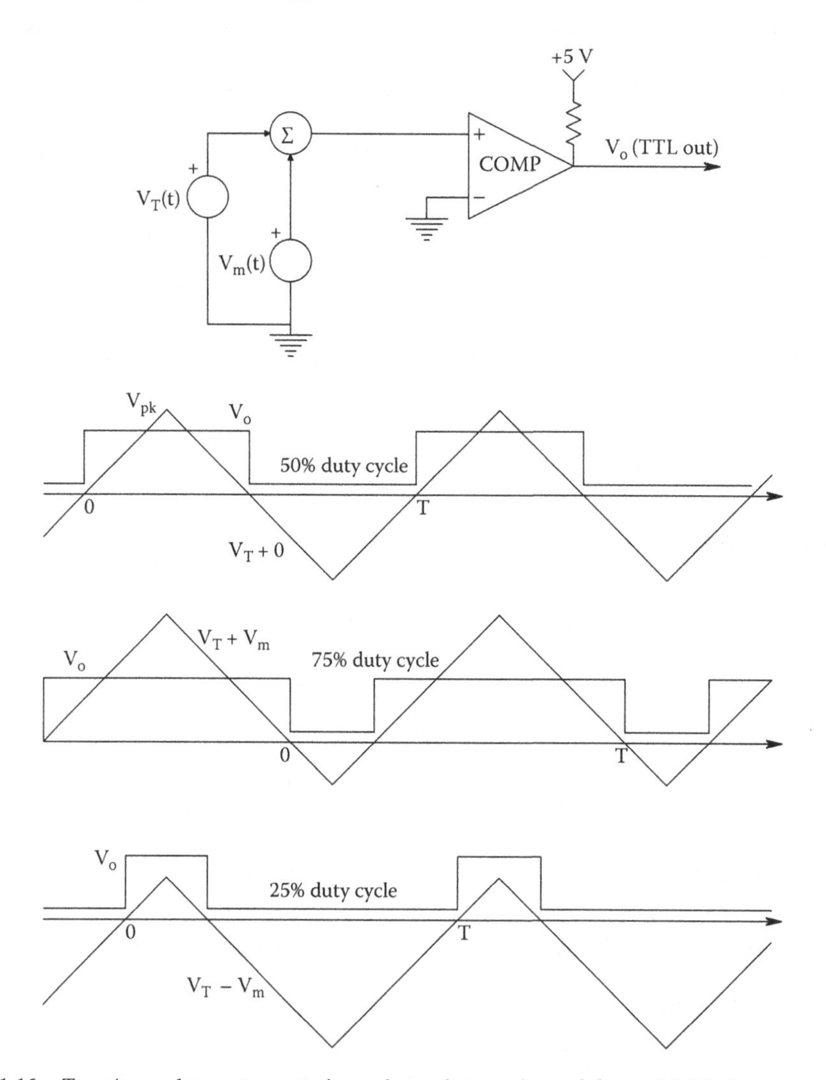

FIGURE 11.16 *Top:* An analog comparator is used as a duty-cycle modulator. A high-frequency, symmetrical, triangle wave carrier is added to the low-frequency modulating signal. *Below:* Waveforms in the modulator for $V_m(t) = 0, +V_m$ and $-V_m$, $V_m < V_{pk}$.

11.6.2 Delta Modulation

Now consider *delta modulation* (DM) and *demodulation*. A delta modulator is also known as a 1-bit, *differential pulse code modulator* (DPCM). The output of a delta modulator is a clocked (periodic) train of TTL pulses with amplitudes that are either HI or LO depending on the state of the comparator output shown in Figure 11.17a. The DM output basically tracks the derivative of the input signal. The comparator output is TTL HI if $e(t) = [v_m(t) - v_r'(t)] > 0$, and LO if $e < 0$. The D flip-flop's (DFF) complimentary output ($\bar{Q} = V_o$) is LO if the comparator output is HI at a positive transition of the TTL clock signal. The LO output of the DFF remains LO until the next positive transition of the clock signal. Then if the comparator output has gone LO, V_o goes high for one clock period (T_c), etc. $v_r'(t)$ is the output of the analog integrator offset by V_{bias} which is one-half the maximum v_r ramp height over one clock period. V_{bias} can be shown to be $1.1T_c/(RC)$ volts. With this V_{bias}, when $v_m(t) = 0$, $v_r'(t)$ will oscillate around zero with a triangle wave with zero mean and peak height $1.1T_c/(RC)$ volts. Note that the $\bar{Q}$ output of the DFF must be used because the integrator gain is negative (i.e., $-1/RC$). That is, a HI V_o will cause v_r' to go negative, and a low V_o will make v_r' go

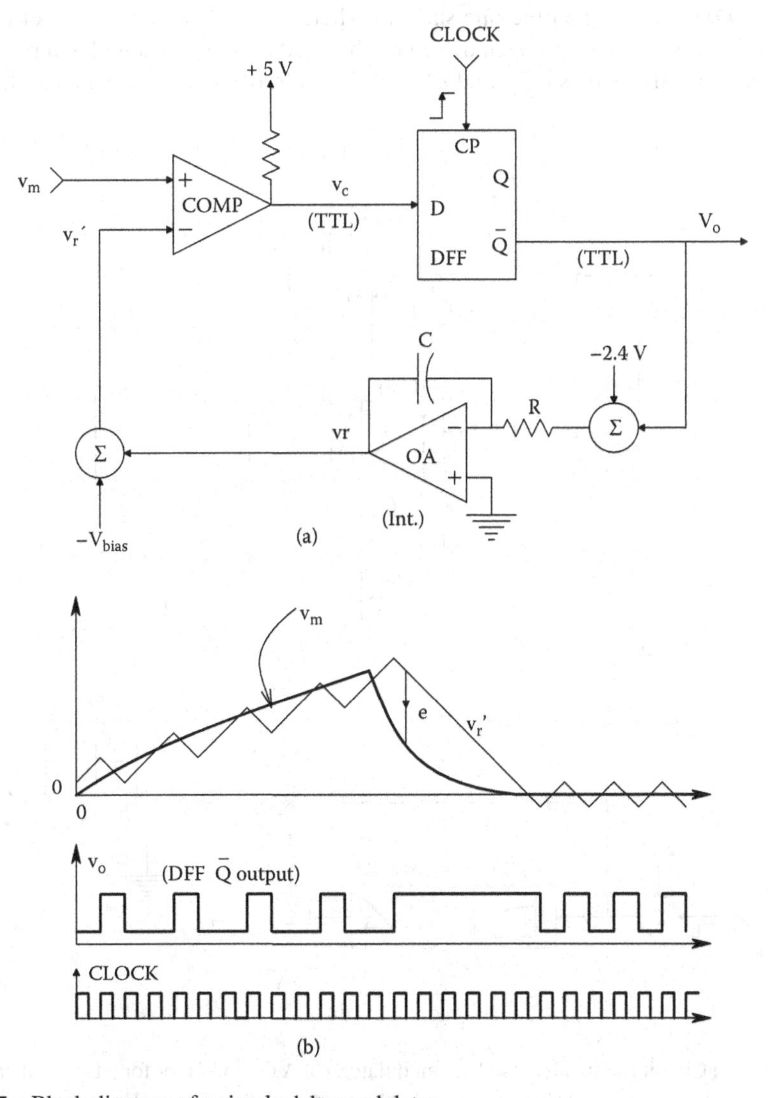

FIGURE 11.17 Block diagram of a simple delta modulator.

positive. Note that $v_r'(t)$ is *slew rate limited* at ± (2.2 V/RC) volts/s, and if the slope of $v_m(t)$ exceeds this value, a large error will accumulate in the demodulation operation of the DM signal. (Slew rate is simply the magnitude of the first derivative of a signal, i.e., its slope.) When a DM system is tracking $v_m = 0$, $v_r'(t)$ oscillates around zero, and the DM output is a periodic square wave, 1-bit "noise."

In *adaptive delta modulation* (ADM), the magnitude of the error is used to adjust the effective gain of the integrator to increase the slew rate of $v_r'(t)$ to better track rapidly-changing $v_m(t)$. One version of an ADM system is shown in Figure 11.18. Note that ideally the comparator should perform the signum operation; hence, we must subtract out the DC value (mean) of the TTL wave before it is filtered, absval'd, and used to modulate the size of the square wave input to the integrator. A conventional analog multiplier is used as a modulator. If a large error occurs as a result of poor tracking due to low slew rate in $v_r'(t)$, the comparator output will remain HI (or LO) for several clock cycles. This condition produces a nonzero signal at v_f, which in turn increases the amplitude of the symmetrical pulse input to the integrator. When the ADM is tracking well so that $v_r'(t)$ oscillates around a nearly constant v_m level, then $v_f \to 0$ and the peak amplitude of the error remains small. In summary, the ADM acts to minimize the mean squared error between $v_m(t)$ and $v_r'(t)$.

There are other variations on DM, such as *sigma–delta modulation,* and other types of nonlinear adaptive DM designs than the one shown earlier. Much of the interest in efficient, simple, low-noise modulation schemes has been driven by the need to transmit sound and pictures over the internet. Medical signals such as ECG and EEG also benefit from this development, because of the

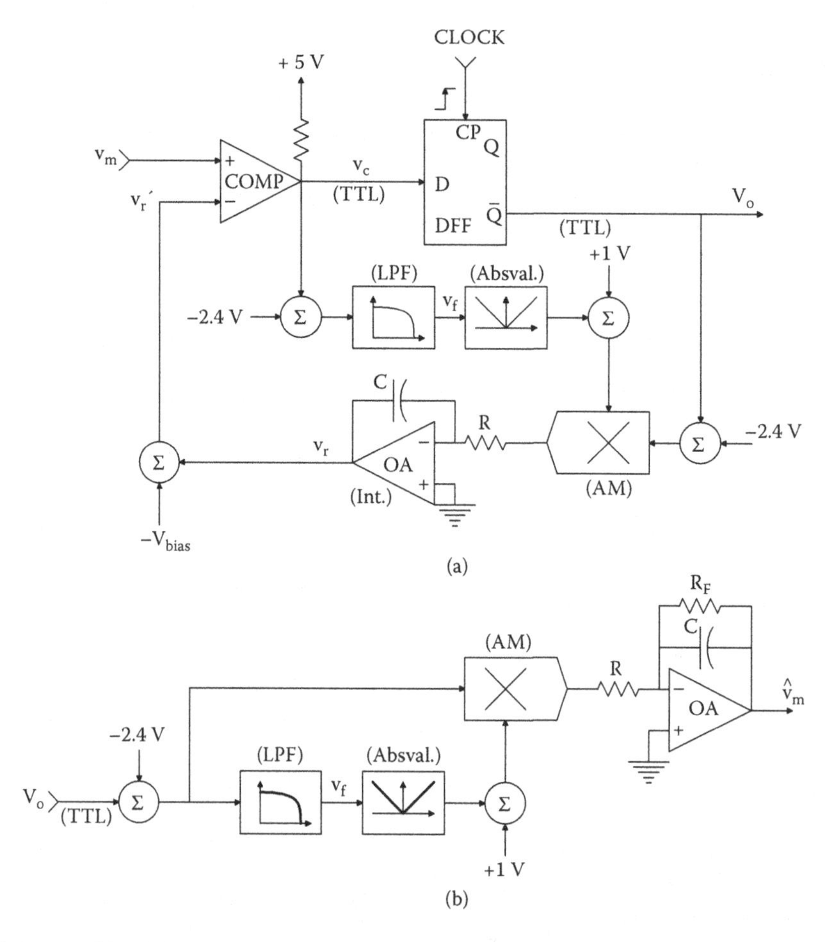

FIGURE 11.18 (a) Circuit for an adaptive delta modulator. (b) A demodulator for adaptive delta modulation. A long time constant, low-pass filter is used instead of an integrator for filtering $\hat{V}_m$.

need to transmit them from the site of the patient to a diagnostician. Biotelemetry is an important technology in the wireless monitoring of internal physiological states, emergency medicine, sports medicine, and in ecological studies.

11.7 CHAPTER SUMMARY

Broadly speaking, modulation is a process whereby a low-frequency modulating signal acts on a high-frequency carrier wave in some way so that the high-frequency, modulated carrier can be transmitted (e.g., as radio waves, ultrasound waves, light waves, etc.) to a suitable receiver after which the process of demodulation occurs, recovering the modulating signal. In the frequency domain, the low-frequency power spectrum of the signal is translated upward in frequency to lie around the carrier frequency. A major purpose of modulation is to permit long-range transmission of the modulating signal by a relatively noise-free modality.

Why transmit modulated carriers? After all, traditional, short distance telephony transmits audio information directly on telephone lines. The answer lies in the signal spectrum. The low frequencies associated with many endogenous physiological signals cannot be transmitted by conventional voice telephony; modulation must be used. The carrier modality can be radio waves, ultrasound, or photons on fiber optic cables. For example, when the modulating signal is an ECG, its power spectrum is too low for direct transmission by telephone lines. However, the ECG can narrow-band, frequency-modulate an audio-frequency carrier that can be transmitted on phone lines, and demodulated at the receiver. In the case where an ambulance is *en-route* carrying a patient, the ECG can directly narrow-band frequency-modulate (NBFM) an RF carrier which is received and demodulated at the hospital's ER.

Subcarrier modulation can be used, as well. Here several low-frequency physiological signals such as ECG, blood pressure, and respiration can each NBFM an audio subcarrier, each with a different frequency. The modulated subcarriers are added together, and used to amplitude of frequency modulate an RF carrier which is transmitted. Subcarrier FM can also be used with ultrasonic "tags" to monitor marine animals such as whales and dolphins. The tag is attached to the animal and reports such parameters as depth, water temperature, heart rate, etc. The subcarriers are separated following detection at the receiver by bandpass filters, and then demodulated themselves.

In the section about AM, the modulation process in the frequency domain was described; examples of selected circuits used in AM and single-sideband AM were given. Double-sideband, suppressed carrier AM was shown to be the simple result of multiplying the carrier by the modulating signal. Examples of DSBSCM were shown to include Wheatstone bridge outputs given ac carrier excitation, and the output of an LVDT. Both broadband and narrow-band FM was examined theoretically, and also circuits and systems used to generate NBFM such as the phase-locked loop (PLL) were described. Integral- and relaxation-pulse frequency modulations were also introduced.

In the section on demodulation, circuits and systems used to demodulate AM, DSBSCM, FM, and NBFM signals were described. Again, the PLL was shown to be a ubiquitous, effective system for demodulation.

Modulation of digital (e.g., TTL, ECL) carriers includes FM and Σ-Δ (sigma–delta) modulation, pulse-width or duty-cycle modulation, and adaptive delta modulation. Means of demodulating modulated digital signals were described.

CHAPTER 11 HOME PROBLEMS

11.1 An analog pulse instantaneous pulse frequency demodulator (IPFD) must generate a *hyperbolic* (not exponential) capacitor discharge waveform to convert interpulse intervals to elements of instantaneous frequency (IF). IF is defined as the reciprocal of the interval between two adjacent impulses in a sequence of pulses. When the $(k + 1)$th pulse in a sequence occurs, the kth hyperbolic waveform voltage is sampled and held, generating the kth element of IF which is held until the (k + 2)th pulse occurs, etc. The capacitor discharge will be a portion of a hyperbola for $t \geq 1$ ms following the occurrence of each pulse. Mathematically, this can be stated:

$$v_c(t) = \frac{C/\beta}{t + \tau_o}$$

where $V_{cmax} = 10$ V, $C = 1$ μF, and $\tau_o = C/(\beta V_{cmax}) = 0.001$ s. It can be shown that if the capacitor is allowed to discharge into a nonlinear conductance so that: $i_{nl}(t) = \beta\, v_c(t)^2$, the hyperbolic $v_c(t)$ above will occur (Northrop 2005). Time t is measured from $(t_k + 0.001)$ seconds (see the timing diagram below the schematic). This means that if $t_{k+1} = (t_k + 0.001)$, $v_c(0) = 10$ V for an IF of 1000 pps. Note that prior to each discharge cycle, C is charged through the diode to +10 V.

In this problem, you are to analyze and design the active circuit of Figure P11.1 that causes $i_{nl}(t) = \beta v_c(t)^2$ and generates the hyperbolic $v_c(t)$ described above. That is, *find* the numerical value of R required, given the parameter values above. Also find the numerical values for β and the peak $i_{nl}(t)$.

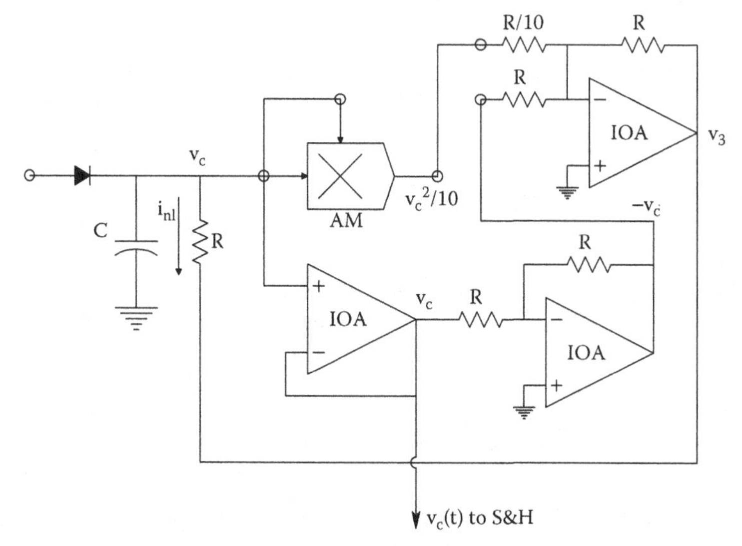

P11.1

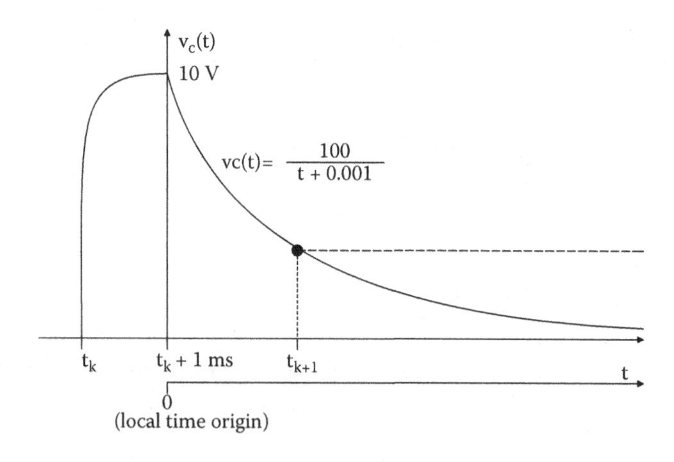

11.2 Show that the PLL circuit of Figure P11.2 generates FM. Show that the phase output of the VCO is true wideband FM. (Hint: find the transfer function, θ_o/X_m.)

11.3 Make a Bode plot of $\boldsymbol{\theta_o/X_m}$ for the system of Figure P11.3. Show the frequency range(s) where FM is generated and where phase modulation (PhM) is generated.

11.4 The system illustrated in Figure P11.4 is an FM demodulator. The $[K_m/s]$ block represents the operation on the phase of the carrier by an ideal FM modulator. *Make a Bode plot* of $\mathbf{V_c/X_m}$ and show the range of frequencies (of $x_m(t)$) where ideal FM demodulation occurs (i.e., where $V_c \infty x_m$).

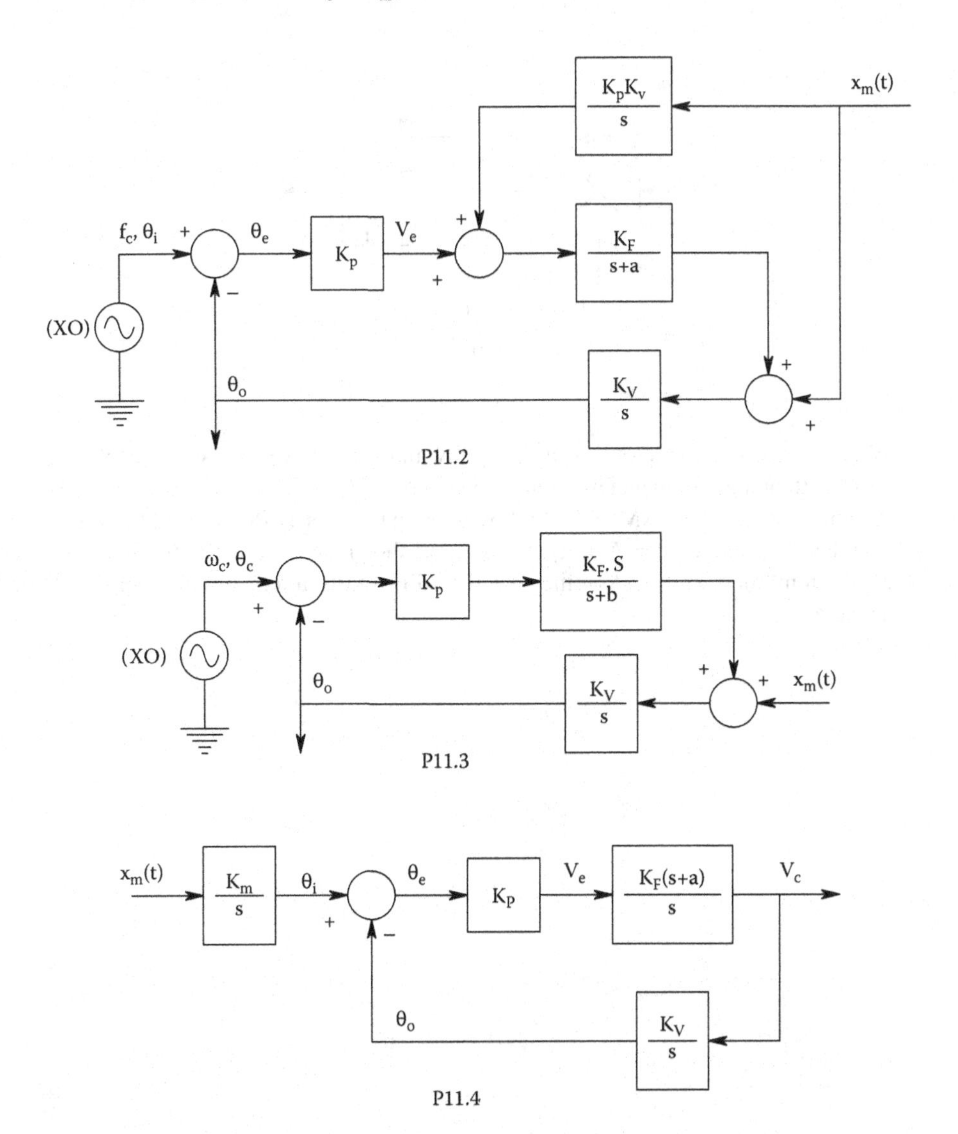

11.5 A quarter-square multiplier, shown in Figure P11.5, is used to demodulate a double-sideband, suppressed-carrier modulated cosine wave. The modulated wave is given by $v_m(t) = A\,x_m(t)\cos(\omega_c t)$.

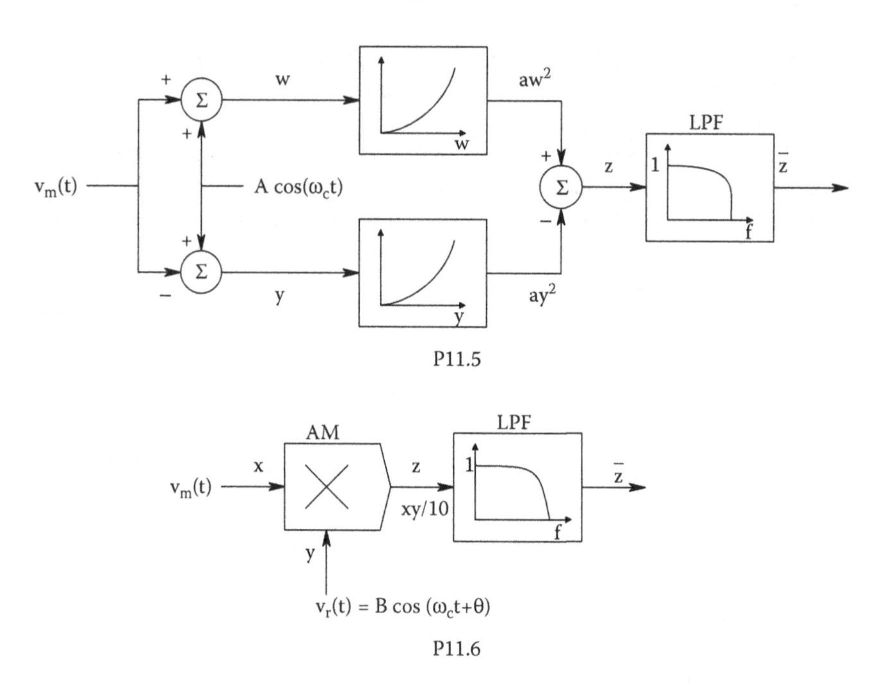

P11.5

P11.6

Write expressions for w, aw^2, y, ay^2, z, andv and show $\overline{z}$ μ $x_m(t)$. Assume that the LPF totally attenuates frequencies at and above ω_c.

11.6 An analog multiplier (AM) followed by a low-pass filter (LPF) is used to demodulate a DSBSC signal, $v_m(t) = A\ x_m(t) \cos(\omega_c\ t)$, as shown in Figure P11.6. Give algebraic expressions for z and $\overline{z}$. Assume that the LPF totally attenuates frequencies at and above ω_c.

12 Power Amplifiers and Their Applications in Biomedicine

12.1 INTRODUCTION

A power amplifier (PA) is intended to deliver electrical energy, generally at a rate of over 0.5 W, to a load. The electric energy can be DC or AC. AC PAs can operate from subsonic frequencies, through the audio- and video-frequency ranges, up through UHF and SHF radio frequencies. The loads that PAs drive can be heaters or thermoelectric coolers, DC servomotors and other motion-generating devices, LEDs, laser diodes (LADs), loudspeakers, piezoelectric ultrasound transducers, and antennas, to name a few.

In the analysis and design of PAs, it is necessary to consider not only the small-signal behavior of the circuit, including its gain and frequency response, but also the circuit's large-signal properties: These include DC biasing, power dissipation, and the heatsinking used to regulate the PA's operating temperature, as well as nonlinearities and output harmonic generation, power supply requirements, efficiency, and input and output impedances.

PAs, like small-signal amplifiers, can be divided into two major classes: Direct-coupled (d-c) PAs, and PAs that are internally reactively-coupled (r-c), and coupled to their loads through transformers or capacitors. The advantage of direct-coupling is that no heavy, expensive output transformer is used, and frequency response extends to DC. PAs typically have a low-power, high input impedance driver stage, which drives the power output stage. Our focus in this chapter will be on PA power output stages, and how they are used in IC power op amp designs.

A power output stage can have a variety of forms; it can use power BJTs, power Darlington BJTs, or power MOSFETs in various circuit architectures. Older PA designs used high-perveance power vacuum tubes (triodes, pentodes) as the output devices. Such vacuum tube circuits had inherently high Thevenin output impedances, requiring the use of transformers to optimally match power transfer to low-impedance loads such as loudspeakers. The modern practice is to use the inherently low output impedance of certain transistor PAs to couple directly to the load impedance and also achieve output impedance reduction through the use of negative voltage feedback. Often a large, series, electrolytic capacitor is used to block DC from the load.

Modern engineering practice is to use one or two power op amps (POAs) to drive a load with direct coupling. Power loads encountered in biomedical engineering range from DC servomotors, fans, pumps, stepping motors, loudspeakers, piezoultrasound transducers, older CRT video displays, readers for RFID tags, and in wireless patient monitoring, RF antennas.

12.1.1 Some Applications and Loads for Power Amplifiers

In biomedical applications, PAs are used to drive a variety of loads; the following list describes some of their applications:

Resistive Loads: In thermal control systems (e.g., for DNA PCR) (heating elements, thermoelectric (Peltier) chillers), battery chargers, incandescent lights used in endoscopes, and X-ray tubes.

Resistive/Inductive Loads: Motion control, including servomotor windings (including stepping motors), solenoids in valves, audio transducers (loudspeakers, headphones). Magnetic CRT beam deflection.

Capacitive Loads: Electrostatic electron beam deflection in small CRTs, electrostatic ion beam deflection in mass spectrometers used in laboratory medicine applications, piezoelectric actuators used below their resonant frequency.

Piezoelectic Transducers: In medical ultrasound imaging systems. (At transducer resonant frequency, the load looks real; off resonance is complex). Sonic energy is also used in the laboratory to lyse cells and emulsify solutions.

LEDs and LADs: Diode loads look real at low- and midfrequencies, otherwise $\mathbf{Z}_L = \mathbf{R}_e - j\mathbf{X}$ due to junction capacitances. Electrical power goes into photon energy and heat.

RF Antennas: Antennas used in wireless patient monitoring. Depending on antenna, coupling transmission line and frequency, the load is generally complex.

12.2 POWER OUTPUT DEVICES

12.2.1 Discrete Power Devices: BJTs

Power BJTs are widely used in standalone PAs and in POA output stages. Power BJTs generally have lower small-signal (s-s) βs (h_{fe}s) and higher output conductances (h_{oe}) than do low-power BJTs. They also can pass considerably more collector current ($\mathbf{I_C}$) than low-power BJTs (i.e., they have high perveances), at much higher collector to-emitter voltages ($\mathbf{V_{CE}}$). Note that the maximum average BJT power dissipation is given by the hyperbolic relation:

$$P_{Dmax} = I_C V_{CE} \tag{12.1}$$

P_{Dmax} for a device is determined by the effectiveness of the transistor's construction and its associated heatsink in keeping its junction temperature below the allowable maximum for that device. P_{Dmax} is usually specified by the manufacturer for a given set of heatsink conditions. In some PA designs, the use of thermoelectric cooling or a fan on the heatsink can extend the actual device $P_D > P_{Dmax}$. Base power input, $P_B = I_B V_{BE}$, is generally neglected.

The hyperbolic P_{Dmax} relation and the device's maximum I_C and V_{CE} define the acceptable operating region for a given power device *and* heatsink. Figure 12.1 shows the $I_C(I_B, V_{CE})$ curves of a typical 60 W power BJT, and the acceptable *operating region* (OR) defined by P_{max}, I_{Cmax}, and V_{Cemax}. Note that this OR is also bounded on the left by the saturation region (**S** in the figure) and the bottom by the I_{CE0} for $I_B = 0$ curve. BJT saturation occurs when the B-E and C-B junctions are both forward-biased (recall that the C-B junction is normally reverse biased). The effect of high junction temperatures is to tip the entire set of $I_C(I_B, V_{CE})$ curves up and to the right. This increases I_C for a given I_B and V_{CE}, and raises h_{oe} in the BJT's common-emitter SSM.

Figure 12.2 illustrates a simple grounded-emitter *npn* BJT coupled to a low-impedance resistive load through a transformer. Recall that a practical transformer has a complicated equivalent circuit (see Figure 12.3) that includes series and mutual inductances of its windings, as well as the resistance of its windings and core losses from hysterisis and eddy currents. Consequently, for pencil-and-paper analysis, we often use the ideal (lossless) transformer model.

In the ideal transformer (IT) shown in Figure 12.4, the input power equals the output power because there are zero losses. The two-port power relations are

$$P_{in} = V_1 I_1 = P_L = V_L{}^2/R_L \tag{12.2a}$$

Also, for an IT,

$$V_L = (n_2/n_1)V_1 \tag{12.2b}$$

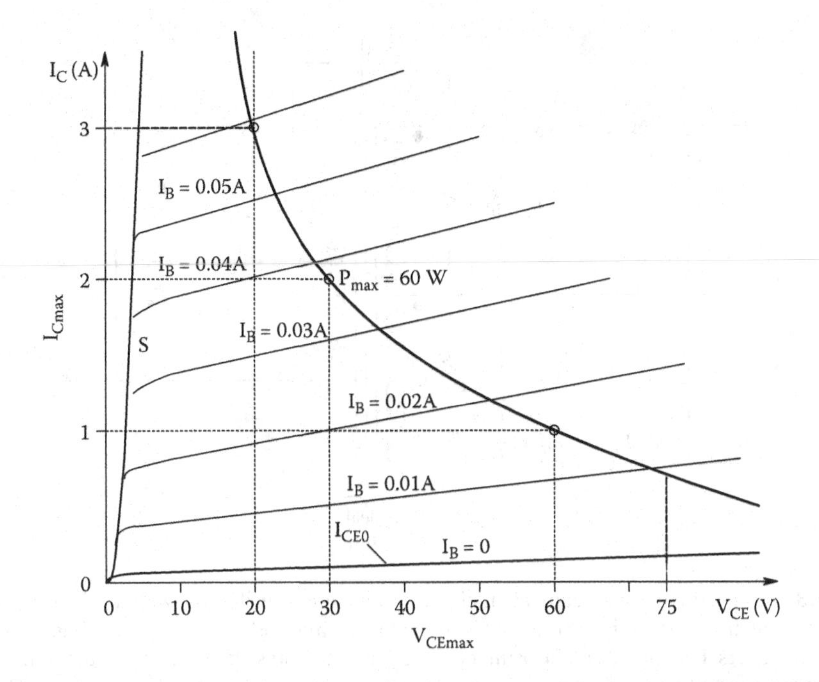

FIGURE 12.1 $I_C(I_B, V_{CE})$ curves of a representative ***npn*** power BJT. The linear operating region is bounded by the Pmax hyperbola, the maximum collector-emitter voltage, the device saturation line S, and the maximum collector current. The BJT's $\beta \approx 50$, high for a power BJT.

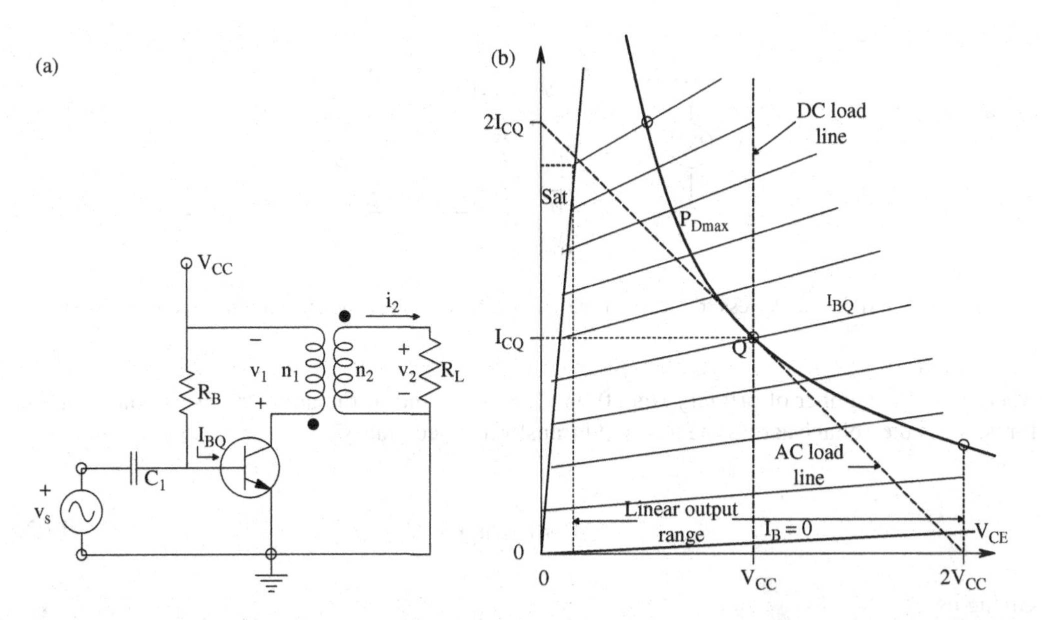

FIGURE 12.2 (a) Ideal transformer-coupled, class A, BJT amplifier. R_B sets the DC operating (Q) point bias, I_{BQ}. Note that the AC load-line slope is set by $R_L = V_{CC}/I_{CQ}$. (b) The DC load-line is drawn vertical because an ideal transformer is assumed. With a real transformer, its slope would be set by the primary winding resistance. The AC load-line slope is $-1/R_L'$, where the R_L' the BJT 'sees' looking into the transformer primary winding is $R_L(n_1/n_2)^2$. Thus to optimally match a given R_L, I_{CQ} is made equal to $V_{CC}/[R_L(n_1/n_2)]^2$. Note that the linear output range is $(2V_{CC} - V_{Cesat})$. The Q point must lie on or below the P_{Dmax} hyperbola.

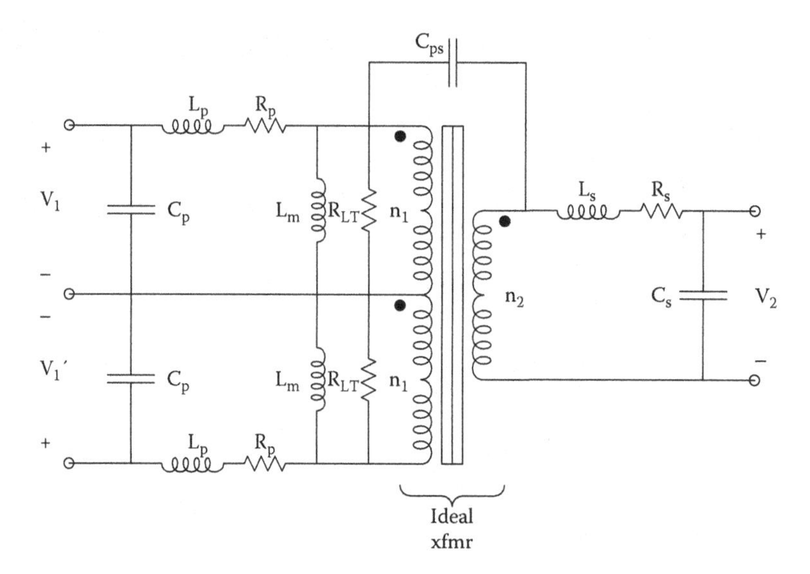

FIGURE 12.3 Lumped-parameter equivalent circuit of an audio transformer with a center-tapped primary winding. An ideal transformer is surrounded with lumped circuit elements representing, in some cases, distributed parameters. For one side of the primary: C_p, L_p, and R_p represent, respectively, the shunt capacitance between primary windings, the primary leakage inductance and the primary winding ohmic (DC) resistance. L_m is the primary magnetizing inductance ($L_m >> L_p$) and R_{LT} the equivalent core loss resistance (from eddy currents and core hysteresis). C_{ps} is the primary-to-secondary coupling capacitance (ideally $\rightarrow 0$), R_s is the secondary winding's DC resistance, and L_s is the secondary leakage inductance.

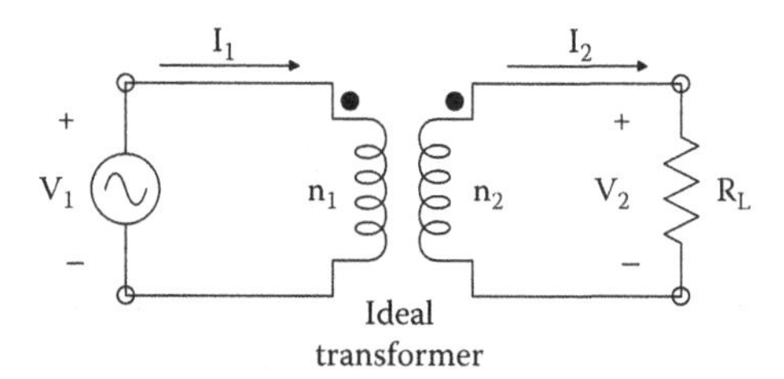

FIGURE 12.4 An ideal, lossless transformer with a load R_L on its secondary winding. See analysis in text.

where n_1 is the number of primary (input) winding turns and n_2 the number of secondary (output) turns. V_L is the voltage across the load (and transformer secondary).
Hence,

$$P_{in} = V_1 I_1 = (n_2/n_1)^2 V_1^2/R_L \tag{12.2c}$$

Giving us,

$$I_1 = (n_2/n_1)^2 V_1/R_L \tag{12.2d}$$

Thus, the resistance, R_L', "seen" by V_1 looking into the transformer's primary is

$$R_L' = V_1/I_1 = (n_1/n_2)^2 R_L \tag{12.2e}$$

Therefore, by manipulating (n_1/n_2), we can present the power stage driving the load with an R_L' that will allow maximum power transfer to the load for a given power device's Thevenin source resistance, R_1.

It is easy to show that the power dissipated in the apparent load, R_L', given a fixed Thevenin V_1, R_1, is

$$P_L = R_L' \frac{V_1^2}{(R_1 + R_L')^2} \text{ W.} \tag{12.3}$$

P_{Lmax} occurs when $R_L' = R_1 = R_L(n_1/n_2)^2$ and is

$$P_{Lmax} = V_1^2/(4R_1) \tag{12.4}$$

Thus, for maximum power transfer with an ideal transformer, it is necessary to make $n_1/n_2 = \sqrt{(R_1/R_L)}$.

In a practical transformer with winding resistances and core losses, the R_L' seen at low frequencies looking into the transformer primary can be expressed by

$$R_L' = R_p + R_{CL} + (R_L + R_s)(n_1/n_2)^2 \tag{12.5}$$

where R_p = primary winding resistance, R_{CL} = core loss equivalent resistance, R_L = secondary load resistance, R_s = secondary winding resistance, n_1 = number of turns on primary winding, and n_2 = number of secondary winding turns.

The C-E *h*-parameter MFSSM of the transformer-coupled BJT amplifier illustrated in Figure 12.2a can be used to find the voltage gain of the amplifier and its power output. The MFSSM for the circuit is shown in Figure 12.5. Using Ohm's law and some algebra, one can write

$$\frac{V_{ce}}{V_s} = \frac{-h_{fe}R_L'}{[h_{ie}(1 + h_{oe}R_L') - h_{re}h_{fe}R_L']} \tag{12.6}$$

To simplify, set $h_{re} \to 0$, giving

$$\frac{V_{ce}}{V_s} = \frac{-h_{fe}R_L'}{h_{ie}(1 + h_{oe}R_L')} \tag{12.7}$$

Now because of the ideal transformer assumption, the power delivered to R_L' is the same power dissipated in R_L.

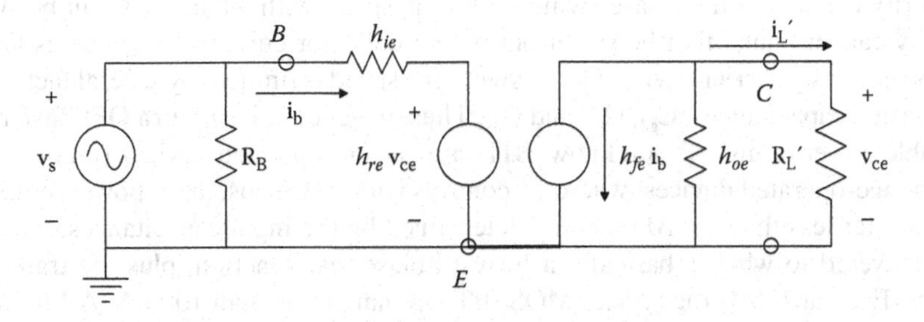

FIGURE 12.5 Small-signal, *h*-parameter model for a simple, grounded-emitter BJT amplifier.

$$P'_L = v_{ce}^2/R'_L = \frac{v_s^2 h_{fe}^2 R'_L}{h_{ie}^2(1 + h_{oe}R'_L)^2} = P_L = v_2^2/R_L \tag{12.8}$$

Emitter-follower circuit geometries are often used in PA output stages, especially in power op amps. Recall the small-signal model of an EF shown in Figure 2.17, in Section 2.3.3. The S-S voltage gain of a simple EF amplifier was found to be

$$K_v = \frac{v_e}{v_s} = \frac{R_L(1 + h_{fe})}{R_L(1 + h_{fe}) + h_{ie} + R_s} < 1 \tag{12.9}$$

It was also shown that the S-S output resistance that R_L "sees" looking up the emitter of an EF is

$$R_{out} = \frac{R_s + h_{ie}}{(1 + h_{fe})} \tag{12.10}$$

where R_L is the emitter resistor (load), h_{fe} is the BJT's S-S current gain, h_{ie} is the base input resistance, R_S = the Thevenin source resistance driving the base node. We assume h_{oe} is negligibly small, and R_B is >> the S-S resistance looking into the BJT' base.

Thus, for optimum power transfer to R_L, R_L must equal R_{out} (or an impedance matching transformer must be used so the emitter "sees" an $R'_L = (R_s + h_{ie})/(1 + h_{fe}) = R_L\,(n_1/n_2)^2$).

Figure 12.6 shows the circuit architectures of four, representative BJT power output stages. (See the caption for details.) Note the use of emitter followers in complimentary-symmetry (CS) architectures *(npn* and *pnp* devices). As we have shown, the voltage gain of an EF amplifier is always <1; however, it has power gain and low Thevenin output resistance, which makes the CS EF architecture suitable for many PA applications. Note that because the EF voltage gain is <1, the power output stages must be driven by a high voltage driver stage to get maximum output.

The Darlington BJT pair and the so-called feedback pair amplifiers were illustrated in Chapter 2 (cf. Figure 2.19a and b). Darlington BJT power transistors have $I_C(I_B, V_{CE})$ curves similar to single BJTs, but have higher h_{fe}s and input resistances (h_{ie}). Most power Darlingtons also include a power diode across the C-E terminals. This diode is reverse-biased under normal operating conditions, and it protects the device from negative voltage transients when it is switching an inductive load.

12.2.2 Power MOSFETs

To better understand power MOSFETs, review Sections 2.43 and 2.5.2 of this Text on FET models. Figure 12.7 shows a simplified, cross-sectional schematic view of an *n*-channel, vertical, double-diffused power MOSFET. (There are many power MOSFET architectures; too many to cover here.) What we will stress is the comparative differences between power MOSFETs and BJTs. BJTs have stored minority carriers in their bases which limit the speed with which they can be switched off. The minority carriers must first be swept out before collector current can go to its OFF level. A MOSFET is a majority carrier device, and its switching speed is limited, by several factors, including its three parasitic capacitances, C_{gd}, C_{gs}, and C_{ds}. Thus, in general, it can turn OFF faster than a BJT of comparable power rating. As you know, BJTs are current-operated devices (i_b controls i_c), while FETs are voltage-operated devices, where v_{gs} controls i_d (or v_{ds}). Thus, drive power requirements for MOSFETs are far less than for BJTs, being determined by the input capacitances, while BJT base current is delivered to what is basically a forward-biased ***pn*** junction, plus the transistor's input capacitances. Even at 125°C the typical MOSFET i_g remains less than 100 nA. A MOSFET begins to turn off as soon as its v_{gs} reaches its threshold voltage, V_T (or V_P).

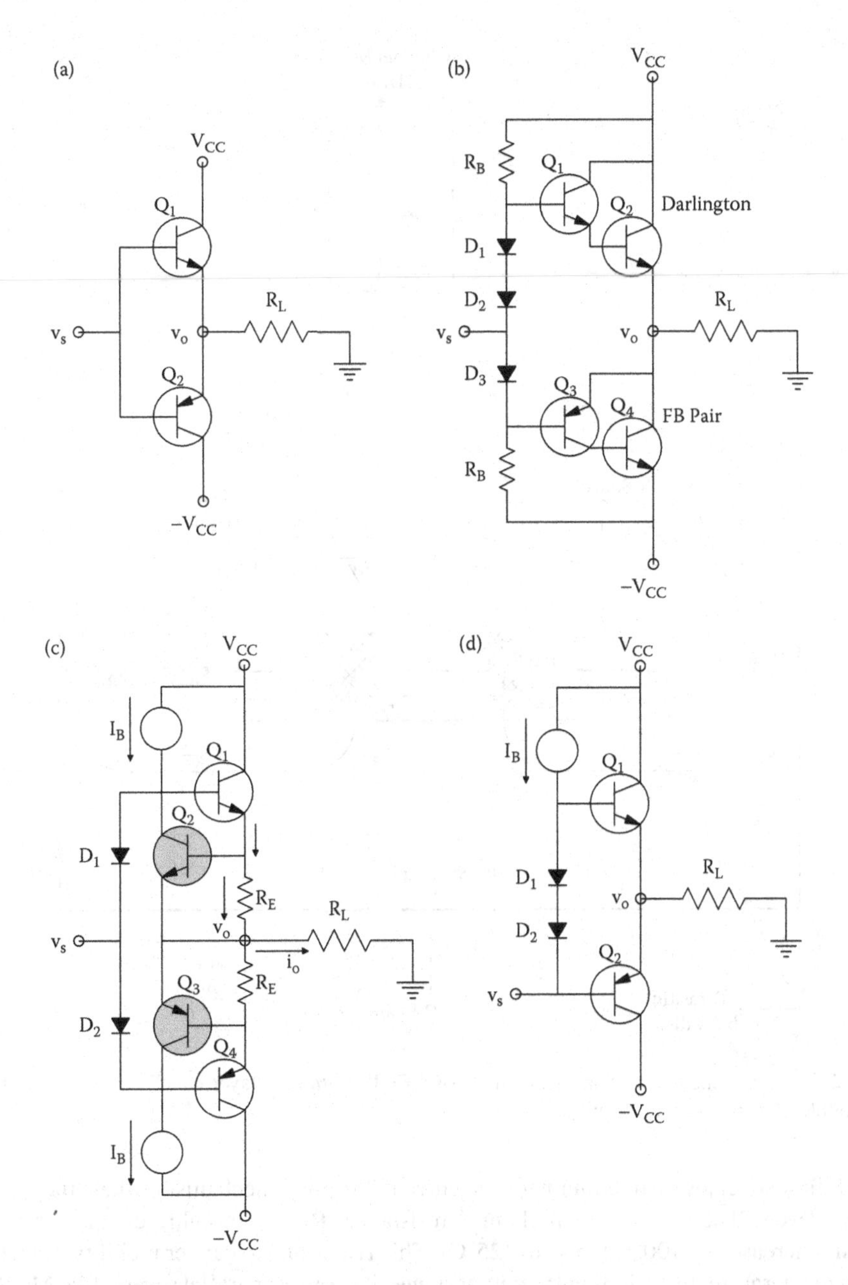

FIGURE 12.6 (a) A simple class B complimentary symmetry (CS), emitter-follower, PA output stage, direct-coupled to a resistive load, R_L. (b) A class AB PA output stage. Q_1 and Q_2 are in a Darlington configuration; Q_3 and Q_4 are in a feedback pair configuration (cf. Section 2.3.4 for a MF SS analysis of the feedback pair amplifier). The feedback pair is equivalent to a single power ***pnp*** transistor. Q_4 is the power transistor and Q_3 is a low power ***pnp*** device. Looking into Q4's collector, we see a low Thevenin resistance because of the feedback. R_B and diodes D_1 and D_2 DC bias the Darlington so that it is just conducting When $V_s = 0$. D_3 and R_B act similarly to bias the FB pair to produce class B or AB operation. (c) A CS PA that uses the two R_Es in conjunction with Q_2 and Q_3 as "base current robbers" to limit the output current, i_o. (For example, if excess i_o flows through Q_1 and its R_E, the voltage drop across R_E turns on Q_2 which "steals" Q_1's base current, limiting i_o. Base current robbers produce symmetrical, soft current saturation.) (d) This is an offset CS PA. Diodes D1 and D2 and the DC biasing current source I_B act to eliminate the dead zone seen in the output of the simple CS circuit of A.

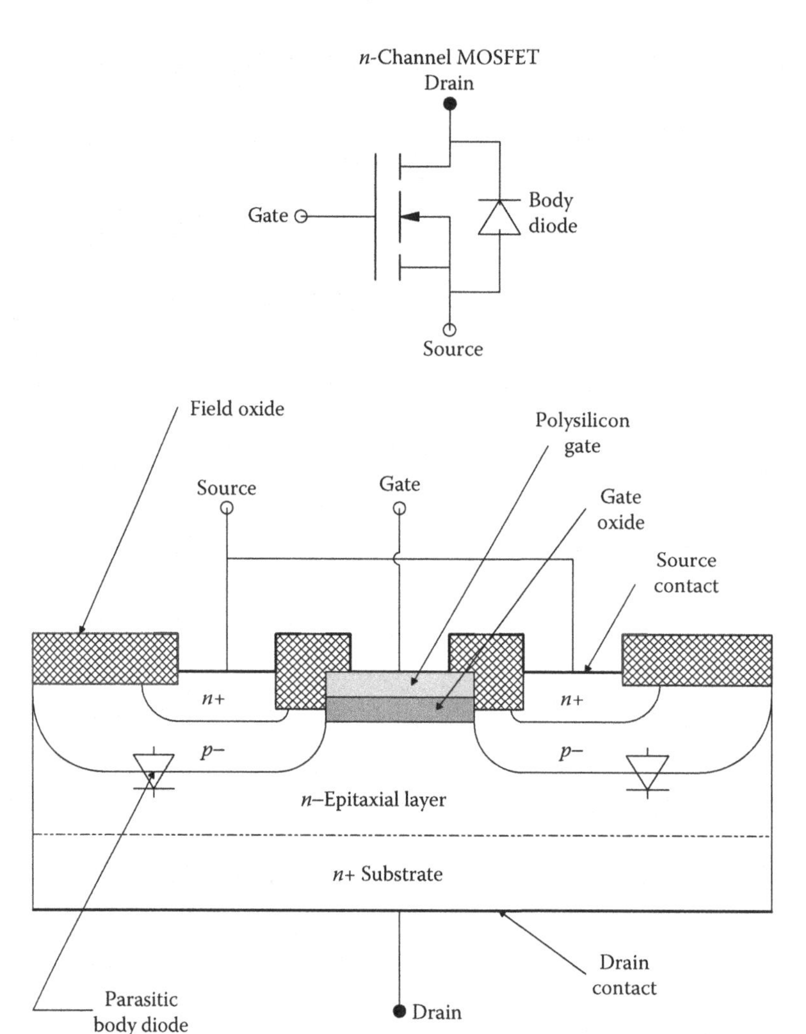

FIGURE 12.7 *Top:* Schematic of an ***n***-channel MOSFET. *Bottom:* "layer-cake" cross-section through a vertical, double-diffused, power MOSFET.

MOSFETs also enjoy a maximum drain current limiting mechanism when they are run a high power levels. The ohmic region channel resistance, $R_{DS(ON)}$, roughly doubles as the device temperature increases by 100°C (25°C to 125°C). This rise is due to carrier mobility reduction with increasing temperature. In designing PA output stages, it is safe to parallel several like MOSFETs; if one tries this with like BJTs, one transistor may have a lower $V_{CE(sat)}$, and will take most of the load current, leading to overheating and device failure.

For a detailed review of the properties of power MOSFETs and their various designs, see the *Application Notes* by Locher (1998) and Barkhordarian (2010).

12.2.3 Power Op Amps

Power op amps are widely used in biomedical applications, including but not limited to: DC motors, solenoid valves, and actuator controls, also for magnetic deflection circuits (in CRTs, mass spectrometer ion beams), audio amplifiers, and ultrasound transducers. They incorporate a high input impedance, high-gain, differential input headstage, high-gain drivers, and a power output stage in a common, heatsinking package: for example, the ubiquitous TO-3. (Other packages include: JDEC MO-127, 7-PIN SIP DK, SIP10, 12-PIN SIP EU, 20-PIN PSOP DK, etc.)

Power op amps differ from ordinary op amps in that they can output considerable average power at high load voltages For example, the Apex PA09 can output 4.5 A peak at $\pm(V_S - 7)$ V, $|V_S| \leq 40$ V. (This is a peak output power of ca. 148 W.) The device itself can dissipate a peak power of 78 W when properly heatsinked and has a 65 W steady dissipation. It has a fast slew rate (200 V/μs), low input noise (JFET input transistors), and a 150 MHz gain-bandwidth product. Its full power bandwidth is 750 kHz. Some applications listed by the manufacturer include: Video distribution and amplification, high-speed deflection circuits, power transducers to 2 MHz, coaxial line drivers, power LED, or laser diode excitation.

The Apex PA03 is another power op amp with primary applications in driving linear and rotary motors, driving CRT yoke/magnetic deflection coils, acting as a programmable regulator in DC power supplies to ±68 V, driving transducers and audio speakers to 1 kW. This amplifier has a peak output current of 30 A, can operate with ±75 V V_Ss, and can swing to $\pm|V_S - 7|$ at a 30 A output. Thus, its peak output power is 2.04 kW. Its slew rate is only 8 V/μs, and its power bandwidth is 30 kHz.

Yet another Apex power op amp is the PA78. It can output 200 mA peak at $V_o = |V_S - 10|$ V, $V_S \leq \pm 175$ V max. (This is a peak output power of ca. 33 W.) This POA can dissipate a steady 23 W when properly heatsinked. It has a slew rate (350 V/μs), and a 1 MHz gain-bandwidth product. Its full power bandwidth is 200 kHz at 300V pk–pk output. The PA78 is recommended for driving piezoelectric positioning and activation systems, electrostatic deflection (CRTs, mass spectrometers, ink jet deflection), deformable mirror actuators, and chemical and biological stimulators. It uses power MOSFETs for its output devices. Figure 12.8 gives a schematic for a push–pull, piezoactuator driver that can use two PA78 op amps. A piezoactuator presents a largely capacitive (reactive) load

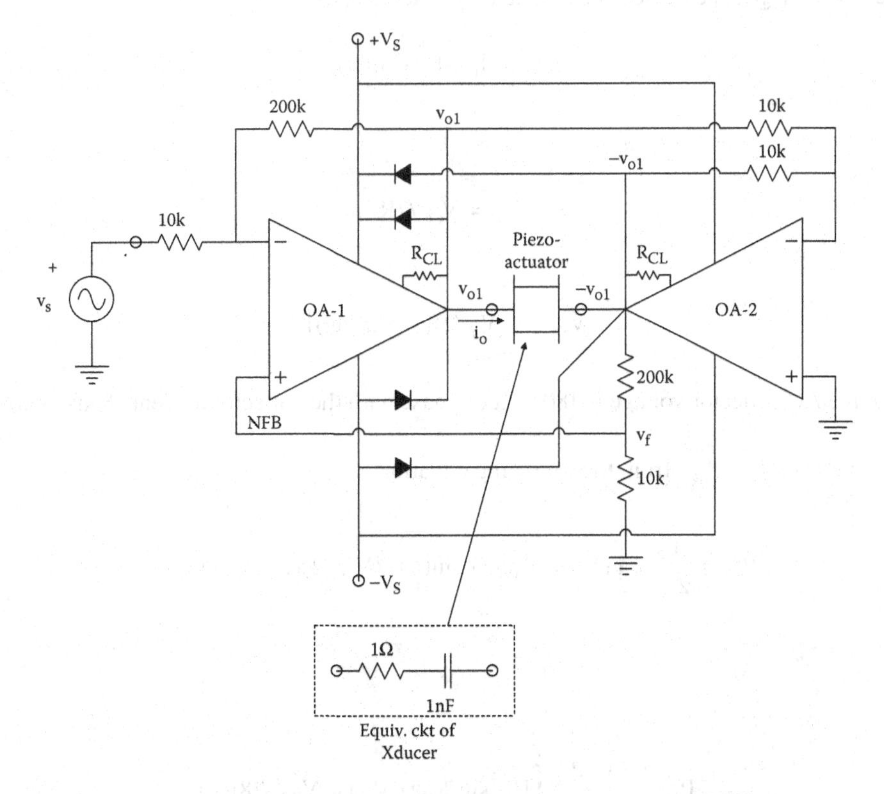

FIGURE 12.8 Schematic of a push-pull, piezo-actuator driver that can use two PA78 power op amps. Note the overall negative voltage feedback to OA-1's noninverting input.

to the amplifiers (1 nF in series with 1 Ω); hence, the real power is dissipated by the op amps. The diodes are high-speed, high voltage types that serve to clamp the op amp outputs between $\pm V_S$ to protect the MOSFET power output stages from voltage spikes generated by unwanted mechanical inputs to the piezoactuator. OA-1 has a voltage gain of –20 for v_s, OA-2 has a gain of –1; thus, the floating load is driven by $2v_{o1}$. There is an overall negative feedback (NFB) loop that feeds back $-v_{o1}/20$ to the noninverting input of OA-1. R_{CL} is the output current limiting set resistor; high-frequency, series R-C compensation networks for each op amp are not shown. It is left as an exercise for the reader to calculate $\mathbf{I_o/V_s}(j\omega)$, assuming ideal op amps.

Note that not all power op amps use MOSFET output stages; some use BJTs in complimentary Darlington circuits, or Darlington and feedback pair architectures. For example, the Apex PA81 POA uses a complimentary BJT Darlington half bridge output circuit.

12.3 CLASSES OF POWER AMPLIFIERS: PA EFFICIENCY

In a class A power amplifier output stage, the device (BJT or FET) conducts throughout an input AC cycle.

The power conversion efficiency, η_p, of a PA is defined as the ratio of the average AC power delivered to the load, P_{AC}, to the average power delivered by the V_{CC} supply (or the $\pm V_{CC}$ supplies), P_{DC}. Needless to say, power efficiency is important in the design of battery-operated, portable electronic equipment such as laptop computers, PDAs, telecommunication equipment, digital cameras, etc.

P_{DC} is independent of the signal level in a class A amplifier, hence to get maximum η_p, one must have a maximum P_{AC}. Maximum P_{AC} occurs when the peak-to-peak swing in V_{ce} and I_c is a maximum. If $V_{CE(sat)}$ is neglected (i.e., made 0), the actual $i_c(t)$ is

$$i_c(t) = I_{CQ}[1 + \sin(\omega t)] \tag{12.11}$$

where

$$I_{CQ} = V_{CC}/2R_L \tag{12.12}$$

$$v_c(t) = (V_{cc}/2)[1 - \sin(\omega t)] \tag{12.13}$$

Note that the AC collector voltage is 180° out of phase with the collector current. Thus, one can find the average

power in the load, P_{AC} $\overline{P_{AC}}$, from the following equations:

$$\overline{P_{AC}} = \frac{1}{2\pi} = \int_{-\pi}^{\pi} (V_{CC}/2R_t)[1 + \sin(\omega t)](V_{CC}/2)[1 - \sin(\omega t)]\, d\omega t \tag{12.14}$$

$$\downarrow$$

$$\overline{P_{AC}} = \frac{V_{CC}^2}{2\pi 4R_L} \int_{-\pi}^{\pi} [1 - \sin 2(\omega t)]\, d\omega t = V_{CC}^2/(8R_L) \tag{12.15}$$

Hence, the maximum power conversion efficiency, η_{pmax}, of the grounded emitted, class A PA is

$$\eta_{pmax} = \frac{\overline{P_{AC}}}{P_{DC}} = \frac{V_{CC}^2/(8R_L)}{V_{CC}(V_{CC}/2R_L)} = 0.25 \tag{12.16}$$

The actual maximum efficiency will actually be less than ¼ for a real class A amplifier because $V_{CE(sat)} > 0$, and the collector leakage current at cutoff. Note that η_{pmax} for an EF PA where $R_E = R_L$, can also be shown to be ¼ (Northrop 1990).

The use of an impedance-matching, coupling transformer in a class A, grounded emitter, BJT PA increases η_{pmax} beyond ¼. In the transformer-coupled, class A BJT amplifier of Figure 12.2 the operating (Q) point was selected to be in the center of the linear operating region, just below the P_{Dmax} hyperbola. V_{CC} is selected to be less than the maximum V_{CE}. n_1/n_2 is made so the BJT's collector "sees" an R_L' value that causes the dynamic load-line to intersect the V_{CE} axis at $2V_{CC}$, and the I_C axis at $2I_{CQ}$. Thus, $R_L' = 2V_{CC}/2I_{CQ} = V_{CC}/I_{CQ} = R_L (n_1/n_2)^2\ \Omega$, and $V_{CC}/I_{CQ} < P_{D(max)}$. The average power from the power supply is $P_{dc} = V_{CC} I_{CQ}$, and the maximum average AC power delivered to the load, $\overline{P_{AC}}$, is the same maximum power delivered to the ideal transformer's primary winding.

Again neglecting the saturation voltage and collector leakage current, one can write the two average power expressions:

$$\overline{P_{AC}} = \frac{1}{2\pi}\int_{-\pi}^{\pi} V_{CC}[1 - \sin(\omega t)]I_{CQ}[1+\sin(\omega t)]\, d\omega t$$

$$\downarrow \tag{12.17}$$

$$\overline{P_{AC}} = \frac{V_{CC}I_{CQ}}{2\pi}\int_{-x}^{x}[1-\sin 2(\omega t)]\, d\omega t = V_{CC}I_{CQ}/2$$

Thus, the maximum class A efficiency approaches

$$\eta_{pmax} = \frac{\overline{P_{AC}}}{P_{DC}} = \frac{V_{CC}I_{CQ}/2}{V_{CC}I_{CQ}} = 0.5 \tag{12.18}$$

This value is double that for a simple class A, GE BJT PA, shown in Figure 12.9a.

As we have shown, a class A PA supplies AC current to the load over an entire AC input voltage cycle. Class AB and B PAs use two devices, as shown in the four PA circuits shown in Figure 12.6. They are often called *push-pull amplifiers.* In a class B amplifier, the positive halves of an AC signal output current cycle are supplied by one device, and the negative halves by the other device. The devices are biased so they are just cut-off at their Q-points to minimize quiescent power drain with no input signal. In class AB biasing, both devices supply power to the load at low AC signal levels, and for large signals, one device is cut-off while the other conducts. Figure 12.10a illustrates a nontuned, BJT class B PA using transformer coupling. The DC and dynamic (AC) load-lines for each device are shown in Figure 12.10b. The AC load-line runs from V_{CC} on the V_{CE} axis to V_{CC}/R_L' on the I_C axis. Of course, $R_L' = (n_1/n_2)^2R_L$, and each BJT "sees" that dynamic load over the half cycle when it conducts. The peak collector current is I_{Cmax}, determined by the intersection of the AC load line with the I_{Csat} line. The maximum efficiency of a class B, push-pull, transformer-coupled PA can be shown to be $\pi/4 = 0.7854$.

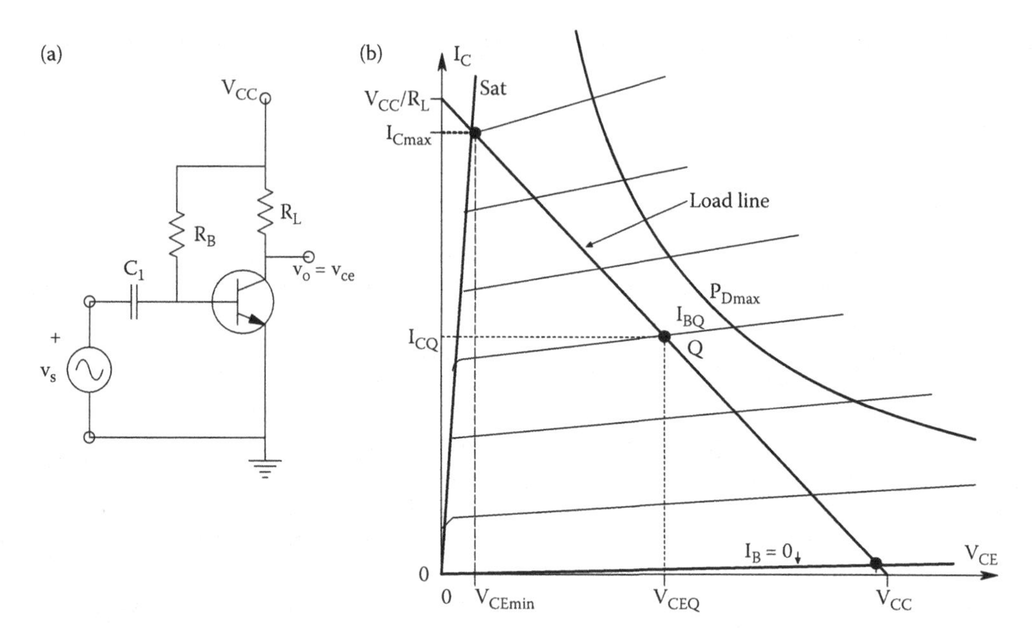

FIGURE 12.9 (a) Schematic of a simple class A, GE BJT PA. (b) Load-line for the BJT PA. Note that it lies well inside the P_{max} hyperbola.

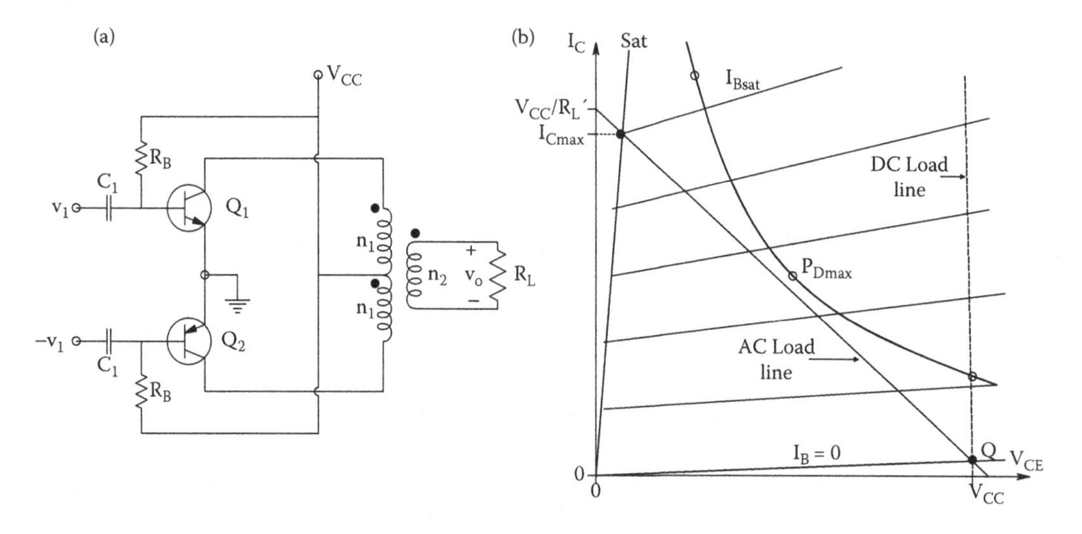

FIGURE 12.10 (a) A nontuned, BJT class B PA using (ideal) transformer coupling. (b) The DC and dynamic (AC) load-lines for each transistor.

12.4 CLASS D POWER AMPLIFIERS

A class D power amplifier works by driving its load with a current that is the time-averaged (low-pass filtered) waveform of a high frequency, pulse-width modulated, bipolar square wave output. Berglund et al. (2006) describe the use of resonant circuits in class D PAs that can work up into the low GHz range. The resonant circuit effectively extracts the fundamental sinusoidal frequency of the switched square wave.

Class D PAs are designed for high operating efficiency and compact packaging. By using power MOSFETs in a switched mode (ON–OFF), their power dissipation can be made very low, leading to amplifier power efficiencies of over 80%. Their principle of operation is simple: the analog (audio) input signal generates high-frequency, high-power, pulse-width modulated pulses. These pulses are averaged by a low-pass filter (LPF) in series with the load to extract the amplified, low-frequency, input modulating signal. Nearly, all the high-frequency power in the filtered output is of negligible magnitude, and is of course, inaudible.

The average power dissipation of a MOSFET is $P_D = I_D V_{DS}$. When a MOSFET is switched OFF at high V_{DS} values, very little drain current, I_D, flows, and the transistor power dissipation is negligible ($P_{D(off)} \rightarrow 0$). When the MOSFET is driven fully ON, into its ohmic region, its I_D is high, but V_{DS} is relatively low, giving a low $P_{D(on)}$. At ON, the MOSFET's operating point lies in its ohmic region where, for an *n*-channel, enhancement-type MOSFET, the drain current can be shown to be (Northrop 1990):

$$I_D = K[2(V_{GS} - V_T)V_{DS} - V_{DS}^2] \quad \text{for} \quad 0 < |V_{DS}| < |V_{GS} - V_T| \tag{12.19}$$

where $V_{GS} = V_T$ is the FET's threshold voltage, where $I_D \rightarrow 0$. V_T is typically a low positive voltage, say 0 to +3V. K is a constant that is a function of the MOSFET's geometry and certain physical constants.

The equation of the line separating the MOSFET's ohmic and saturation operating regions is the parabola:

$$I_{DB} = K_V V_{DS}^2 \tag{12.20}$$

See Figure 12.11 for a plot of a typical *n*-channel enhancement MOSFET's $I_D(V_{GS}, V_{DS})$ curves. *p*-channel MOSFETs have similar characteristics as *n*-channel devices, except the signs of their parameters (I_D, V_{GS}, V_{DS}, V_P, and V_T) are the opposite.

The instantaneous power dissipation of an ON *n*-channel MOSFET assumed to be in its ohmic region is the product of I_D given by Equation 12.19 above times $V_{D(HI)}$, found from its load-line.

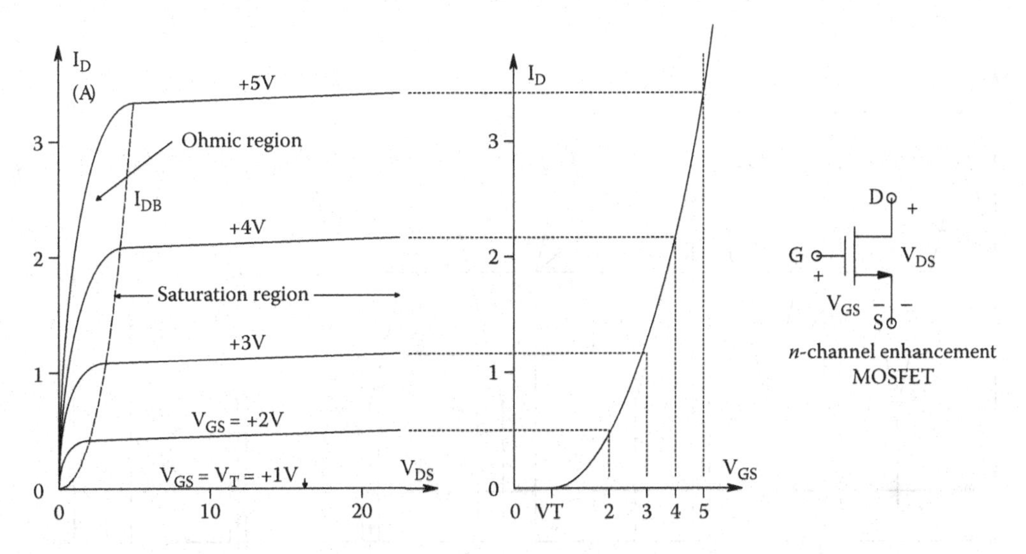

FIGURE 12.11 *Left:* Characteristic $I_D(V_{GS}, V_{DS})$ curves with operating regions delineated. *Center:* $I_D(V_{GS})$ curve. *Right:* Device schematic for an *n*-channel enhancement MOSFET.

Most class D PAs use pulse-width modulation (PWM) at a constant carrier frequency to drive the switching MOSFETs (see Section 11.61 and Figure 11.16 in this Text). Figures 12.12 and 12.13 illustrate PW modulated signals. Figure 12.14 illustrates a single-ended, class D PA. A high-speed analog comparator is used in conjunction with a high-frequency triangle wave, v_T, to generate a TTL PWM carrier. For an audio amplifier, the frequency of v_T can range from 200 kHz to over 1 MHz. The audio signal, v_s, may have a bandwidth from ca. 50 to 20 kHz. After conditioning by a class D switching PA IC, a high-voltage, bipolar, PWM signal, v_o', is generated. When v_o' is averaged by an RLC low-pass filter, the amplified signal, v_o, is recovered and is the input to the output transducer (loudspeaker or headphones). Note that when $v_s = 0$, v_o' is a symmetrical, high-voltage square wave with a 50% duty cycle, and no average power is delivered to the loudspeaker load ($v_o = 0$).

Other forms of pulse modulation for class D PA output stages include *pulse density modulation* (PDM), in which the number of pulses in a given time window is proportional to the average value

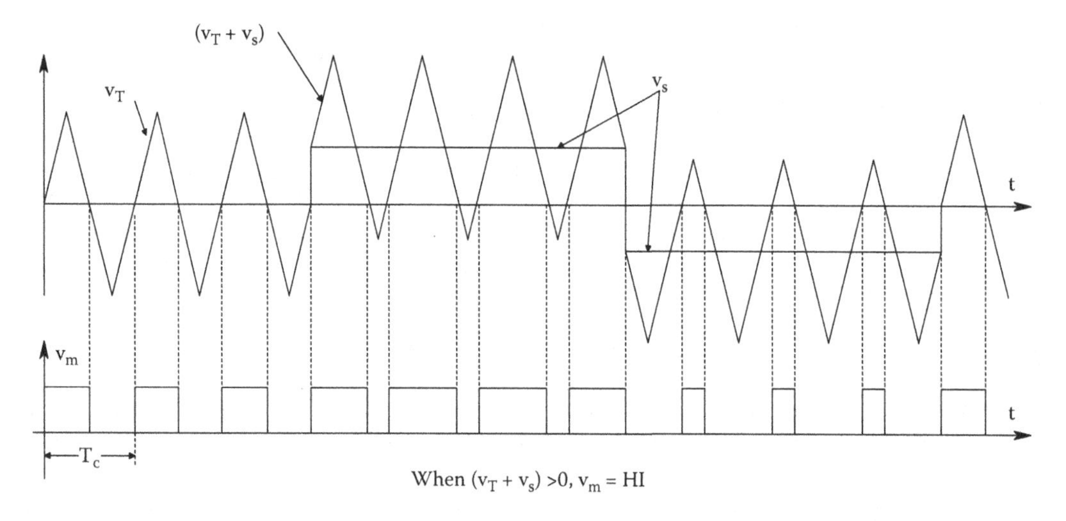

FIGURE 12.12 Waveforms in the generation of a pulse-width-modulated (PWM) signal; the input is a square wave. Note the duty cycle of the output pulses.

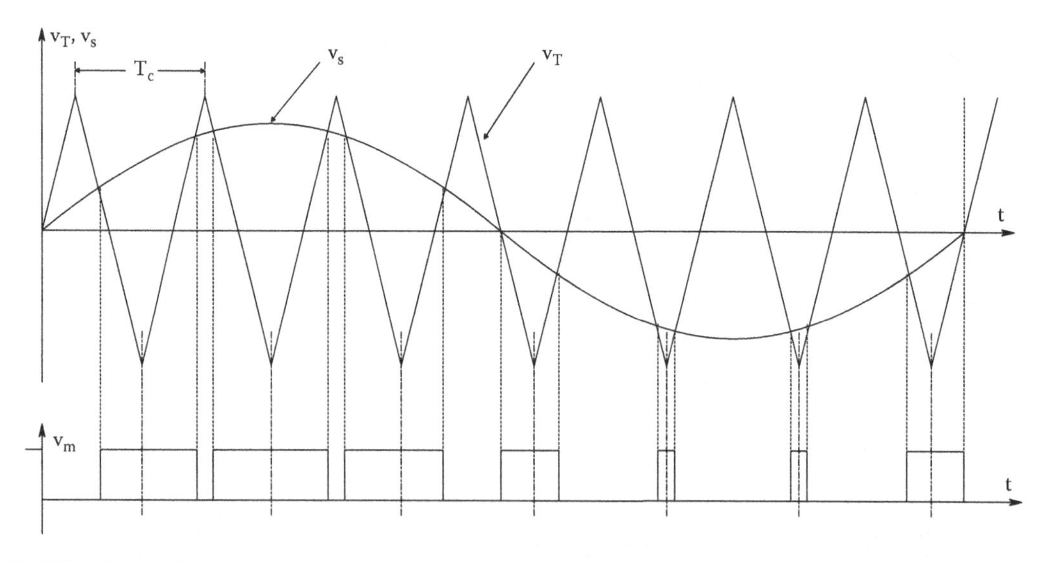

FIGURE 12.13 Same as Figure 12.11, except the modulating signal is a sine wave.

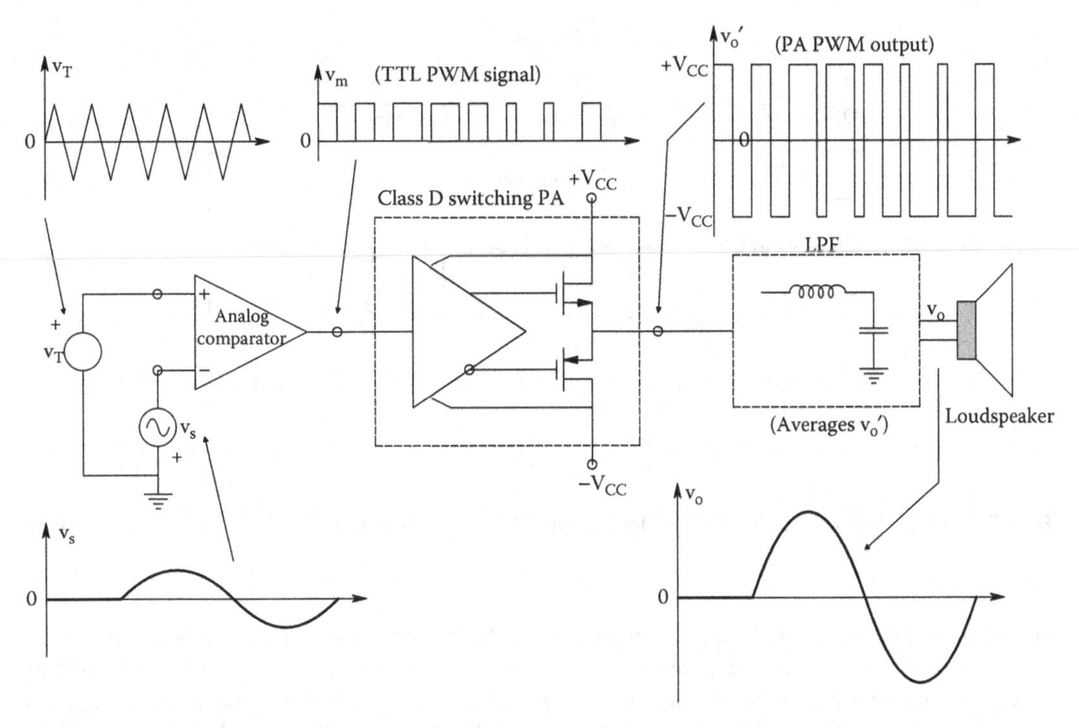

FIGURE 12.14 Block diagram of a class D, PWM audio amplifier. See text for description.

of $v_s + c$ (c is a DC level required for ($v_s + c$) to be non-negative). Individual pulse widths are not infinitely variable as in PWM (described in Figure 12.13), but are quantized to multiples of the PDM clock period, T_c. One-bit delta–sigma modulation (see Section 10.5.6 of this Text), and adaptive delta modulation are forms of PDM. Typical Δ-Σ and PDM clock frequencies lie between 2 and 6 MHz.

By using a push-pull, class D output stage (see Figure 12.15), the class D output power is doubled. This class D PA configuration is also called a full H-bridge switching circuit (Gaalaas 2006). The two half-bridge switching circuits alternately supply pulses of opposite polarity to the two, L-C LPFs. Two *p*-MOSFETs (Q_1 and Q_3) have their sources connected to + V_{CC}, and the two low-side, *n*-MOSFETs (Q2 and Q4) have their sources connected to V_{SS}, which can be zero or negative.

The choice of output MOSFETs in the full H-bridge PA requires consideration of a number of factors: Considering the load impedance of the output transducer (loudspeaker in this case), what is $\mathbf{Z}_L(j\omega)$, and what is the maximum audio power, $PA_{(max)}$, to be delivered to it? Z_L and $PA_{(max)}$ determine the maximum I_D(ON) and V_{DD} and V_{SS}. To ensure that the transistor power dissipation stays low, V_{DS} must be small when conducting large I_D. This requires an ON resistance of ca. 0.1 to 0.2 Ω; consequently, these large devices will have large gate input capacitance (C_G). This large C_G places a power burden on the transistors diving the power switches that is μ $C_G f_s$. Gaalaas (2006) observed:

> Power transistor manufacturers try to minimize the $R_{ON} \times C_G$ product for their devices to reduce overall power dissipation in switching applications, and to provide flexibility in the choice of switching frequency [f_s].

Because PWM class D PAs use carriers in the range of hundreds of kHz to low MHz, and the RLC LPFs are imperfect, the filtered output current contains electromagnetic interference (EMI) that lies at and around the triangle-wave clock frequency, f_T. The residual EMI through the load is inaudible; it can cause AM-band radio interference, however. This EMI and its harmonics can

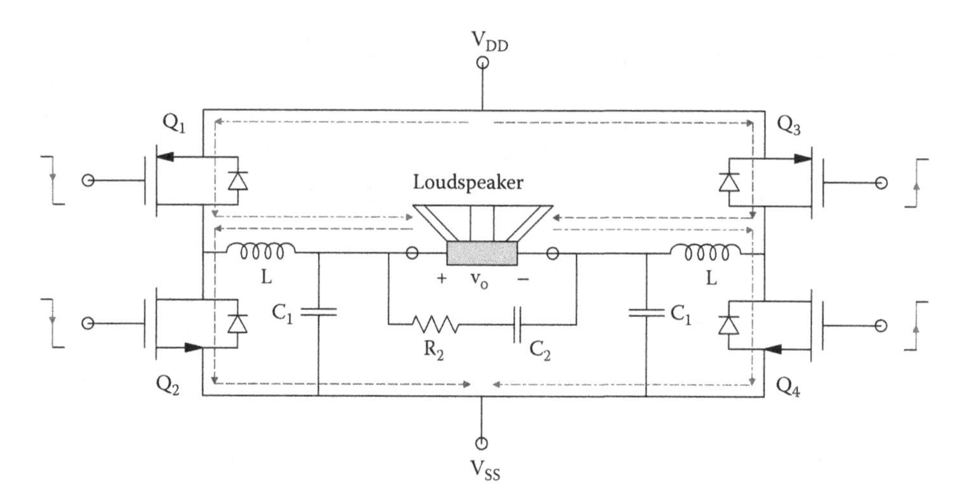

FIGURE 12.15 A switched MOSFET bridge used to drive a loudspeaker. This is also called a full H-bridge, class D PA.

be radiated from unshielded leads from the PA to the loudspeakers, and the PA's power supply wires. Remedies for this radio-frequency interference (RFI) include proper grounding and shielding practices, and the use of ferrite beads, radio-frequency chokes, and bypass capacitors in the power supply leads. Also, the use of low-loss, shielded toroidal inductors in the output L-C low-pass filters can reduce RFI. For an 8 Ω (nominal) loudspeaker impedance, one can obtain a −3dB corner frequency at 41 kHz using a 22 μH inductor with a quality 0.68 μF capacitor in the LPF (Gaalaas 2006). Beyond 41 kHz, the LPF attenuation rolls off at 40 dB/decade.

Many manufacturers make class D PA ICs. For example, the Analog Devices' AD1994 has two independent class D channels including two input, programmable-gain amplifiers (PGAs), two Σ-Δ modulators and two power output stages to drive two, full H-bridge-tied loads. The AD PA is intended for use in home theater, automotive, and PC audio applications. It generates switching waveforms that can drive stereo speakers (through external L-C LPFs) at up to 25 W per speaker, or 50 W to a single, monophonic speaker. This IC PA has integrated protection against output stage abuses such as overheating, overcurrent, and shoot-through current. Total harmonic distortion (THD) at full power output is an amazingly low 0.001%. It has a 105 dB dynamic range, and over 60 dB *power supply rejection* (PSR). It uses 1-bit, Σ-Δ modulation specially designed for class D application, and a +5 V supply for the PGA, modulator, and digital logic. A high-power supply from 8 to 20 V is required for the power stages. When driving 6 Ω loads, with 5 V and 12 V supplies at the 1 W level, the AD1994 dissipates 710 mW. With no signal input, it dissipates 487 mW.

National Semiconductor makes the LM4651 PWM driver IC and the LM4652 H-bridge power MOSFET IC. With proper heatsinking, these chips can be used to make a single channel, 170 W audio PA (Hobby 2010). This chipset has a thermal cut-out to protect the LM4652, which comes in a TO-220 package.

Another interesting class D PA IC is the Maxim MAX9700 (Maxim 2007). This PA boasts a "filterless output" architecture. Figure 12.16 illustrates the simplified system. Two comparators are used to generate differential switching signals for the full H-bridge MOSFET PA. Waveforms are shown in Figure 12.17. When both comparator outputs are LO, each output of the class D PA is HI ($+V_{DD}$), and the NOR gate output, R, goes HI. R going HI is delayed a few nanoseconds by the R_{on}-C_{on} LPF at its output. When the delayed output reaches the HI for the two MOS signal switches (SW1 and SW2), they close, this causes both outputs (v_1 and v_2) to go LO and remain LO until the

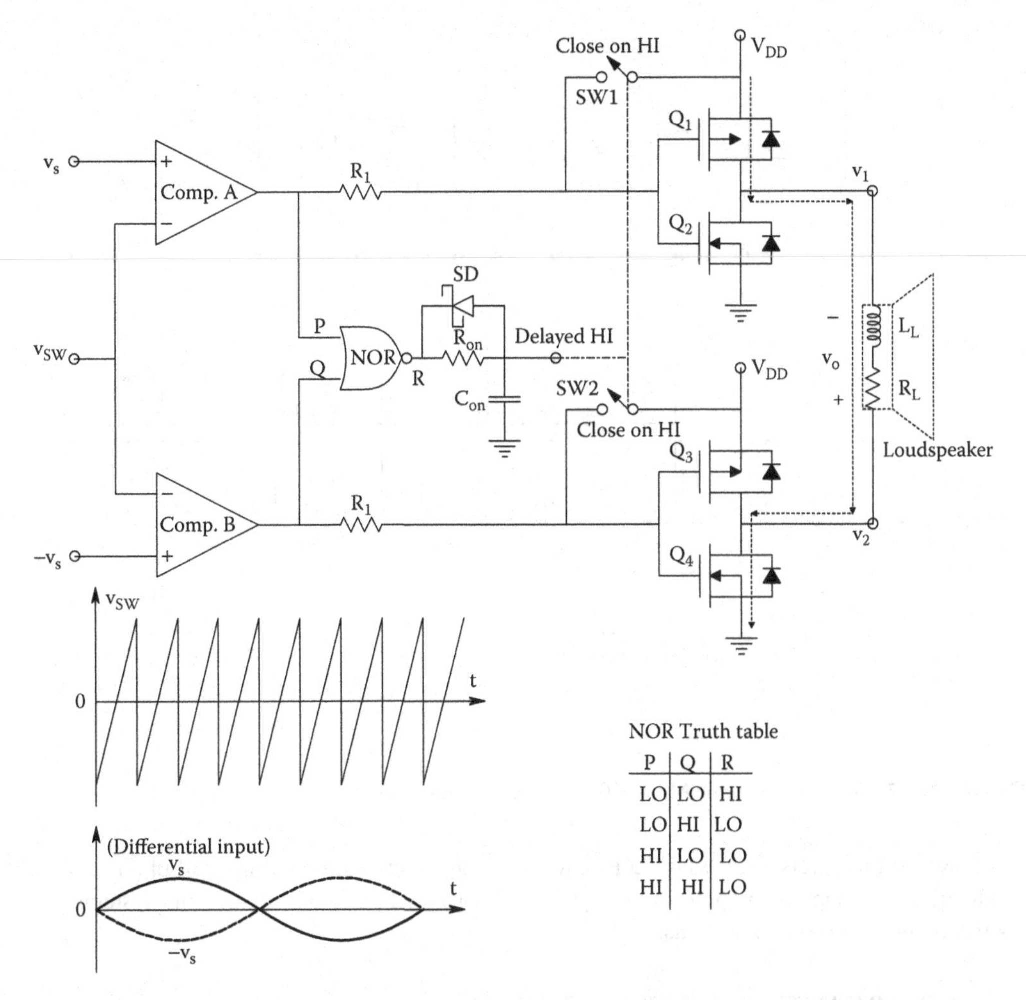

FIGURE 12.16 Simplified schematic of the Maxim MAX9700, filterless output class D PA IC. Note that no low-pass filters are used between the switched FETs and the loudspeaker, such as seen in Figure 12.15.

next sampling period begins. This protocol causes both outputs to be ON for a minimum amount of time, $t_{ON(min)}$, which is set by $R_{on}C_{on}$. When $v_s = 0$, the outputs are in phase, and their pulse widths are $t_{ON(min)}$, so $v_o = v_1 - v_2 = 0$. When $v_s > 0$, v_1 has PWM pulses, while v_2 produces a train of narrow, $t_{ON(min)}$-width pulses. Similarly, when $v_s < 0$, v_2 has the PWM pulses and v_1 produces the train of narrow, $t_{ON(min)}$-width pulses. The MAX9700 class D amplifier makes use of the inherent inductance (L_L) of the loudspeaker's voice coil and its series resistance (R_L) to form a first-order LPF to smooth the pulses in the bipolar current i_o waveform in the loudspeaker voice coil. (Voice coil deflection force is proportional to i_o.) The −3dB frequency of this LPF is easily seen to be $f_o = R_L/(2\pi L_L)$ Hz. By making the frequency of the sawtooth wave about 1.4 MHz, it is possible to recover the audio signal and also prevent excessive amounts of high-frequency switching energy from being dissipated in R_L. Clearly, when using this amplifier, the loudspeaker's **Z** should be inductive at the carrier wave's frequency.

As with other PWM, full-H PAs, "filterless" class D amplifiers generate RFI, and must be properly shielded and bypassed to minimize this interference.

Modern class D PAs have good linearity, high power efficiency, and low PC board space requirements.

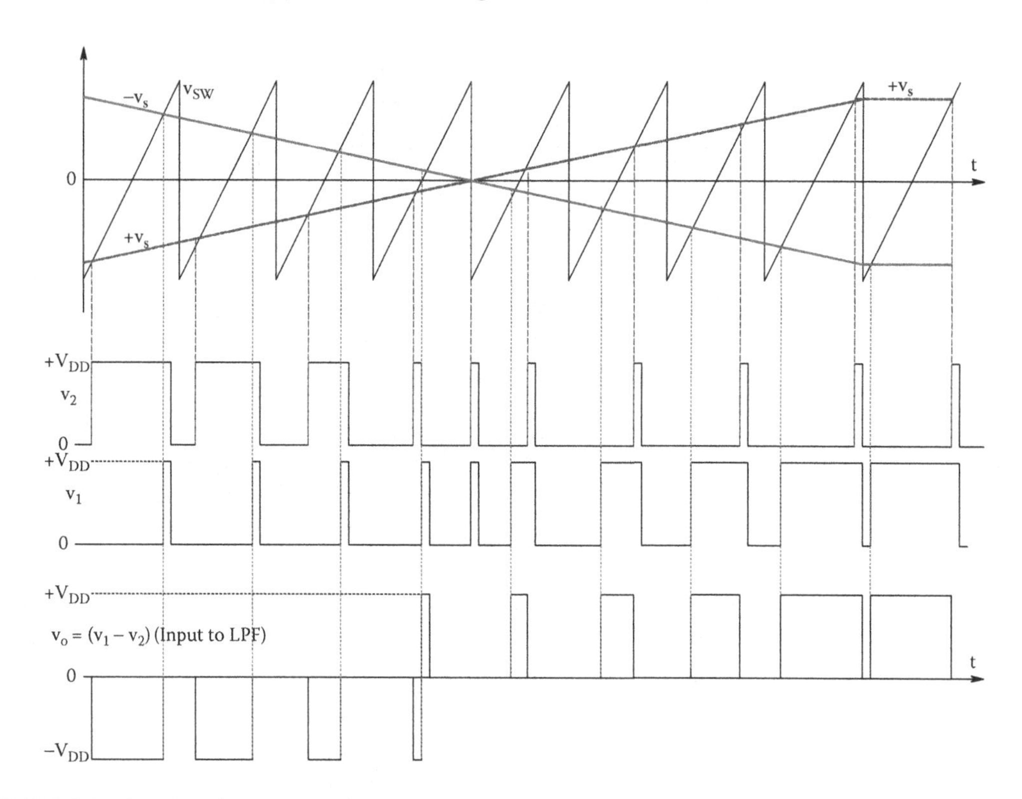

FIGURE 12.17 Waveforms in the MAX9700. See text for description.

Many manufacturers make class D PAs for many applications, including: cell phones, portable audio equipment, laptop computer sound systems, flat-panel TVs, automotive sound systems, and of course, home stereo sound systems.

12.5 NONLINEARITY AND DISTORTION IN PAs

Depending on the transistor biasing used, the nonlinear (static) transfer curve of a PA alone can have both a pronounced deadzone *and* saturation (see Figure 12.18). Such nonlinear transfer curves can generate unwanted harmonics in v_o. Even though classes AB and B PAs create more distortion in the output voltage, they are widely used because of their greater efficiencies, and the fact that overall negative voltage feedback can reduce the total harmonic distortion (THD) at the output. Total harmonic distortion and its reduction were described in Section 4.3.2 of this text. To illustrate how negative voltage feedback can markedly reduce THD, especially in power op amps, consider Figure 12.19a, which illustrates the circuit of a simple, single-loop, negative voltage feedback system using an op amp to drive a resistive load, R_L. Figure 12.19b illustrates a simple, midfrequency, block diagram/Thevenin circuit of the POA output and its THD voltages, v_{thd}, driving the load. In general, v_{thd} is an increasing function of the Thevenin signal output voltage, v_{os} (see Figure 4.3c in this text). All of the THD is assumed to arise in the power output stage. From this circuit and system, we can write

$$v_i' = v_s\alpha + v_o\beta \tag{12.21}$$

$$v_o = \gamma(-K_v v_i') + \gamma\, v_{thd} \tag{12.22}$$

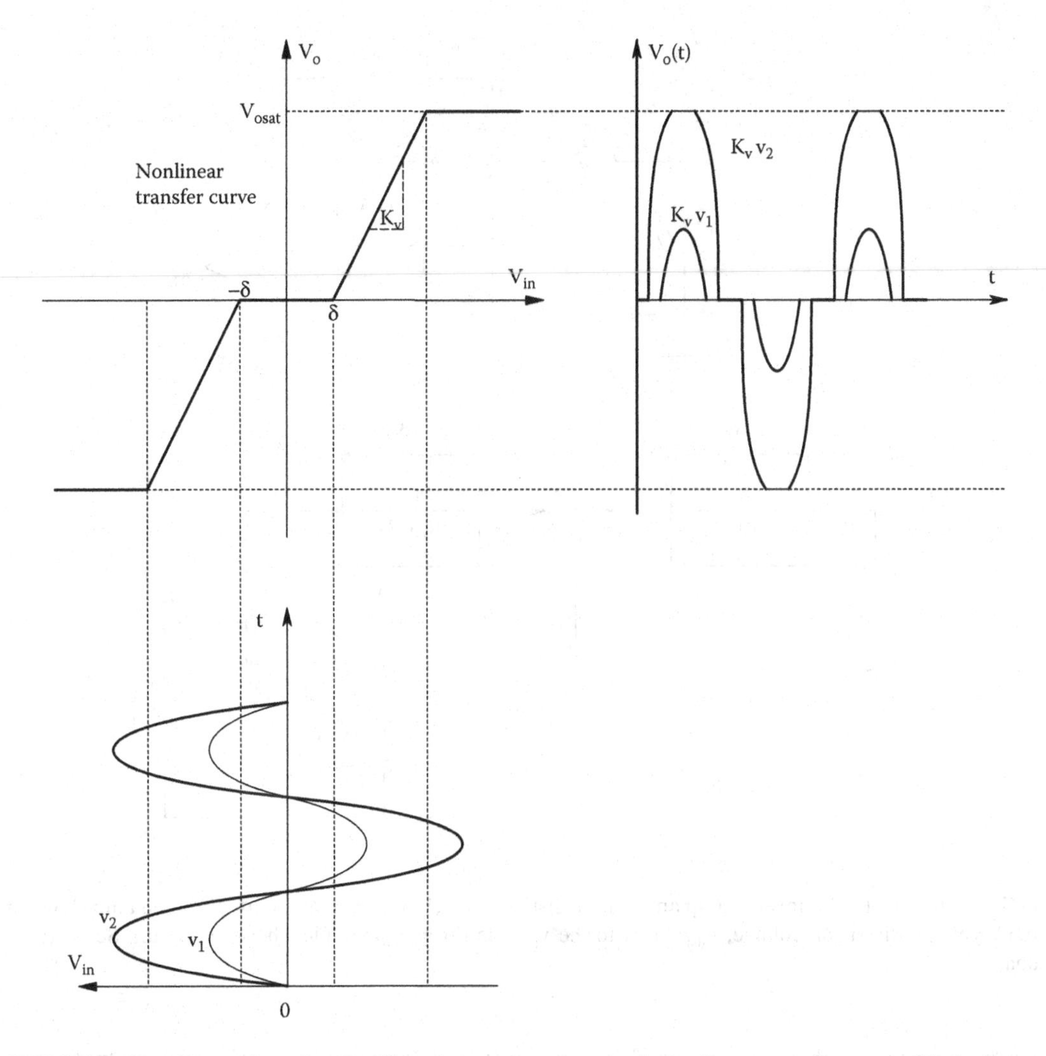

FIGURE 12.18 Generation of output distortion products by a static, nonlinear transfer curve with dead-zone and saturation in a PA.

where $\alpha \equiv \dfrac{R_2}{R_2 + R_1}$, $\beta \equiv \dfrac{R_1}{R_2 + R_1}$, and $\gamma \equiv \dfrac{R_L}{R_L + R_s + R_s'}$ (from the resistor voltage dividers)

Combining Equations 12.21 and 12.22, and using superposition, v_o is solved for

$$V_o = \frac{-v_s \gamma K_v \alpha}{(1 + \gamma K_v \beta)} + \frac{v_{thd}\ \gamma}{(1 + \gamma K_v \beta)} \tag{12.23}$$

Now assume $\gamma K_v \beta >> 1$. The negative voltage feedback amplifier's output voltage can be written as

$$v_o \cong -v_s (R_2/R_1) + v_{thd}/(K_v \beta) \tag{12.24}$$

The inverting signal gain is determined by R_2/R_1, and the THD voltage is reduced by dividing it by the feedback amplifier's *return difference* $(1 - \mathbf{A}_L(j\omega))$, in this case $(1 + \gamma K_v \beta) = [1 + \gamma K_v R_1/(R_1 + R_2)]$, generally a very large number. Although a simple op amp example was used here, the

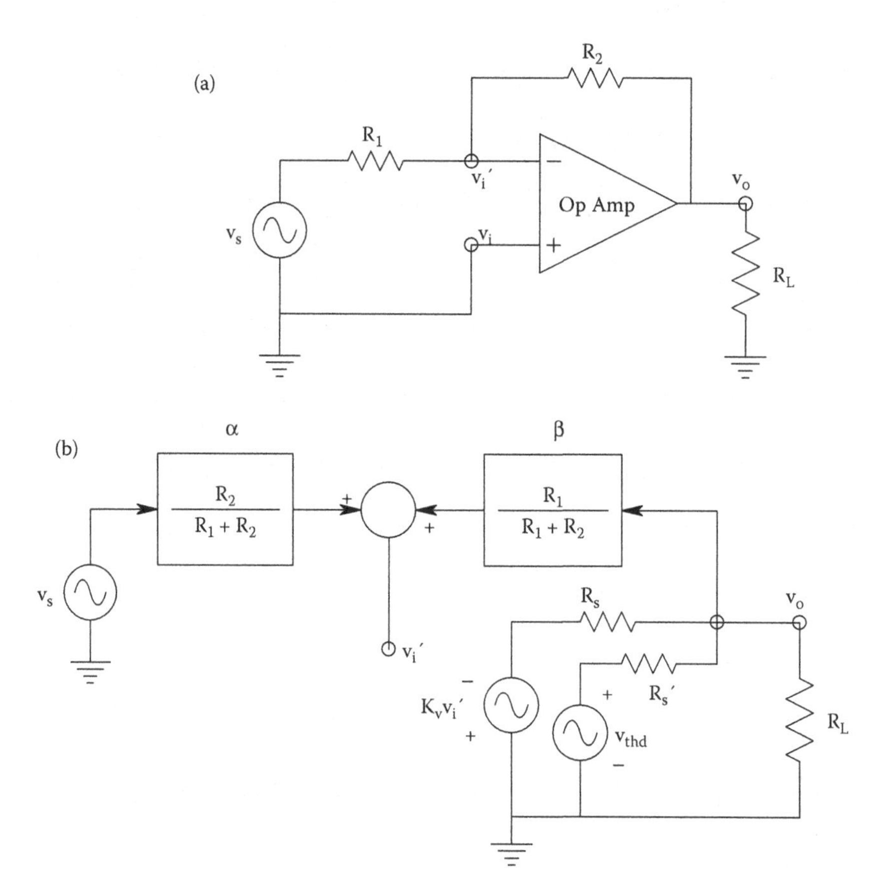

FIGURE 12.19 (a) An inverting op amp with resistive load. (b) Equivalent circuit of the op amp showing the harmonic distortion voltage, v_{thd}, input to the v_o node through a simple Thevenin circuit. See text for analysis.

general principle is that because the THD voltages may be assumed to occur in the output stage, negative voltage feedback will always reduce THD at the output by a factor of $1/|1 - \mathbf{A}_L(j\omega)|$. It may be easily shown that if distortion arises in the input stage of a PA, such reduction does not occur because it is effectively in series with the input signal.

12.6 IC VOLTAGE REGULATORS IN MEDICAL ELECTRONIC SYSTEMS

12.6.1 Introduction

Nearly, all medical electronic systems, including op amps, power amplifiers, ADCs, DACs, logic chips, microcomputers, IC thermometers, analog multipliers, ECG amplifiers, SpO_2 monitors, etc. are operated from regulated DC power supplies. Such medical systems also include battery-operated electronics (used for isolation). As batteries are drained of energy, their open-circuit EMFs drop, and their Thevenin equivalent internal resistances rise; in sum, they become less and less like ideal voltage sources. Consequently, some sort of IC voltage regulator is generally put between the battery and the circuit it supplies to provide a constant output voltage through a very low dynamic output (Thevenin) impedance.

DC power supplies that operate off 120 VAC generally consist of an isolation-type, step-down power transformer, a full-wave rectifier, and capacitor low-pass filter. The DC voltage at this point generally has some 120 Hz ripple, and its average value can change proportionally with the mains voltage. Thus, a voltage regulator IC is used to "purify" the basic rectifier's output voltage, as well as to remove output voltage changes due to variations in the load current, I_L.

12.6.2 Zener (Avalanche) Regulators

Zener diode regulators are simple, inexpensive, low-power, passive voltage regulators. Figure 12.20 shows a generic zener diode volt–ampere curve. Note that in the zener region, the curve has a finite slope, giving the zener a small, small-signal, Thevenin series resistance, r_z. The zener is generally operated at a Q-point, I_{zo}, V_{zo}, to obtain minimum r_z. Figure 12.21a shows the basic circuit of a simple zener diode regulator, typically used for powering a few low-voltage ICs (e.g., +5V logic chips) on a circuit board. In the circuit, R_L is the effective load resistance; it is equal to V_z/I_L by Ohm's law. From Ohm's law, one can see that the required value of the series resistor, R_S, is

$$R_S = \frac{V_S - V_{zo}}{I_{zo} + I_L} = \frac{R_L(V_S - V_{zo})}{I_{zo}R_L + V_{zo}}$$

The required wattage of $R_S = (V_S - V_{zo})(I_L + I_{zo})$. (This analysis neglected r_z.) Under zero load conditions, only R_S limits the current through the zener, and this Resistor must be large enough

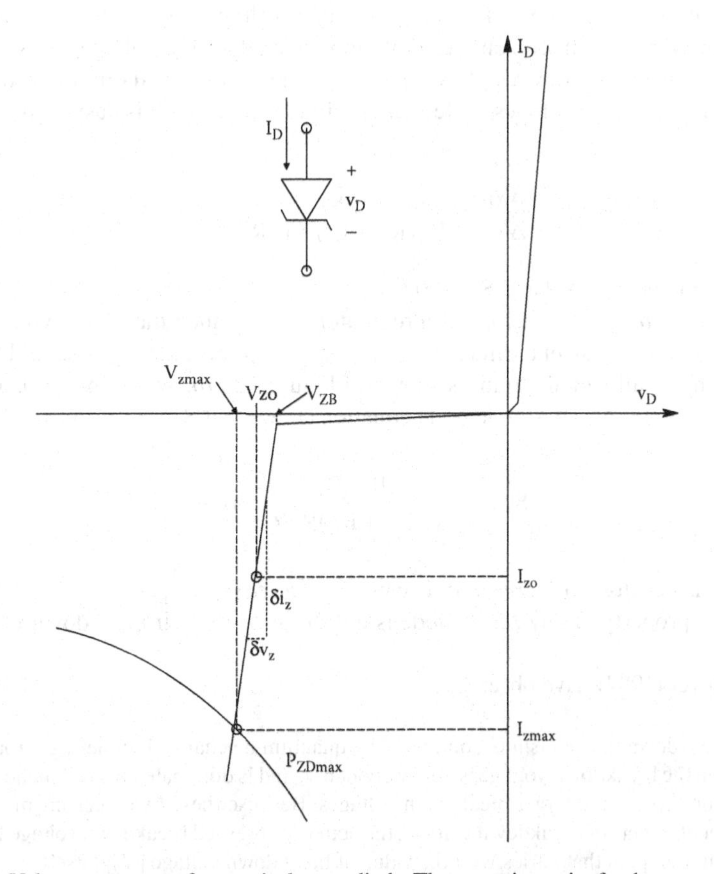

FIGURE 12.20 Volt–ampere curve for a typical zener diode. The operating point for the zener diode is at I_{zo}, V_{zo}.

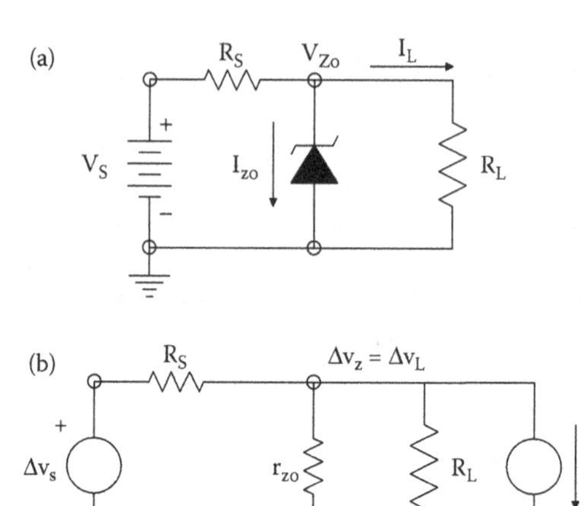

FIGURE 12.21 (a) Basic circuit for a zener diode-regulated DC source. (b) DC small-signal model for the zener regulator used to derive input and output sensitivities.

to prevent the zener power from exceeding the maximum dissipation for the diode. That is, $[(V_S - V_{Zmax})/R_S]V_{Zmax} < P_{Zmax}$. Often an electrolytic or tantalum capacitor is placed across the load for low-pass filtering V_o.

An important figure of merit for any regulated voltage supply is its *small-signal input sensitivity*. That is, given a fixed zener circuit, how much does the voltage across R_L, V_L, vary as the result of a change in the raw supply voltage, V_S? The small-signal circuit used in this analysis is shown in Figure 12.21b. From a simple voltage-divider relation, it is easy to show that the input sensitivity is

$$\frac{\Delta V_L}{\Delta V_S} = \frac{r_{zo} R_L}{R_S(R_L + r_{zo}) + r_{zo} R_L} = S_{in}$$

If the diode were ideal, $r_{zo} \to 0$ and $S_{in} \to 0$.

The *small-signal output sensitivity* of a regulator is how much the output voltage varies as the result of a change in load current; dimensionally, it is a resistance; ideally, it should be zero. That is, $\Delta V_o/\Delta I_L \to 0$. The small-signal circuit is shown in Figure 12.21b. We set $\Delta v_s = 0$, and consider the change in V_L caused by Δi_L. A simple node equation shows that $S_{out} = \Delta v_L/\Delta i_L$ is

$$S_{out} = -\frac{R_S r_z R_L}{r_z(R_L + R_S)R_S R_L} \text{ ohms}$$

The minus sign is because an *increase* in I_L causes a *decrease* in V_L.

An important property of any zener diode is the variation of their breakdown voltage, V_{ZB}, with temperature.

Gray and Meyer (1984) have observed:

> The actual breakdown mechanism is dominated by quantum mechanical tunneling through the depletion layer when the breakdown voltage is below about 6 V, and is dominated by avalanche multiplication in the depletion layer at the larger breakdown voltages. Because these two mechanisms have opposite temperature coefficients of breakdown voltage, the actually observed breakdown voltage has a temperature coefficient [tempco] that varies with the value of breakdown voltage [V_{ZB}] itself.

The zero tempco V_{ZB} is seen to be about 5.3 V; above 5.3 V, the tempco increases rapidly, being ca. 5.5 mV/°C at $V_{ZB} = 10$ V. The use of zero tempco zener diodes is desirable in generating stable internal voltage references for IC regulators.

One need not use a zener diode, *per se,* for a regulated reference supply. The reverse-biased, emitter-base diode of a BJT can also be used. The unregulated DC supply is attached to the emitter with an appropriate series resistor, R_S, and the base and collector are grounded. A typical V_{ZO} (from emitter to ground) for a small-signal *npn* BJT is ca. 6.2 V at 10 mA.

Zener diodes come in a wide range of voltages, P_{Zmax}s, and packages, permitting simple supplies that can supply mA to amps to a load at V_{ZO}.

12.6.3 Active IC Regulators

An active, IC voltage regulator is seen simply as a high-gain, d-c amplifier that uses negative voltage feedback to force its DC output voltage to remain constant in spite of variations in output current or DC source voltage. Its dynamic output impedance is made very low by the high loop-gain negative feedback. However, like an op amp, its performance deteriorates with the increasing frequency of its load current.

Most IC regulators are series regulators, i.e., they are put between the raw, higher voltage source, V_S, and the lower, regulated, DC voltage across the load, $V_o = V_L$. Some have fixed V_os, others allow V_o to be adjusted. Negative and positive V_o regulators exist. For example, the TO-220 flat heatsinked package is used to house the popular LM78XY and LM79XY regulators. The "78"s are positive regulators, and the "79"s supply negative V_os from negative V_Ss. The "XY" gives the magnitude of the nominal regulated output voltage; i.e., the LM7905 gives −5 V out. The LM78XY and LM79XY regulators can supply as much as 1.5 A at their rated V_o. Generally the TO-220 package must be attached to a heatsink; the approximate power dissipation of one of these regulators is $P_R = (V_S - V_o)I_L$ Watts. For example, an LM7805 supplying 1 amp and driven from a + 15 V V_S will produce over 10 W. that must be dissipated so the internal power transistor junctions do not exceed ca. 160°C.

Figure 12.22a illustrates the circuit of a basic series, positive output, low-dropout, IC regulator. Note that a series regulator varies the voltage across its series element(s) $(V_S - V_o)$, in order hold V_o constant in the face of changes in V_S and I_L. Negative voltage feedback is used to maintain a constant V_o; V_o is subtracted from a fixed, internal, DC reference voltage, V_R to generate an error voltage, V_e. (V_R can be generated from an internal, zero-tempco, zener source.)

Some IC regulators feature output current limiting in which the output voltage falls to zero rapidly as $I_L > I_{Lmax}$. For example, the LP2952 regulator will source at least 250 mA without current limiting as long as $1.25 \le V_o \le 29$ V, and the input voltage V_s is $\ge 0.8 + V_o$.

The differential amplifier in the simple series regulator schematic of Figure 12.22a must have a high differential gain, similar to an op amp, for good regulation. V_R is compared to βV_o, if an increase in regulator I_L causes βV_o to drop below V_R, an increase in the DA output voltage causes an increase in base current in Q1, which in turn turns on Q1 more, causing the emitter current in Q2 to increase and its V_{CE} to decrease, restoring V_o. Figure 12.22 also illustrates three popular series element circuit architectures that are driven by the *npn* Q1. The circuit of **B** is the simplest; a series *pnp* power transistor, Q2, used in *low dropout* (LDO) regulators that typically supply $I_{Lmax} = 1$ A. The feedback pair circuit is shown in **C**. It is used in "Quasi-LDO" regulators that supply ca. $I_{Lmax} = 7.5$ A. The standard series regulator element is shown in **D**. It uses a feedback-pair/Darlington architecture. Here, $I_{Lmax} \cong 10$.A.

The electrical characteristics of IC series regulators are typically specified at a standard temperature of 25°C. For the ubiquitous LM7805, +5 V, 1A regulator, they include but are not limited to.

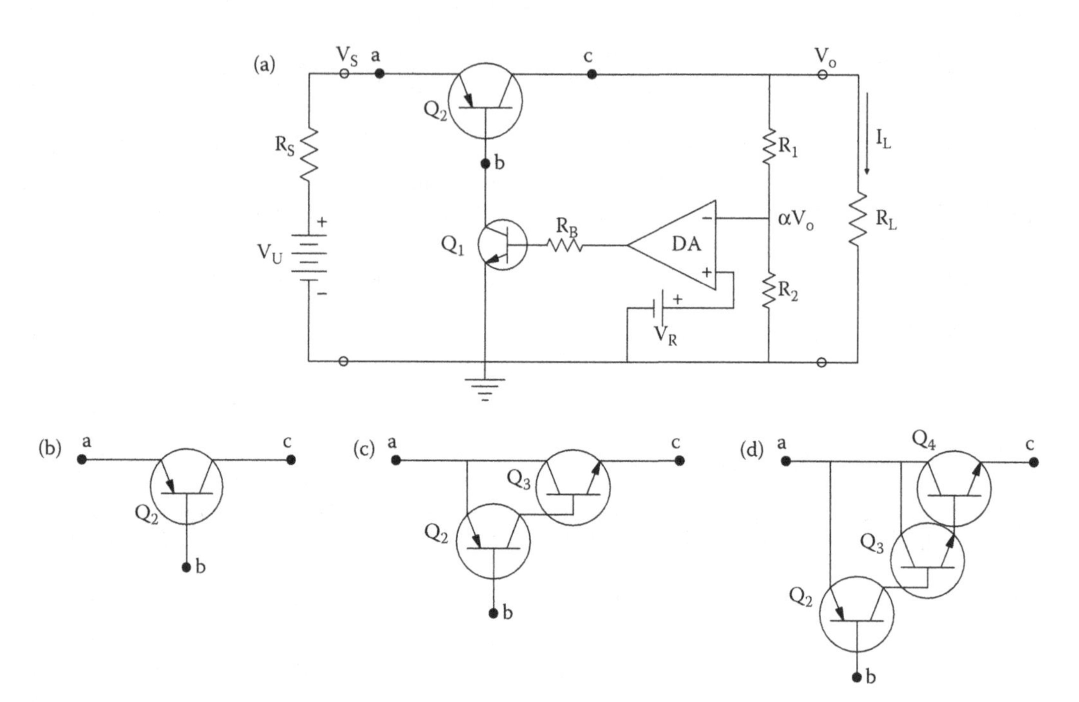

FIGURE 12.22 (a) A simplified schematic for a low dropout, series voltage regulator. The regulator's performance deteriorates at high frequencies of I_L because of the high frequency response attenuation of the DA and transistors. (b) *pnp* series regulator BJT used in a positive-output voltage, low-dropout (LDO) regulator. (c) A feedback pair series regulator used in a quasi-LDO positive regulator. (d) A feedback pair-Darlington series regulator architecture.

TABLE 12.1
Summary of the Electrical Characteristics of the Fairchild KA7805 3-terminal, 1A, Positive Voltage Regulator IC

Parameter	Symbol	Conditions	Typical Value	Unit
Output Voltage	V_o	5 mA ≤ Io ≤ 1.0 A, 25°C	5.0	V.
Line (input) regulation	Regline		4	mV/V
Load (output) regulation	Regload	I_o = 5ma to 1.5 A	9	mV/A
Quiescent (0 load) input current			5	mA
Output voltage drift	$\Delta V_o/\Delta T$	Io = 5 mA	−0.8	mV/°C
Output noise voltage	V_N	10 Hz ≤ f ≤ 100 kHz, 25°C	42	μV/V_o
Ripple rejection	RR	f = 120 Hz, Vo = 8 – 18V	73	dB
Dropout voltage ($V_S - V_o$)	V_{Drop}	I_o = 1A, TJ = 25°C	2	V.
Output resistance (small-signal)	r_o	f = 1 kHz	15	mΩ
Short-circuit current	I_{SC}	V_S = 35 V, 25°C	230	mA
Peak current	I_{PK}		2.2A	A.

Note: Note that Regload has the dimensions of milliohms; it is in effect, the Thevenin output resistance of the regulator (mV/A = mΩ)

In summary, there are many kinds of linear series voltage regulators; Most output fixed positive or negative DC voltages at current ranges from 1 A to over 10 A. Just as PAs have used the class D, switched output to minimize amplifier power dissipation, *Switching regulators* such as the National Semiconductor LM2575 also use the same principle to minimize regulator power dissipation. The LM2575 accepts +7 to 40 V unregulated DC inputs, and outputs +5 V @ 1A. Because its raw output is a square wave with a variable duty cycle, it is low-pass filtered by an external L-C low-pass filter (L = 330 μH, C = 330 μF). Switching regulators are available in various circuit configurations: flyback, feed-forward, push-pull, and nonisolated single polarity types. They can also operate in any of three modes: step-down, step-up, or polarity inverting. For example, the LM2577 switching regulator can accept a +5V unregulated input and deliver +12V @ ≤ 0.8 A. All switching regulators use external components: electrolytic capacitors, resistors, a zener diode, and an inductor (generally a small toroidal coil about 2 cm in diameter).

The underlying principle of all regulators is the use of a high-gain, negative feedback loop in which the regulated output voltage is subtracted from a stable, DC reference voltage (V_R) to generate an error voltage (V_E) that is used to vary the current in a series pass amplifier, correcting for drops in V_o due to changes in I_L. Like all high-gain, d-c feedback systems, IC series regulators have a high frequency response limitation. In general, the magnitude of a regulator's small-signal output impedance increases from a low, real value (r_o in milliohms) to a larger, complex value of $\mathbf{Z}_o(j\omega)$ as the frequency of the load, $\mathbf{I}_L(j\omega)$ increases. To compensate for this increase of $|\mathbf{Z}_o|$ with increasing ω, designers often connect a tantalum electrolytic capacitor to ground at the regulator's output node. Thus, the regulator's net output admittance is $\mathbf{Y}_o'(j\omega) = j\omega C + \mathbf{Z}_o^{-1}(j\omega)$; as ω increases, the decrease in $\mathbf{Z}_o^{-1}(j\omega)$ is offset by increasing ωC. Also, broadbanding techniques are used in the design of the error voltage-generating DA.

12.7 HEATSINKING

A frequent cause of electronic power amplifier, IC series voltage regulator, and DC power supply failures is high transistor temperatures caused by running the system at full power output when poor attention has been given to the design of the heatsinks and the heat dissipation system associated with the power transistors. With power BJTs, excess junction temperature can shift the power devices' Q points upward so thermal runaway may occur.

To approach the problem of heatsink design, a simple DC circuit analog describing a heat-dissipating system will be used: DC voltage will represent temperature, electrical resistances will represent thermal resistances (Θ degrees Celsius/watt), and current sources will represent heat (power) sources. Figure 12.23 illustrates an analog DC circuit model for heat flow for a power device (BJT, MOSFET, and POA) on a heatsink. $\mathbf{T_J}$ is the device junction temperature (all temperatures are modeled as voltages). $\mathbf{T_{J(max)}}$ is the manufacturer's specified maximum temperature for the device's junctions (if it is a BJT), or its channel (if it is a MOSFET). $\mathbf{T_C}$ is the device's case temperature (the case is in intimate contact with a heatsink), $\mathbf{T_H}$ is the heatsink temperature (assumed to be uniform), and $\mathbf{T_A}$ is the fixed, ambient air temperature. Θ_{jc} is the thermal resistance of the device to its case,

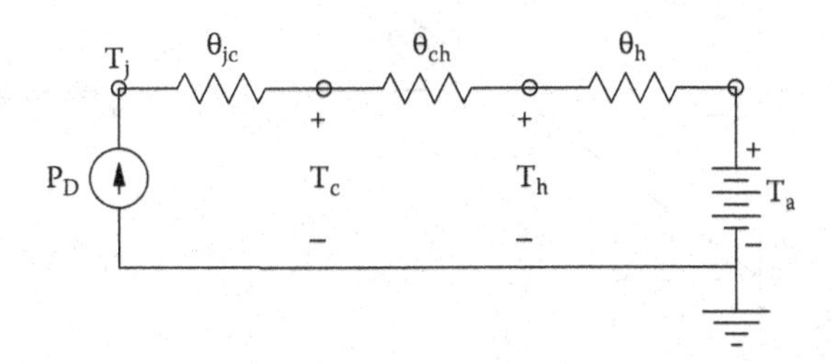

FIGURE 12.23 Electrical analog circuit for heat generation and flow in a transistor-heatsink system. See text for analysis.

Θ_{ch} is the thermal resistance of the device case to the heatsink, and Θ_h is the thermal resistance of the heatsink itself. (Note that the units of thermal resistance are degrees K per watt.) The device heat source, represented as a DC current source in the analog circuit, is $\mathbf{P_D}$ watts.

Good thermal design involves choosing a heatsink with Θ_h small enough to satisfy

$$T_{J(max)} \leq P_D(\Theta_{jc} + \Theta_{ch} + \Theta_h) + T_A \tag{12.25}$$

Or equivalently,

$$\Theta \leq \frac{T_{J(max)} - T_A - P_D(\Theta_{jc} + \Theta_{ch})}{P_D} \tag{12.26}$$

To obtain a low Θ_h, designers make heatsinks from a metal with high thermal conductivity and add fins to heatsinks to enhance radiation and convection, and also they make use of small fans for heatsink cooling. In some applications, thermoelectric (Peltier) cooling is used, but this just moves the device heat to the Peltier hot junctions, which can be heatsinked outside of the electronics package.

Often manufacturers of power devices supply a power derating curve, $\mathbf{P_D(T_C)}$. A typical derating curve is shown in Figure 12.24. Safe device operation lies under the derating curve, and to the left of $\mathbf{T_{J(max)}}$. Note that when the case temperature reaches $\mathbf{T_{J(max)}}$, device failure is immanent and it should be turned off. Often in Hi-Fi equipment, and regulated power supplies, temperature-sensing switches are put on the heatsinks to turn off the system when $\mathbf{T_H \approx T_{J(max)}}$ Some modern POAs also shut down automatically when $\mathbf{T_C \approx T_{J(max)}}$.

A simultaneous solution of the derating curve of Figure 12.24, $\mathbf{P_D} = f(\mathbf{T_C})$ with the temperature difference $(\mathbf{T_C} - \mathbf{T_a})$ from Figure 12.23 can be written as

$$P_D = \frac{T_C}{(\Theta_h + \Theta_{ch})} + \frac{T_A}{(\Theta_h + \Theta_{ch})} = f(T_C) \tag{12.27}$$

The solution is shown graphically in Figure 12.24. Where the $\mathbf{f(T_C)}$ curve crosses the derating curve yields the equilibrium case temperature, $\mathbf{T_{eq}}$. It is clear that the more efficient the heatsink is, the lower $(\Theta_h + \Theta_{ch})$ will be, the lower $\mathbf{T_C = T_{eq}}$ can be, and the higher the permitted $\mathbf{P_D}$ can be.

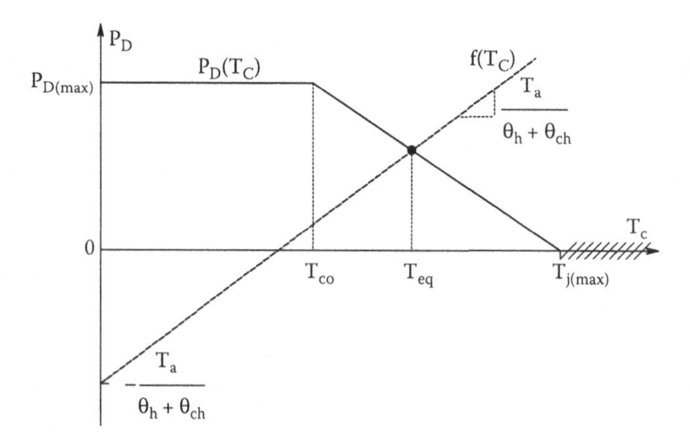

FIGURE 12.24 Simultaneous solution of the device derating curve, $P_D(T_C)$, and the thermal resistance "load-line," $f(T_C)$, giving the device equilibrium temperature, T_{eq}. See text for details.

From Figure 12.24 and Equation 12.27, we can write an expression for the maximum $(\Theta_h + \Theta_{ch})$ that will allow $\mathbf{P_D} = \mathbf{P_{D(max)}}$, given any $\mathbf{T_A} < \mathbf{T_{co}}$. This is

$$(\Theta_h + \Theta_{ch}) \leq \frac{T_{co} - T_A}{P_{D(max)}} \tag{12.28}$$

Equation 12.28 tells us that the thermal resistances $(\Theta_h + \Theta_{ch})$ must be less than the right-hand side of Equation 12.28 in order for the device to be run at its maximum power rating, $\mathbf{P_{D(max)}}$.

Heatsinks are usually located outside on the cases of audio power amplifiers and power supplies. This location offers two advantages: It keeps the internal low-power electronics cooler, and it also allows cooling by free-air convection; fans are seldom used. When heatsinks are used *inside* the case on the motherboard, one or more mini-fans are generally used to circulate outside air through the case (this design is widely seen in desktop and laptop computers). In laptops, the fan can be activated when the CPU temperature reaches some preset limit.

12.8 CHAPTER SUMMARY

In this chapter, we first considered non-tuned applications for power amplifiers in biomedicine. Then, we described the volt–ampere characteristics of power output devices, including high-perveance BJTs, MOSFETs, and power op amps. Power amplifier efficiency was considered, and classes A, AB, B, C, and D PAs were described and analyzed. The important IC voltage regulator was next introduced, including the simple zener supply. Lastly, we considered the important topic of heatsinking in PA designs. Device cooling can be by radiation/convection using finned heatsinks, or fans, thermoelectric (Peltier) cooling, or in extreme cases (some X-ray tubes) water cooling.

CHAPTER 12 HOME PROBLEMS

12.1 A Thevenin source, V_S, R_S, is coupled to a resistive load, R_L, through an idea transformer with turns ratio n_1/n_2. Find an expression for the turns ratio that will maximize the power transfer from the source to the load.

12.2 A ***pnp*** emitter-follower is used as a PA. *Let:* $V_{CE(sat)} = 0$, $R_L = 100\ \Omega$, $\beta = 19$, $V_{CEQ} = -10$ V, and $v_1 = V_1 \sin(\omega t)$. See Figure P12.2.

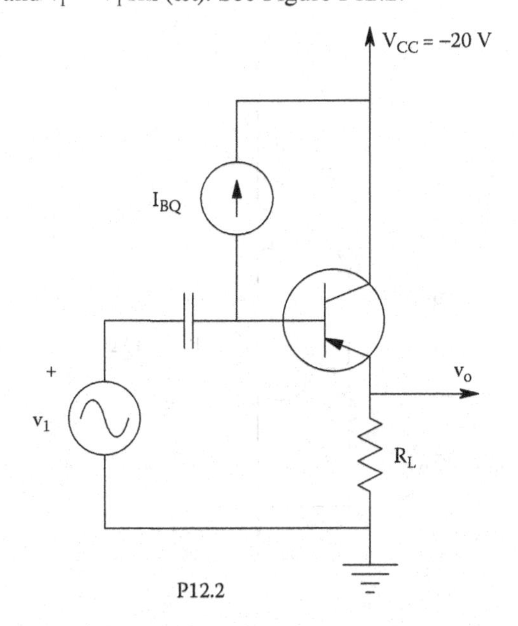

P12.2

(A) Find I_{BQ} required for DC quiescent biasing.
(B) Find the DC power dissipated in R_L under quiescent conditions.
(C) Find the maximum average undistorted power in R_L under sinusoidal operating conditions.

12.3 The peak undistorted sinusoidal output voltage of a certain power op amp is 35 V; the peak undistorted sinusoidal output current is 5 A. The POA is used to drive a 700 Ω load, R_L. Let $v_i = V_1 \sin(\omega t)$.
(A) Find the maximum average undistorted AC power in R_L in Figure P12.3A.

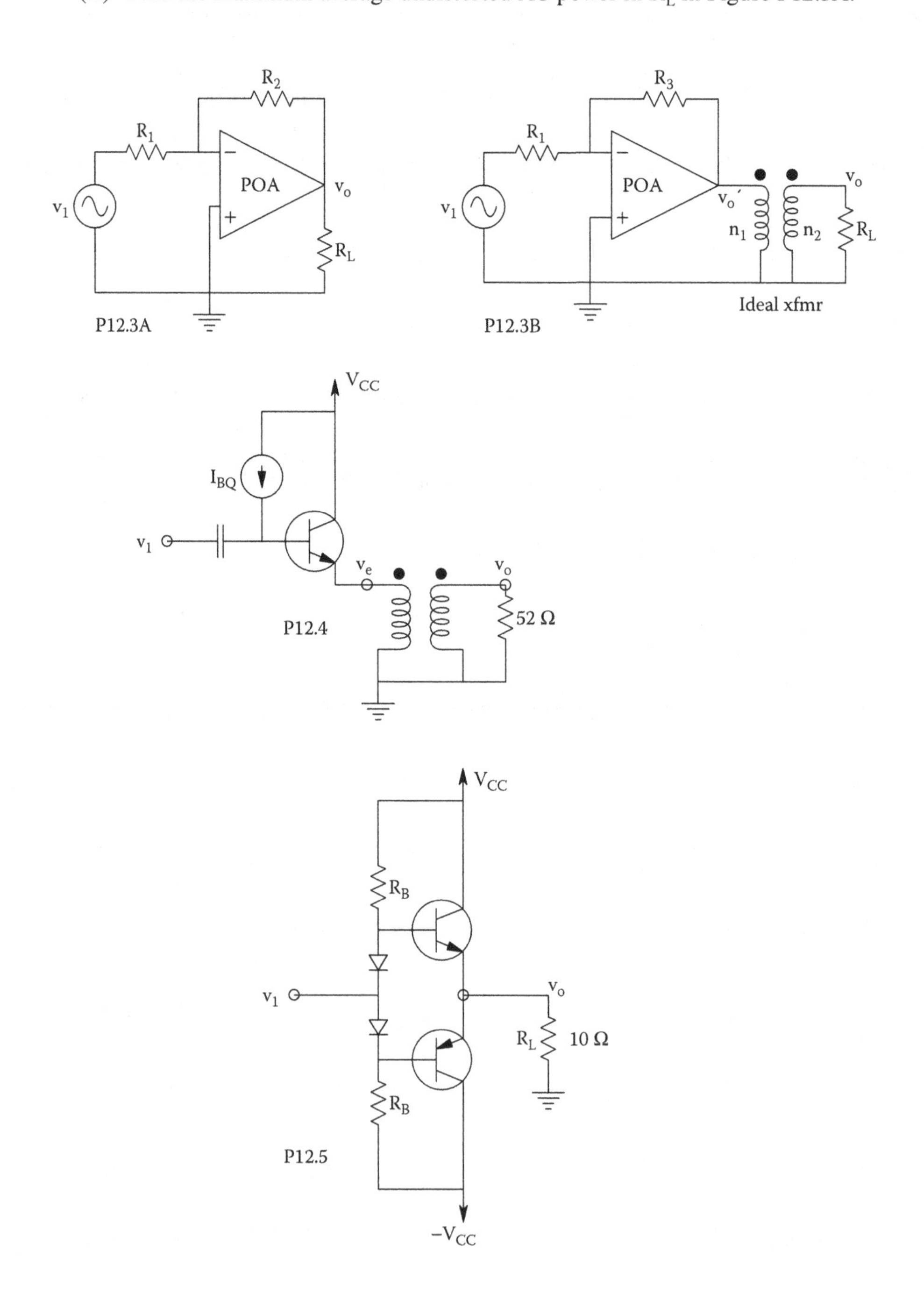

(B) In Figure P12.3B, the load is now coupled to the power op amp with an ideal transformer to improve power transfer efficiency. What turns ratio, n_1/n_2, is necessary to obtain maximum average undistorted AC power in R_L?

12.4 An ***npn*** BJT emitter-follower is coupled to a 52 Ω load with an ideal transformer. The power transistor has $\beta_o = 29$, $h_{oe} = h_{re} = 0$, and is biased so that $I_{CQ} = 0.1$ A. Assume $hie \cong 1/40I_{BQ}$. See Figure P12.4.

(A) Assume small-signal sinusoidal operation. Find the Thevenin source resistance the transformer's primary is driven by at the BJT's emitter.

(B) Use the MFSSM to find an expression for v_e/v_1.

(C) Use the MFSSM to find an expression for v_o/v_1.

(D) Find n_1/n_2 required for maximum power transfer to R_L under small-signal conditions.

12.5 A class B, complimentary-symmetry power output stage drives a 10 Ω load (see Figure P12.5). Assume $V_{CE(sat)}$ for the transistors is 0. The PA stage is to deliver 50 W maximum average power to the 10 Ω load. Let $v_1(t) = V_1 \sin(\omega t)$.

(A) Find the smallest V_{CC} that can be used.

(B) Find the peak sinusoidal output voltage for which Q_1 and Q_2 dissipate maximum average collector power, P_C.

$$\overline{P_C} = \overline{V_{ce}(t)I_c(t)}. \text{ Find } P_{C(max)}.$$

(C) Find the maximum average power that must be supplied by the positive and negative V_{CC} supplies.

12.6 A class B, complimentary-symmetry power output stage uses matched transistors with $|V_{CE(max)}| = 80$ V and $|I_{C(max)}| = 5$ A. (Refer to Figure P12.5.) With proper heatsinks, each transistor can safely dissipate $\overline{P_{CE}} = 50$ W.
Let $V_{CE(sat)} = 0$ V.

(A) What is the maximum average output power that the amplifier can deliver with a sinusoidal signal?

(B) Specify the values of $\pm V_{CC}$ and R_L needed to obtain the output power in part A. (Note: $V_{CE(max)} = 2V_{CC}$.)

(C) Find the maximum P_{CE}.

12.7 In Figure P12.7, a BJT complimentary-symmetry, class B PA stage generates 13.10 VRMS of total harmonic distortion at its output when driven by a pure sinusoidal input signal so that the RMS fundamental frequency output is 17.68 V. No feedback is used ($\beta = 0$). This power stage is to be driven by a high-gain, linear, differential amplifier (not an op amp) with output given by $v_o = K_v(v_1 - v_1')$. Overall negative voltage feedback is to be used.

(A) What loop gain, $-K_v\beta$, is required to reduce the closed-loop system's output THD to 0.03% when the RMS fundamental frequency output is again 17.68 V?

(B) Find K_v and β required so that V1 = 100 mVRMS produces an average fundamental frequency power of 10W in R_L.

12.8 The simple PA shown in Figure P12.8 uses 3 identical BJTs with $\beta_o = 50$, $V_{BE(ON)} = 0.7$ V, and $V_{CE(sat)} = 0.3$ V.
Sketch and dimension $v_o(t)$ for a sinusoidal input. Assume v_1 is large enough so that the output clips show saturation and crossover voltage levels. Also, derive an expression for the dead- (crossover-) zone angle.

12.9 In Figure P12.9, a class B, complimentary-symmetry, *bridge PA* is used to drive a 25 Ω, floating resistive load. The transistors Q_1 and Q_3, and Q_2 and Q_4 are driven in phase. Q_2 and Q_4 are driven 180° from Q_1 and Q_3, however.

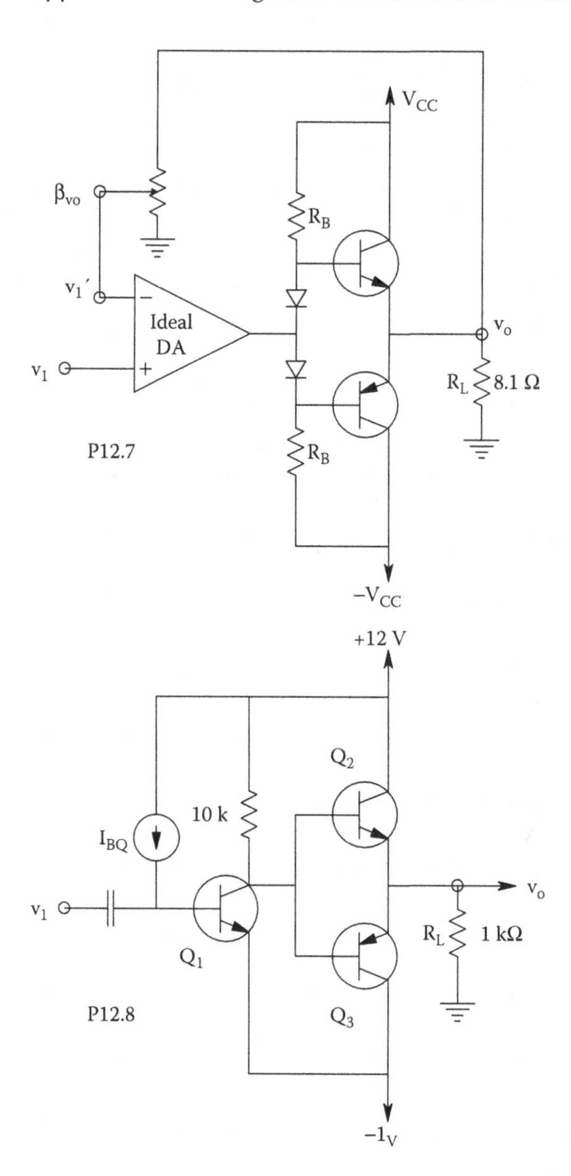

(A) Assume all $V_{CE(sat)} = 0$. Find the peak power dissipated in R_L.
(B) Find the maximum average undistorted AC power in R_L.
(C) Find the maximum average undistorted power dissipated in any one transistor.
(D) What Thevenin source resistance does R_L "see" when the transistors are in their linear operating regions?

Assume the transistor bases are driven by ideal voltage sources; use MFSSM CE *h*-parameter analysis.

(E) Calculate the bridge amplifier's efficiency, η.

12.10 In Figure P12.10, a class A, push-pull, emitter-follower PA drives a 20 Ω resistive load. Assume $Q_1 = Q_2$, $V_{CE(sat)} = 1$ V, $h_{fe} >> 1$, and $I_{EQ} = 0.95$ A (DC sinks). For peak positive v_1, Q_1 is just saturated, and Q_2 is cut off.

(A) Find the maximum peak undistorted power in R_L.
(B) Find the maximum average undistorted power in R_L.

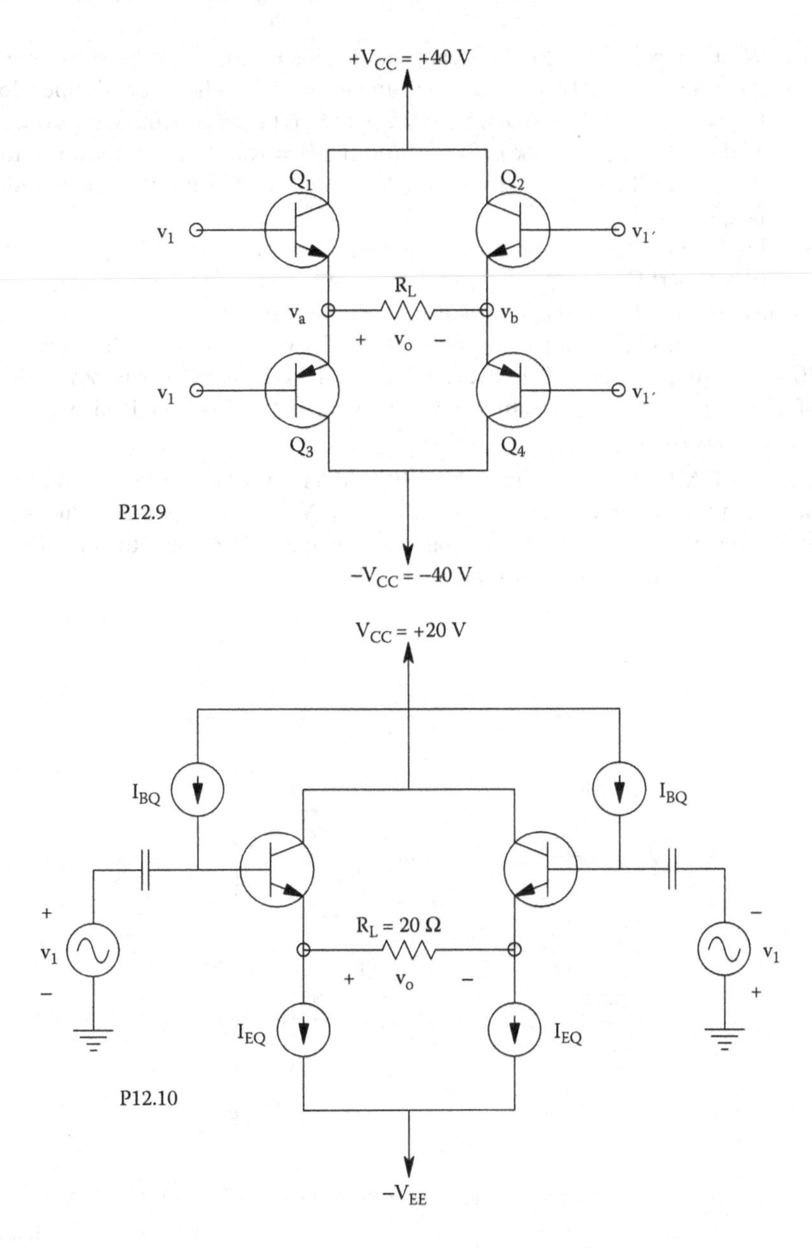

(C) Find the maximum average collector power dissipation in Q_1 and Q_2 for the conditions of part B.

(D) Find the maximum average power the 20 V DC source must supply for the conditions of part B. Calculate the amplifier's efficiency, η.

12.11 The complimentary pair of power VMOSFETs in Figure P12.11 is used to make a class B PA output stage driven by an op amp. Overall negative feedback is used. Q_1 is an enhancement ***n***-channel device; Q_2 is an enhancement ***p***-channel device. Both Q_1 and Q_2 are biased to have very small quiescent drain currents and equal V_{DS}s so that $V_L = 0$ under quiescent conditions.

(A) Assume that for $v_1 > 0$, Q_1 is operating in its linear (saturated drain) region, and Q_2 is cut-off. Similarly, Q_1 is cut-off and Q_2 is linear for $v_1 < 0$. *Write an expression for the steady-state Thevenin source resistance R_L sees.*

(B) Write an expression for the steady-state voltage gain of the PA stage, $A_v = v_o/v_1$.

(C) Assume $r_d = 200\ \Omega$, $g_m = 0.750$ S, and $R_L = 10\ \Omega$. The op amp's open-loop gain $K_{vo} = v_1/v_i' = -10^4$. When $V_o = 25$ VRMS (at the fundamental frequency), the THD *without feedback* is 20%. Find the $\beta = R_1/(R_1 + R_2)$ required to reduce the output THD to 0.02% when V_o is again 25 VRMS at the fundamental frequency.

(D) Find the overall voltage gain of the amplifier with feedback, v_o/v_s, for the condition of part C.

12.12 An analog audio PA is designed using two identical power op amps using the circuit of Figure P12.12. The op amps have slew rates of 20 V/μs, open-loop differential gains of 100 dB, a first pole at 45 Hz, a second pole at 1 MHz, a maximum power dissipation of 48 W, and a maximum (saturation) output current of 5 A. The loudspeaker presents a 10 Ω resistive load.

Use an ECAP (e.g., Microcap™, SPICE™, MATLAB™, etc.) to describe the amplifier's small-signal frequency response $(\mathbf{V_2} - \mathbf{V_3})/\mathbf{V_s}$ over a range that includes the upper and lower 0 dB points. Vary the input amplitude and frequency to demonstrate slew-rate limiting and output distortion in $(\mathbf{V_2} - \mathbf{V_3})$.

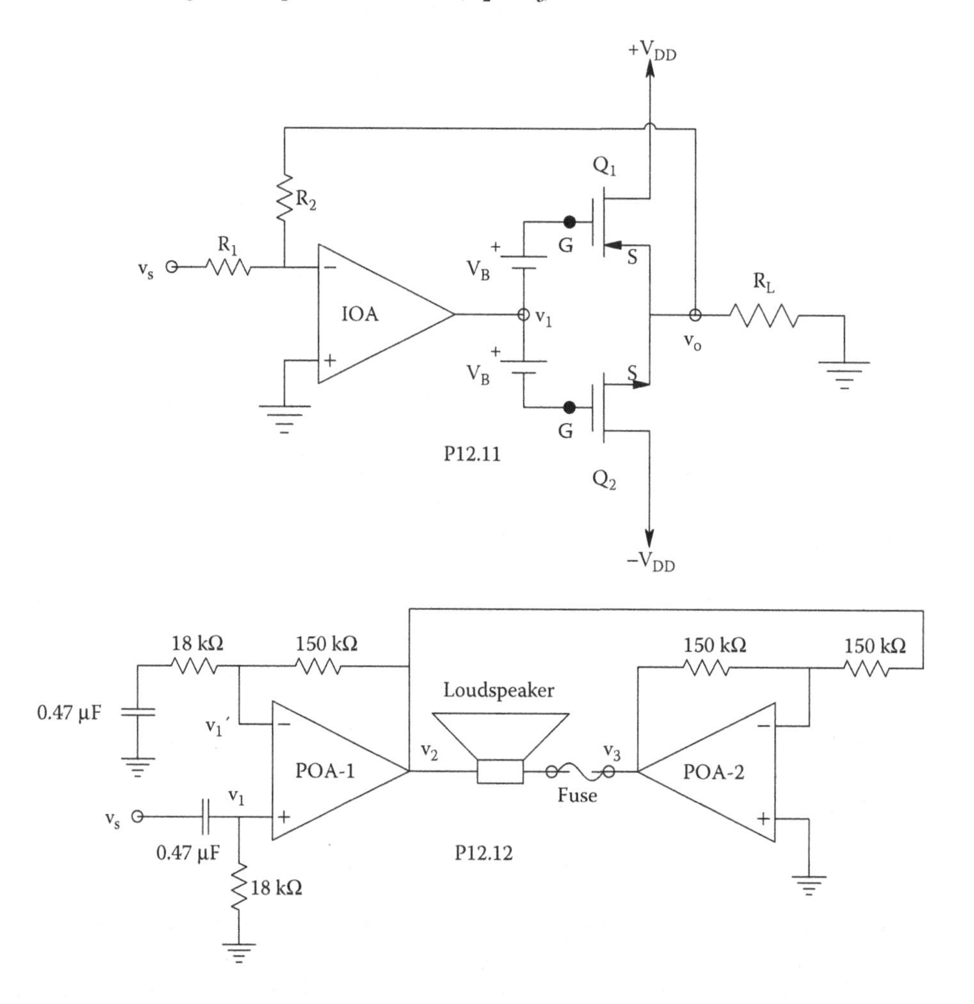

12.13 A class D PA drives a special, high-impedance loudspeaker with a bipolar, PWM square wave, as shown in text Figures 12.16 and 12.17. Assume a single sinusoidal voltage source drives a series R-L equivalent circuit of the loudspeaker's voice coil. I_L is the force-generating current through the loudspeaker's coil. $L_c = 0.01$ H, $R_c = 100\ \Omega$.

(A) Derive the frequency response function, $(I_L/V_s)(j\omega)$, in time constant form. Assume $v_s(t) = V_s \sin(\omega t)$.

(B) Using A, plot 20 log vs f for f = 30, 300, 3000, and 1.4×10^6 Hz (a Bode magnitude plot). (1.4×10^6 $|I_L/V_s|$ Hz is the fundamental frequency of the modulated square wave.)

12.14 A class D PA is used to deliver power to a 10 Ω resistive load. The signal has a bandwidth from 30 Hz to 3 kHz. A 1 MHz, PWM, bipolar square wave is filtered by a simple L-C LPF, shown in Figure P12.14.

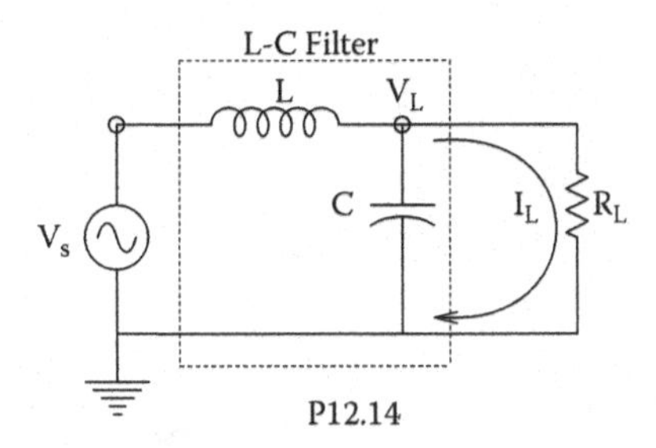

P12.14

(A) Derive the frequency response function, $(I_L/V_s)(j\omega)$, in time constant form. Assume $v_s(t) = V_s \sin(\omega t)$.

(B) Calculate the damping factor, ζ, of the circuit. Assume $R_L = 10\ \Omega$, L = 0.1 Hy and C = 1 μF.

(C) Using A, plot $20 \log|I_L/V_s|$ vs f for f = 30, 300, 3000, and 10^6 Hz (a Bode magnitude plot). (10^6 Hz is the fundamental frequency of the modulated square wave.)

13 Wireless Patient Monitoring

13.1 INTRODUCTION

Wireless patient monitoring (WPM), (or wireless medical telemetry services (WMTS)), is a rapidly growing technology applied to the monitoring of the vital signs of patients in all hospital departments (OR, RR, ICU, etc.), as well as ambulatory patients undergoing physical therapy and exercise. Analog sensors attached to patients measuring parameters such as blood pressure (BP), ECG (various leads), EEG (various leads), blood O_2 saturation and heart rate, body temperature, etc. send their output signals to IC battery-powered digitizers, modulators, and RF transmitters, generally operating around 600 MHz, 1.4 GHz, or in the wireless local area networking (WLAN) bands at 2.4 and 5.1 GHz. These RF data transmissions are received at central stations where they are displayed in real time for nurses and clinicians and stored as part of a patient's permanent medical record. They are screened by computer for unacceptable physiological values, which if present, sound alarms.

WPM offers the flexibility of data interception by authorized nursing staff, residents, and attending physicians on their RF-equipped portable computers, as well as the ability to collect data from ambulatory patients as they exercise. Physicians can also access patient's electronic health records (EHRs) with their laptops and mobile PDAs, also by an RF link using protocols such as *WiFi* or *Bluetooth.*

13.2 SENSORS AND SENSOR SIGNALS COMMUNICATED IN WPM

The sensors used in WPM are basically those used in conventional, wired patient monitoring. For example, in the recovery room and intensive care facility, critical parameters such as blood pressure (BP), % oxygen saturation of hemoglobin (PsO_2), pulse rate, ECG, respiratory effort, respiration rate, and body temperature are frequently measured. The ECG, respiratory effort, and temperature can be displayed continuously as time signals on a monitor; other parameters are quasi-periodic and require at least one period to determine the instantaneous rate, which is generally displayed as numbers on the monitor. If the BP is measured by a catheter sensor or a servo finger cuff, it can also be displayed continuously.

Heart rate can be measured continuously, beat-by-beat, by *instantaneous pulse frequency demodulation* (IPFD) of the QRS complex of the ECG waveform (Northrop 1966; Northrop et al. 1967). A cardiac IPFD works by first generating a logic pulse sequence by passing a waveform generated by the beating heart (e.g., ECG QRS waves, pulse oximetry waveform, blood pressure waveform) through a comparator "window" circuit. The window circuit output consists of a train of narrow logic pulses at the cardiac frequency. The *instantaneous frequency* of a pair of window output pulses, r_i, is defined as the reciprocal of the time interval between any pair of pulses, that is,

$$r_i \equiv 1/(t_i - t_{i-1}) = 1/\tau_i, \quad 1 \le i \le \infty \tag{13.1}$$

where r_i is the ith element of instantaneous frequency (a number) defined only over the interval, τ_i. t_i is the time of occurrence of the present (ith) pulse, t_{i-1} is the time of occurrence of the previous pulse. The first pulse in the sequence occurs at $t = t_0$.

An IPFD "machine" generates a continuous, stepwise, analog output signal, q(t), described by the equation

$$q(t) = k\sum_{i=1}^{\infty} r_i[U(t - t_i) - U(t - t_{i+1})] \tag{13.2}$$

where $U(t - t_k)$ is a unit step function, defined as zero for $t < t_k$ and 1 for $t \geq t_k$, r_i is the ith element of instantaneous frequency (a number) defined above, and k is a positive scaling constant. The analog voltage $q = kr_i$ is held until $t = t_{i+1}$. Note that the first pulse input to the IPFD "machine" occurs at time $t = t_0$.

(The circuit for and waveforms found in an IPFD designed by the author can be found in Section 7.2.3 in Northrop, 2005.)

Pulse oximeters (POs) generate a smooth, sawtooth-shaped, periodic analog voltage waveform at heart rate. A PO measures the relative % O_2 saturation of a patient's hemoglobin (Hb), SpO_2. The waveform is periodic because at systole, the heart forces fresh, arterial blood into the capillaries, being illuminated by the PO's LEDs. In the interval between the systoles, the Hb gives up some O_2 to the adjacent tissues, and the measured SpO_2 drops fairly linearly. Details of pulse oximeter designs and operation can be found in Section 15.8 in Northrop (2002). By appropriate signal processing, the quasi-periodic PO output waveform can also give heart rate.

One basic, noninvasive means of generating an analog signal proportional to respiratory effort makes use of an elastic, conductive belt around the chest or abdomen in which the belt resistance increases with strain. When the patient breathes in, the resistance of the belt increases as the chest/abdomen expands. The belt is made one arm of a Wheatstone bridge that is balanced to give zero output at maximum exhale. The unbalance signal of the bridge is thus proportional to chest/abdomen expansion during breathing. This signal is quasi-periodic and can be noisy because breathing is modulated by activities such as coughing, movements, crying, or speech.

Blood pressure (BP) is traditionally noninvasively measured by an inflatable, pneumatic, sphygmomanometer cuff placed on the upper arm. The cuff is used manually by the health-care giver inflating it to a pressure above the suspected systolic BP, and then slowly releasing the cuff pressure while listening for the well-known Korotkoff sounds, made by the elastic brachial artery as the heart begins to force blood through the artery collapsed by the pressure from the cuff (Guyton 1991). The pneumatic pressure of the cuff (indicated on an aneroid pressure gauge or mercury manometer) at the first Korotkoff sound defines the (brachial) systolic BP (SBP). The cuff pressure at the last sound heard before smooth (soundless) flow in the artery gives the diastolic BP (DBP). This process can also be done automatically by a computer: The cuff is inflated through a solenoid valve and then slowly deflated through another. The cuff pressure measured by an electronic pressure sensor is continuously converted to digital form and fed to the computer's digital input interface. A microphone is used to pick up the Korotkoff sounds, they, too, are digitized, and the filtered digital audio signal is processed to derive the systolic/diastolic BP numbers. Another means of detecting arterial flow pulses is by Doppler ultrasound measurement on the brachial artery. Alternately, oscillometry can be used; the output of the electronic pressure sensor on the cuff bladder is passed through a high-pass filter to extract the small pressure modulations caused by the pulsatile flow in the collapsed brachial artery (see Section 5.2 in Northrop, 2002). The positive pressure "blips" are passed through threshold logic to extract the systolic/diastolic BP numbers using a proprietary algorithm (the average cuff pressure is also sensed) (Kennedy 2009). Use of an automatic cuff sphygmomanometer can yield a numerical BP measurement every inflation-deflation cycle, about a minute in duration.

The Marshall Astro Finger F-88® system measures BP in the left index finger oscillometrically. A small air bladder 3 cm wide (diameter 2.5 cm; circumference 7.8 cm) that encircles the left index finger is put around the first phalange. Pressure is applied until the bladder completely blocks arterial flow in the index finger. A LED/photodiode photo-plethysmograph detects new blood flow as pressure in the ring cuff is automatically bled off. As with a brachial cuff sphygmomanometer, the first detected pulse signifies (the finger's) systolic BP, the last pulse gives the diastolic finger blood pressure (FBP), and then the automatic cycle of inflation/deflation is repeated (Iryiboz 1990). The Astro F-88 system was found to measure systolic FBP lower compared to brachial BP with a mean of 2.3 mmHg and SD of 14.9 mmHg. It measured diastolic FBP low with a mean of 2.9 mmHg and a SD of 14.5 mmHg. (Iryiboz did not recommend the Astro F-88 system for the clinical evaluation of BP.)

More reliable, beat-to-beat estimates of BP in finger arteries (FBP) can be obtained with a finger BP cuff used with the Finapres® Model 2300 BP monitor. The mechanism by which the Finapres® system works is based on the servo-plethysmograph (volume-clamp) design of Peñaz (1973), Wesseling et al. (1995), and Holejšovská et al. (2003).

Figure 13.1 illustrates a block diagram of one possible configuration of a Finapres-type system. The finger plethysmograph has an elastic, inflatable cuff that fits over a phalange, and has a simple, infrared photoplethysmograph on the inside. During open-loop initialization, the cuff is inflated with fluid to the mean arterial pressure in the finger (FMAP). The IR level at FMAP is made the set-point in the system's servo loop (V_{REF}), and then the servo loop is closed. In the closed-loop, volume clamp mode, the controlled cuff pressure keeps the IR level constant. At systole, more blood enters the finger and more IR light is absorbed than at diastole. As a consequence, the output of the photoplethysmograph's photodiode *decreases.* This analog output is compared to the set point, and the resultant error signal is conditioned and used to force fluid into the finger ring cuff to oppose the initial increase in finger artery blood volume. The elastic cuff is actively deflated during the decreasing phase of the FBP cycle to keep the photodiode output constant. Thus, rapid fluid servo action over each cardiac cycle maintains a constant photoplethysmograph output. The cuff pressure is thus proportional to the finger's arterial BP(t) (Lemson et al. 2009). Wesseling et al. (1995) devised a Finapres® operating mode in which the MAP setpoint was updated after every 70 cardiac cycles.

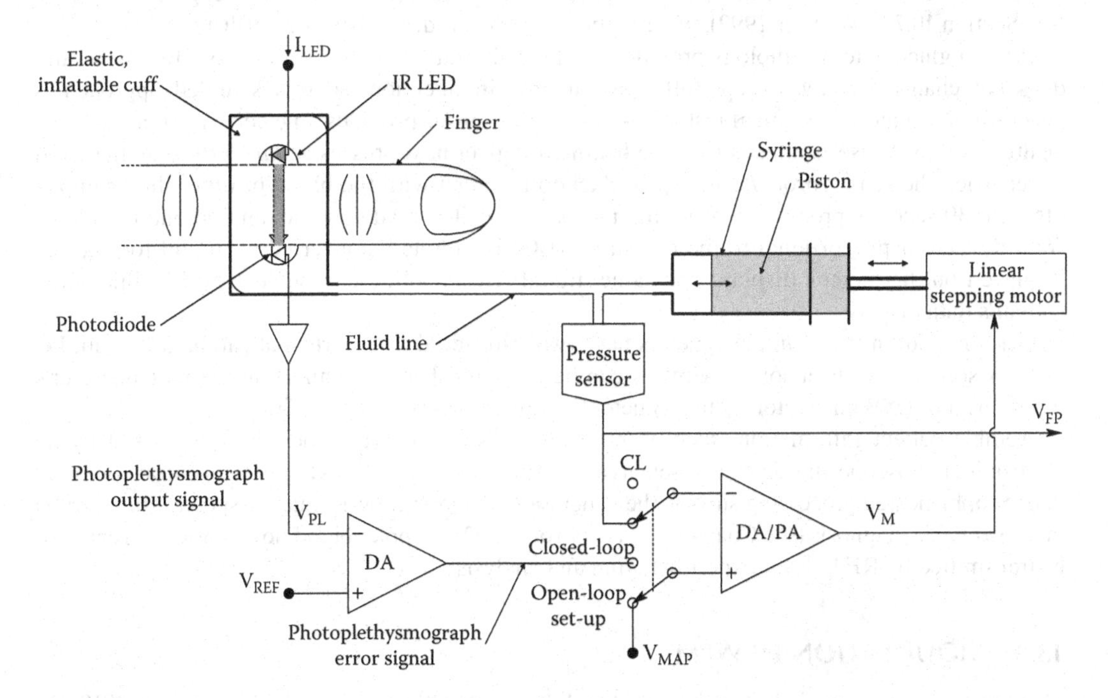

FIGURE 13.1 Block diagram of a closed-loop, Finapres®-type finger blood pressure measuring system. In the closed-loop mode, the linear motor/syringe air pump is driven so that the photoplethysmograph maintains a constant output signal regardless of the influx of arterial blood during each cardiac pumping cycle. The output of the pneumatic pressure sensor is proportional to the finger's arterial pressure.

The output of the Finapres® pressure sensor is a voltage proportional to the instantaneous BP in the finger to which it is attached. This waveform rises abruptly from a minimum (diastolic pressure) value to a peak systolic pressure then falls almost linearly to the diastolic pressure value at the end of the cardiac cycle. Thus, the waveform approximates two triangles with a base at P_{dias} and a common peak at P_{syst}. Thus, the FBP(t) can be processed to find the mean finger arterial pressure (FMAP) using this simple triangular approximation to FBP(t). FMAP can be shown to be

$$\mathrm{FMAP} = P_{dias} + 1/3\ (P_{syst} - P_{dias}) = (2P_{dias} + P_{syst})/3 \tag{13.3}$$

A new FMAP value can be computed using the formula above at the end of every cardiac cycle from the most recent values of P_{syst} and P_{dias}, then averaged over several cardiac cycles (Raamat et al. 2000, 2003).

In surgical and critical care scenarios, an electronic sensor on the tip of an invasive, pressure-measuring catheter may be used in a convenient artery, yielding a continuous BP signal giving systolic, diastolic, and mean arterial pressure. Such catheter-derived data is the "gold standard" of BP measurement. A conventional arm-cuff, inflatable plethysmograph using a mercury manometer (as opposed to an aneroid or chip pressure sensor) is *not* a gold standard for BP measurement, but has clinical reliability and acceptance; its accuracy depends, in part, on the expertise of the human operator.

The *blood glucose concentration* (BG) is important to measure in diabetic patients undergoing surgical procedures or in intensive care. Unfortunately, after many years of research on the problem, no one has been able to develop a truly noninvasive, continuous, reliably accurate means of measuring (BG). The present state-of-the-art in measuring (BG) requires a microliter quantity (a drop) sample of blood (or plasma, urine, saliva, etc.) to measure the glucose concentration. One means is based on an electrochemical redox reaction (fuel cell), using the enzyme, glucose oxidase (see Section 10.7 in Webster 1992), or catalytic metal electrodes (Pasta et al. 2010).

Present glucometer technology provides sampled, digital readouts. Fortunately, [BG] generally does not change rapidly, except following an insulin injection, so this sampled approach is generally adequate. A chemical test strip-based [BG] sensor provides an electrical signal when a health-care giver inserts a test strip. The heath-care giver next presses a *start button* on the [BG] meter when the sensor probe/test strip is placed in contact with the blood or other fluid sample; after ca. 30 seconds processing time, the meter signals it is ready, and an analog output voltage from the sensor proportional to the measured [BG] is sampled, converted to digital format and displayed on the meter's display. The same digital [BG] reading can be sent by RF link to the patient's data display.

Certain modern test-strip glucometers have two-wire serial data ports that can be used with PC or PDA software. Conversion to wireless can be accomplished by connecting the manufacturer's 9-pin serial or USB connector, or to a Bluetooth wireless interface (Baisa 2005).

Audible patient information, such as breath sounds and heart sounds, can be sensed by an electronic stethoscope, digitized, and sent as a real-time data stream by RF link to a central computer where sophisticated processing such as the generation of a joint time-frequency spectrogram can be made to enable diagnosis (see Chapter 3 in Northrop, 2002). Doppler blood flow sonograms can also be transmitted by RF link for expert listening and analysis.

13.3 MODULATION IN WPM

Most physiological signals have relatively low bandwidths (see Section 1.1 in Northrop, 2010). In general, the bandwidths (equivalent frequency content) of endogenous physiological signals can range from nearly DC (ca. 1.2×10^{-5} Hz (or 12 μHz), a period of 24 h) to several kHz (Stefanovska 2007). Many endogenous hormones, neuromodulators, and behavioral parameters have circadian (ca. 24 h) cycles. Cardiac pumping spans 0.6–4 Hz, respiratory effort lies in a 0.145–0.6 Hz bandwidth (BW). Other neurogenic mechanical rhythms in the digestive system have even lower BWs. Bioelectric signals recorded from the skin surface have higher bandwidths: these include the EEG, EOG, ECoG, EMG, ECG, etc. Sounds emitted by organs recorded through the skin with microphones include heart valves and blood vessel turbulence sounds, sounds from the respiratory tract (e.g., rales), and sounds from arthritic joints. Such sounds generally require an audio signal conditioning bandwidth, typically from 10 Hz to 3 kHz or so. Details on the bandwidths required to condition and reproduce physiological signals and their amplitudes can be found in Northrop (2002), and descriptions and analyses of modulation and demodulation schemes for biomedical signals are given in detail in Chapter 11 of this text.

Because the majority of physiological signals (x_m) recorded and transmitted in WPM have very low frequencies, the modulation scheme used must have frequency response to DC. Frequency modulation (FM) and narrow-band FM (NBFM) are ideal for this purpose. FM and NBFM signals can easily be demodulated using phase-locked loops (see Section 11.5.3 of this text). Another modulation scheme that supports a DC or low frequency signal is double-sideband, suppressed-carrier modulation (DSBSCM) (see Section 11.5.4 in this text). Duty cycle or pulse-width modulation (PWM) of the RF carrier can also convey DC information. Detection is by rectification and low-pass filtering of the PWM RF, and then subtracting out the DC level when the RF pulse duty cycle is 50% (for $x_m = 0$).

13.4 RF COMMUNICATIONS PROTOCOLS USED IN WPM

Wi-Fi™ is a trademark of the Wi-Fi Alliance that manufacturers may use to brand certified products that belong to a class of *wireless local area network* (WLAN) devices based on the IEEE 802.11 standards. The IEEE 802.11b standard defines 11 RF channels for Wi-Fi communications in the ISM 2.4 GHz band; the center frequencies are separated by 5 MHz, and are at: 2.412, 2.417, 2.422, 2.427, 2.432, 2.437, 2.442, 2.447, 2.452, 2.457, and 2.462 GHz. The absolute spectral width of each Wi-Fi channel is 22 MHz, so channels overlap (see Wiki 2010c, 2010d, for a summary of Wi-Fi protocols). Because of channel overlap, Wi-Fi user density, RF emissions from Bluetooth devices, baby monitors, cordless telephones, microwave ovens, etc., interference issues have arisen for Wi-Fi users. These have been called "Wi-Fi pollution" (Wiki 2010d).

There are more than 220,000 public Wi-Fi "hotspots" where Wi-Fi equipped laptops can access the internet. Wi-Fi is also used for wireless internet connections in tens of millions of homes, corporations and university campuses worldwide. Embedded Wi-Fi systems have been used in portable (ambulatory) ECG monitors to permit home recording of a patient's ECG and its wireless transfer to the internet, thence to a hospital. The current version of Wi-Fi Protected Access encryption (WPA2) as of 2010 is considered secure, provided that a strong passphrase is employed by users. The range of Wi-Fi communications using the 802.11b or 802.11g standards can be 32 m indoors and 95 m outdoors, using a standard antenna. In the new 802.11n standard, these ranges are effectively doubled.

Zigbee is another established set of specifications governing wireless personal area networking (WPAN) systems using digital radio communications. Zigbee uses the 868–870 MHz, and the 915 (902–928) MHz and 2.4 (2.4–2.5) GHz, ISM RF bands. Maximum data rates allowed on these bands are: 250 kbps @ 2.4 GHz, 40 kbps @ 915 MHz, and 20 kbps @ 868 MHz. Zigbee protocols have been standardized by the IEEE 802.14.4 Wireless Networking Standard. The Zigbee protocol's data bandwidth is only approximately one fourth that of Bluetooth (1 Mbps); this allows replacement of cables for many serial data applications, lower costs and longer battery life (Zigbee 2010). Zigbee applications include, but are not limited to: personal, home and hospital care, home automation, telecommunications, commercial building automation, etc. Zigbee devices can go from sleep to active mode in 15 ms or less, while Bluetooth wake-up delays are typically approximately three seconds. There are three different types of Zigbee devices (Wiki 2010b): (1) The *Zigbee Coordinator*

(ZC) forms the root of the network tree and can bridge to other networks. There is only one ZC in each network. It stores information about the network, including acting as the Trust Center and repository for security keys. (2) The *Zigbee Router* (ZR): As well as running an application function, the ZR can act as an intermediate router, passing on data from other devices. (3) The *Zigbee End Device* (ZED) can just talk to the parent node (either the ZC or ZR), but cannot relay data from other devices. This protocol allows the ZED to be asleep for a significant amount of time, giving longer battery life. A ZED requires the smallest memory, and therefore can be less expensive to manufacture than a ZR or ZC.

Bluetooth RF networking is rapidly becoming a preferred technology for WPM (Baisa 2005). It uses a radio transmission protocol called *frequency-hopping spread spectrum* which chops the data being sent into packets and transmits it on up to 79 bands of 1 MHz width in the range of 2.402–2.480 GHz (this is in the global Industrial, Scientific & Medical (ISM) 2.4 GHz band that requires no licensing). In classic Bluetooth, the modulation is Gaussian frequency-shift keying (GFSK). It can achieve a gross data rate of up to 1 Mbit/s (1 Mbs). Other modulation schemes give extended data rates of 2 and 3 Mbit/s (Wiki 2010a; Bluetooth). Bluetooth provides a secure way to connect and exchange information between devices such as mobile phones and their accessories, faxes, telephones, laptops, PCs, printers, GPS receivers, digital cameras, and WPM devices. Bluetooth system specifications are developed and licensed by the Bluetooth Special Interest Group (BSIG). The BSIG is comprised of more than 13,000 companies. Bluetooth transmitters are classified by radiated power: Class 1 has a maximum permitted power of 100 mW and an effective range of ca. 100 m. Class 2's max. power = 2.5 mW; its range is ca. 10 m. Class 3 radiates 1 mW and has a range of ca. 1 m.

The Bluetooth protocol of frequency-hopping spread spectrum makes a Bluetooth signal difficult to eavesdrop on.

13.5 UHF TRANSMITTERS AND ANTENNAS

13.5.1 UHF Oscillators

At UHF frequencies, conventional passive components (R, L & C) cannot be treated by simple lumped-parameter models. Resistors have distributed capacitance to ground, and their leads have self-inductance. Capacitors have leakage and equivalent loss resistances as well as lead inductance, and even simple air-core inductors, have distributed capacitance between turns, capacitance to ground, and resistance from the wire.

Even wires have distributed resistance (from skin effect), capacitance (to ground and other wires and components), and self- and mutual inductances. From my perspective, the design of stable, functional UHF amplifiers and oscillators is an art as well as a science. Even the metal box a circuit is housed in is important for its performance.

Fortunately for the UHF faint-of heart, monolithic (chip) VCOs are available at 2.4 GHz. Maxim™ offers the MAX2753 2.4 GHz monolithic voltage-controlled oscillator with differential outputs. This L-C oscillator is tunable from 2.4 to 2.5 GHz using a bias voltage applied to two, nose-to-nose varactor diodes across a tank inductance on the chip. The push-pull output signal is buffered to have a 50 Ω output impedance. Over a $0 \leq V_{TUNE} \leq 3.0$ V range, the output frequency ranges from ca. 2.2 to 2.6 GHz, respectively. The VCO chip works for $+2.7 \leq V_{CC} \leq +5.5$ V. Maxim™ has also gone several steps further and offers a monolithic 2.4 to 2.5 GHz, RF transceiver, PA, and Rx /Tx/antenna diversity switch system that meets the 802.11g/b standards. This MAX2830 chip is intended for 2.4–2.5 GHz wireless local area network (WLAN) applications, including Wi-Fi, PDA, VOIP, and cellular handsets, wireless speakers and headphones, and general 2.4 GHz ISM radios.

Figure 13.2 illustrates the schematic for a 2.4 GHz, Si-Ge low phase-noise VCO IC. Again, the tuning is by varactor diode, voltage-variable capacitances (see Equation 15.30 in this text). Many

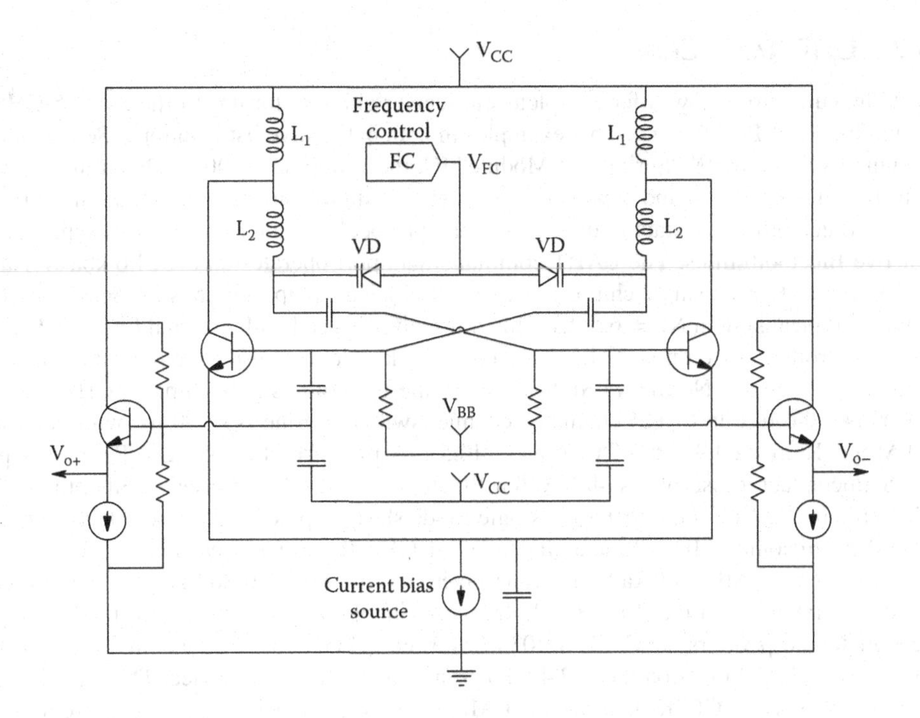

FIGURE 13.2 Simplified schematic for a 2.4 GHz, Si-Ge low phase-noise VCO IC. The tuning is by varactor diode (VD), voltage-variable capacitances changing the resonant frequency of the L-C tank circuit (Lai et al. 2003).

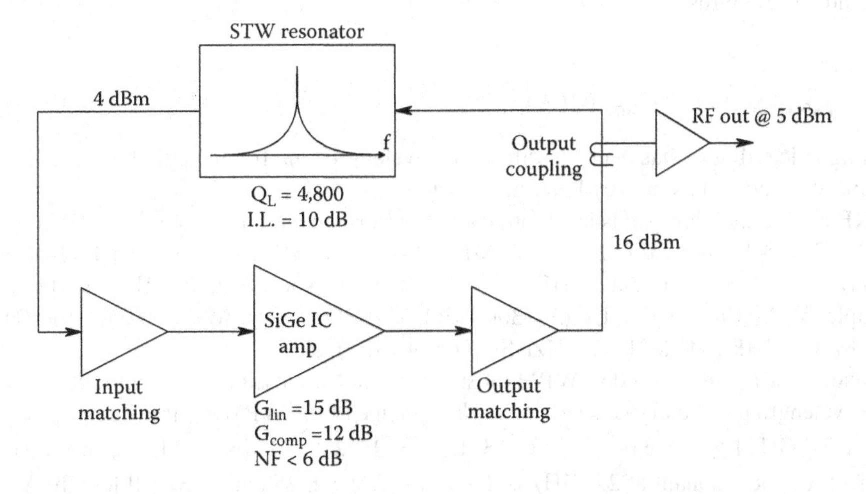

FIGURE 13.3 A block diagram of a surface transverse wave (STW) resonator, PFB oscillator described by Hay et al. (2004). Resonator center frequency was ca. 2.4 GHz.

other VCO designs exist for the 2.4–2.5 GHz range, see for example the 2.4 GHz IC oscillator design described by Xu et al. (2009), and the 900 MHz VCO design by Zhu (2005). Another successful design that used a surface transverse wave (STW) resonator was described by Hay et al. (2004). A block diagram illustrating their approach is shown in Figure 13.3. A tuned, STW device with a high Q (=4800) was used to set the oscillator's center frequency.

13.5.2 UHF Radio Chips

Many IC manufacturers now offer complete transceiver chipsets for use in the 2.4–2.5 GHz ISM band, suitable for WPM. We cite some examples (not an exhaustive list): National Semiconductor® has designed a Bluetooth™ "Serial Port Module" IC, the LMX9820 (2004). This transceiver measures 10.1 × 14.0 × 1.9 mm and contains in addition to a digital smart radio, all circuitry required for 2-way, Bluetooth (v.1.1 stack) communications protocol. Its internal memory supports up to three active Bluetooth links. The UART command/data port operates up to 921.6 kbaud. National also offers the LMX3162 single chip transceiver (2000). This chip radio has RF sensitivity to –93 dBm, with a typical system NF = 6.5 dB. This transceiver is used with external filters and an external microcontroller. An on-board, 1.3 GHz phase-locked loop is used for both modulation and demodulation functions. Nordic VLSI ASA offers the nRF2401 single chip 2.4 GHz transceiver (2003). This radio has up to 125 channels; channel switching time is <200 μs, with data rate up to 100 Mbps. Runs on 1.9–3.6 VDC, draws ≤10.5 mA pk. current at –5 dBm RF output power. Nordic Semiconductor also offers (4/20/09) a Bluetooth™ 2.4 GHz transceiver line, the μBlue™. The first chip in this line is the nRF8001 single-mode slave chip, ideal for wearable sensors. (Visit http://nordicsemi.com/). Micro Linear makes a 2.4 GHz Radio Chipset: The ML2712 2.4 GHz radio transceiver, the ML2713 Radio IF transceiver, and the ML7730 802.11 Baseband Processor. This system is intended for the IEEE 802.11 frequency-hopping spread spectrum standard. Cypress Semiconductor Corp. offers the CYRF69103 low power, 2.4 GHz radio on a chip (2010). This is an 8-bit flash based MCU function and a 2.4 GHz transceiver in a single device. The radio has DSSS rates up to 250 kbps, a GFSK data rate of 1 Mbps, –97 dBm receiver sensitivity, programmable output power up to +4 dBm, automatic gain control (AGC), etc. The radio has a dual-conversion, low IF architecture optimized for power and range/robustness; it supports up to 98 discrete 1 MHz channels. Atheros Communications offers a single-chip, AR5007EG IEEE 802.11b/g WLAN transceiver operating in the 2.3–2.5 GHz ISM band. This transceiver is compliant with the IEEE 802.11b, –g, –d, and –i standards.

13.5.3 Antennas Used in WPM

Electromagnetic radiation has been classified by wavelength (and frequency); the Table 13.1 denotes the commonly accepted frequency band designations.

The RF communication bands are more exactly described as: ULF ($10^7 \leq \lambda \leq 10^8$ m), ELF (10^5–10^7 m), VLF (10^4–10^5 m), LF (10^3–10^4 m), MF (10^2–10^3 m), HF (10–10^2 m), VHF (1–10 m), UHF (10^{-1}–1 m), SHF (10^{-2}–10^{-1} m), and EHF (10^{-3}–10^{-2} m). Other sources define RF bands by frequency, for example: VLF (10–30 kHz), LF (30–300 kHz), MF (300 kHz–3 MHz), HF (3–30 MHz), VHF (30–300 MHz), UHF (300 MHz–3 GHz), SHF (3–30 GHz), etc.

The size of the antennas used in WPM must be as small as possible, subject to the constraints of the RF wavelength used, and the designed working range of the WPM device. Recall that the wavelength of a 2.4 GHz EM wave is $\lambda_{(meters)} = 0.3/f_{(GHz)} = 0.3/2.4 = 0.125$ m = 12.5 cm. A conventional two-element dipole resonant at 2.4 GHz is $2 \times \lambda/4 = \lambda/2 = 6.25$ cm in overall length. As you will see in Section 14.3.2 in this text, efforts to shrink the effective size of antennas in WPM and RFID applications have led to various planar antenna designs that can be etched onto PC boards. Such designs include the various meander and fractal antenna geometries described in Section 14.3.2.

When a WPM modulator/transmitter (M/T) is implanted in an animal's or a person's body, or is swallowed, the RF wavelength in the body is shorter because the RF propagation velocity (**c**) in tissue is slower than in air. One implantable M/T described by Hashemi (2009) that used a center frequency of 915 MHz had a simple, optimum, λ/4, bent-single-wire antenna length of 8 cm in air, but the implanted device required a 5 cm, λ/4, bent-wire antenna, a 37.5% reduction in length. Of course, the conductive, water-containing tissue surrounding the antenna attenuated the broadcast RF.

TABLE 13.1
The EM spectrum

Band	Wavelength, λ	Frequency	Photon energy
Cosmic rays	1 pm	300 EHz	1.24 MeV
Gamma rays	10 pm	30 EHz	124 keV
Gamma and X-rays	100 pm	3 EHz	12.4 keV
Far UV, X-rays	1 nm	300 PHz	1.24 keV
Near ultraviolet (NUV)	10 nm	30 PHz	124 eV
Visible light	100 nm	3 PHz	12.4 eV
Near infrared (NIR)	1 μm	300 THz	1.24 eV
Mid infrared (MIR)	10 μm	30 THz	124 meV
Far infrared (FIR)	100 μm	3 THz	12.4 meV
Extra high frequency (EHF)	1 mm	300 GHz	1.24 meV
Super high frequency (SHF)	1 cm	30 GHz	124 μeV
Ultra high frequency (ULF)	10 cm	3 GHz	12.4 μeV
Very high frequency (VHF)	1 m	300 MHz	1.24 μeV
High frequency (HF)	10 m	30 MHz	124 neV
Medium frequency (MF)	100 m	3 MHz	
Low frequency (LF)	1 km	300 kHz	
Very low frequency (VLF)	10 km	30 kHz	
Ultra low frequency (ULF)	100 km	3 kHz	
Super low frequency (SLF)	1000 km	300 Hz	
Extra low frequency (ELF)	10^4 m	30 Hz	
Extra low frequency	10^5 m	3 Hz	

EHz = ExaHertz = 10^{18}, PHz = PetaHertz = 10^{15}, THz = TeraHertz = 10^{12}, GHz = GigaHertz = 10^9, MHz = Mega Hertz = 10^6. Photon energy is important at shorter wavelengths because of its role in initiating chemical reactions and breaking chemical bonds.

13.5.4 Power Sources for WPM Sensors

Clearly, WPM sensors can be powered by compact, rechargeable batteries, such as lithium-ion. A WPM receiver's software can be programmed to detect loss of signal and give an alarm, should a battery fail or a sensor become disconnected from the patient.

An emerging technology of "energy harvesting" power sources that derive their power from ambient or "free energy" promises to create ultra-reliable sources for WPM sensors. Energy Harvesting ICs can be powered from thermoelectric generators (TEGs). TEGs are simply thermopiles consisting of many *n*- and *p*-type semiconductor (e.g., Bi_2Te_3) pellets arranged as series thermocouples sandwiched between two, flat, ceramic, heat-conductive plates. The Seebeck effect produces open-circuit EMFs on the order of 10 to 50 mV/ΔT°C, depending on the TEG size and the temperature difference, ΔT, between the two plates in contact with either the "hot" or "cold" junctions. Note that in WPM sensor applications, $\Delta T \cong 38 - 21 = 17°C$, using the temperature difference between the human body and the hospital room as the energy source. Figure 13.4 illustrates a simplified schematic of the Linear Technology Corp LTC3108-1 energy harvester chip, showing its use to power a wireless patient sensor. Note that in the LTC3108-1, the low DC voltage from the external TEG is converted to a higher AC voltage by chopping and use of a 1:100 step-up transformer, and then the AC is rectified, regulated, and filtered. A battery can be connected to the V_{STORE} input terminal to provide backup, as shown in the figure. The maximum power output of the LTC3108 is in the range of 200 μW to 1 mW, depending on the specific TEG used, the ΔT, the TEG's $V_{max} \times I_{max}$ product, and the chopper transformer turns ratio. The LT3108-1 can be

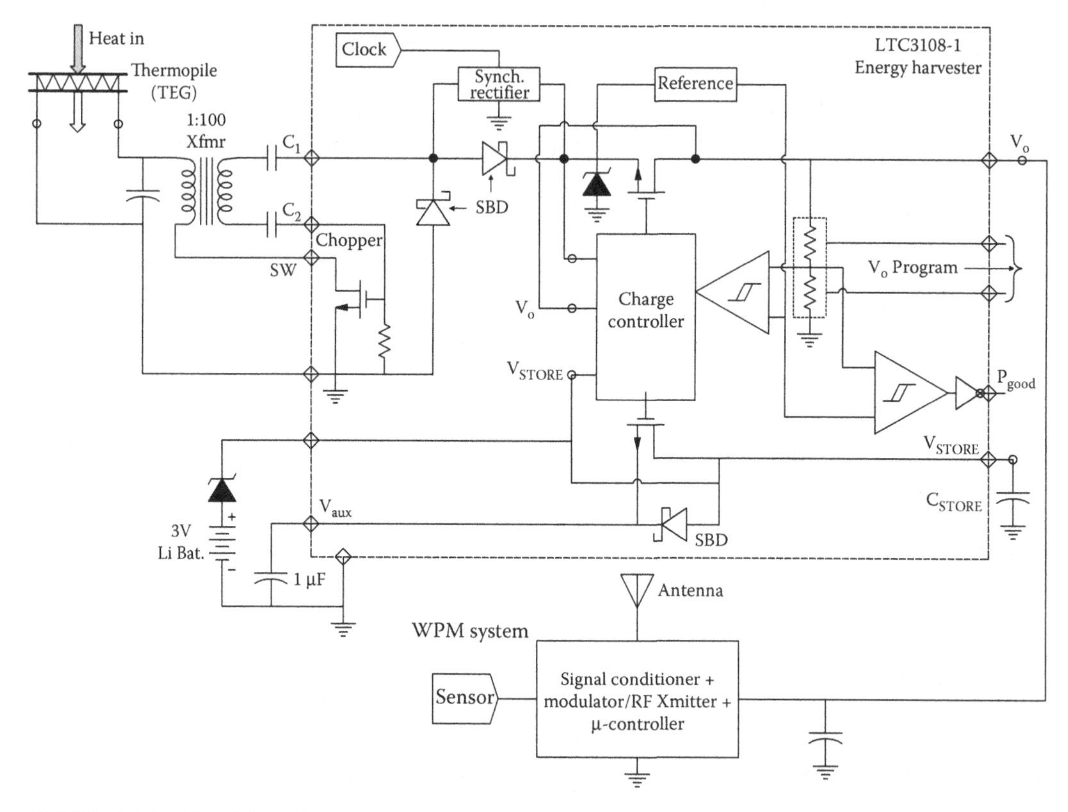

FIGURE 13.4 Simplified block diagram of an LTC3108-1 energy harvester IC using a thermoelectric generator for a power source. It can use patient body heat to power a WPM sensor/transmitter module.

programmed to output 2.5 V, 3.0 V, 3.7 V, or 4.5 VDC to power the WPM sensor, microcontroller, and RF transmitter.

Details of energy harvester ICs which can be powered by TEGs, piezoelectric generators, and solar sources may be found in the Linear Technology *Journal of Analog Innovation,* LT (2010).

13.6 WPM SYSTEMS

13.6.1 Commercial WPM Systems

Remote and Wireless Patient Monitoring Systems are a rapidly growing, competitive area of medical electronics (Kalorama 2010). Many corporations offer WPM product lines, most are for fixed hospital/clinical settings, and a few are portable systems intended for emergency medicine (field use). A nonexhaustive list of WPM system manufacturers is given below:

Aerotel Medical Systems: e-CliniQ™ system. The RF-linked Tele-Cliniq™ family is designed for individual patient use at home or clinic: (www.aerotel.com/en/products-solutions/ medical-parameters-monitoring/index/php (Accessed 5/5/11).
BioWatch Medical™, Inc., Columbia, SC. Vital Signs Transmitter (VST™): www.biowatchmed.com/index.php?option=com_content&task=view&id=36&Itemid=87 (Accessed 5/6/11).
CardioNet: Conshohocken, PA. WPM Systems. Mobile Cardiac Outpatient Telemetry (MCOT™) systems: www.cardionet.com (Accessed 5/6/11).

GE Healthcare: ApexPro® CH telemetry works seamlessly with CARESCAPE™ Enterprise Access. It can monitor two V-leads on each patient, and continuous ECG, SpO_2, and episodic monitoring of noninvasive BP and temperature. Up to 438 patients can be monitored, using the 600 MHz and 1.4 GHz bands, sending data to the CARESCAPE CIC Pro Clinical Information Center. Data on up to 16 patients can be viewed on each display: www2.gehealthcare.com/portal/site/esen/gehchome/ (Accessed 5/6/11).

LifeScan, Inc., Milpitas, CA. IRMA SL Blood Analysis System.
Life Watch Services, Inc: (LifeWatch AG is parent company.) PMP4® Wireless Healthcare System. LifeStar™ ACT Ambulatory Cardiac Telemetry service: (www.lifewatch.com/siteFiles/1/545/6438.asp) (Accessed 5/5/11).
Medtronic: CareLink® Network for cardiac device patients; LIFENET® BLUE telemetry from the LIFEPAK® 12 defibrillator/monitor: www.medtronic.com/ (Accessed 5/6/11).
NuPhysicia® LLC: (A private telemedicine company associated with the University of Texas Medical Branch at Galveston.) They offer the portable B3Zero® Telemedicine Suitcase System for emergency diagnostic medicine, specifically targeted for use on offshore oil rigs. Also the T-cart® clinical telemedicine system: www.nuphysica.com/ (Accessed 5/5/11).
Ortivus AB: CoroNet™ cardiac monitoring system. To hospital's LAN: ECG, SpO_2, invasive BP: www.ortivus.se/en-gb/Products (Accessed 5/6/11).
Phillips wireless patient monitoring systems: (www.heathcare.philips.com/main/products/index.wpd (Accessed 5/5/11).
Remote Diagnostic Technologies (RDT): Basingstoke, UK. Makes the Tempus IC™ portable telemedicine diagnostic system: www.remotemedical.com/Tempus-IC-Telemedicine-Device/ (Accessed 5/5/11).
Roche Diagnostics UK: Makes the Accu-Chek® Inform II blood glucose monitoring system with wireless link to the hospital's patient information system using the cobas® IT1000 POC data management software: www.selectscience.com/product-news/roche-diagnostics-uk/wireless-blood-glucose-monitoring-system-helps-to-improve-patient-care/artID=176428/ (Accessed 5/5/11).
Welch Allyn: EMR Connectivity. Connex® Electronic Vitals Documentation System: www.welchallyn.com/wafor/hospitals/emr_connectivity/default.htm (Accessed 5/5/11).
Viterion TeleHealthcare, a subsidiary of Bayer HealthCare Diabetes Care: Viterion® 200 wireless monitor for patient's weight, SpO_2, BP, and pulse rate. Uses Bluetooth technology: www.viterion.com/web_docs/V200Ad.pdf/ (Accessed 5/5/11).
Voxiva, Inc: Washington, DC. HealthConnect℠ Platform (uses the Web, phone lines or RF links): www.voxiva.com/services/technologyPlatform.html (Accessed 5/6/11).

GE Healthcare's Carescape™ Enterprise Access™ operates in two protected frequency bands; 600 MHz and 1.4 GHz for wireless medical telemetry service (WMTS). Quoting GE Healthcare (2009):

> Hospitals using GE Heathcare ApexPro CH telemetry transmitters have the flexibility to leverage the existing 600 MHz frequency band transmitters and expand into the 1.4 GHz frequency band with the CARESCAPE Telemetry T14 Transmitter on CARESCAPE Enterprise Access.

The Swedish company, Ortivus AB, makes WPM devices to monitor patient ECG (up to 12 leads), impedance-based respiration, BP monitoring (invasive and NI), pulse oximetry, CO_2, and myocardial ischemic dynamic analysis. Up to 36 patients' data can be viewed on four flat-screen monitors, and mobile transport monitors are used to view the signs of single patients, in transit.

The *Tempus IC*™ telemedicine system by *RTD* (a UK company) finds use on commercial aircraft, cruise ships, tankers and other commercial ships, oil rigs, etc. where medical emergencies may occur but the time to transport the patient to hospital may be on the order of hours, and a trained physician may not be aboard. This is a compact, portable, modular instrument that requires only a minimum of emergency medical training to use. Its purpose is to transmit real-time medical data via Wi-Fi, Bluetooth, mobile or satellite (e.g., Iridium, Inmarsat) RF links to an ER or casualty center. The physiological parameters transmitted include: blood pressure, hemoglobin oxygen saturation (SpO_2), 12-lead ECG, respiration rate, tympanic (LIR) temperature, blood glucose concentration, plus pictures from an integral digital camera (stills and real-time streaming video) can be sent, as well as two-way voice communication with the remote ER or response station doctors. The Tempus IC™ is a portable diagnostic system, and has an integral digital library of first-responder therapies available as helpscreens. It has a (rechargeable) six-hour, active battery life. A three-hour training course is offered for individuals or groups purchasing the Tempus IC™ system.

The NuPhysicia® B3Zero® portable telemedicine monitor is designed for use on offshore oil rigs (Anscombe 2010). It has the following features: A metal, rolling travel case; a 5" multifunction display for video inputs; a medical quality videoconferencing system with a desktop microphone and TCP/IP (H.323) connection capability; a digital stethoscope (CareTone® Telephonic Stethoscope) with chest microphone and noise-canceling headphones; and a multipurpose medical scope (with digital camera), fiber optic illumination, and attachments (otoscope, dermoscope, and laryngoscope). It has the ability to operate with either 120 or 240 VAC power. It can be partnered with wireless computer networks (BlueTooth, Wi-Fi, etc), satellite VSAT technology, and laptop computers. The B3Zero® system can run on either 120 VAC or 240 VAC power.

The American TeleCare® company offers a family of CareTone® Telephonic Stethoscopes that allow transmission of real-time heart, lung, and bowel sounds over a standard analog or digital telephone line. It uses +12V power from a wall-mount (plug-in) power supply. It has two frequency ranges: Bell pickup—20 Hz–250 Hz; Diaphragm pickup—20 Hz–500 Hz. See www.americantelecare.com/prod_caretone.html (Accessed 9/13/10).

13.7 HOW WPM REDUCES THE PROBABILITY OF PATIENT MICROSHOCK

Webster (1992) gave several examples of how ground faults in wired patient monitoring and care systems can lead to fatal cardiac microshock. (All of these scenarios involved patients with cardiac catheters used for pacing or BP measurement.) It is seen that by using a wireless ECG monitor, all conductive pathways for microshock are broken. The initial scenario posed by Webster is shown in Figures 13.5a and b. A patient in the ICU is connected to a conventional, line-powered, ECG machine while at the same time, the patient's left ventricular BP is being measured by a saline-filled, intracardiac catheter connected to a line-powered, metallic BP sensor which is grounded through ICU ground line B. The patient's left leg is connected to the ECG machine's ground, which is connected to the hospital ground through ICU ground line A. In one Webster scenario, a floor polisher is used in an adjoining ICU room using a three-prong mains plug that connected to ground line A. The polisher has a severe ground fault (which does not stop its motor) that injects 5A into the A ground line between the ECG monitor and the main hospital ground. The resistance between the A ground line and the main ground is 0.1 Ω. The 5A flowing in the A ground line puts the ECG ground 500 mV above the hospital ground and ground B. From the equivalent circuit of Figure 13.5b, we see that the patient's left leg is effectively driven by a 500 mV, 60 Hz voltage source. The left leg-to-heart resistance is ca. 300 Ω, and the heart-to-catheter ground resistance is 50 kΩ, so the microshock current through the heart is simply $I_s \cong 0.5/5E4 = 10\ \mu A$, just below the fibrillation danger threshold. If the catheter resistance was lower or the ground line resistance was higher, the patient would probably go into cardiac fibrillation.

Clearly, if the ECG system were wireless (battery-powered), *there would be no conductive path from hospital ground line A to the patient, and no shock hazard.* Also, modern hospital electrical safety practice places ground fault interrupters (GFIs) at utility power outlets used in wet areas for machinery such as polishers and bed motors. An egregious 5A ground fault current from a polisher would instantly cause the GFI to shut down the power to the machine. Obviously, GFIs *are not used* on outlets powering critical care and patient life support equipment, such as respirators, external pacemakers, etc. Also note that a modern, insulated, solid-state pressure sensor on the catheter would have a very high resistance to ground, on the order of 10s of megohms. The mandatory use of MIAs and medical-grade, isolating power supplies also protects against cardiac microshock.

Webster (1992) pointed out that for safety, every power outlet and metal object in the patient's room (e.g., bed frame. door frame, sink, window frame, etc.) should be connected to a common,

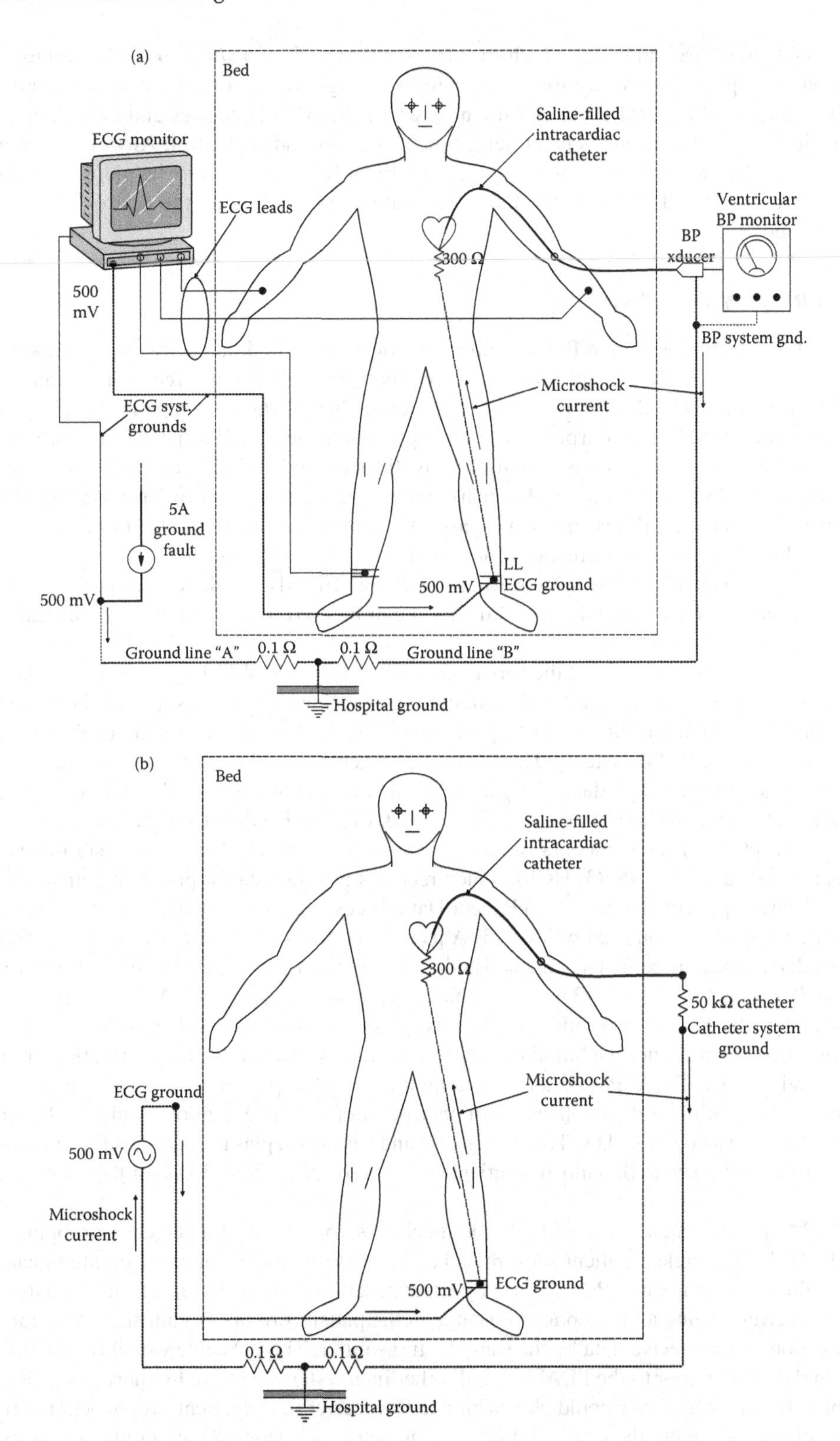

FIGURE 13.5 (a) Illustration of how a 5A ground fault current can give a patient with a cardiac catheter a microshock. The problem lies in the grounding circuits in the hospital. (b) A schematic showing the microshock current path through the heart. See text for discussion.

local (isopotential) ground plate, which in turn, is connected by a *single wire* to a robust, reference grounding plate that is, in turn, connected by a single thick copper cable to the building's ground. This forces all local grounds (green wires) of the AC receptacles and all exposed metal surfaces in the patient's room to be at nearly the same (ground) potential. Any electric machinery (polishers, bed motors, etc.) used in proximity to an ICU patient must be plugged in through GFI-protected outlets. The single ground wire strategy will eliminate the microshock scenario described above.

13.8 PRIVACY IN WPM

Because the information in a WPM system is broadcast as a modulated RF signal (albeit short-range), it is theoretically possible for a clandestine, "eavesdropping" receiver to intercept it, demodulate, and download it for nonmedical purposes. Such invasion of a patient's privacy could be used for various nefarious purposes. For example: In business, will a sick CEO or other executive be returning to work soon, or remain an invalid; how will this affect stock prices and corporate structure? In government, will a heart attack cause a politician to have to resign? In life insurance, will a chronic illness make a high-profile entertainer uninsurable? In military combat situations, how many persons are casualties? How bad are their wounds? An enemy could also jam a military hospital's WPM system to create chaos. Illicitly obtained patient medical information is generally only valuable in so far that it can be converted to financial, political and/or strategic gain.

Leister et al. (2008) considered the threat assessment issues in WPM systems used in hospitals (diagnostics, surgery, recovery, and intensive care settings), nursing homes, private homes, and by paramedics (civilian and military). They gave specific recommendations to "harden" the security of hospital and other WPM systems. They described a generic WPM system model that contained: (1) A patient source of WPM data; the patient is identified by a code number known only in the hospital's central Health Care Information System (HCIS). The RF data from patient sensors is generally unencrypted. (2) A patient data collector (PDC) which collects data from one or more patient sources and forwards it to the (3) HCIS, which receives patient data for processing and/or storage and may forward patient data to the (4) Patient Data Accessing Unit (PDAU), which presents these data to the medical staff on secure links. (5) A patient ID-data mapper uses primary data from the PDC and determines the patient's name and address, admission data, etc. and sends this information to the HCIS and PDAU. Figure 13.6 shows a block diagram of a typical WPM system based on the Leister model. One of the more vulnerable points to eavesdrop on patient data is the low-power RF link from the patient to the PDC module. One would have to have a priori information on patient location and identity. The WPM data received by the eavesdropping receiver could be stored in it, or rebroadcast to an illicit data collector. Another point of data interception would be the RF link from the PDAU to a doctor's PDA. The doctor's ID and password, plus the patient's ID and password would have to be known to download a patient's data to the physician's PDA, or the eavesdropping receiver.

A WPM system design that could provide much less opportunity for RF eavesdropping eliminates the RF! The wireless patient sensors and signal conditioners would now communicate with a patient data accessing unit (PDAU) first by a frequency-modulated IR link from the patient to a local IR receiver driving a fiber optic (FO) cable in the patient's room. A vital signs monitor in the patient's room could receive data by the same IR transmitter. The FO cable would run inaccessibly buried in the wall or floor to the PDAU, and all other intersystem links are by short-range IR and/or FO cables. If some malefactor could plant a hidden IR receiver in the patient's room near the IR data transmitter (line-of-sight), they could, of course, intercept data. However, certainly not as easily as picking up RF data from a patient's room. A disadvantage of an IR/FO cable wireless data link is that it is more easily interrupted by persons walking around the patient's room. Redundant FO cable IR receivers could mitigate this problem.

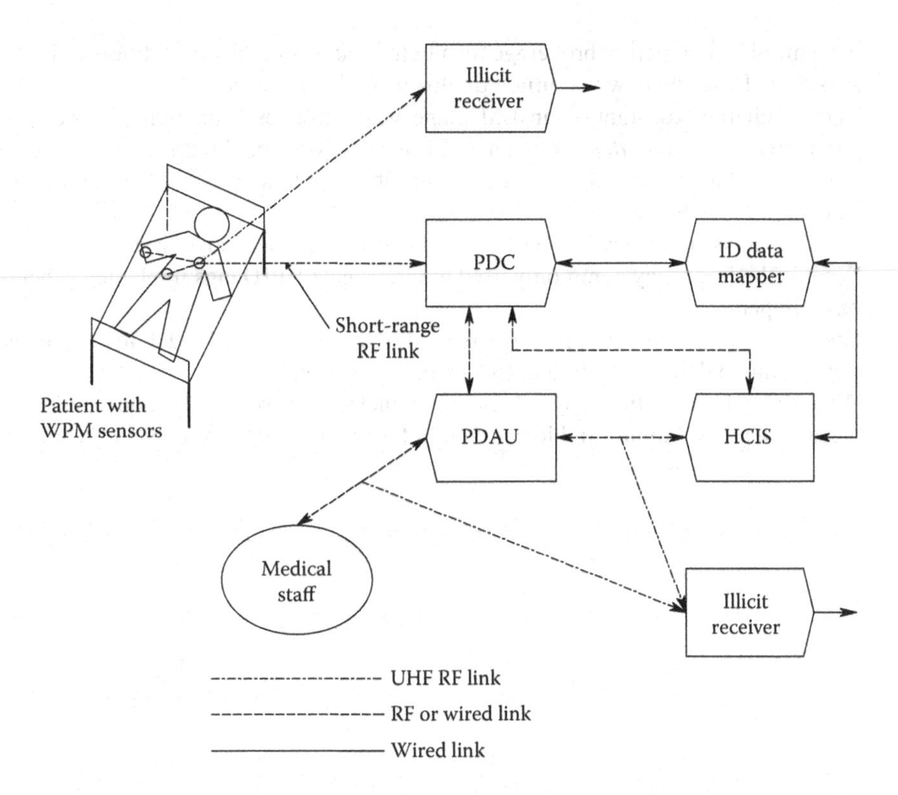

FIGURE 13.6 Signal flow paths in a typical WPM system, showing "soft" paths where patient information could be acquired illicitly.

13.9 CHAPTER SUMMARY

In this chapter, we examined the needs for, the architecture of, and the applications for wireless (RF) patient monitoring. We first described the sensors typically used in WPM systems found in surgery, recovery rooms, and intensive care units. Next we described the modulation schemes used in WPM, and the communications protocols used to link patient transmitters with a central data acquisition station (e.g., ZigBee, Bluetooth, Wi-Fi, and global satellite radio services such as *Iridium* and *Inmarsat*).

We described the basic architecture of UHF oscillators, UHF radio chip-sets, and UHF antennas. Listed were a number of manufacturers of WPM systems and emergency telemedical systems. Lastly, we considered the overall architecture of WPM data collection systems and how they may be vulnerable to illicit eavesdropping.

The use of thermoelectric generators and "energy harvester" ICs to power patient-located, WPM sensors was introduced.

CHAPTER 13 HOME PROBLEMS

13.1. Describe and discuss the relative merits and disadvantages of the current noninvasive means of blood glucose measurement.

13.2. What audio signal bandwidth is required to transmit the following sounds? (A) Heart sounds. (B) Lung and airway sounds. (C) Doppler-shifted blood flow sounds from carotid arteries.

13.3. The CFO of a major brokerage house has passed out during a board meeting and has been taken to a major hospital that uses WPM. You are a private investigator and have been hired by competing brokerage firm to find out his medical condition and prognosis ASAP. Describe how you might do this using RF devices.

13.4. The attenuation constant of an EM plane wave in a lossy medium is given by the parameter α. The *skin depth* δ of an EM wave in a lossy medium is defined as the distance $\delta = \alpha^{-1}$ it must travel in order to reduce its amplitude by $e^{-1} = 0.368 = 36.8\%$ (see Balanis, 1989; Chapter 4).
Plot δ in m. vs frequency in kHz for sea water and for soft body tissues.

13.5. What is the frequency commonly used to interrogate RFID tags implanted subcutaneously in pets?

13.6. Discuss the pros and cons of using infrared light instead of UHF RF to couple patient sensor data to data acquisition units in a patient's room.

13.7. What critical care patient physiological parameters are commonly monitored?

13.8. Design an apnea monitor in block diagram format. How will you detect breathing?

14 RFID Tags, GPS Tags, and Ultrasonic Tags Used in Ecological Research

14.1 INTRODUCTION

Radio-frequency identification (RFID) tags, along with optical barcodes, allow our complex society to identify, track, sort, locate, and price goods, as well as identify animals and even people. An RFID system consists of the following: (1) a class of objects to be identified (e.g., cattle, pets, books, shipping containers, controlled substances), (2) the physical tags (which can be classified as either active (self-powered), or passive), and (3) a tag-reading system (basically a radio transmitter/receiver with an RF output link to a computer that compiles data and does statistics on the tags read). All RFID tags work basically in the same way: (1) Identification (ID) data is stored in the tag's on-board ROM, waiting to be read. (2) The tag's antenna receives electromagnetic energy from the tag's RFID reader system. (3) Using power from its internal battery, or power derived from the reader's RF signal, the tag sends modulated RF back to the receiver for processing and storage.

RFID tags themselves consist of three major electronic subsystems: (1) A compact antenna that receives a tag reader transmitter's RF energy. This energy is detected and "wakes up" the tag, and in the case of passive tags, it provides it with DC power. The antenna also transmits the tag's signature RF response that allows its identification. (2) A digital section that pulse-codes the tag's signature response. (3) An RF modulator and transmitter that broadcasts the tag's response via the receive/transmit antenna. Battery-powered ("active") tags require an RF input to "wake them up," and because their power is internal, they have greater output range, and in some cases, in addition to broadcasting their ID signature, they can store and transmit data on environmental conditions (e.g., temperature, humidity, mechanical shock), or past reading history (when, where, who).

The distance over which the reader-tag system can operate varies and depends on the reader-tag system's RF operating frequency, its antennas, and the RF power levels transmitted from the reader (and tag). Self-powered tags can be read as far away as 100 m, while passive RFID can work up to 6 m, but usually no more than to 0.6 m.

14.2 APPLICATIONS OF RFID TAGS

RFID tags have many uses: *in biomedicine,* they can be used to identify and locate patients and hospital staff, do inventory control on controlled substances, track laboratory specimens, and identify laboratory animals (with tag implants). An RFID tag can be attached to a patient's "hospital bracelet" and read by a caregiver's PDA/tag reader to verify the patient's ID and his/her scheduled, prescribed drugs that must be administered.

A controversial future RFID tag application is the implantation of passive tags in humans. On the good side, these could serve as electronic dog tags for soldiers in combat (coding the wearer's ID, blood type, allergies, etc.), or as medic alert devices for persons with drug allergies, food allergies, or chronic diseases such as Alzheimer's, epilepsy, or diabetes. Another biomedical application is the wireless delivery of UHF RF energy to an implanted tag antenna, whose output can be rectified and used to signal and/or power implanted devices such as drug delivery pumps, neural stimulators, etc. (see the thesis by Soora, 2005). On the dark side, implanted tags in humans could permit a controlling central government to track its citizens, the antithesis of privacy. Such tracking would require an immense, expensive, tag reading, and data-processing support bureaucracy.

Elsewhere, RFID tags are used for a broad spectrum of applications: One finds passive RFID tags competing with barcodes in inventory control. RFID tags are now also used to prevent theft in a variety of stores (e.g., selling books, DVDs and music CDs, clothing), also to prevent theft in libraries and museums, identification of stolen or lost domestic animals, to prevent forgery of passports and identify passport owners through stored biometric data (such as fingerprints), to prevent forgery of currency (the Euro), to enable rolling vehicle identification, fare collection and passage through toll gates, to enable rapid and automatic fare collection on subways, trains, ferries (they can be embedded in credit cards and disposable paper tickets), to restrict access to certain secure areas, to track and sort airline baggage, and to track shipments of controlled drugs (e.g., opioids). The US Department of Defense uses active RFID tags on all of its million-plus shipping containers that travel outside of the continental United States.

RFID tags are often used along with or as replacements for Universal Product Code (UPC) bar codes. Bar codes require the laser scanner to have direct, proximal, line-of-sight to them to be read. An RFID tag does not need to be facing the reader to respond; it can be out of sight or hidden. A tag and a tag reader generally are more expensive than a UPC label and reader, however.

RFID tags are also used for vehicle toll collection on highways, tunnels, and bridges worldwide. A well-known example of toll transponders is the *E-ZPass*™ unit, made by Mark IV Industries Corp., IVHS Division. *E-ZPass* transponders are used in the toll systems of 14 states in the Northeastern United States. The battery-powered units are interrogated by a 915 MHz RF signal sent at 500 kbps using the IAG protocol in 256-bit packets. A transmitter/reader antenna is usually located over a vehicle lane in a toll plaza. The vehicle unit's response informs the reader of the vehicle's ID, its type (passenger car, 18-wheeler, etc.) and the owner's account number to be debited. The unit stores the location, time, and date where it was last interrogated so the next reader can calculate the toll, which is automatically billed. Similar vehicular transponders are in use and are being adopted in other states (e.g., *FasTrak* in CA; *K-Tag* in KS; *SunPass* in FL; *TxTag* in TX).

Passive RFID *implants* are currently being used to identify valuable domestic animals including dogs, cats, ferrets, cows, sheep, goats, pigs, and horses, as well as zoo animals including llamas, alpacas, bears, bison, rabbits, deer, elk, lizards, alligators, turtles, etc. The chips are about the size of a large grain of rice and are coated with a bioinert plastic, or are covered with a biocompatible glass made from soda lime. Tags in dogs and cats are usually located subdermally, on the midline between the shoulder blades. Tags in large farm animals are often placed subdermally in the neck, located on collars, or clipped to their ears.

Because the interrogating RF energy must penetrate skin and soft tissue, very low frequencies around 125–134.2 kHz are generally used to minimize the tissue absorption of RF energy. The tag reader antenna also must be in close proximity (<5 cm) to the animal. Animal RFID tags operate in the nearfield, where RF energy is coupled as a magnetic field to a tag's coil antenna or tank coil. The resonant RF voltage across the L-C tank circuit is rectified, and the DC obtained is used to power the tag's data ROM and logic.

Most manufacturers of animal RFID chips comply with International Organization for Standardization (ISO) standards. ISO standards 11784 and 11785 specify how a transponder tag is activated and how the stored information is transferred to the interrogating transceiver. ISO 14223 specifies the structure of the RF code for advanced tags for animals.

14.3 DESIGN OF RFID TAGS

14.3.1 Sizes and Cost

One of the limitations of RFID tag size is the antenna dimensions required at a given RF operating frequency. The electronics can be made very small. The smallest tag (without antenna) may be Hitachi's *Mu Chip*™; it is 0.4 mm square × 60 mm thick and can store 10^{38} unique IDs using a 128-bit ROM (Hitachi 2011). The *Mu* tag's readable distance is small, however, <40 cm, because of the UHF operating frequency (2.45 GHz) and its small antenna. There is great advantage to using RFID operating frequencies in the ranges of hundreds of MHz, or low GHz, as the effective antenna size requirements shrink with decreasing RF wavelength, also the shorter read distances of UHF RFID tags ensures a modicum of privacy. From inspection of several Hitachi RFID products using the 2.45 GHz *Mu Chip,* the insulated wire antenna length is about 70 mm long. The mu chip with an antenna attached on a substrate sells for US$ 0.43 in lots of 70,000 or more.

As you will see in the next section, the use of planar fractal antenna designs has enabled further size reduction of RFID tags. Most passive RFID tag ICs cost between 5 and 50 US cents; active and semipassive tags cost more.

14.3.2 Tag RF Frequencies and Antennas

Tag operating frequencies have a wide range, depending on application and design. Worldwide, low frequencies (LFID) (125–134.2 kHz and 140–148.2 kHz) can be used without license. High-frequency RF (HFID) 13.56 MHz can also be used worldwide without license. There are restrictions on UHF use, however, because of potential interference with communications bands, aircraft instrumentation, etc. In North America, UHF in the range of 902–928 MHz (915 ±13 MHz) can be used unlicensed for RFID with power restrictions; 2.4–2.5 GHz is also used. In Europe, the unlicensed RFID UHF band is 856–868 MHz. In Australia and New Zealand, 918–926 MHz are free for RFID, but power restrictions apply. (A comprehensive list of standards for RFID transmissions can be found in Wiki, 2010a; Bluetooth.)

Active RFID tags can be found that operate at frequencies including 303, 315, 418, 433, 868, 915, and 2400 MHz with read ranges of ca. 18.3 to 91.4 m. *Wi-Fi* active RFID tags are designed to operate in the unlicensed ISM bands of 2.4 to 2.4835 GHz or 5.8 to 5.825 GHz.

Some low-frequency (LF) (9-135 kHz) RFID tags operate in the nearfield by capturing the reader's RF signal with a multiturn, loop antenna that responds to the magnetic field component of the RF electromagnetic signal. At high frequencies, the nearfield loop antenna is usually a printed-circuit coil consisting of continuous, concentric turns etched on a thin circuit board. Such tags are used in seaports to track shipping containers; they do not need to be miniature. The nearfield distance is ca. 380 m (Scharfeld 2001).

Most conventional HF and VHF antennas use designs that employ $\lambda/2$ elements. (Recall that $\lambda/2 = c/2f$, where λ is in meters, c is the velocity of EM waves *in vacuo* (3E8 m/s) and f is the RF frequency in Hz.). Thus, $\lambda/2$ for a 915 MHz, UHF carrier is 16.4 cm, far too large for conventional, miniature tag antenna designs (including $\lambda/2$ monopole-ground plane radiators, dipoles, or folded dipoles). Consequently, most UHF RFID tags now use some form of antenna design that uses far less space (volume) than conventional linear dipoles and arrays. These include "compressed" designs such as meander ("crank") dipoles (see Figure 14.1 for a straight, $\lambda/4$ dipole and two, typical meander element designs). Meander dipoles are usually printed on a flexible plastic (polyester) dielectric using conductive (colloidal silver) "ink," or can be etched from a thin, copper-clad, fiberglass, printed-circuit (PC) board wafer, then gold plated. Low-frequency, nearfield, current loop antennas can also be etched on fiberglass PC boards as a flat spiral coil with over a dozen "turns." The tag electronic chip is often located in the center of the current loop antenna.

In Table 14.1, we summarize the radio frequencies used in RFID tag technology.

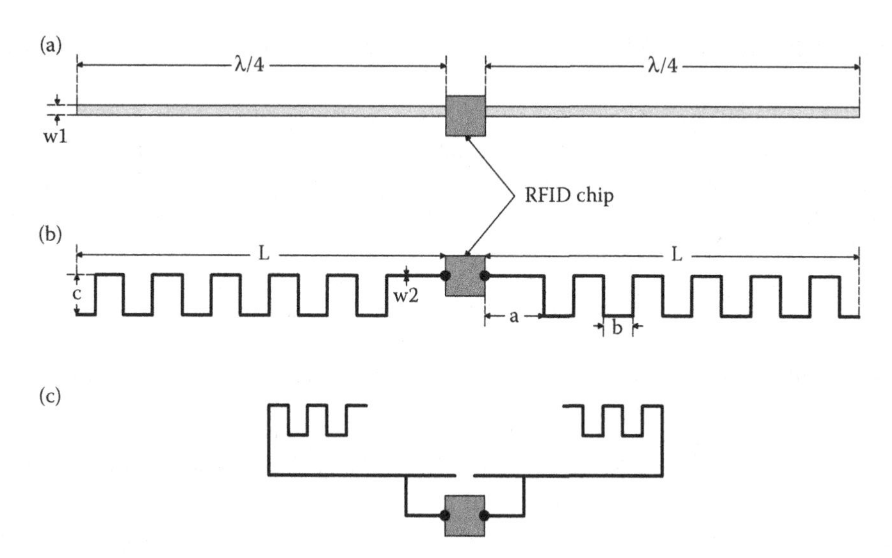

FIGURE 14.1 (a) An RFID chip with a conventional, dual, λ/4 dipole. (b) and (c) Two versions of a *meander dipole*. Note that in general, L <λ/4.

TABLE 14.1
Frequencies used for RFID tag technology

Frequency range	Comment	Allowed field strength/ transmission power
<135 kHz	Low-frequency, inductive coupling; used in animal implants.	72 dB μA/m max.
3.155 – 3.400 MHz	Electronic article surveillance (EAS)	13.5 dB mA/m
6.765 – 6.795 MHz	Medium frequency (ISM), inductive coupling	42 dB mA/m
7.400 – 8.800 MHz	Medium freq., used for EAS only	9 dB mA/m
13.553 – 13.567	Medium freq (13.56 MHz, ISM), inductive coupling, widely used for smartcards, smart-labels and item management	60 dB mA/m
26.957 – 27.283 MHz (HF)	Medium frequency (ISM), inductive coupling, special applications only	42 dB mA/m
433 MHz (UHF)	UHF ISM, backscatter coupling	10–100 mW
865.6 – 867.6 MHz	UHF RFID only, listen before talk	2 W ERP (=3.8 W EIRP) (Europe only)
902 – 928 MHz	UHF SRD, backscatter coupling	4 W EIRP-spread spectrum. US and Canada only.
2.400 – 2.483 GHz (SHF)	SHF ISM, backscatter coupling	4 W spread spectrum. US and Canada only.
2.446 – 2.454 GHz	SHF RFID and automatic vehicle ID	0.5 W EIRP outdoor, 4 W EIRP indoor.

14.3.2.1 Fractal Antennas

Obviously, all RFID tags require antennas, and there is a general need for antenna designs that are small (have dimensions <λ/4) and are planar (fit on a PC board). Nathan Cohen (1997) was probably the first person to put a fractal antenna design to practice (in 1988), in an attempt to shrink his ham radio antenna. Since then, fractal space-filling antenna designs have proliferated in all areas of RF communications, including WPM, cell phones, RFID tag designs, and GPS systems operating in the UHF frequencies (Wiki 2010g).

Fractals are iterative, self-replicating geometries found throughout nature and science. Mathematically, a deterministic fractal is a broken curve generated by repetitively applying a *generator function* (GF) with successive decreases in scale to an *initiator.* The initiator can be a straight line, or a geometric area such as a triangle, circle, ring, cross, a Haar wavelet doublet, or a square. Deterministic fractals in two and three dimensions are also generated by mathematical formulas, e.g., the Mandelbrot set equations, the Julia set equations, and Ferguson's *Sterling* fractal-generating computer program (Wiki 2010f).

Random fractals are found in nature: for example, tree dendrition, a lightning bolt's branching, certain plants (e.g., ferns, romaneso broccoli), frost crystals on glass, etc. They can be generated on a computer by introducing random perturbations (noise) into a fractal-generating formula's constants.

There is growing use of various fractal antenna (FA) designs for applications such as RFID tags, mobile communications (e.g., cell phones, laptop computers), GPS receivers, etc. Fractal antennas are also referred to as multilevel, patch antennas, and space-filling curves. The major feature of a FA is the repetition of a geometrical motif over several scale sizes (usually no more than four). They generally operate on the radiated electromagnetic (EM) field of the tag reader in the far-field (at 915 MHz, the far-field exists greater than 5.2 cm from the antenna (Scharfeld 2001)).

Many FA element designs are planar monopoles, i.e., they exist on a two-dimensional plane ("patch"). The FA's ground plane is generally orthogonal to the planar monopole radiation element, giving the entire antenna a three-dimensional domain. (See Werner and Ganguly (2003) for an in-depth review of FA designs.) The evolution of a fifth-order, *space-filling,* Hilbert fractal pattern antenna element is shown in Figure 14.2 (Mitchell 2001; Wiki 2010e; Wolfram 2010). In this case, the generator function is the same as the initiator. The gold-plated conductor pattern is laid down on a dielectric substrate such as glass, ceramic, or fiberglass.

One linear FA design, illustrated in Figure 14.3, generates a 2-D fractal in a plane by repetitively applying a triangular generator to a straight-line initiator with successive reductions in scale. This von Koch fractal process generates elements that can be used as dipoles or multielement FAs. Generally, from three to four iterations of the simple von Koch linear fractal algorithm are used. Zainud-Deen et al. (2009) gave a thorough analysis and evaluation of two, third iteration (K3) Koch fractal elements connected in series as a monopole ($2L_e = 7.35$ cm, $\alpha = 70^o$), sandwiched between two dielectric layers. The antenna center frequency was ca. 910 MHz. Two K3 von Koch fractals were connected as a dipole antenna and the behavior studied by Ibrahiem et al. (2006). They reported that their antenna had two resonances; one at 868 MHz and the other at 2.45 GHz. von

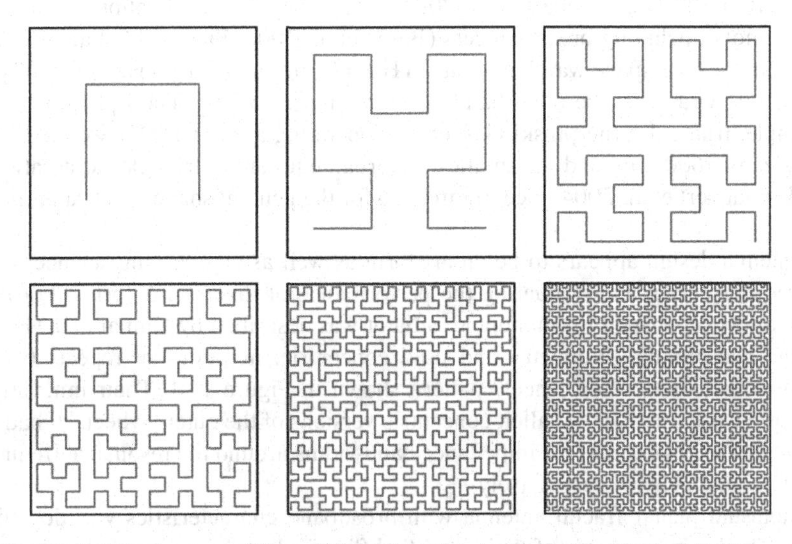

FIGURE 14.2 Evolution of an area-filling, Hilbert fractal antenna design. Upper left, the generator. Lower left, the third iteration. Five iterations are shown.

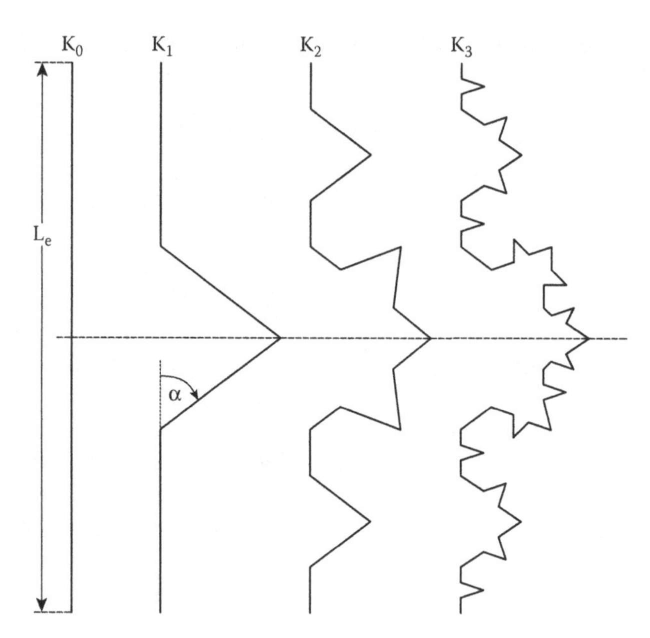

FIGURE 14.3 Evolution of a third-order, linear koch fractal.

Koch fractal monopoles and dipoles are, in general, more effective antennas than meander dipoles, shown in Figure 14.1.

A general property of FAs is that they tend to be broadband, i.e., have effective radiation properties over a relatively broad band of operating frequencies. Conventional linear dipoles and multi-element arrays tend to have "tuned" or narrowband characteristics, although the log-periodic antenna array, such as used in broadcast TV reception, are relatively broadband. Log periodic antennas have been called "fractal" (Wiki 2010g), and log-periodic elements have been "fractalized" using von Koch triangular generators (see Karim et al. 2010) in order to reduce antenna size at a given frequency (by 26% for a series iteration having two triangle "bumps"/element).

Another property of fractal antennas is that they are scaleable; they are even useful at THz frequencies (0.1–10 × 10^{12} Hz) (Gaubert et al. 2004) where they find application in imaging *ex vitro* and *in vitro* tumors, including breast cancers (Berry et al. 2004; Fitzgerald et al. 2006; Townsend 2008). Note that the free-space wavelength at 1 THz = 0.3 mm, and a 1 THz "photon" carries only 4 meV of energy. X-rays, on the other hand, are ionizing radiations. Their photons carry 10^3–10^4 eV. For example, triangular Sierpinski Gasket FAs operating around 1 THz were designed with a major edge size of 1600 mm, and the smallest, internal, equilateral triangles at iteration 4 are 100 mm on a side (Gaubert et al. 2004). See Figure 14.6 for the general shape of a triangular Sierpinski Gasket FA.

Fractal antenna design appears to be an art form as well as engineering science; many papers have appeared presenting and evaluating the performance of diverse FA forms. For example, an unusual, planar, wheel-shaped FA monopole radiator was described by Kumar and Malathi (2009). Their antenna had circular symmetry and used concentric, iterations or repeats (wheels inside wheels) of the outer, basic "cog wheel" pattern shown in Figure 14.4. Their innovative "wheel" fractal used three, progressively smaller, concentric versions of the outer "wheel." It had resonances at 1.34, 2.575, and 4.22 GHz and the impedance bandwidths around the resonance frequencies were 40.77%, 19.02%, and 26.94%, respectively.

Another unusual planar fractal antenna with broadband characteristics was described by Liu et al. (2006). The basic geometry of their modified Sierpinski fractal monopole antenna is shown in Figure 14.5. The basic monopole consists of two, vertical, 60° metal triangles (88.9 mm high,

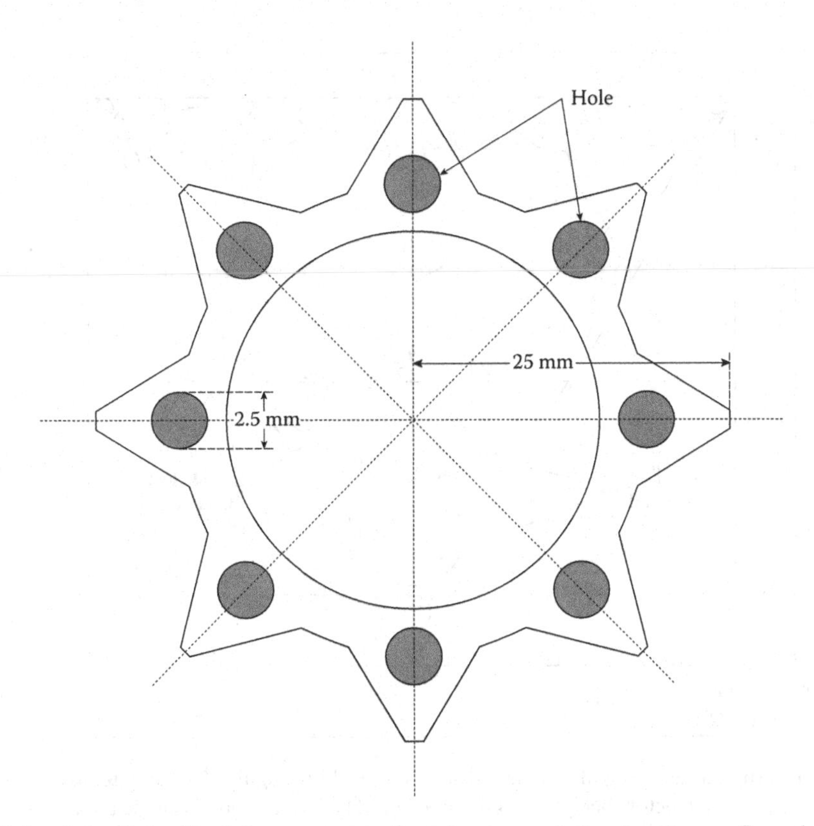

FIGURE 14.4 Outer "wheel" of the concentric fractal antenna design by Kumar, R. and Malathi, P., *International Journal of Recent Trends in Engineering.* 2(6): 98–100, 2009. Three progressively smaller "wheels" were placed inside the outer wheel. See text for description of performance.

51.3 mm base) on a 200 × 200 mm ground plane. The authors show the resonance spectra when one large metal circle (the F1 generator) is added between the triangles, then three smaller circles plus the first circle, then nine even smaller circles are added, and finally in the fourth iteration, 27 small circles are clustered in groups of 3 around each of the 9 even smaller circles. The fourth iteration Sierpinski fractal antenna is usable from 1 to 10 GHz.

Puente-Baliarda et al. (1998) described yet another fractal monopole antenna. This fractal antenna is shown in Figure 14.6. Shown in the upper left is the fourth-order evolution (S4) of the Sierpinski triangle gasket applied to a metal (m), vertical triangular monopole initiator (tip down) (the other 2/3 of the figure shows the (S3) design). Each triangular area added to the metal initiator is dielectric (d in the figure). In each iteration, the triangles are one-half the size of those in the preceding iteration. Puente-Baliarda et al. tested a fifth-order (S5) version of the triangular Sierpinski gasket monopole antenna, the smallest triangles of which were 1/32 the size of the original (S0) triangular monopole. This monopole fractal antenna was useful over a broadband UHF range of ca. 0.5 to 14 GHz.

Figure 14.7 illustrates a second-order, space-filling fractal element based on crosses (Werner and Ganguly 2003). (The crosses are metal strips laid down on a dielectric substrate.) The F0 initiator is the big cross, the F1 iteration adds four cross pieces, and F2 adds 12 smaller cross pieces. An F3 (not shown) iteration can be obtained by crossing each of the 12 smaller cross pieces, giving 36 small crosses. The cross-fractal tree element can be used as a monopole radiator with a ground plane or a dipole.

A comprehensive comparison of UHF fractal antenna designs and their performances at various frequencies seems to be lacking in all of the extensive, available, current literature on the design and evaluation of FAs. There are a bewildering variety of FA shapes and geometric evolutions. One

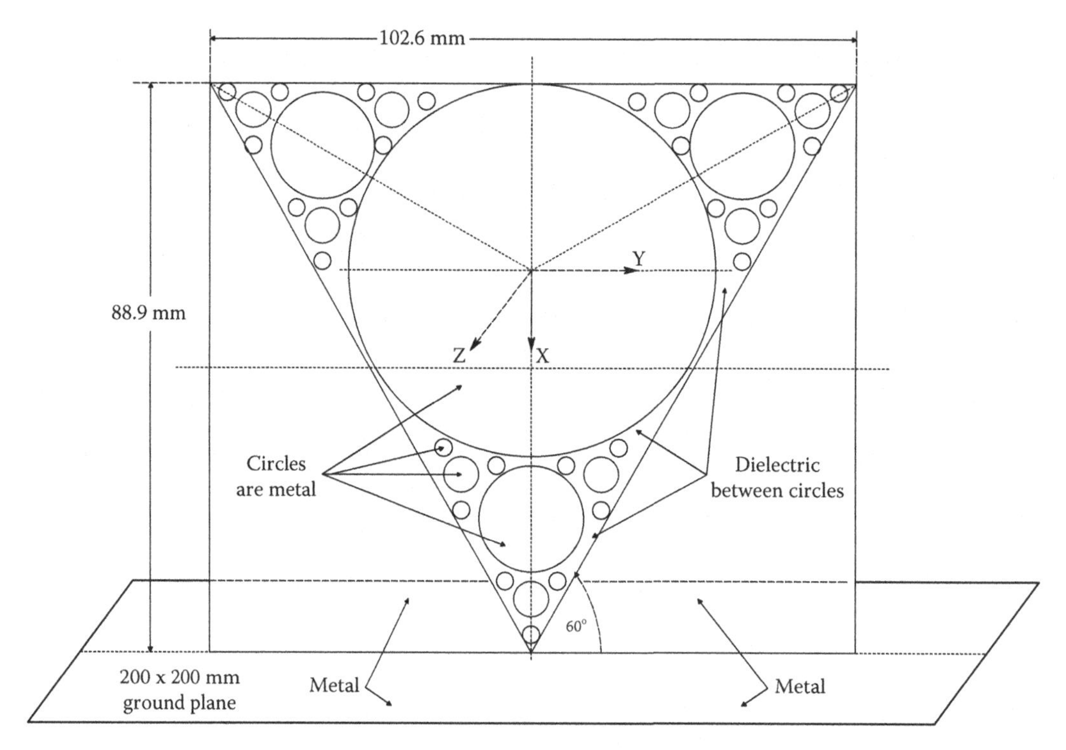

FIGURE 14.5 An unusual triangular, space-filling, Sierpinski triangular fractal antenna. The triangle is a dielectric on a square conductor sheet over a ground plane. The circles in the triangle are metal.

principle does emerge, however; the higher the order of the fractals and the more space-filling that is used results in broader useful bandwidths and smaller antennas at a given frequency than unfractalized designs.

14.3.3 Tag Modulation Schemes

14.3.3.1 Introduction

Every basic, passive RFID tag must have a memory chip (ROM) in which is stored its unique identification (ID) code. When the tag receives an RF input of the correct frequency from the reader (with the correct gating sequence, if so required), its RF response is activated; it broadcasts back to the reader its coded ID sequence, i.e., its electronic product code (EPC). Since the reader is, in general, in sight of the container, animal, etc. that holds the tag, unique identification is possible. Even if the tagged object is not in sight, its presence is inferred by the reader's response to the tag's ID signature.

Because the tag's response may be received by other readers, there are security and privacy concerns. A simple cryptographic circuit can be added to the tag to deny public access to its response. However, this addition makes the tag circuit as well as the reader circuit more complicated and consequently more expensive. Also, the simple encryption is relatively easy to break. It is possible to prevent UHF RFID tags from being read (or at least responding) by wrapping them in metal foil or inserting them in a metallized Mylar antistatic bag (used for electronic components). For protection against *skimming* (e.g., using an RFID reader to get someone's passport data without them knowing it), US passports have a metallized shield between the passport's cover and first page. The passport's UHF RFID tag can only be read (at ranges less than ca. 10 cm) when the cover is open.

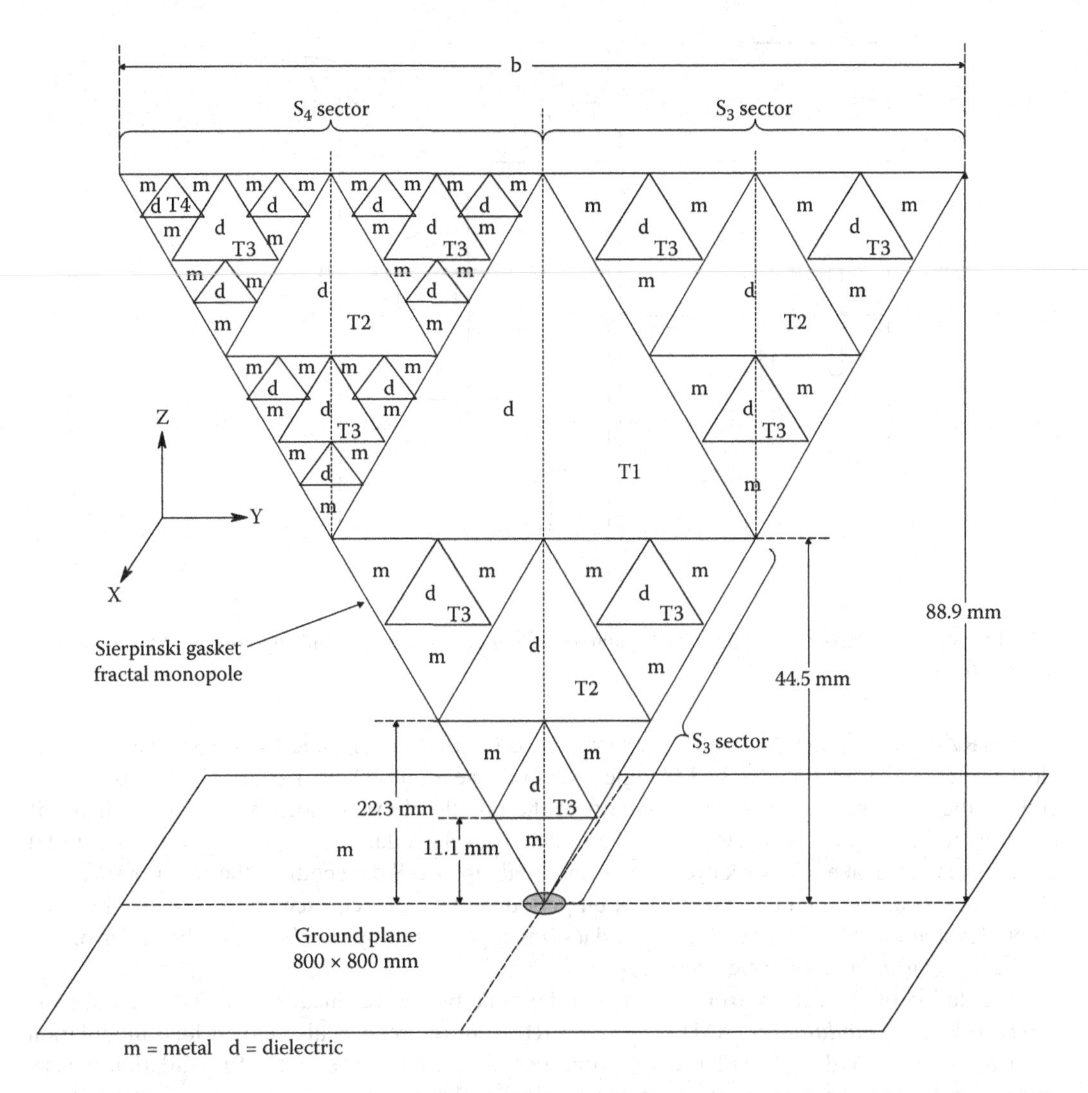

FIGURE 14.6 Another vertical, Sierpinski triangle antenna over a ground plane. m is metal, and d is dielectric.

Privacy concerns have been generated by the fact that RFID tags attached to products (e.g., clothing, laptop computers) remain functional even after being taken home, and theoretically could be used at long range for surveillance. To overcome this potential problem, a Clipped Tag design was devised by IBM researchers, which allows the purchaser to tear off a portion of the tag's antenna. This transforms a long-range tag to a proximity tag that only can be read at a few centimeter. The clipped tag may still be used later for returns, recalls, or recycling.

What we will examine in the next section are the general means by which the basic tag responds, and how its information is stored and encoded.

14.3.3.2 Tag Operation

All RFID tags have built-in clocks that drive their data encoding circuits and modulation systems. The clock frequency is always some fraction of the radio frequency used. Encrypted RFID tag digital data can be encoded by nonreturn to zero-level (NRZ-L), biphase-L (Manchester), or differential biphase-S coding protocols (Sorrells 1998).

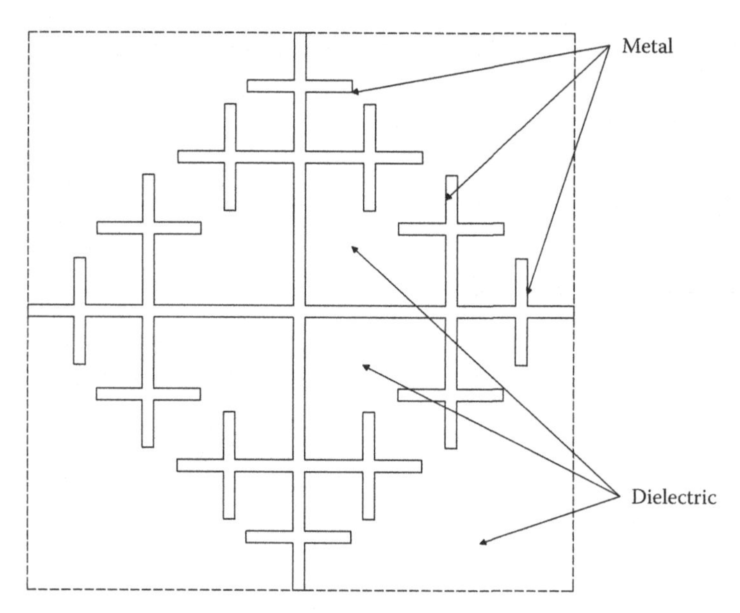

FIGURE 14.7 A third-order, planar fractal antenna using crosses as space-filling conductors. See text for description.

In NRZ-L data coding, a data "1" is represented by a HI coder logic level over one (or more) clock cycles, and a "0" is coded by LO logic level over one (or more) clock cycles. In biphase-L data coding, the coder output level change occurs at the middle of every clock bit period: A data 1 is represented by a high-to-low level change at midclock cycle; a data 0 is represented by a LO to HI coder level change at a midclock cycle. In Differential biphase-S data coding, the coder output level change occurs at the middle of every clock bit period: A data 1 is represented by a change in coder output level at the start of a clock cycle; a data 0 is represented by *no change* in the coder output level at the start of a clock cycle.

Modulation of RF energy from the tag can be done by several means; the *simplest means is direct amplitude modulation* (AM) of the CW RF from the reader, also called load modulation for nearfield tags, and backscatter modulation for far-field tags. The level of modulation is very small and depends on tag/reader geometry. Typically, the data voltage is ca. 60 dB down from the transmitted voltage on the reader coil (a 0.1 V peak drop in a 100 V peak-to-peak RF signal). This drop is caused by the modulated switching of a load across the tag's (receiving) antenna, increasing its admittance. This change in the loading of the tag antenna is reflected as an RF load increase on the inductively coupled reader's antenna circuit, causing the RF voltage across the reader's antenna to drop. Since the clock frequency is a tenth or less of the reader's RF frequency, the modulation can be recovered by detecting and low-pass filtering the reader's antenna voltage, then amplifying and passing the filtered output through comparators to regenerate the modulation square wave.

A second means of modulating tag data is by frequency shift keying (FSK), a form of FM. FSK is only practical on active tags using NRZ encoding. The modulated tag data causes the tag's RF output to change frequency; f_c for a 1 and $f_c + \Delta f$ for a 0 (see Stark, Tuteur, and Anderson, 1988).

Still another modulation scheme for active tag data is by phase shift keying (PSK). Here the modulator shifts the phase of the tag's output, and the carrier frequency stays the same. The RF output phase is changed by 180° between modulated 1s and 0s. Two common types of PSK are: Change carrier phase for the duration of any 0 or change phase at any data change ($0 \rightarrow 1$ or $1 \rightarrow 0$).

> PSK provides fairly good noise immunity, a moderately simple reader design, and a faster data rate than FSK. Typical applications utilize a backscatter [tag] clock of $f_c/2$. (Sorrells 1998)

Figure 14.8 illustrates a simplified circuit of a passive RFID tag design (Dudenbostel et al. 1997). In the Dudenbostel design, 4 MHz, CW, nearfield, RF energy was coupled into the tag's L_2 loop antenna from the reader's antenna and then rectified and regulated to make DC to operate the tag's CMOS circuits (e.g., clock and modulator). The tag's modulator generates a return signal by simply closing and opening a CMOS switch that loads and unloads antenna L_3. Loading the parallel resonant circuit, L_3-C_3, causes the load on the transmitting antenna to increase (by mutual inductance coupling, M_{13}); this in turn causes the RF voltage, v_1, across L_1 to drop for several RF cycles. This drop in v_1 is sensed by the reader as a logic LO. When the modulator switch is open, v_1 has a higher amplitude; this is sensed as logic HI. This process is called load modulation. It is generally used with LF and HF passive RFID tags running at 125 to 135 kHz, and 4 MHz. The EM field energy in load modulation decays as $1/r^6$ (r is the distance from antenna to antenna).

When passive tags are operated in the far-field, the modulation process is called backscatter modulation. The tag architecture is essentially the same as in the load modulation system (see Figure 14.9). By causing the modulator to switch a resistive load in and out across the receiving antenna, the receiving antenna's characteristic impedance, $\mathbf{Z_a}$, is modulated. Incident EM waves at carrier frequency will be reflected back from the tag's antenna to the reader's antenna with higher and lower amplitudes, encoding the data. The major difference is that in the load modulation scheme, the load is coupled to the reader's antenna by mutual inductance, while in far-field operation, it is the reflected RF energy (due to impedance mismatching) that carries the information that must be decoded by the reader. Far-field tags have the property that the far-field EM field decays as $1/r^2$.

Active RFID tags generally operate in the unlicensed SHF ISM bands of 2.4 to 2.4835 GHz or 5.8 to 5.825 GHz, or in the HF band at 13.56 MHz, and in the UHF bands including 303, 315, 418, 433, and 915 MHz. Figure 14.10 illustrates the simplified architecture of a typical active RFID tag.

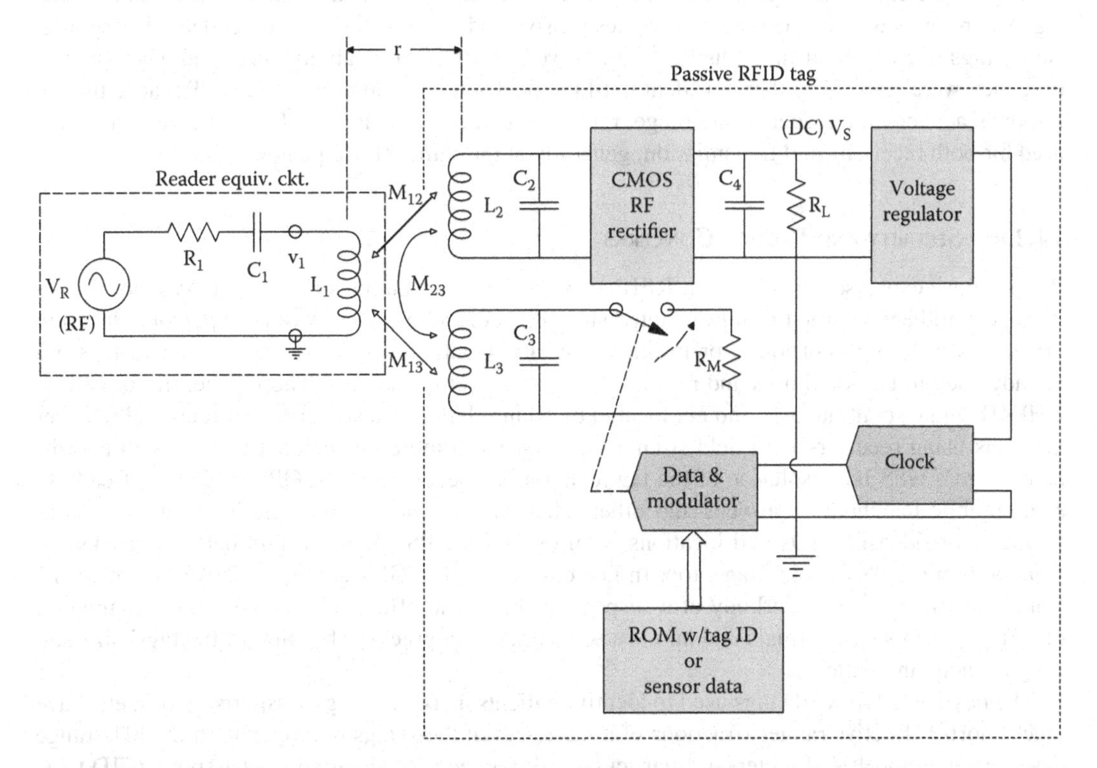

FIGURE 14.8 Simplified circuit of a passive RFID tag design by Dudenbostel, D. et al., *Proceedings of the 1997 International Conference on Solid-State Sensors and Actuators*, Chicago, 1997. This tag operated at 4 MHz. Modulation is done by the tag varying the load its receiving antenna presents the tag reader. Increased load causes a drop in v_1 in the reader, which is detected.

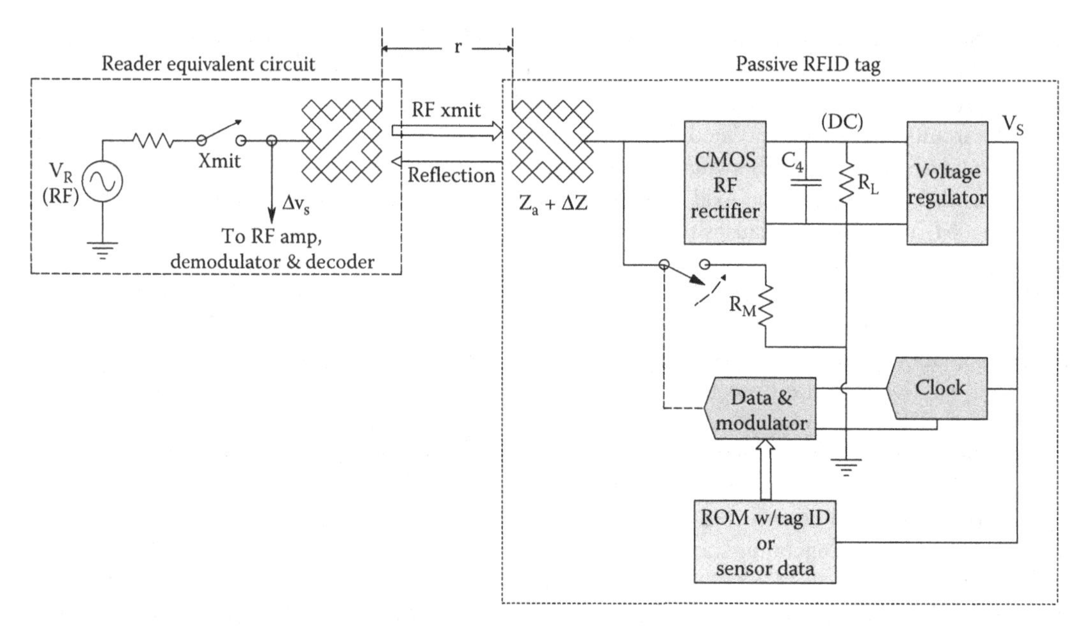

FIGURE 14.9 Another passive RFID tag designed for far-field operation. Again, the load on the tag's receiving antenna is modulated, and reflected energy is detected by the reader.

The tag generally operates on standby (MOS switch in the "R" position) until it receives an appropriately coded transmission from the reader. The reader can send ID, date, and location data for the tag to store in its RAM. The reader now goes passive and 'listens' for the tag's coded RF response. Active tags transmit their individual ID data as well as information about where and when the last time they were read. They then go silent until the next time they are interrogated. Because the tag responds actively, the reader-to-tag range, r, can be as much as a 100 m. The same tag antenna is used for both receiving and transmission, generally at the same RF frequency.

14.3.4 Security and Privacy Concerns

Persons have expressed concern that RFID tags implanted in humans or in a person's clothing or luggage could enable illicit or unwarranted surveillance, and pose a risk to both personal location privacy as well as to corporate or military security. Continuously broadcasting, active tags are already used to track animals and reptiles in wildlife ecology studies. These generally broadcast VHF ID signals continuously and are located by triangulation of a signal with directional receiver antennas using receivers with field strength meters. By combining such active tags with coordinates from a GPS IC, resolution of the tag location has become trivial. GPS chips are already in some mobile telephones. Parolees and other released criminals wear ankle bracelets with continuously broadcasting IDs and locations from on-board GPS chips. Certain delivery trucks are equipped with GPS tracking tags, too. In law enforcement, a GPS-equipped active tag "beacon" can be attached to the underbody of a suspect's vehicle and effectively tracked. Bioimplantation of active tags in small animals and humans is generally not practical because of the tags' size and weight (including battery).

The passive, UHF RFID tags used to identify patients, pets, clothing, passports, goods, etc. have much shorter effective ranges (fractions of a meter), even those tags that operate in the kHz range have ranges in the 10s of meters. Of particular risk for security violation are passport RFID tags. However, to be effectively illicitly read (skimmed), the illegal reader has to be nearly the same distance from the passport's tag as the immigration and custom's enforcement (ICE) agent's reader. Also, passport data are encrypted. Passport tag data can include a biometric identifier unique to the

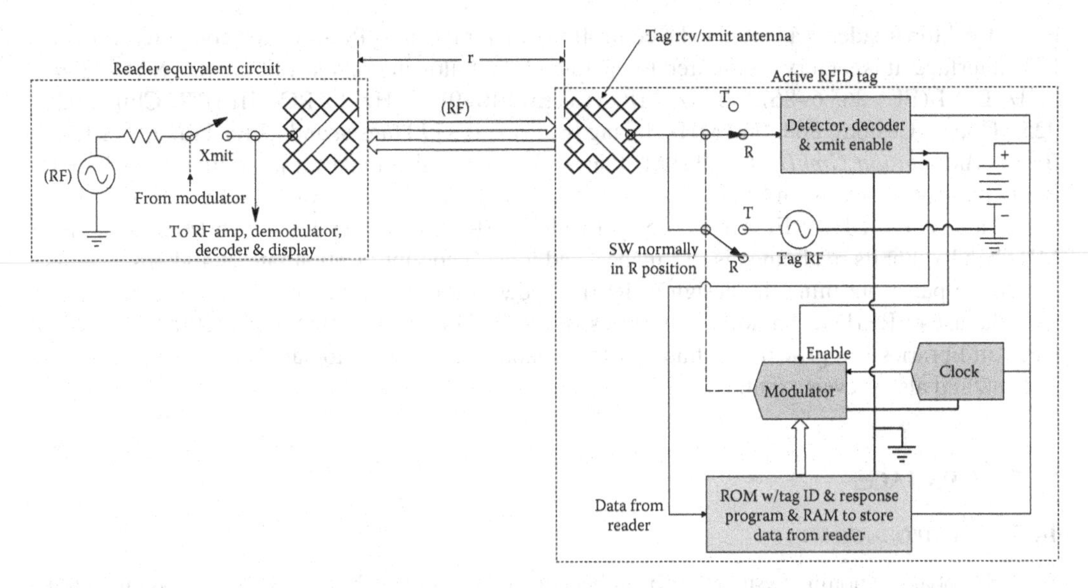

FIGURE 14.10 Block diagram of an active RFID tag. The tag, having received its coded, specific, "wake-up" signal from the reader, actively broadcasts its ID data (and other information) back to the reader.

passport holder, such as a fingerprint or a digital photograph that will permit face recognition technology to be used at ports-of-entry/departure. One answer to the passport tag privacy and skimming problem has been to read the passport's tag inside a shielded booth. On the other hand, the data on a passive UHF RFID tag in a credit card or an ATM card could be skimmed by a concealed, illegal reader near the ATM or point of sale.

It would be virtually impossible to read a UHF passive RFID tag implanted in a person's clothing or luggage unless the illicit reader were less than a half meter from the tag. Hence, tracking the detailed movements of a person wearing such an UHF passive tag would be highly difficult if not impossible. Fixed tag readers would have to be located at airports, train and bus stations. *Implanted* LF (134.2 kHz) tags of the type used in pets have reading ranges less than half a meter and thus present a challenge for detailed, long-range tracking. Active toll tags on vehicles, such as the *E-ZPass*™, can easily be tracked and continuously broadcasting GPS tags on trucks and taxis are meant to be tracked.

In conclusion, privacy concerns about passive RFID tags implanted in passports, ATM and credit cards is warranted; on the other hand, it would be nearly impossible to precisely locate a human with a passive, UHF or LF RFID tag except at "choke points," such as gates at airports, train and bus stations, sporting events, ATM machines, or hospital ERs.

14.4 TAG READERS

Passive tag readers are either handheld or fixed. They are radio transceivers; they first broadcast a continuous wave (CW) signal to the tag to activate its circuitry, then a coded and modulated burst of RF energy appropriate for the class of tags they are reading. Upon receiving this enabling code from the reader, the tag then responds with its unique ID code using backscatter modulation of the reader's broadcast CW RF signal.

An important design consideration is that the reader has a compact, sensitive, and directional antenna. Ukkonen et al. (2007) described the design of Koch fractal-based patch antennas for an UHF tag reader giving it a read range of 1–2 m. Their reader broadcast 50 mW at 869.525 MHz.

All RFID tag manufacturers make readers. For example, *ThingMagic, Inc.* of Cambridge, MA, makes a number of different tag reader designs, both fixed and handheld. For example, their USB

RFID Desktop Reader is adapted to be controlled by a typical host PC or laptop computer through a USB interface. It is factory configured to operate in the following regions: FCC (NA, SA) 902–928 MHz; ETSI (EU) 865.6–867.6 MHz; MIC (Korea) 910–914 MHz; SRRC-MII (P.R. China) 920–925; "Open" (Custom) 860–960 MHz. Its tag read rate is ≤190 tags/s, and its read range is ≤31 cm. *Brooks Automation GmbH* of 95490 Mistelgau, Germany, also makes a large line of 13.56 MHz RFID readers for cards and tags. Another company, *SkyeTek®, Inc.,* of Westminster, CO, USA, makes a desktop, UHF RFID reader (SkyeReader™ SR70) that operates at 916 MHz with an 88 MHz bandwidth; its read range is ≤12 inches, and it has a communication rate of 40 kbps.

See the paper outlining the design of RFID readers for retail stores by Chalasani et al. (2005). Also the use of RFID technology in libraries is described in a paper by Shahid (2005). The use of RFID in libraries is a growing technology that enables the rapid, automated checking of books in and out, and also prevents theft.

14.5 GPS TAGS

14.5.1 Introduction

The US Global Positioning System (GPS) has been in existence since the early 1980s. It was put in place by the US DoD as a response to cold war threats. Twenty-four satellite vehicles (SVs) were put into overlapping, medium Earth orbits at 26,562 km above the Earth's center. There are six orbital planes, each with four equally spaced satellite vehicles (SVs). Three of the 24 SVs are nonactive "spares." The orbital period of each SV is 11h, 56 min. All GPS SVs carry four atomic clocks; two cesium vapor maser clocks and two rubidium vapor maser clocks. Synchronized precision time keeping between all GPS SVs is essential to precisely triangulate a GPS receiver on the Earth's surface. The cesium beam clocks run with an error of $\pm 2 \times 10^{-12}$, amounting to an error of several ns/day. (See Section 7.3.3.1 in Northrop (2005) for details on the GPS SVs and how the UHF L1 and L2 signals are coded.)

Early GPS receivers had position (circle radius) accuracies of ca. 15 m. Differential GPS developed by the US Coast Guard using fixed shore stations, gives ship position accuracies of ca. 0.75 m. WAAS (WAGPS) was developed in the 1990s for aircraft navigation. It also uses surveyed ground stations to mitigate errors, but instead of transmitting the error to the moving receiver, it uploads the processed error data from many surveyed base stations to a geosynchronous SV [at an orbital altitude of 35,786 km (22,236 mi)] from which it is downloaded to the receiver. WAAS receivers with postprocessing now can realize errors as small as 10 cm! To further explore GPS technology, see the excellent tutorial on GPS satellite navigation available online from ublox (2009a).

A GPS receiver requires simultaneous signals from four (overhead) orbiting SVs to determine its position in longitude, latitude, and altitude (and time). From this data, the receiver can also supply a course vector (speed, direction). Position calculation requires that the atomic clocks onboard the GPS SVs, and the receiver, be synchronized in order that the propagation time of the RF signal from an SV to the receiver is precisely known. (An error in propagation time, $\Delta\tau$, of only 1 μs can give a position error of 300 m!) The determination of the four unknowns in receiver position [longitude (X), latitude (Y), height (Z), and time error ($\Delta\tau$)] require the simultaneous solution of four nonlinear equations for which the four SVs provide input data. Quoting from the ublox (2009a) GPS tutorial:

> The details displayed and calculations made by a GNSS [GPS] receiver primarily involve the WGS-84 (World Geodetic System 1984) reference system. The WGS-84 coordinate system is geocentrically positioned with respect to the center of the Earth. Such a system is called ECEF (Earth Centered, Earth Fixed). The WGS-84 coordinate system is a three dimensional, right-handed, Cartesian coordinate system with its original coordinate point at the center of mass (= geocentric) of an ellipsoid, which approximates the total mass of the Earth.

Figure 14.11a illustrates a receiver at point **P** in Cartesian coordinates (x, y, z) on an ellipsoid. Spheroidal polar coordinates (R_N, λ, φ) are transformed to latitude, longitude, and height in the final

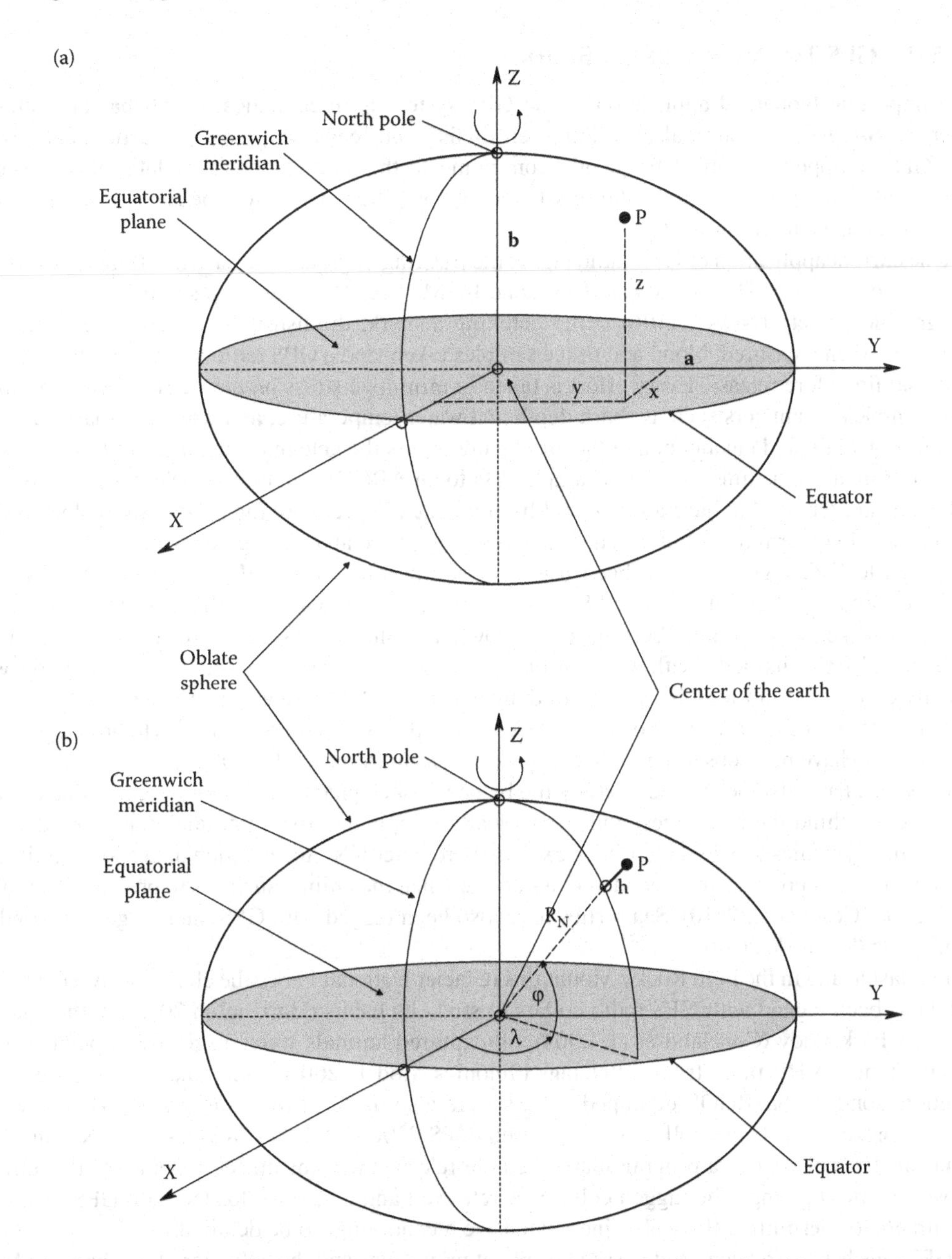

FIGURE 14.11 GPS coordinate systems: (a) GPS receiver at point P on the surface of an oblate spherical coordinate system (on the Earth). (b). Coordinates showing spherical location of the GPS receiver (RN + **h**, φ, λ) and its equivalent latitude and longitude. **h** is the receiver's height above the Earth's surface.

GPS display, shown in Figure 14.11b. **h** is the receiver's height above the (ideal) ellipsoid surface. The semimajor axis **a** of the ellipsoid Earth model is 6,378.137 km. The semiminor axis of the ellipsoid is **b** = 6,356.752 km. Clearly, the Earth is an spheroid, flattened at the poles by ca. 21,385 km relative to the mean equatorial radius, **a**. This 0.3353 % distortion of the Earth's volume (hence mass) from an ideal sphere causes slight, unique distortions in each of the SVs' ideally circular orbits which must be compensated for in calculating the receiver's position, given the four SVs' time and ID signals. The actual algebra of coordinate transformations and position determination are beyond the scope of this section. The interested reader should read the clear tutorial paper by ublox (2009a).

14.5.2 GPS Tag Applications in Biology

One important biological application of the GPS system is in ecological and behavioral studies where GPS-tagged wild animals, including certain fish, cetaceans, seals, and sea turtles are tracked. The GPS-equipped tags must frequently communicate the animal's position data, plus recorded behavioral measurements, via a radio link to a data-compiling station (on the Earth's surface, or to a satellite, thence to an Earth station).

One current application of GPS radio tags is the tracking of great white sharks off the Californian and Mexican coasts. This work has been done by Michael Domeier, sponsored by the National Geographic Society (NOAA 2010). After catching a shark, the fish is lifted from the water and unhooked, then measured, blood and tissue samples taken, and a GPS radio tag is literally bolted to its dorsal fin before release. Every effort is taken to minimize stress on the shark. The tag periodically samples parameters such as shark depth and water temperature, and when the shark surfaces with its dorsal fin and tag antenna in the air, the tag senses the antenna is in air and it broadcasts its GPS coordinates plus time, date, and sample data to an ARGOS satellite vehicle (SV). These GPS radio tags are reported to have a functional lifetime of ca. 6 years, giving behavioral biologists and ecologists a long-term record of a shark's feeding, migration, and mating behavior.

Long-life GPS tags have also been used to track ocean sunfish (*Mola mola*) in the Western Atlantic (Sims et al. 2009). These GPS tags transmit to the ARGOS satellite system when on the surface. Unlike the releasable PAT tags (see below), the sunfish GPS tags were attached behind the fish's dorsal fin to its body with a 1.5 m long permanent monofilament tether. The tag body was roughly conical, 15 cm long by 80 mm in diameter; the ARGOS satellite antenna was 17.1 cm in length. Sunfish like to bask at the ocean surface, giving the tag good opportunities to broadcast data, but they also have been observed to dive as deep as 472 m (Sims et al. 2009).

GPS tags have also been used to study the behavior of elephant seals in the ocean. Glued to the seal's neck behind the head, these tags periodically sample and record animal depth and data on swimming dynamics supplied by X, Y, Z axis accelerometer ICs. Acceleration data and the animal's depth record and position are uploaded to a satellite when the animal surfaces to breathe (Tremblay et al. 2009; Costa et al. 2010). Sea turtles have also been tagged with GPS data loggers epoxied to their shells (Seaturtle 2010).

In Alaska, and in the high Rocky Mountains (Glacier National Park), the elusive wolverine *(Gulo gulo)* has been tagged with GPS radio collars to study its habits (Harrington 2010). In the Glacier National Park study (Copeland et al. 2004), all captured animals were surgically implanted with intraperitoneal VHF radio transmitter tags (Telonics Models 200 for kits and 400 for adults) In addition, some GPS/ARGOS equipped collars were also used. In the Alaska study (Lewis et al. 2008), store-on-board GPS collar tags were used (GPS-3300S, by Lotek Wireless Inc., Newmarket, Ontario). The collars had a programmable, remote-release mechanism, set to come off the animal 24 weeks after tagging. The tagged collar was retrieved and data downloaded with GPS locations and time/date, permitting the wolverine's extensive meanderings to be detailed.

GPS tags have also been used to study elephant migrations and the behavior of elephants in Mali in Africa (Kiger 2010).

Before the era of GPS tagging, pop-up archival tags (PATs) were used exclusively to investigate the behavior of large fish, such as sharks. A PAT tag is ca. 17 cm in length, and has a float and antenna on one end. A thin, flexible line with a plastic dart that is imbedded into the back of the fish is attached to the thin end of the tag opposite the float and antenna. The PAT streams behind the fish as it swims. At a preprogrammed date and time, the tag stops data collection and separates itself from the line, then floats to the ocean surface. There, antenna upright, it broadcasts its ID and a summary of its stored data to an ARGOS polar-orbiting satellite from which it is relayed back to an Earth receiver. One configuration of PAT samples the fish's depth, ocean temperature and light intensity every minute, and stores this data in RAM. The very approximate latitude and longitude of the shark's position is estimated (during the day) from the light level data acquired by the tag. The total day length gives an approximation to the shark's latitude. The time of midday can also be estimated from light level data and be used to calculate the shark's longitude (Praxmayer 2010). If the floating tag is recovered, a detailed data download is possible. Clearly, the dorsal fin-mounted GPS tag on sharks offers a significant improvement in terms of position precision in long-term tracking, and in tag life (6 years).

A Telonics™ ST-18 GPS tag measures 12 × 5 cm and weighs ca. 200g in air. The Telonics ST-14 GPS tag is larger, 16 × 10 cm and weighs ca. 750 g (bigger batteries). Other companies offer GPS tags: the Sirtrack KiwiSat 101™ is 18 × 6 cm. Wildlife Computers, Inc. offers several models of ARGOS-compatible tags. GPS tags are not inexpensive—for example, the Widlife Computers' SPOT5 tag costs $1,350 or more, depending on custom features (see www.wildlifecomputers.com/products.aspx?ID = 2 Accessed 11/11/10).

On land, a continuously-broadcasting, "beeper" RF tags affixed to an animal by a collar or other means permits the animal's position to be triangulated using directional receiving antennas at known map coordinates. Two or more receiver positions determine directional vectors, the intersection of which on the map estimates the tagged animal's approximate location. More sophisticated GPS collar tags have been used to track elephant migrations, and wolverine behavior (Harrington 2010; Kiger 2010).

Clearly, GPS tags are more complicated and expensive than "beeper" beacon tags, but they also provide precise location data for ecological and behavioral studies, *and only one receiver is needed.* They are also more easily retrieved if they become detached from the animal.

An interesting family of underwater data storage tags (DSTs) is made by Star-Oddi, an Icelandic company [see http://star-oddi.com/products/ (Accessed 5/02/11)]. These tags are normally implanted internally in larger fish, and some can record up to 87,217 measurements of time/date and certain of various physical parameters including temperature, depth, roll and pitch, and salinity. This family of tags does not broadcast their stored data by RF or ultrasound; the tag must be retrieved from a caught fish to be read out. One Star-Oddi DST tag has the capability of receiving ultrasonic GPS coordinate data from a special Simrad sonar system located on a research/fishing vessel. The GPS coordinates of the vessel are stored in the DST tag's ROM, along with time/date and certain physical data, giving fisheries biologists an approximate location (a 4 km radius circle around the fish) of the fish at a certain time/date.

14.5.3 GPS Signals

Broadcast from the GPS SVs, the GPS L1 carrier is at 10.2300 MHz × 154 = 1.57542 GHz, the L2 carrier center frequency is at 10.2300 MHz × 120 = 1.22760 GHz. The new L5 ("Safety of Life") channel center frequency is at 10.2300 MHz × 115 = 1.17645 GHz. The L5 civilian-use signal is being implemented in new GPS SVs launched during and after 2010. The L1, L2, and L5 carrier frequencies are derived from a master clock in the SV by phase-lock loop techniques.

Modulation of the GPS L1 and L2 signals is complicated, as is their demodulation and position calculation by the receiver. Figure 14.12 illustrates the modulation process used on the L1 and L2 SV carriers: NM is the "navigational message" data, which also modulates the L1 and L2 carriers. The NM code describes an SV's orbit, clock corrections and other arcane system parameters. The C/A code is a Gold Code of register size 10, which has a binary sequence length of 1023 and a clocking rate of 1.0230 MHz, thus repeats itself every 1 ms. The C/A code is used by the receiver for SV acquisition and ID. The P code is used for high-precision position determination.

14.5.4 GPS Tag Hardware

A GPS tag antenna must have a compact, broadband design; such a design will usually use a fractal or other space-filling geometry. The GPS L signals from the antenna are conditioned by a low-noise preamplifier and sent to an integrated GPS receiver chip for processing. Siakavara (2007) presented the design for a compact, fractal microstrip antenna composed of the union of four

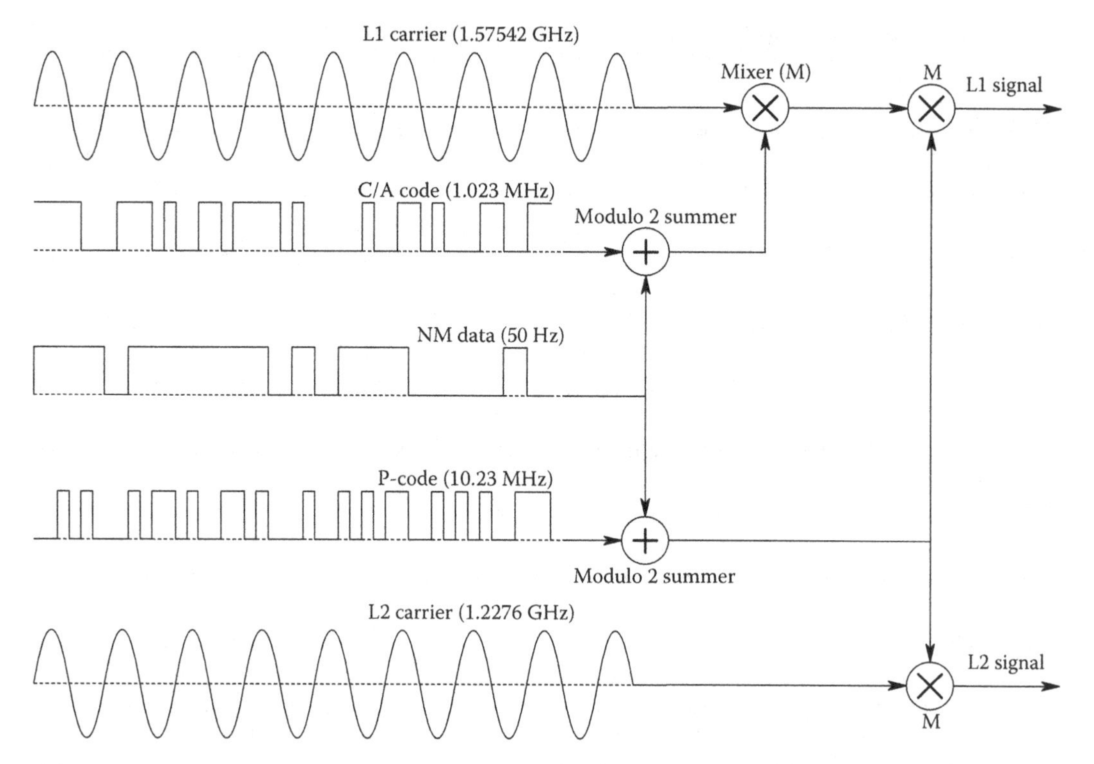

FIGURE 14.12 The GPS modulation process used on the L1 and L2 SV carriers. See text for description.

inverse Koch fractal patches. This broadband antenna operates in three frequency ranges (GPS L bands, Digital Cellular System-DCS1800, and 2.7 GHz). In the GPS bands, the antenna generates a circularly polarized field with the maximum strength at the broadside direction. Another planar fractal antenna design for the GPS L1 (1.57542 GHz), GSM (1.850 GHz), and Wi-Fi (2.440 GHz) bands was described by Azaro et al. (2007). Their antenna, before the Koch triangle "nibbles" were taken, measured 4.5 × 4.5 cm. An excellent tutorial paper summarizing and evaluating various GPS antenna designs can be found at ublox (2009b).

There are several other antenna designs used with GPS receivers other than planar fractal geometries. Perhaps the simplest GPS antenna is the two-element (2 × λ/4) dipole at the L1 frequency, each λ/4 arm of the dipole is 4.761 cm. This dipole size can be shrunk by making the dipole in 2-D; using a flat "meander" pattern, such as the Greek key "crank," on the arms.

If design space permits, greater omnidirectional sensitivity can be found using the quadrifilar helix antenna (QHA) design described in ublox (2009b). For the GPS L1 frequency, if the QHA antenna is surrounded with air, its outline will be ca. 6 cm high x 4.5 cm in diameter; if gold wire is deposited on a high dielectric constant ceramic, the size can be shrunk to 1.8 cm high x 1.0 cm diameter without loss of performance. Because of its omnidirectional sensitivity, the QHA can pick up F1 signal reflections from terrain and vehicles such as aircraft, often causing degraded navigational performance. Many other passive GPS antenna designs exist (e.g., chip antennas, loop antennas, planar inverted F antennas, patch antennas, etc.), too many to describe here.

The so-called active GPS antennas are used when the antenna must be placed over a few cm from the receiver, such as on the roof of a metal vehicle. Basically, a low-noise amplifier (LNA) is located directly at the antenna terminals and is used to condition the received GPS L-signals (gain typically ca. 15 dB), and drive a transmission line/coaxial cable of up to ca. 5 m at its characteristic impedance (e.g., 52 Ω) to prevent standing waves. The LNA typically may have a noise factor F ≅ 2 dB (see Section 9.4 of this text). A SAW bandpass filter can be used to enhance the SNR at the receiver chip.

In GPS tags used for tracking animals, the antenna is often a space-saving, planar fractal design, on or near the PCB carrying the GPS chip set.

The electronic circuitry bulk required for GPS receiver functions has been steadily shrinking, driven by the need to embed GPS in mobile telecommunications and computer systems, and also by the need to actively track vehicles, goods, and animals from a distance. Several manufacturers offer compact GPS chips for size-critical applications.

A laptop computer can be turned into a GPS system with the *GSAT*™ USB Dongle GPS receiver, model ND-100S. This device is the size of a large flash drive (6.55 × 2.3 × 1.1 cm) and contains a SiRFstarIII® chip; it runs with all popular OSs (Windows 98/2000/XP/Vista/7, Mac OS8/9/10, and Linux RedHat 7.8/8.0/9.0).

The Swiss corporation, ublox AG, makes a complete line of GPS and Galileo receivers, chipsets, and antennas (ublox 2009b). Their UBX-G6000 series GPS chips contain an RF front end with a low-noise amplifier (LNA), and have the following characteristics/specifications: The receiver has 50-channels and receives GPS L1 C/A code, also adapted to GALILEO L1 open service (with upgrade, Europe). Maximum update rate up to 5 Hz-ROM, 2 Hz-flash memory; Accuracy (all SV signals ≥ –130 dBm): Position, 2.5 m CEP; SBAS 2.0 m CEP. Acquisition times with TCXO: cold starts—28 s, warm starts—28 s, hot starts—1 s. RF sensitivity (with crystal osc.): Acquisition –160 dBm; Tracking –160 dBm; cold start -147 dBm. Operational limits: Velocity 500 m/s (972 knots); altitude 50,000 m. Serial interfaces: 1 UART (UBX-G6010), 2 UARTS (UBX-G6000), 1 USBv.2.0 12 Mb/s, 1 DDC (I^2C compliant), 1 SPI. Power consumption (important for animal tagging): 59 mW continuous, 30 mW @ 1.8 V power save mode. Supply voltages, single voltage supply: 1.8 V or 2.5–3.6 V; dual voltage supply: 1.4/1.8 V or 1.4/2.5–3.6 V or 1.8/2.5–3.6 V. (*ublox* makes several other single-chip and 2-chip GPS systems (e.g., UBX-G5010, G5000/G0010, etc.), as well as a variety of GPS antennas.)

One of the smallest GPS chip sets is made by *Rakon,* a New Zealand company [see www.gps-fortoday.com/small-gps-tracking-chips/ (Accessed 5/02/11)]. Originally designed to go into cell phones, one Rakon chip measures only 2.5 × 2.0 mm. Its small size makes the Rakon chip attractive for animal GPS tag designs. Clearly, an effective antenna for the Rakon chip would have to be larger than the chip, a case of the "tail wagging the dog."

A survey of GPS chip receivers may be seen at: http://gpstekreviews.com/2007/04/14/gps-receiver-chip-performance-survey/ Accessed 5/02/11).

14.6 ULTRASONIC TAGS IN FISHERIES BIOLOGY

Tagging fish that do not ordinarily surface for the purpose of behavioral and ecological studies presents several problems: First, GPS signals do not penetrate water. A second is whether to use a LF radio tag (RFID, active or passive), or an ultrasonic ID tag. A third is where to attach the tag: externally, clipped to a fin or flipper, or internally (e.g., swallowed, or surgically implanted just below the skin). A fourth is how to locate precisely the tagged fish, including its depth. A detailed examination of these problems can be found in an on-line, tutorial paper by the Arizona Game & Fish Dept. (2010). A problem for RFID is that high radio frequencies do not propagate well in water, especially salt water (Balanis 1989), limiting the effective reader/tag range, **r**.

We have described that in some ecological applications, where marine mammals such as whales and sharks periodically come to the surface, an externally attached active RFID tag with a GPS chip can sense the surface, and broadcast ID, time and exact location data to an ARGOS satellite receiver, along with a sampled history of depth, temperature and sampling times, profiling the animal's behavior. In this section, we will discuss self-powered acoustic tags used in marine fisheries studies where the fish do not surface to permit RF transmission. Sound travels well in water (unlike RF energy) and two or more sensitive, directional hydrophones can triangulate the position of a sonically tagged fish and read its tag data. Tracking fish in rivers and estuaries is effective because arrays of radio-linked, fixed hydrophones can be sited along the shore at known locations to listen for tags on fish. Then trigonometric algorithms can be applied to the received signals to estimate fish position in x, y, z coordinates. The shorter the sound wavelength, the more precise the fish location can be, but the greater the sound attenuation with distance will be. For example, the sound attenuation in 10°C sea water is 0.02 dB/km at 0.5 kHz, rising to 0.92 dB/km at 20 kHz (Kaye and Laby 2008).

Fish location in three, Cartesian dimensions is made possible by having a precisely located array of *four* hydrophones, and by knowing the speed of sound in the water, **c** (a function of frequency, temperature and salinity; for example, *c* in 10°C sea water is ca. 1490 m/s. At 30°C it is ca. 1546 m/s). For the number one hydrophone, the time the sound takes to travel from the fish to the hydrophone, τ_1, can be expressed as

$$\tau_1 = (1/c)\sqrt{(x_1 - x_f)^2 + (y_1 - y_f)^2 + (z_1 - z_f)^2} \quad (14.1)$$

where $\mathbf{x_f}$, $\mathbf{y_f}$, and $\mathbf{z_f}$ are a tagged fish's location in x,y,z space; x_1, y_1, and z_1 give the #1 hydrophone's exact known location in a common x,y,z coordinate volume. **c** is the velocity of sound in water of a certain salinity and temperature.

Note that one can never know τ_1, *per se,* only the *differences* in pulse arrival times between the closest (#1) hydrophone and the three others, $(\tau_2 - \tau_1)$, $(\tau_3 - \tau_1)$, and $(\tau_4 - \tau_1)$, can be measured. Consider a second hydrophone at known coordinates x_2, y_2, and z_2. The absolute time it takes the same sound pulse to reach hydrophone 2 is

$$\tau_2 = (1/c)\sqrt{(x_2 - x_f)^2 + (y_2 - y_f)^2 + (z_2 - z_f)^2} \quad (14.2)$$

Although the actual values of τ_1 and τ_2 are not known, their difference, $\delta t_{21} = (\tau_2 - \tau_1)$ can be measured. This difference is

$$\delta t_{21} = (1/c)[\sqrt{(x_2 - x_f)^2 + (y_2 - y_f)^2 + (z_2 - z_f)^2} - \sqrt{(x_1 - x_f)^2 + (y_1 - y_f)^2 + (z_1 - z_f)^2}] \quad (14.3)$$

Thus, one has one equation and three unknowns, $\mathbf{x_f}$, $\mathbf{y_f}$, and $\mathbf{z_f}$. It is clear that for a total of *four hydrophones*, there will be three, distinct difference equations, albeit nonlinear, which can be solved numerically for the fish's three location coordinates, $\mathbf{x_f}$, $\mathbf{y_f}$, and $\mathbf{z_f}$, given **c**, and the hydrophone coordinates, x_k, y_k, and z_k, k = 1, 2, 3, 4.

If it is assumed the sonic-tagged fish are in a shallow river or estuary, we can neglect depth, **z**. Figure 14.13 illustrates such a scenario. Note that now only three hydrophones are needed. The equations to be solved are now:

$$\delta t_{21}c = \{\sqrt{(x_2 - x_f)^2 + (y_2 - y_f)^2} + \sqrt{(x_1 - x_f)^2 + (y_1 - y_f)^2}\} \quad (14.4)$$

$$\delta t_{31}c = \{\sqrt{(x_3 - x_f)^2 + (y_3 - y_f)^2} + \sqrt{(x_1 - x_f)^2 + (y_1 - y_f)^2}\} \quad (14.5)$$

To simplify, set hydrophone #1 at x,y coordinates 0,0. The equations now become

$$\delta t_{21}c = \{\sqrt{(x_2 - x_f)^2 + (y_2 - y_f)^2} + \sqrt{(x_f{}^2 + x_f{}^2}\} \quad (14.6)$$

$$\delta t_{31}c = \{\sqrt{(x_3 - x_f)^2 + (y_3 - y_f)^2} + \sqrt{x_f{}^2 + y_f{}^2}\} \quad (14.7)$$

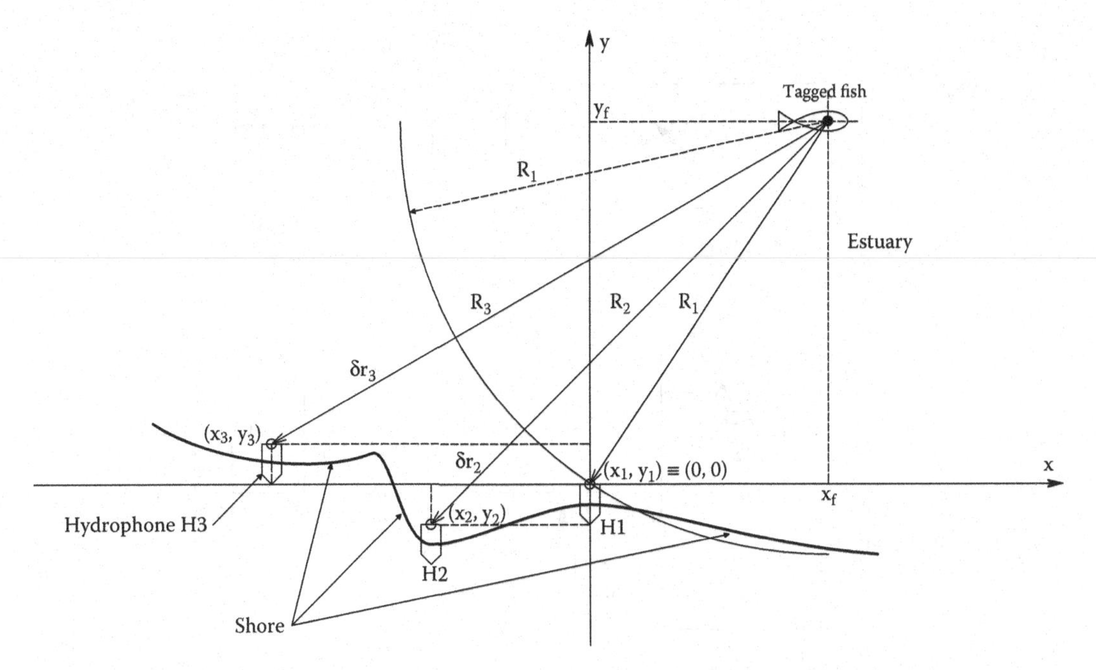

FIGURE 14.13 Plan view of three hydrophones on the bank of an estuary used to locate an ultrasonically-tagged fish by differences in sound pulse arrival times. See text for analysis.

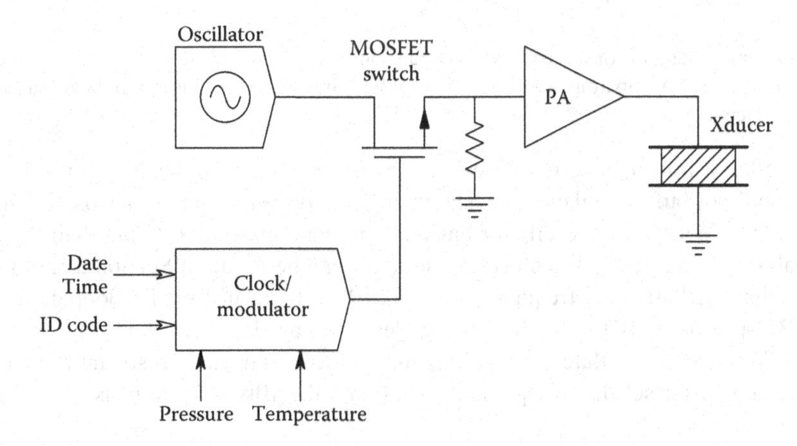

FIGURE 14.14 Block diagram of a basic, pulsed, ultrasonic fish tag.

where *it is* assumed that δt_{21}, $\delta t_{31,}$ and **c** are known, and x_2, x_3, y_2, and y_3 are known relative to hydrophone #1.

These nonlinear, simultaneous, quadratic equations are solved by computer. No simple algebraic solution exists.

The architecture of an active fish tag is relatively simple. Figure 14.14 illustrates the basic organization of a sonic fish tag. The modulator generates pulses of oscillator voltage which are amplified by the power amplifier (PA) and transmitted into the water by the resonant piezo-transducer. Transmitted are the tag's ID code, a date plus time code, and coded dated on pressure and temperature if the tag is so equipped. The modulator is programmed to set the interpulse (data sampling) interval. Ultrasonic acoustic energy is generated by an appropriate transducer, generally a high-output piezo-ceramic such as barium titanate, lead zirconate-titanate (LZT), or lead metaniobate (see Section 6.4.3 in Northrop (2005) on piezoelectric transducers) and coupled into the water.

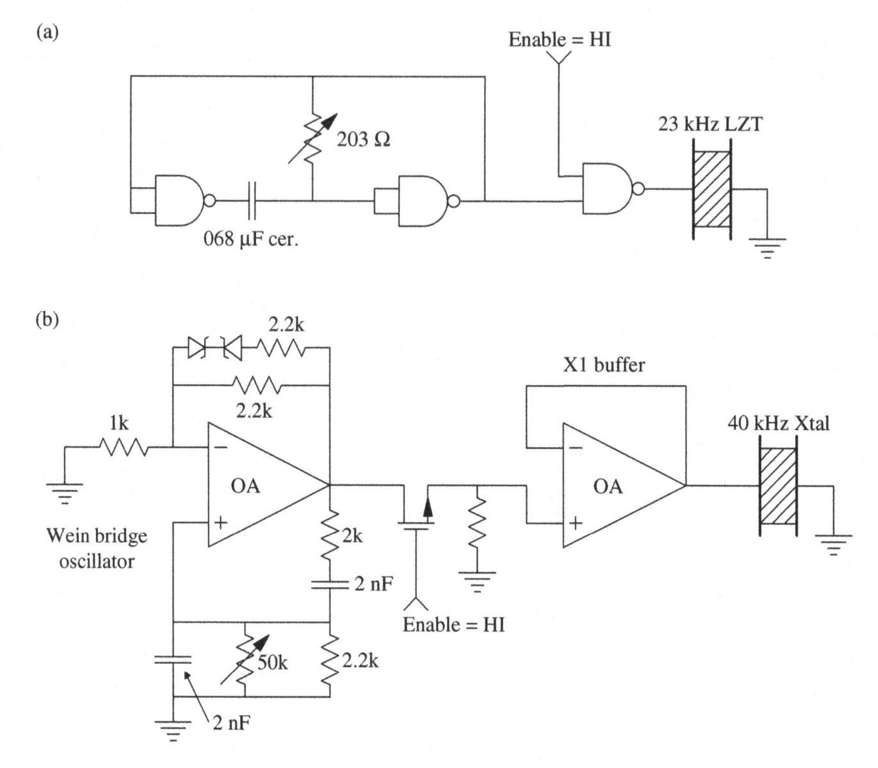

FIGURE 14.15 (a) Schematic of a basic, NAND gate pulse oscillator used to drive a low-power, 23 kHz ultrasound transducer. (b) An op amp, 40 kHz, Wien bridge, sinusoidal oscillator with buffer used to drive an ultrasound transducer.

Two simple oscillator-transducer circuits designed by the author are shown in Figure 14.15. A simple NAND gate oscillator-buffer-Xtal circuit is shown in A; an op amp Wien bridge oscillator and buffer is shown in B. The Wien bridge oscillator has a much more sinusoidal output than the gate multivibrator. Analysis of an op amp Wien bridge oscillator can be found in Section 5.5.3 of this text. It can be shown that oscillations of frequency $f_o = 1/(2\pi RC)$ Hz occur for a DC loop gain, A_v, > + 3.

A basic BJT-piezo oscillator for a fish tag designed by Thorson et al. (1969) is shown in Figure 14.16. This circuit oscillated at 134 kHz and drove a transducer resonant at that frequency. The 5M variable resistor set the interpulse interval, and the 10k variable resistor set the 134 kHz pulse duration.

The piezotransducer is generally located inside the tag capsule, although some early designs have located it separately; the tag body being internal to the fish, and the transducer located externally (on a fin) to avoid sound attenuation by tissues (Thorson et al. 1969). The tags described by Thorson et al. used lead zirconate disk transducers that oscillated at 134 kHz; they varied the pulse duration and the interpulse interval to code five different fish tags. Their tag used a 7 V, 160 mAH battery, giving a tag life of ca. 2000 h or 12 weeks. They placed their hydrophones 150–200 ft. apart, at a depth of 4–6 ft. mounted ca. 1 ft. above the stream bottom.

Although it is common to find disk transducers used in sonic fish tags, hollow cylindrical piezoresonators have also been used. They oscillate by radial expansion-contraction. (A detailed analysis of the properties of piezoelectric transducers can be found in Section 6.4.3 of Northrop, 2005.)

Ehrenberg and Steig (2003) described a tag that emitted at 307 kHz. The tags were encapsulated in an inert epoxy resin, and measured 18 mm x 6.6 mm (0.71 × 0.26 in) and weighed 1.5g (0.053 oz) in air, less than 1 g in water. Their tag's transmitted acoustic power was ca. 155 dB re 1 μPa at 1 m range. Nominal interpulse intervals (between coded bursts) ranged from 1 to 6 s. Transmitted, coded, pulse duration was 0.5 to 3 ms. Useful tag life was over 30 days. Ehrenberg

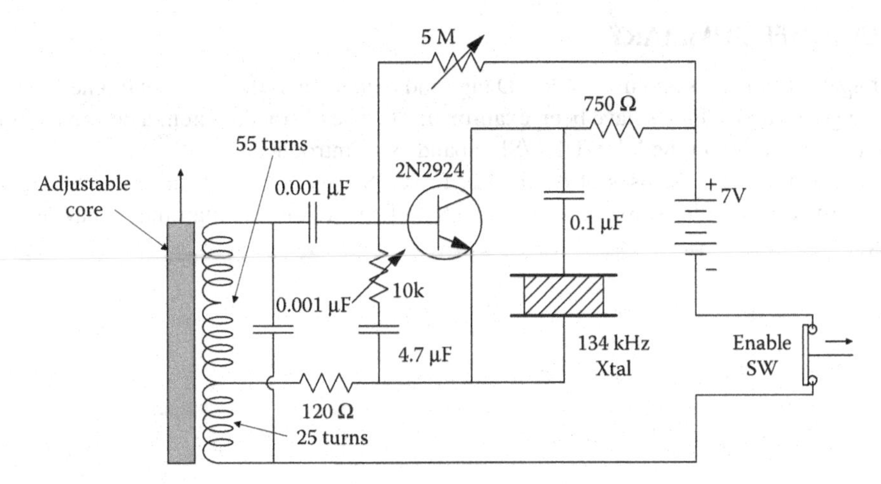

FIGURE 14.16 A basic BJT-piezo-oscillator for a fish tag designed by Thorson, T., Esterberg, G., and Johnson, J., *Ultrasonic Shark Tag Monitoring System Technical Report,* 1969. Faculty Publications in the Biological Sciences, University of Nebraska, Lincoln. Available at: http://dig-italcommons.unl.edu/cgi/view-content.cgi?article=1006&context=bioscifacpub&sei-redir=1#search=%22Thorson,+Esterberg+1969+%22Ultrasonic+Shark+Tag+Monitoring+ System%22%22 (Last accessed 8 June 2011). Driven at its resonant frequency, the resonant Xtal presents a nearly real load to the transistor.

and Steig claimed that up to 50 tagged fish can be simultaneously tracked without ambiguity. The interpulse intervals (pulse rep. rate) and pulse durations were used to discriminate tags (and fish). A more sophisticated system might modulate the tags' chirps with an ID code, similar to that used with RFID tags.

A well-known manufacturer of sonic fish tagging systems is the Canadian company, Vemco (a division of Amirex Systems) (www.vemco.com/ Accessed 5/02/11). Vemco has been designing and marketing acoustic fish tracking equipment since 1979, including sonic tags (of different sizes and frequencies, giving ID, temperature and depth information), hydrophones, and receivers giving automated data collection, also, real-time, high-resolution position information). For example, the Vemco V6 coded tag emits at 180 kHz (tags that emit at over 200 kHz are less effective in salt water due to attenuation). The V6 is a self-contained capsule that measures 16.5 mm in length and ca. 6 mm in diameter; it weighs 0.5 g in water. Its full sonic pressure output is 140 dB (re 1 μPa @ 1 m). Its small size make it useful for tracking the migration of salmon smolts, and other juvenile fish released from hatcheries. The V6 tag has a programmed emission schedule: When first activated (after surgical implantation in a fish) it transmits one day at low power; it then goes silent for a period of 9 days (for postsurgical recovery). At day 10, it transmits at full power for 45 days; this allows fisheries biologists to track the fish in their migration. At day 55, the tag again switches to low-power transmission for 200 days, allowing researchers to study fish behavior in "... a more residency type setting."

Fish tag receivers consist of a hydrophone, preamplifier, synchronized master clock, and data processing module (DPM) which gives a tag's ID, time and date for downloading to a computer. The DPM also supplies time-coded pressure and temperature data from tags that have this capability. The central computer calculates the fish position either in 3-D (from 4 hydrophones) or 2-D Cartesian coordinates (3 hydrophones). To do this, there must be the same electronic delay from each receiver to the computer. Linkage from each receiver's DPM to the computer can be by coaxial cables of the same length, or by RF links or fiber optic cables (in which case the transmission delay will be negligible compared to sonic delays).

14.7 CHAPTER SUMMARY

In this chapter, the designs and uses of RFID tags and readers, and their uses in biomedicine as well as tracking goods and vehicles have been examined. The use of fractal antenna designs to miniaturize radio tags operating in the VHF/UHF/SHF bands was introduced.

Also considered were the uses of miniature, IC, GPS tags in ecological research. The designs and uses of underwater ultrasonic tags in research on fish and marine mammal behavior were also described.

15 Examples of Special Analog Circuits and Systems Used in Biomedical Instrumentation

15.1 INTRODUCTION

As a biomedical engineer, there are many specialized integrated circuits you may be expected to be familiar with, understand their operation, and be able to effectively incorporate them into biomedical instrumentation system designs. These integrated circuits include, but are not limited to:

- IC thermometers
- Phase detectors
- Phase-lock loops
- Phase-sensitive rectifiers
- True-RMS converters
- Voltage- and current-controlled oscillators

Most designers and vendors of analog ICs such as Analog Devices, Burr-Brown, Exar, Maxim, National, Texas Instruments, etc. make one or more of the aforementioned special-function ICs. In describing them in this chapter, applications as well as designs will be stressed.

15.2 THE PHASE-SENSITIVE RECTIFIER

15.2.1 INTRODUCTION

The *phase-sensitive rectifier* (PSR) is also known as the *phase-sensitive detector*, the *synchronous rectifier* or *detector*, or the *balanced demodulator*. Its primary role is to recover the modulating signal in a *double-sideband, suppressed-carrier* (amplitude) modulated (DSBSCM) *carrier* (see Section 11.1 in this text). The PSR is also at the heart of the *Lock-In Amplifier*, which is widely used in photonics and in certain applications in physics and engineering to recover a low-frequency modulating signal buried in noise. A PSR will also demodulate ordinary AM. There are *four* major embodiments of the PSR: (1) The analog multiplier/low-pass filter (LPF) PSR. (2) The switched op amp PSR. (3) The electromechanical chopper PSR. (4) The balanced-diode bridge PSR. The analog multiplier PSR will be examined first.

15.2.2 ANALOG MULTIPLIER/LPF PSD

Just as a DSBSCM signal can be made by multiplying a high-frequency sinusoidal carrier by a low-frequency modulating signal, the DSBSCM signal can be demodulated by multiplying the modulated carrier by a carrier frequency reference signal of the correct phase (refer to Figure 15.1). Let the coherent modulating signal be a low-frequency sinusoid:

$$v_m(t) = V_m \sin(\omega_m t) \tag{15.1}$$

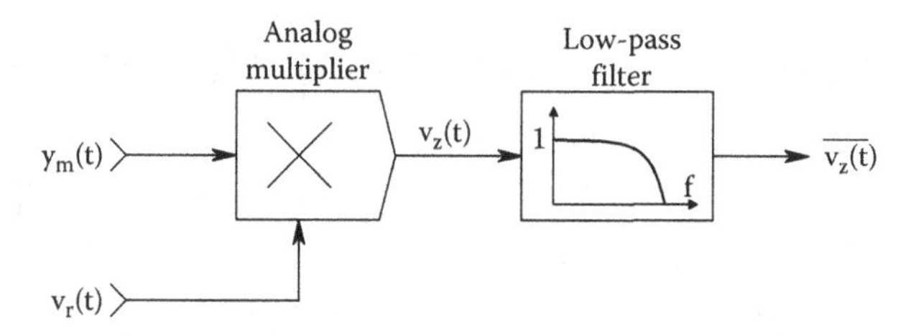

FIGURE 15.1 Block diagram of an analog multiplier—low-pass filter demodulator for DSBSCM signals. See text for analysis.

The carrier is

$$v_c(t) = v_c \cos(\omega_c\ t),\ \omega_m \ll \omega_c \tag{15.2}$$

And the modulated carrier, $v_{cm}(t)$, is found by trigonometric identity:

$$v_{cm}(t) = (v_m V_c/2)\{\sin[(\omega_c + \omega_m)t] + \sin[\omega_c - \omega_m)t]\}\ \text{DSBSC} \tag{15.3}$$

The *reference signal* is of the same frequency as the carrier but in general differs in phase by a fixed angle, $(\pi/2 + \varphi)$ radians. By trigonometric identity, this is

$$V_r(t) = v_r \sin(\omega_c t + \varphi) \tag{15.4}$$

The analog multiplier output is thus

$$\begin{aligned} v_z(t) = \{v_r(t)v_{cm}(t)\}/10 = (V_m V_c V_r/20)\ \{&\cos[\omega_m t - \varphi] - \cos[(2\omega_c + \omega_m)t + \varphi] \\ &+ \cos[\omega_m t + \varphi] - \cos[(2\omega_c - \omega_m)t - \varphi]\} \end{aligned} \tag{15.5}$$

(Note that the output of a transconductance-type analog multiplier IC is the product of the two voltage inputs divided by 10.) A unity-gain low-pass filter removes the two, $2\omega_c$ terms, leaving

$$\overline{v_z(t)} = (v_m V_c V_r/20)\ \{\cos[\omega_m t - \varphi] - \cos[\omega_m t - \varphi] + \cos[\omega_m t + \varphi]\} \tag{15.6}$$

From the trigonometric identity $\{\cos\alpha + \cos\beta\} = 2\cos[½(\alpha + \beta)]\cos[½(\alpha - \beta)]$ we find

$$\overline{v_z(t)} = (V_m V_c V_r/10)\cos(\omega_m t)\cos(\varphi) \tag{15.7}$$

In the development above we assumed that $0 < \omega_m << \omega_b < < \omega_c$, where ω_b is the LPF's break frequency. Note that the recovered modulating signal is maximum when the reference signal is *in-phase with the quadrature carrier* of the DSBSCM signal ($\varphi = 0$). Thus, an analog multiplier can not only form DSBSCM signals, but can demodulate them, returning a signal $\alpha\ v_m(t)$.

15.2.3 Switched Op Amp PSR

Figure 15.2 illustrates a PSR that uses three op amps and a digitally controlled, analog MOS switch to demodulate DSBSCM signals. The MOS switch, when closed, has a very low resistance. When it is open, its resistance is on the order of megohms. The switch is controlled by the signum function, $\text{sgn}\{V_r \sin(\omega_c t)\}$, which is +1 when $\sin(\omega_c t)$ is ≥ 0, and -1 when $\sin(\omega_c t) < 0$. The output, $v_z(t)$, is a full-wave rectified $y_m(t)$, which goes negative when the sign of the modulating signal, $v_m(t)$ goes

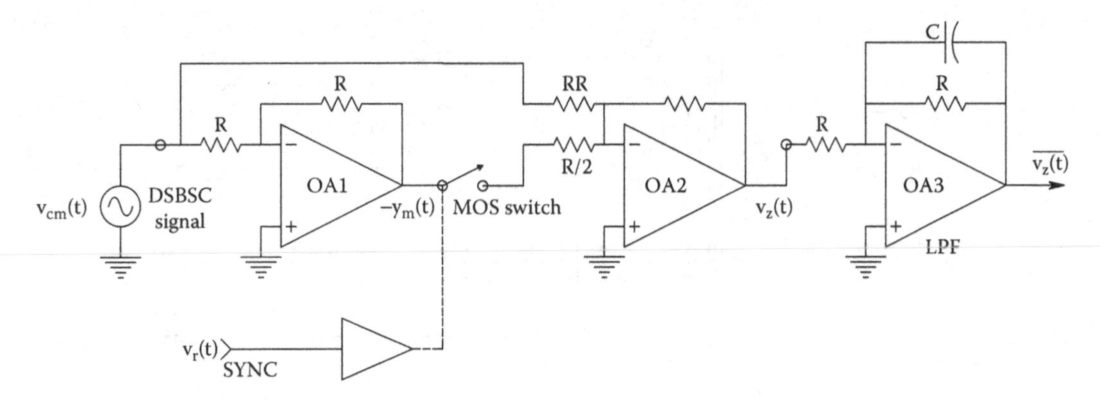

FIGURE 15.2 (a) switched op amp demodulator for DSBSCM signals, also known as a phase-sensitive rectifier (PSR). See text for analysis.

negative. It is easy to see that after low-pass filtering, $v_z(t)$ is α $v_m(t)$. The average (DC value) of a full-wave rectified sine wave is $\pi V_{pk}/2$. Note that the action of the switch is to effectively multiply the DSBSCM input signal by a ±1 peak value square wave of frequency $\omega_c/2\pi$ Hz.

15.2.4 Chopper PSR

Figure 15.3a illustrates the circuit of an *electromechanical chopper.* Electromechanical choppers are basically SPDT switches commutated by a driver coil at switching frequencies from 50 to 400 Hz. They were developed in the WWII era as modulator/demodulators for power-line frequency DSBSCM signals used in servomechanisms. They are now an obsolete technology. The same SPDT action can be obtained using appropriately buffered MOS switches that can be commutated in the 100s of kHz, or by photoelectrically turning on and off phototransistors in a photoelectric chopper. The basic electromechanical chopper used a center-tapped signal transformer to couple the DSBSCM carrier to the switch points. Figure 15.3b illustrates the raw switch output, $v_z(t)$. This signal must be low-pass filtered to recover $v_m(t)$. Note that a phase shift φ between the sinusoidal input and the chopper square wave causes some of the chopped signal to be negative over φ radians of the cycle. When averaged, this negative area subtracts from the output signal. It can be shown that the phase error φ in the reference signal effectively multiplies the averager output by cos(φ). Thus, if the reference signal is 90° out of phase, the low-pass filtered output will be zero.

15.2.5 Balanced Diode Bridge PSR

Still another circuit which can be used to demodulate DSBSCM signals is the balanced diode bridge PSR, illustrated in Figure 15.4. The modulated signal, $v_m(t)$, and the reference signal, $v_r(t)$, are coupled to the diode bridge by two center-tapped transformers. The transformer on the left is called the *signal transformer,* the one on the right the *reference transformer.* To understand how the diode bridge PSR works, refer to Figures 15.5 and 15.6. Assume $v_r(t) > 0$, diodes *a* and *b* conduct current i_{r+}, and *c* and *d* are cut-off (treated as open circuits). The positive signal voltage at node B causes a current i_{ma} and i_{mb} to flow through diodes *a* and *b,* respectively. Assume that $i_{ma} > i_{r+}$ so diode *a* continues to conduct. The currents i_{ma} and i_{mb} flow through both halves of the reference transformer secondary, combine, and flow to ground through the resistor R. Note that it is the top half of the signal transformer that supplies i_{m+}.

The raw output voltage is $v_z(t) = i_{m+}(t)R$ for positive $v_r(t)$ and positive (or negative) $v_m(t)$. During the negative half cycle of $v_r(t)$, diodes *c* and *d* conduct, and *a* and *b* are reverse biased. Now the lower half of the signal transformer secondary delivers signal current i_{m-} to the load R in the same

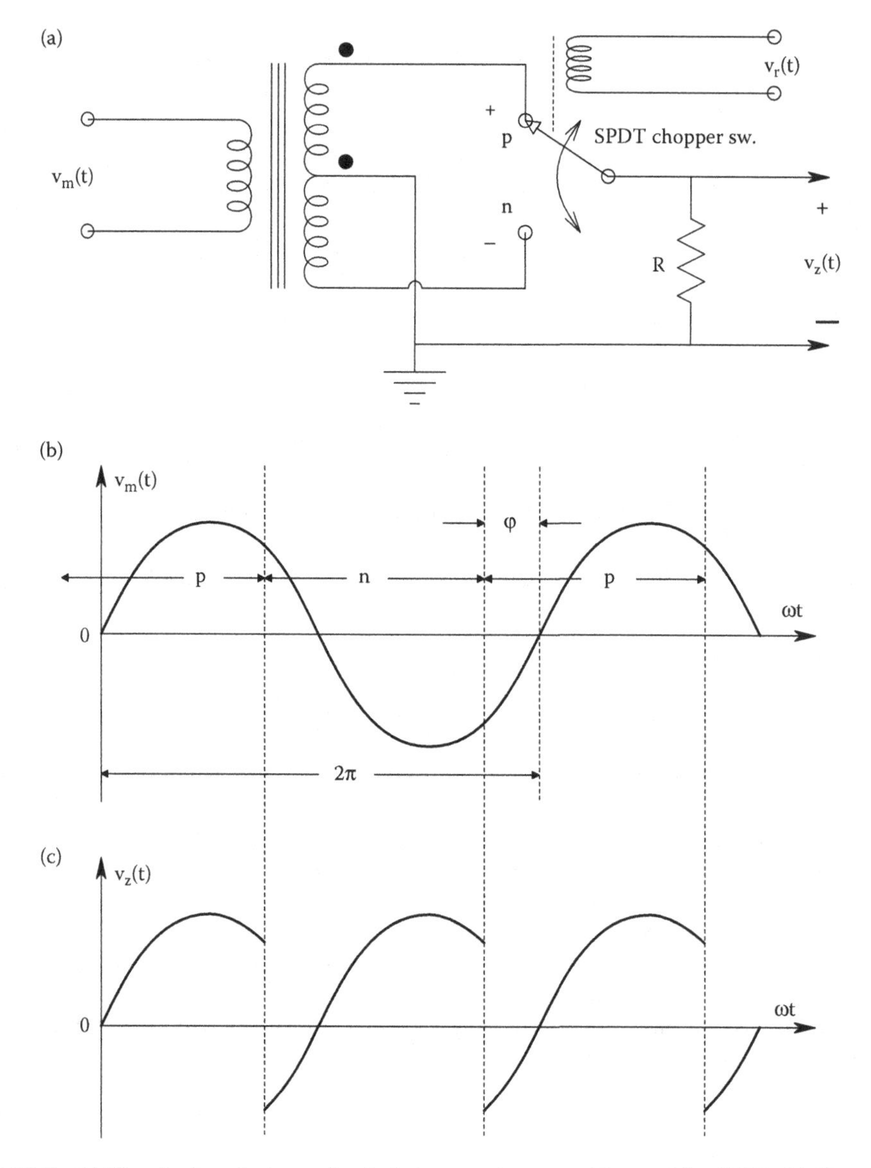

FIGURE 15.3 (a) Circuit of an electromechanical chopper phase-sensitive rectifier (PSR). (b) Chopper input. ***p*** and ***n*** denote the intervals the chopper switch dwells on the + or – contacts, respectively. (c) Chopper output when the switch control sync voltage, $v_r(t)$, is out of phase with $v_m(t)$ by φ radians. Perfect full-wave rectification is not achieved.

direction as i_{m+}, producing phase-sensitive rectification. Note that if the phase of $v_m(t)$ changes by 180°, the sign of the rectified $v_z(t)$ also changes, giving a negative output.

The output of the balanced diode bridge PSR (BDBPSR) has a relatively high output impedance and therefore must be buffered before $v_z(t)$ is passed through a low-pass filter for averaging. The permissible upper carrier frequency of the BDBPSR is determined by the type of diodes used; *Schottky diodes* switch extremely fast because they are majority carrier devices and there is no minority carrier storage at the junction. Schottky diodes will give satisfactory results well into the 100s of MHz (Yang 1988).

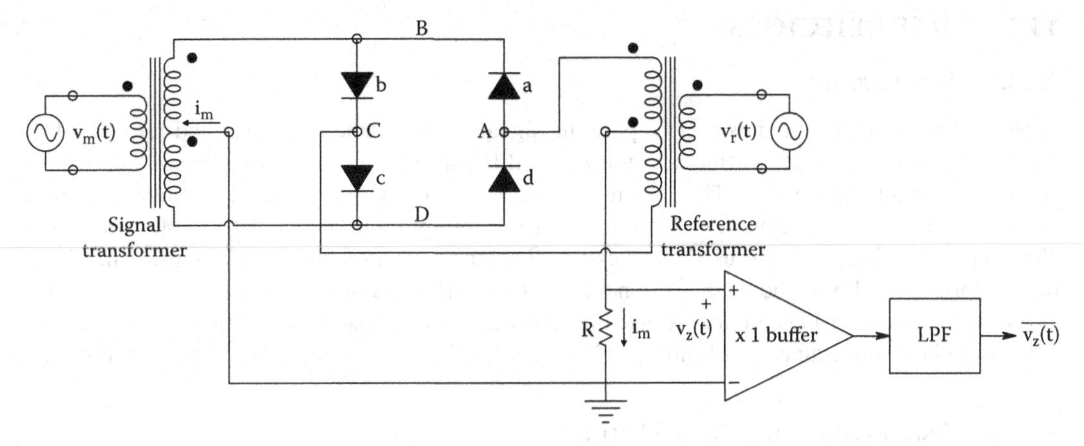

FIGURE 15.4 A balanced-bridge diode PSR.

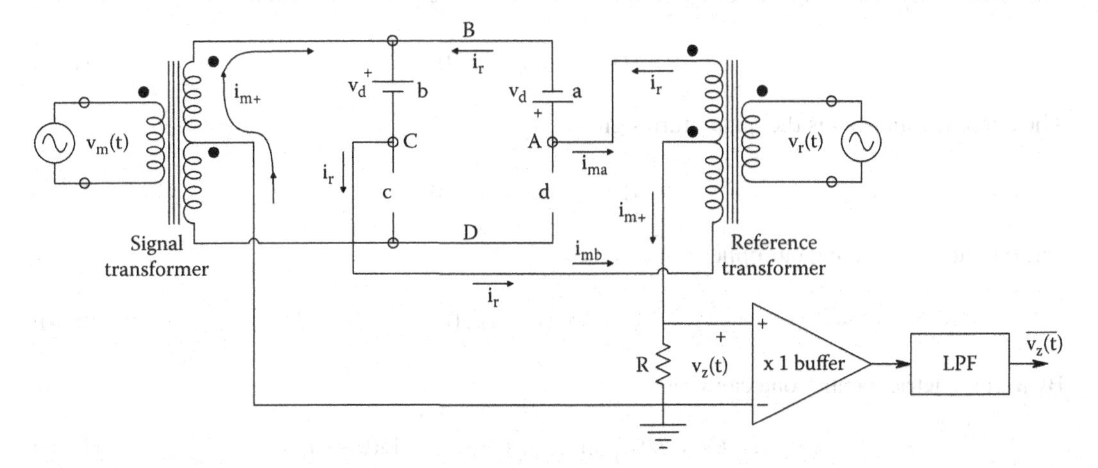

FIGURE 15.5 The diode bridge PSR when diodes **a** and **b** are conducting, and **c** and **d** are blocking current flow.

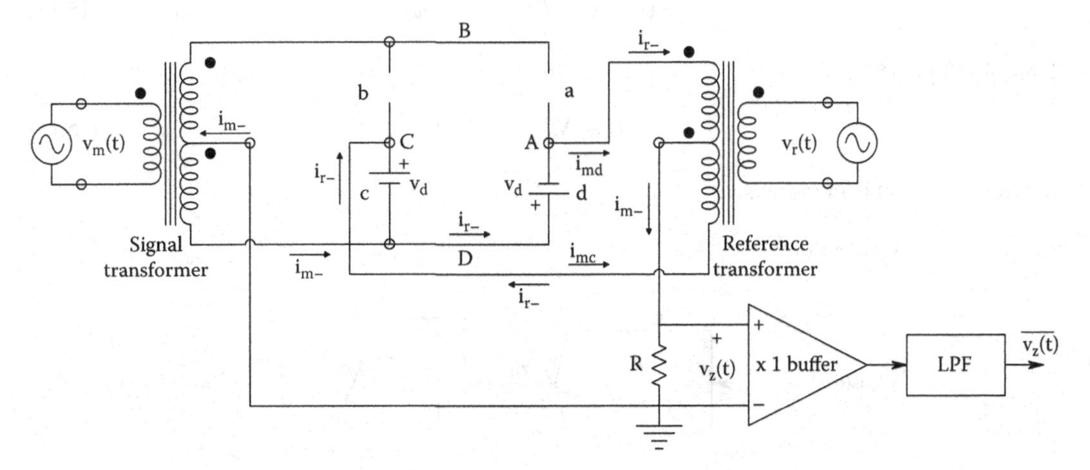

FIGURE 15.6 The diode bridge PSR when diodes **c** and **d** are conducting, and **a** and **b** are blocking current flow.

15.3 PHASE DETECTORS

15.3.1 Introduction

A phase detector (PD) operates on two periodic signals of the same frequency and returns a DC signal voltage which is proportional to the phase difference between the two signals. PDs have several important applications: They are used in lock-in amplifiers to ensure the reference signal retains the correct phase relation with the input carrier for optimum demodulation (McDonald and Northrop 1993). They are also used as an essential component in all phase-lock loops, which have many applications. It was shown in Section 6.6.6 that a PD is necessary in a phase-locked laser radar (LAVERA) system. A PD can also be used in impedance bridges and autobalancing bridges used to measure body impedance or admittance. PDs can be subdivided into analog and digital designs.

15.3.2 Analog Multiplier Phase Detector

Perhaps, the simplest *analog phase detector* is the ubiquitous analog multiplier followed by a low-pass filter, as shown in Figure 15.7. The input sinusoid whose phase we wish to measure is

$$v_s(t) = V_s \sin(\omega_c t + \theta) \tag{15.8}$$

The reference sinusoid is the quadrature signal:

$$v_r(t) = V_r \cos(\omega_c\ t + \phi) \tag{15.9}$$

The output of the analog multiplier is given by

$$v_z(t) = v_r(t) v_s(t)/10 \tag{15.10}$$

By trigonometric identity one can write

$$v_z(t) = (V_r V_s/20)\{\sin(2\omega_c t + \theta + \phi) + \sin(\theta - \phi)\} \tag{15.11}$$

The unity-gain LPF attenuates the $2\omega_c$ frequency term; its output simply estimates the average of $v_z(t)$:

$$\overline{v_z(t)} = (V_r V_s/20)\sin(\theta - \phi) \tag{15.12}$$

Thus, for $|\theta_e| < 15°$,

$$\overline{v_z(t)} \cong (V_r V_s/20)(\theta_e) \tag{15.13}$$

where $\theta_e \equiv (\theta - \phi)$ is in radians.

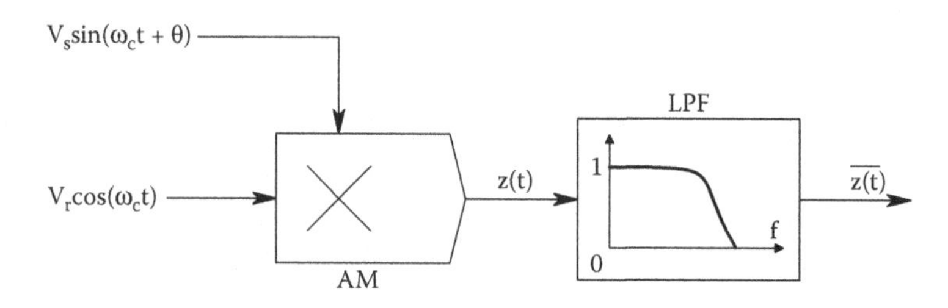

FIGURE 15.7 Block diagram of an analog multiplier phase detector. This circuit architecture is also used to demodulate DSBSCM carriers.

A systems approximation for the analog multiplier PD is shown in Figures 15.8b and c. Note that for small phase error, the PD is linear, but exhibits periodic, nonlinear behavior for $|\theta - \phi| > 15°$. Because the two coherent signals must be 90° out of phase for the AM PD to work, it is called a *quadrature PD.*

As in the case of the switched op amp PSR, one can have a switched op amp or transistor PD in which the input analog signal $v_s(t)$ given by Equation 15.8 is effectively multiplied by a ±1 reference quadrature square wave given by the $\text{sgn}\{V_r \cos(\omega_c t)\}$ operation. To demonstrate that the switched PD gives the same result as the analog multiplier PD, recall that a unity square wave can be expressed by its *Fourier series*. The Fourier series for a periodic time function, f(t), can be written as the infinite harmonic sum (Northrop 2010):

$$f(t) = a_0 + \sum_{n=1}^{\infty} \{a_n \cos(n\omega_c t) + b_n \sin(n\omega_c t)\} \tag{15.14}$$

where the fundamental (or carrier) frequency is defined as

$$\omega_c \equiv 2\pi/T \text{ r/s} \tag{15.15a}$$

$$a_0 = \text{the average value of f(t)} \tag{15.15b}$$

$$T = \text{period of f(t)} \tag{15.15c}$$

The coefficients of the Fourier series are given by the well-known integrals:

$$a_n \equiv \frac{2}{T} \int_{-T/2}^{T/2} f(t) \cos(n\omega_c t)\, dt \tag{15.16}$$

(a)

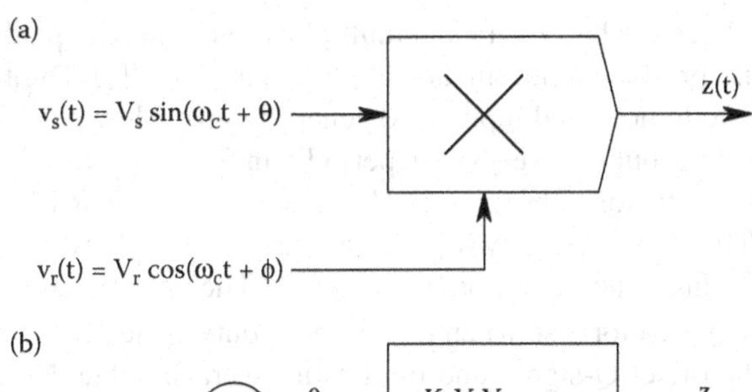

(b)

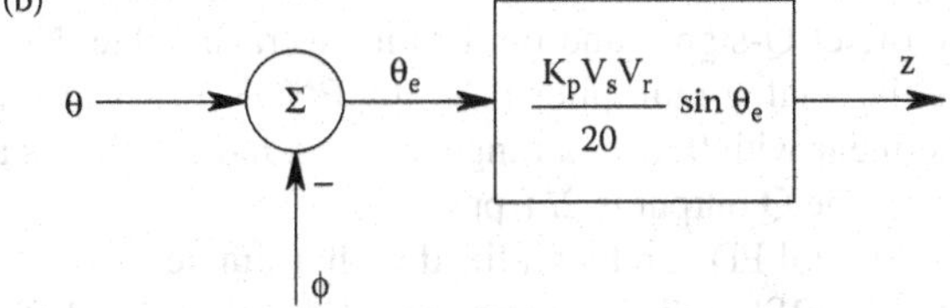

(c)

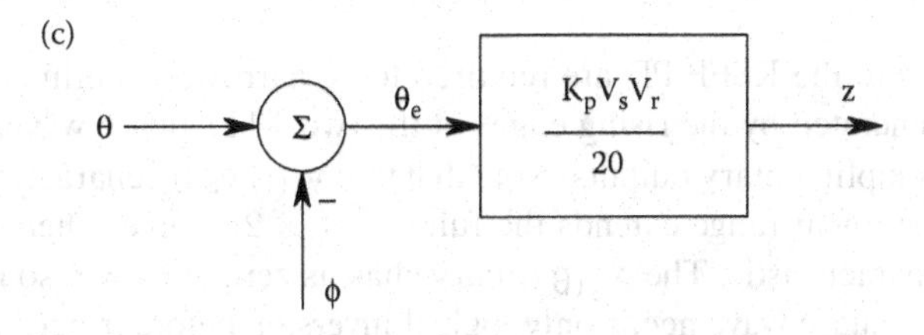

FIGURE 15.8 (a) Analog multiplier quadrature phase detector without the LPF. (b) $\sin(\theta - \phi)$ approximation to analog multiplier quadrature phase detector without the LPF. (c) When $|\theta - \phi| < 15°$, then $z \propto (\theta - \phi)$.

$$b_n \equiv \frac{2}{T}\int_{-T/2}^{T/2} f(t)\sin(n\omega_c t)\,dt \tag{15.17}$$

To show that the product, $v_z(t) = V_s \sin(\omega_c t + \theta_e)$ **sgn**$\{V_r \cos(\omega_c t)\}$, when averaged, gives us phase detection, we only need to use the fundamental frequency (n = 1) term in the *F*-series for the cosine square wave, **sgn**$\{V_r \cos(\omega_c t)\}$. The higher-order harmonics in the F-series lead to output frequencies, which are multiples of ω_c and which are therefore filtered out. Note also for **sgn**$\{V_r \cos(\omega_c t)\}$, that $a_0 = 0$, and $b_n = 0$ because f(t) is an even function. Thus, f(t) is approximated by

$$f_1(t) \cong (4/\pi)\cos(\omega_c t) \tag{15.18}$$

Thus,

$$v_z(t) = (4V_s/\pi)\sin(\omega_c t + \theta_e)\cos(\omega_c t) = (2V_s/\pi)[\sin(2\omega_c t + \theta_e) + \sin(\theta_e)] \tag{15.19}$$

After low-pass filtering, we have the desired output:

$$\overline{v_z(t)} = (2V_s/\pi)\sin(\theta_e) \cong (2V_s/\pi)(\theta_e), \quad (\theta_e) \text{ in radians} \tag{15.20}$$

The latter term in Equation 15.20 is valid for the phase difference between input and output waves, $|\theta_e| < 15^o$. Note that this PD has the same sin(q) nonlinearity as the pure analog multiplier PD. This type of phase detector is used in many IC phase-lock loop designs.

15.3.3 Digital Phase Detectors

Note that analog phase detectors based on ideal multiplication require a quadrature reference signal and a low-pass filter and produce a nonlinear output given by $\sin(\theta_e)$. Digital phase detectors, on the other hand, accept two logic signal inputs and generally give a low-pass filtered output which is linear over some range of θ_e, but is nevertheless periodic in θ_e.

The first digital phase detector to be examined is the *exclusive NOR* PD, illustrated with waveforms in Figure 15.9. This PD accepts two TTL square waves with 50% duty cycles, having the same frequency but differing in phase by some amount, θ_e. The op amp has two functions: (1) It subtracts ca. 1.7 V from the Q waveform so when Q has a 50% duty cycle, the average output, $\bar{V}_z(t) = 0$. (2) It low-pass filters the offset Q-signal and outputs its average value. Note that $\bar{V}_z(t) = 0$ when $\theta_e = \pm k\pi/2$, k odd. Like the analog multiplier PDs, the ENOR PD is also a quadrature PD. Note that the average output is linear with θ_e over a range of 0 to π radians, but is also periodic in θ_e with period 2π. The frequency of the Q output is 2/T pps.

Another simple, linear, digital PD can be realized with a simple *R-S flip-flop* (RSFF), as shown in Figure 15.10. Note that the RSFF PD uses the same DC offset and LPF op amp circuit as the ENOR PD.

However, the inputs to the RSFF PD are required to be narrow, complimentary pulses, such as those which can be generated by the rising edges of the two TTL square waves triggering the one-shot multivibrators' complimentary outputs. Note that the $\overline{V_z}(t)$ vs θ_e characteristic is also periodic with period 2π, but the linear range extends the full $0 \angle \theta_e \angle 2\pi$ range. There is no negative slope portion of this PD's characteristic. The $\overline{V_z(\theta_e)}$ curve has its zero at $\theta_e = \pi$, so it is not a quadrature system. The reference square wave needs only logical inversion before triggering the one-shot.

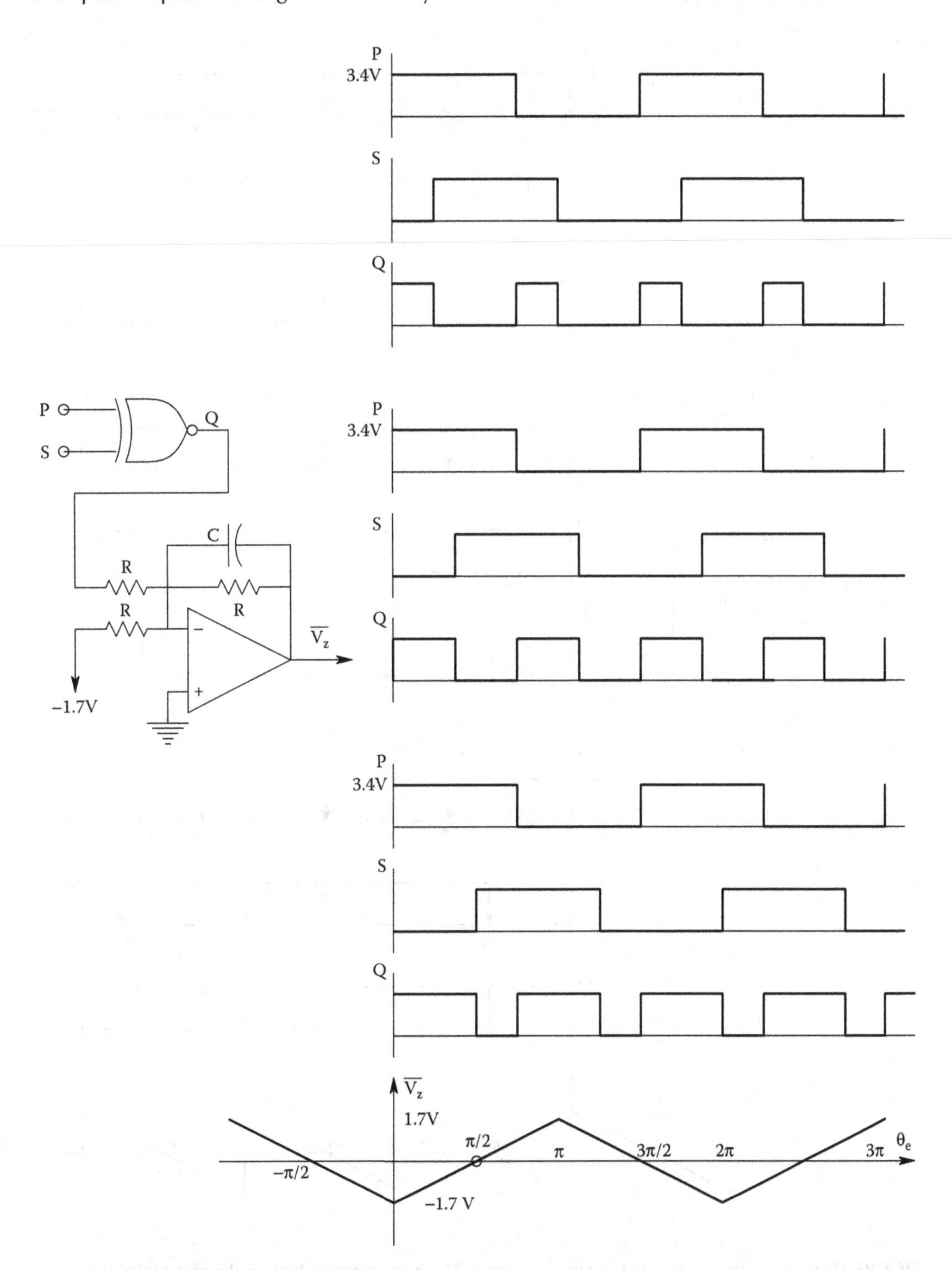

FIGURE 15.9 An exclusive NOR digital phase detector and examples of its waveforms. The bottom graph shows a plot of the (offset) average output voltage of this PD vs the phase difference between TTL inputs P and S. Note the zeros are at odd integer multiples of (π/2).

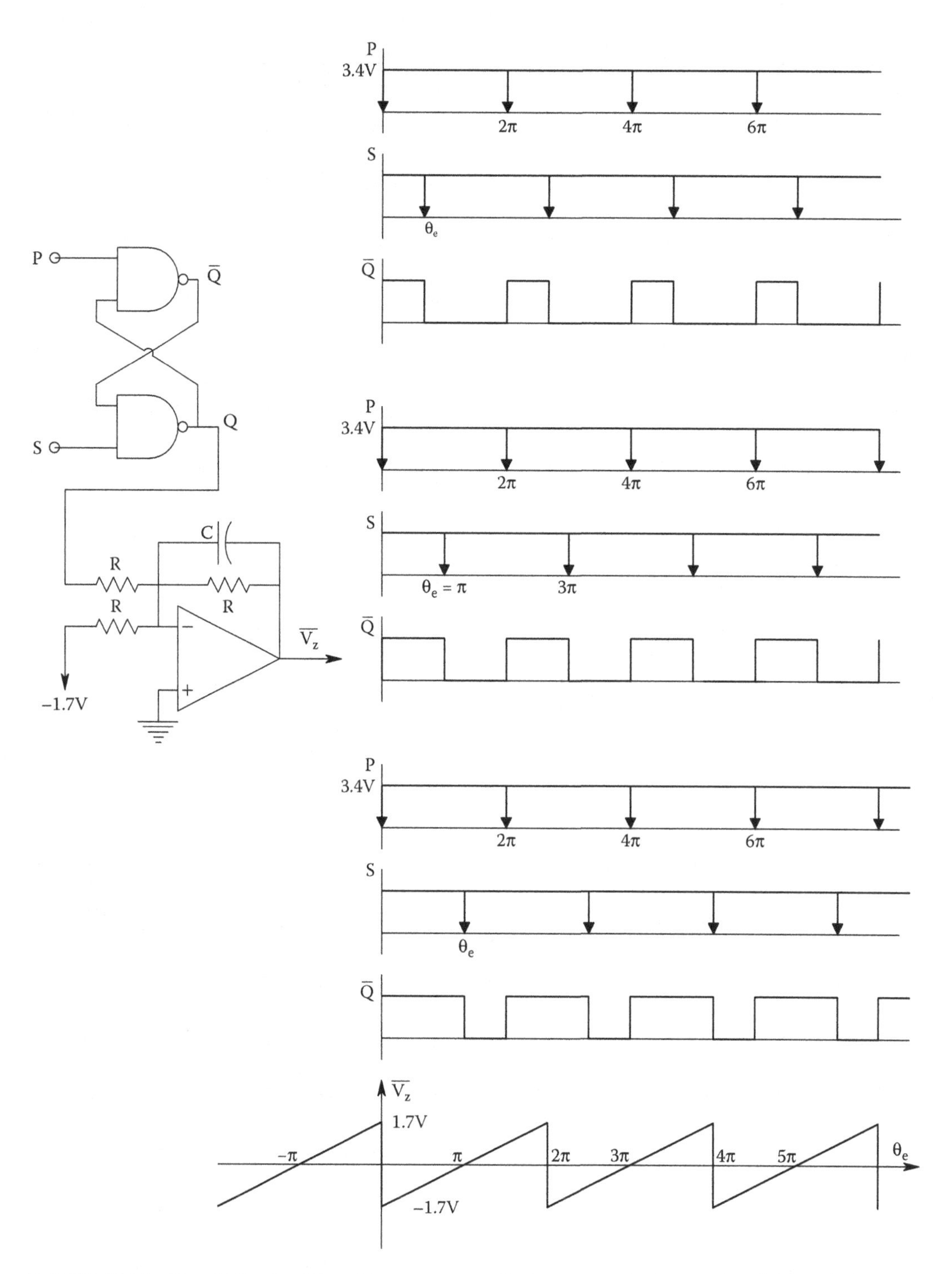

FIGURE 15.10 The RS flip-flop PD and its waveforms. The bottom graph shows a plot of the (offset) average output voltage of this PD vs the phase difference between TTL inputs P and S. Note the significant zeros are at odd integer multiples of π.

More complex, linear, digital phase detectors have been devised. One design, based on the venerable Motorola MC4044 phase-frequency detector IC, is shown in Figure 15.11. This PD's architecture is made up from various NAND gates. Note the two RS flip-flops in the center of the left-hand column. Figure 15.12 illustrates the input and output waveforms at nodes R, V, U, and D, respectively. The digital waveforms for V lagging R (top set) and below for V leading R (middle set) are shown. When U is subtracted from D by a simple op amp DA, and the difference is low-pass filtered to recover the average output, $\overline{V_z}$, shown in Figure 15.12, we obtain a linear output voltage vs θ_e over a full $\pm 2\pi$ interval, as shown in Figure 15.13.

Still another logic chip-based, digital PD is shown in Figure 15.14 (Northrop 1990). This circuit uses a 7495 (or Fairchild 9300) 4-bit, bidirectional shift register. As a PD in a PLL, it can detect lock ($\omega_p = \omega_r$) by Q_0 = LO, Q_2 = HI, and Q_1 has the TTL phase signal similar to the RSFF output. If $\omega_p > \omega_r$, then Q_0 = LO, Q_1 = LO and Q_2 has a duty cycle proportional to $(\omega_p - \omega_r)$. If $\omega_p < \omega_r$, then Q_1 = HI, Q_2 = HI and Q_0 has a duty cycle proportional to $(\omega_r - \omega_p)$.

Note that this *phase-frequency detector's* phase difference output on Q_1 is not periodic in θ_e, like other digital PDs, it saturates LO for $\omega_p > \omega_r$, and saturates HI when $\omega_p < \omega_r$. Q_1 has a 50% duty cycle when $\omega_p = \omega_r$ radians, giving $\overline{V}_z(\theta_e) = 0$. Note that the P and R inputs must be narrow, complimentary pulses, derived from the $\overline{Q}$ (complimentary) outputs of one-shots.

Because of their linearity, digital PDs are useful in instrumentation schemes where phase difference must be measured. Note that it is possible to run two, noise-free sinusoidal signals through comparators with hysteresis to generate two digital signals that can be measured with a simple, linear, digital PD.

A microcomputer-based, frequency-independent, digital phase meter with one millidegree resolution was designed and tested by Du (1993), working in the author's laboratory. The reference digital input channel was also the input to a Signetics NE564 phase-lock loop which used a divide-by

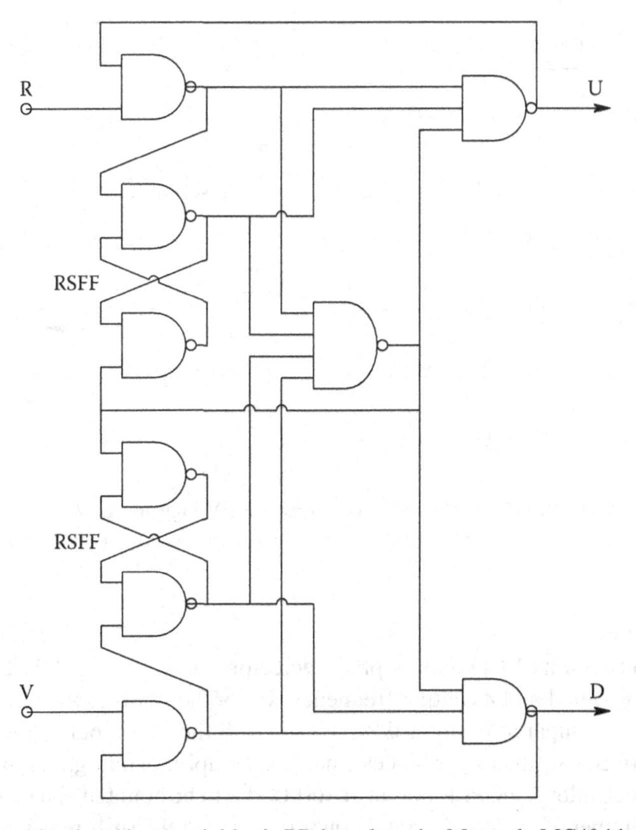

FIGURE 15.11 A combinational/sequential logic PD based on the Motorola MC4044 digital PD IC.

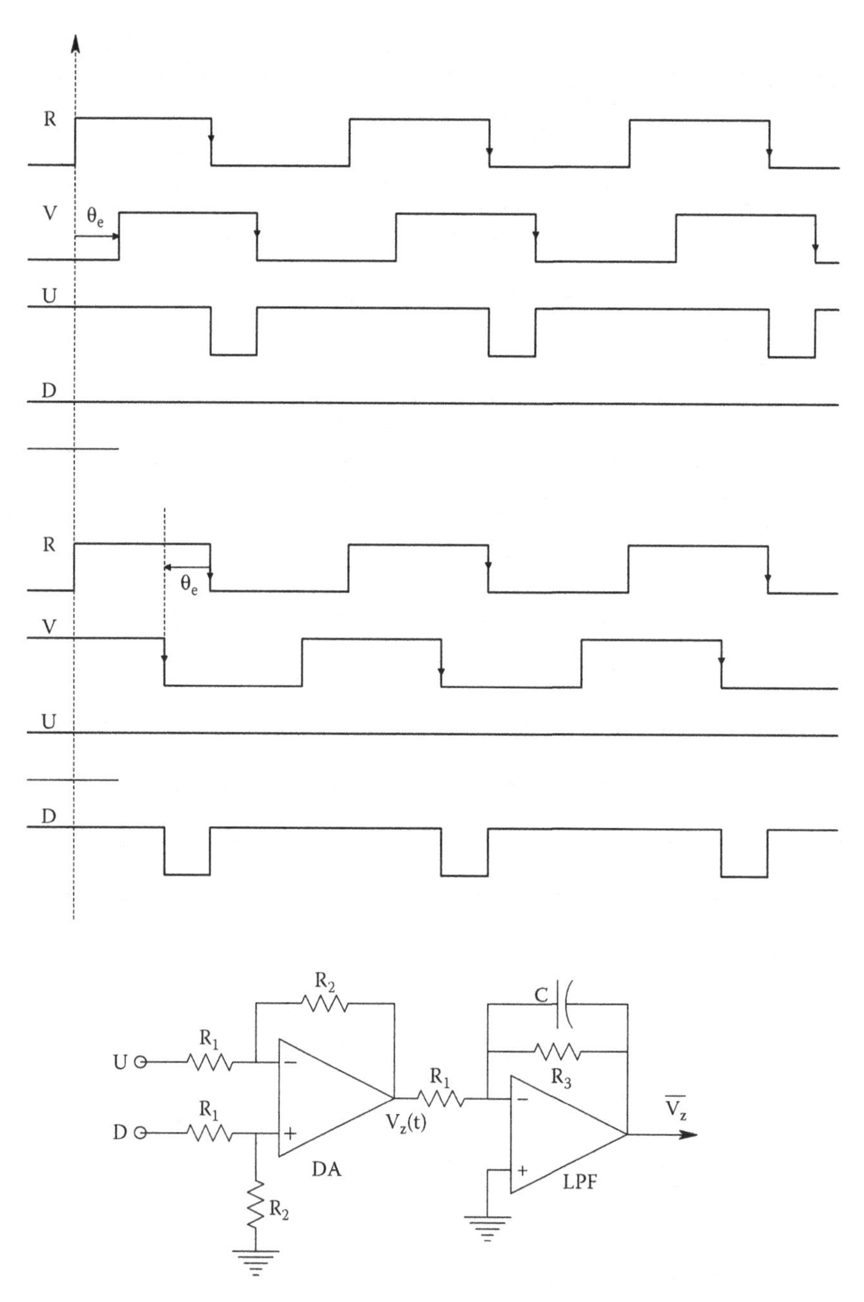

FIGURE 15.12 *Top*: Example of the 4044 PD's waveforms for V lagging R. *Mid*: Example of the 4044 PD's waveforms for V leading R. *Bottom*: Op amp DA and low-pass filter used to condition the 4044 PD's outputs, U and D.

360,000 counter between its VCO and its phase detector. Thus, the VCO TTL output was phase-locked to the input R signal and its output frequency was 360,000 times the input frequency, f_o. The high level of the $\bar{Q}_R$ comparator output is NANDed with the Q_S output of the signal comparator. Any phase shift between V_R and V_S produces a narrow, complimentary gating pulse at the output of the NAND gate which allows the PLL output at $360,000\ f_o$ to be counted. The count occurs once per cycle for a preset number of cycles. The total count is stored in the shift registers (74F299) and then

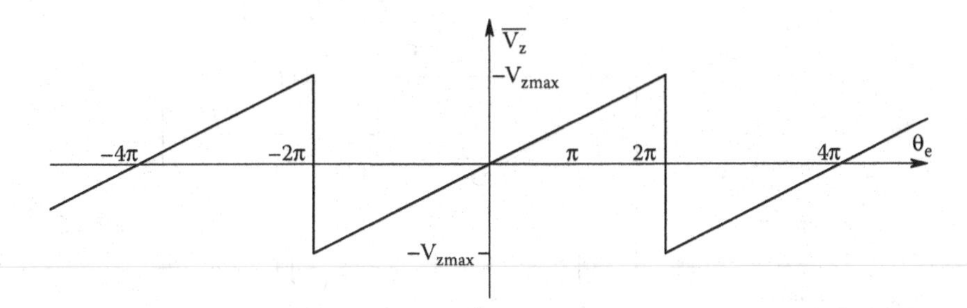

FIGURE 15.13 Average output voltage vs input phase difference for the 4044 PD with the op amp signal conditioner in Figure 15.12. Note each linear segment spans a full ±2π radians, and has zero output for zero phase difference between R and V.

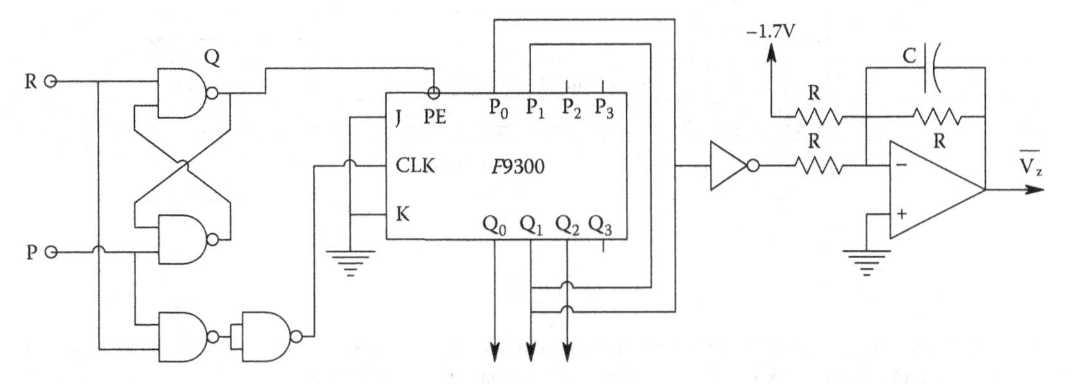

FIGURE 15.14 A shift-register-based digital phase-frequency detector.

downloaded into a PC for averaging. Each count is the phase lag between V_R and V_S in millidegrees and is independent of the frequency of the inputs.

Du's phase meter worked with input frequencies, f_o, of up to 100 Hz, and gave a numerical output of θ_e, and its statistics. Figures 15.15 and 15.16 illustrate the architecture of the millidegree phase meter and the PLL used as a × 360,000 frequency multiplier. Du's system was used in dielectric materials measurements where it was desired to measure minute phase shifts caused by dielectric losses at power-line frequencies.

15.4 VOLTAGE AND CURRENT-CONTROLLED OSCILLATORS

15.4.1 Introduction

The voltage-controlled oscillator (VCO) or current controlled oscillator (CCO) is an important subsystem in many electronic devices and systems. As you will see, it is a key component system in the phase-lock loop, as well as certain communication and instrumentation systems. VCOs and CCOs can have sinusoidal, triangular or TTL outputs of constant amplitude. The frequency of a VCO or CCO, *in its linear range*, can be expressed by

$$f_o = K_V V_c + b \text{ Hz} \tag{15.21a}$$

or

$$f_o = K_C I_C + b \tag{15.21b}$$

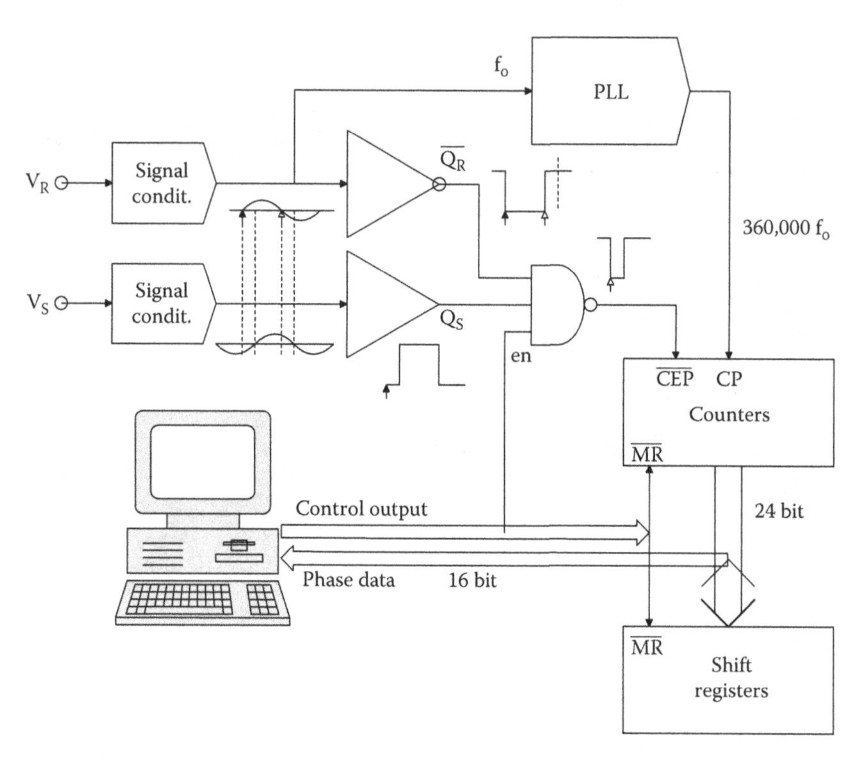

FIGURE 15.15 Architecture of the millidegree phase detector devised by Du (1993). The system is based on a phase-lock loop whose clock runs 360,000 times faster than the input frequency.

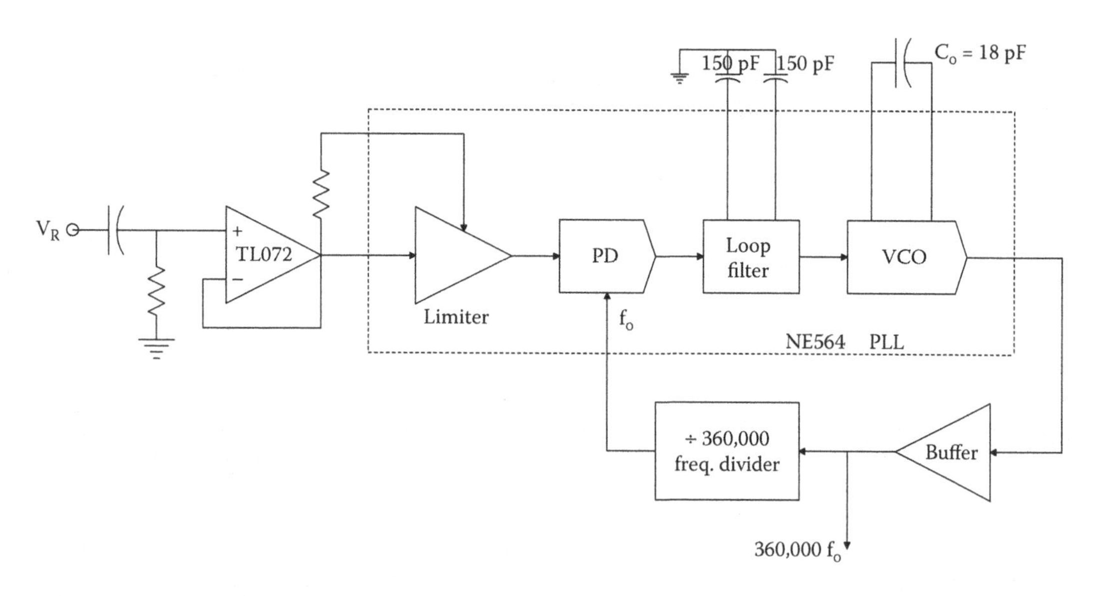

FIGURE 15.16 Block diagram of Du's PLL.

The frequency constants K_V and K_C can have either sign, as can the intercept, b. It is desirable that a VCO have a wide *linear operating range* $\equiv [(f_{omax} - f_{omin})/(f_{omax} + f_{omin})]$, low noise (phase and amplitude), low-*frequency tempco* $\equiv (\Delta f_o/\Delta T)(1/f_o)$, and a high-spectral purity (low THD) if it produces a sinusoidal output (many VCOs produce TTL outputs and/or triangle wave outputs). There are many architectures for VCOs. The first we examine below is a "linear amplifier" oscillator in which f_o is tuned by two variable-gain elements, which can either be analog multipliers or multiplying digital-to-analog converters (MDACs).

15.4.2 An Analog VCO

Figure 15.17 shows the schematic of an electronically tuned VCO based on the use of linear circuit elements connected in a *positive feedback loop* (Northrop 1990). The block diagram below the schematic illustrates the transfer functions of the two minor loops whose poles are set by the $\mathbf{V_C}$ DC voltage input to the two analog multipliers. After reducing the two minor loops, the oscillator's loop gain can be written as

$$A_L(s) = \frac{+\,s\,kV_C\,/\,(10RC)}{s^2 + s\,2V_C/(10RC) + V_C{}^2/(10RC)^2} \tag{15.22}$$

From Section 5.5 on oscillators, we see that the root locus diagram for this oscillator is a circle centered on the origin. The locus branches for the closed-loop poles begin at $\mathbf{s} = -V_C/(10RC)$ r/s, cross the jω axis in the s-plane at $\mathbf{s} = \pm j\omega_o$ when k = 2, hit the positive real axis at $\mathbf{s} = +\omega_o$, then one branch approaches the zero at the origin while the other branch goes toward + ∞ as k increases.

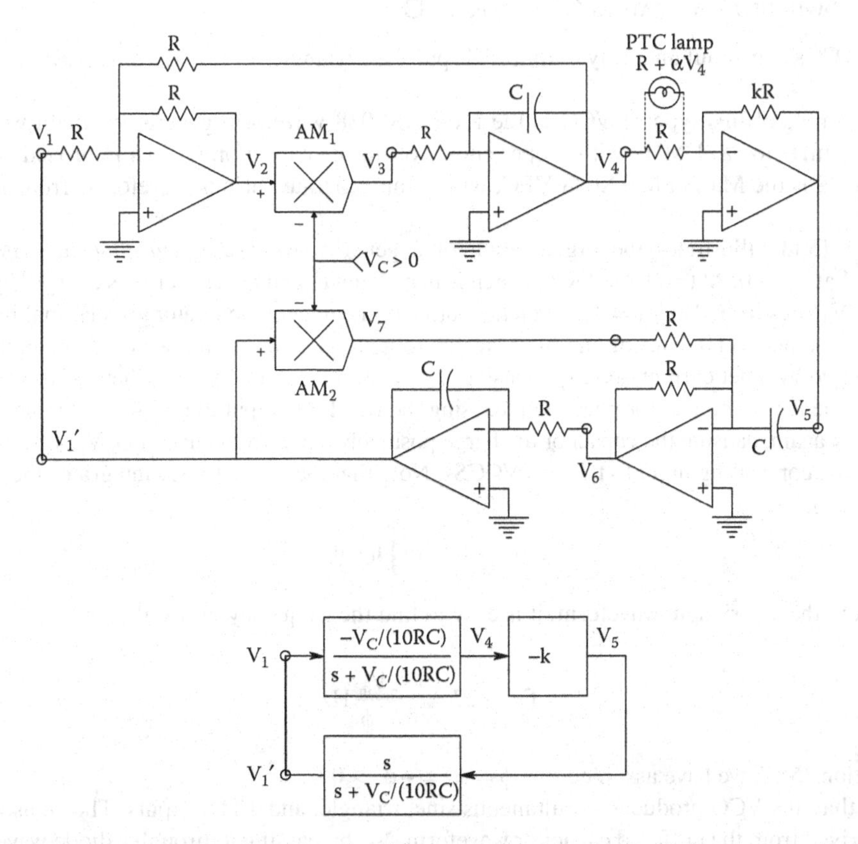

FIGURE 15.17 Schematic of a voltage-tuned oscillator using positive feedback. The tungsten filament lamp is used to limit and stabilize oscillation amplitude. A systems block diagram of the linear part of the oscillator is shown below the schematic. See Text for analysis.

Let us use the venerable Barkhausen criterion for oscillation on this oscillator (Millman 1979). Set

$$A_L(j\omega_o) \equiv 1\angle 0^\circ = \frac{j\omega_o k V_C/(10RC)}{[-\omega_o^2 + V_C^2/(10RC)^2] + j\omega_o 2V_C/(10RC)} \tag{15.23}$$

Clearly, the real term in the denominator must be equal to zero. This condition gives us the radian oscillation frequency:

$$\omega_o = V_C/(10RC) \text{ r/s} \tag{15.24}$$

and also, the minimum gain for oscillation, k = 2. Thus, $\mathbf{V_C}$ can set ω_o over a wide range, e.g., 0.01 $\leq V_C \leq$ 10 V, or a 1:1000 range. For practical reasons, we make k > 2 and use a positive temperature coefficient (PTC) tungsten lamp instead of the input R to the third op amp. Now, the overall gain of this stage is

$$\frac{V_5}{V_4} = -\frac{k R}{R + \alpha V_4} = -2 \tag{15.25}$$

If we set k = 4, then the steady state, equilibrium value of V_4 is found to be R/α for any ω_o. Making k = 4 allows the oscillations to grow rapidly to the equilibrium level.

15.4.3 Switched Integrating Capacitor VCOs

Certain VCOs can simultaneously output TTL pulses, a triangle wave and a sine wave of the same frequency.

An example of this type of VCO is the Exar XR8038 waveform generator, which works over a range of mHz to ca. 1 MHz with proper choice of timing capacitor, C_T. An improved version of the XR8038 is the Maxim MAX038 VFC, which can generate various waveforms from 1 mHz to 20 MHz.

Figure 15.18 illustrates the organization of a generic *switched integrating capacitor* VCO. Assume that $V_{in} > 0$. At t = 0, the MOS switch is in position ***u***, and the capacitor is charged by current $G_m V_{in}$ so V_T goes from 0 to $V_T = \phi_+$, when the output of the upper comparator goes HI making the RS flip-flop Q output go HI, causing the MOS switch to go to position ***d***. In position ***d***, the capacitor C_T is discharged by a net current, $-G_m V_{in}$, causing V_T to ramp down to $\phi_- < 0$. When V_T reaches f_, the output of the lower comparator goes high, causing the RSFF Q output to go LO, switching the MOS switch to ***u*** again, causing the capacitor to charge positively again from current $G_m V_{in}$, etc.

V_{in} is the controlling input to the two VCCSs. Note that the capacitor C_T integrates the current:

$$V_T = (1/C_T)\int i_C \, dt \tag{15.26}$$

Thus, from the V_T triangle waveform, it is easy to find the frequency of oscillation:

$$f = 1/27 = \frac{G_m V_{in}}{4C_T\phi} \text{ Hz} \tag{15.27}$$

In Equation 15.27, we have assumed that $\phi = \phi_+ = -\phi_- > 0$.

Note that this VCO produces simultaneous sine, triangle, and TTL outputs. The sinusoidal output is derived from the buffered capacitor waveform, V_T, by passing it through a diode wave-shaper, sin(*) NL. This type of VCO IC is often used as the basis for inexpensive laboratory function generators.

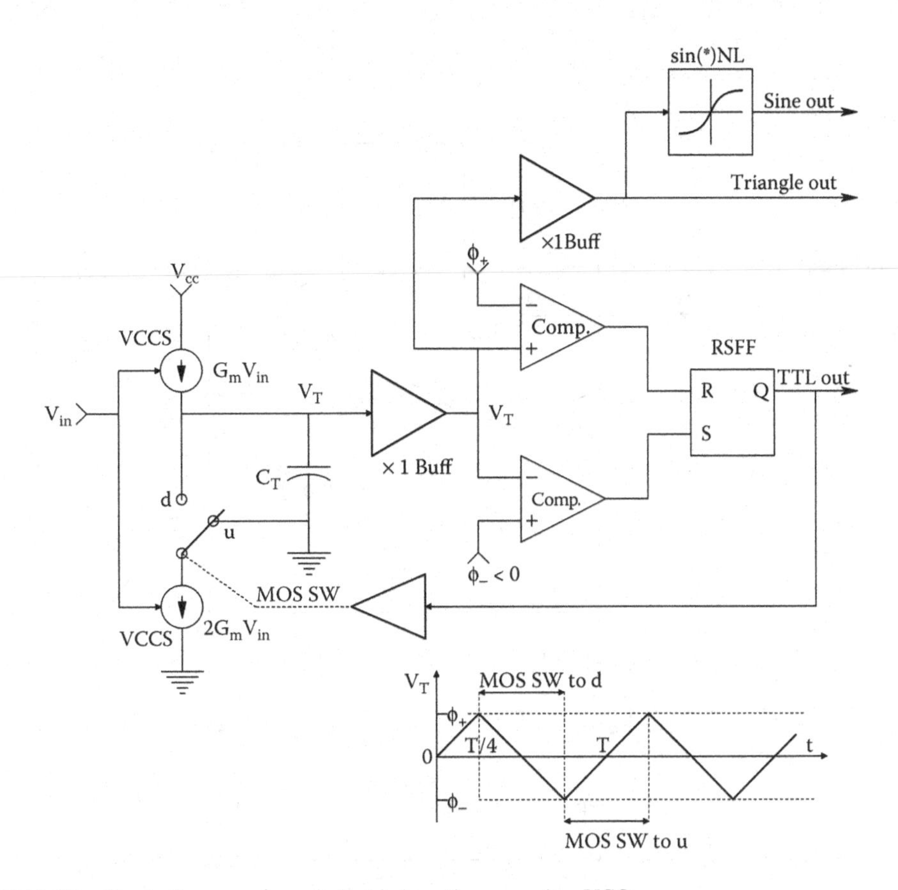

FIGURE 15.18 Block diagram of a switched integrating capacitor VCO.

15.4.4 Voltage-Controlled, Emitter-Coupled Multivibrator

Figure 15.19 illustrates the simplified schematic of another popular VCO architecture. This astable, emitter-coupled multivibrator (AECMV) derives its frequency control from the transistors Q_5 and Q_6, which act as VCCSs and control the rate that C_T charges and discharges, hence the AWCMV's frequency. This architecture gives an inherently high-frequency oscillator, and versions of it using MOSFETs have been used to build a VCO with an 800 MHz tuning range that operates in excess of 2.5 GHz (Herzel et al. 2001).

The heart of this VCO is the free-running, AECMV, which alternately switches Q_1 and Q_2 on and off as the timing capacitor charges and discharges. Detailed analysis of this circuit can be found in Franco (1988), and also in Gray and Meyer (1984). Analysis is helped by considering the circuit of Figure 15.20 and the waveforms of Figure 15.21.

To analyze the operation of the AECMV, its frequency can be calculated by first assuming that Q_1 is turned off and Q_2 is turned on. The circuit for these conditions is shown in Figure 15.20. Assume the current I_{c2} is large so that the voltage drop $I_{c2}R$ is large enough to turn on diode D_2. This causes the base of Q_4 to be one diode drop below V_{CC}, and the emitter is two diode drops below V_{CC} and the base of Q_1 is two diode drops below V_{CC}. If one neglects the base current of Q_3, its base is at $\approx V_{CC}$ and its emitter is one diode drop below V_{CC}. Thus, the emitter of Q_2 is two diode drops below V_{CC}. Since Q_1 is off, a current $I_1 = [g_mV_{in}]$ is charges the capacitor so that the emitter of Q_1 is becomes more negative. Q_1 turns on when the voltage at its emitter becomes equal to three diode drops below V_{CC}; the resulting collector current in Q_1 turns on D_1. As a result, the base of Q_3 moves in a negative direction by one diode drop, causing the base of Q_2 to also move negatively by one

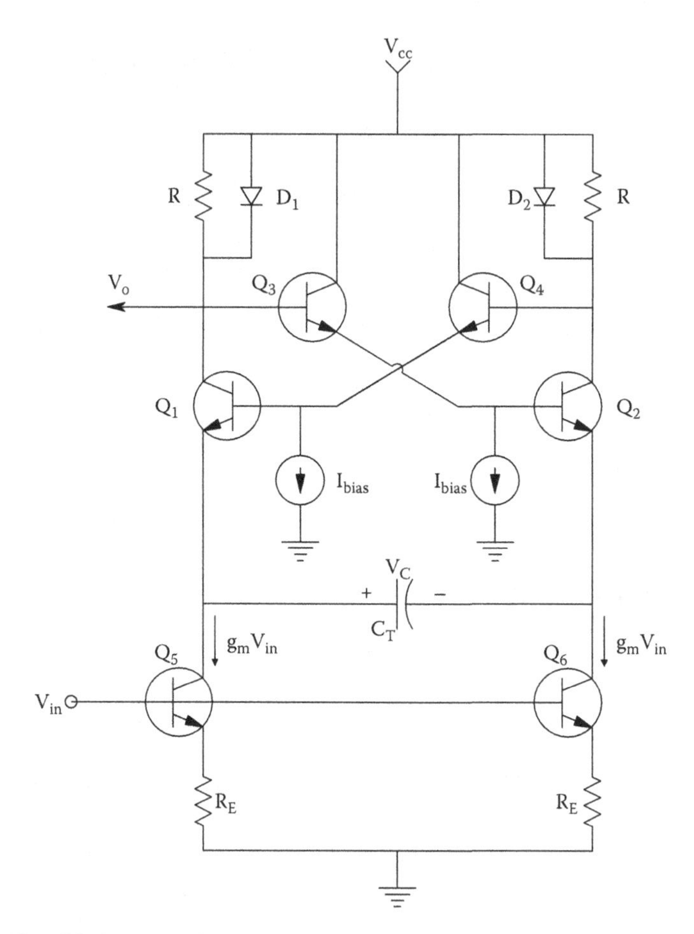

FIGURE 15.19 Simplified schematic of a voltage-controlled, emitter-coupled, (astable) multivibrator (VCECM).

diode drop. Q_2 then turns off, causing the base of Q_1 to move positive by one diode drop because D_2 also turns off. As a result, the base-emitter junction of Q_2 is reverse-biased by one diode drop because the voltage on C_T cannot change instantaneously. The current $[g_m V_{in}]$ must now charge the capacitor voltage in the negative direction by an amount equal to two diode drops before the circuit will switch back again. Since the circuit is symmetrical, the half period is given by the time required to charge the capacitor, and is

$$T/2 = Q/(g_m V_{in}) = \frac{C_T 2V_{BE(on)}}{g_m V_{in}} \tag{15.28}$$

where $Q = C_T \Delta V = C_T 2V_{BE(on)}$ is the charge on the capacitor. The frequency of the AECMV oscillator is thus

$$f = \frac{1}{T} = \frac{g_m V_{in}}{4C_T V_{BE(on)}} \tag{15.29}$$

Note the similarity between Equations 15.29 and 15.27. Note that the AECMV is a regenerative, positive feedback circuit when it is switching. The complimentary state changes of Q_1 and Q_2 are made more rapid by the positive feedback.

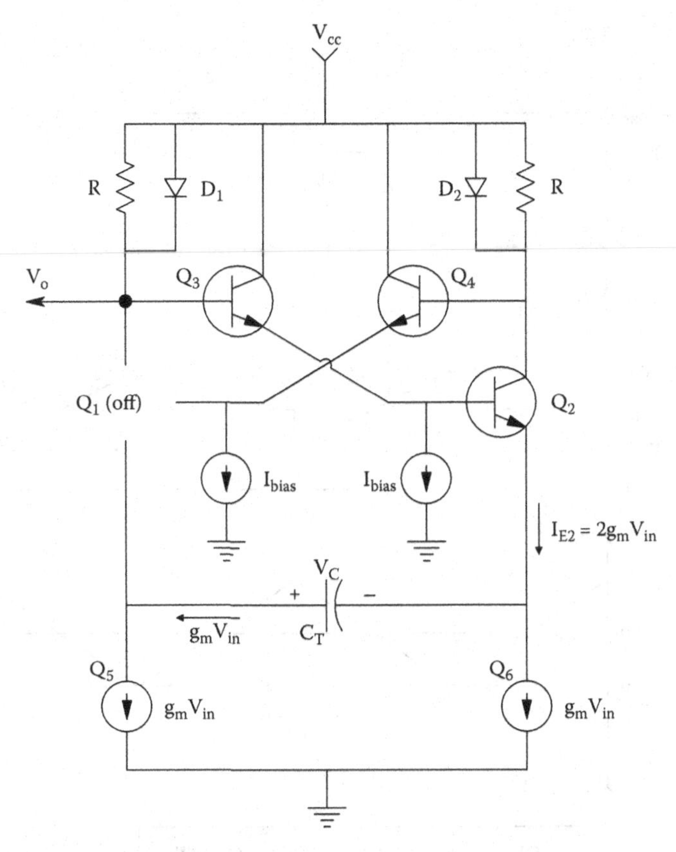

FIGURE 15.20 The VCECM charging CT with Q1 OFF.

Figure 15.22 illustrates the use of two nose-to-nose varactor diodes (also called epicap diodes by Motorola) to tune a MC1648 emitter-coupled multivibrator VCO. (Also see the 900 MHz, varactor diode-tuned, emitter-coupled MV described by Zhu in his (2005) PhD dissertation.)

A varactor diode (VD) is a *reverse-biased*, Si, *pn* junction diode, characterized by a *voltage-variable depletion capacitance,* C_v, modeled by Equation 15.30:

$$C_v = \frac{C_{vo}}{(1 - V_D/\psi_o)^\gamma}, V_D < 0 \tag{15.30}$$

where C_{vo} is the varactor diode's junction capacitance at $V_D = 0$, ψ_o is the "built-in barrier potential," typically on the order of 0.75 V for a Si diode at room temperature, and γ is the capacitance exponent. γ can vary from ca. 1/3 to 2, depending on the doping gradients at the junction boundary. γ can be shown to be $\cong 0.5$ for an abrupt (step) junction (Gray and Meyer 1984).

The output of the MC1648 oscillator is an emitter-coupled logic (ECL) square wave; frequencies as high as 225 MHz can be obtained with this IC, which can serve as the VCO in a PLL. In the circuit shown, the tuning range lies between $V_D = -2$ to -10 V (or $2 \leq V_c \leq 10$ V). The actual $f_o(V_c)$ curve is sigmoid but can be approximated by the linear VCO relation

$$f_o \cong 15V_c + 20 \text{ MHz} \tag{15.31}$$

over the range of V_c shown. Note that two VDs are used in series to halve their capacitance seen in the resonant "tank" circuit. A Motorola MV1404 VD's capacitance goes from 160 pF at $V_D = -1$ to ca. 11 pF at $V_D = -10$ V.

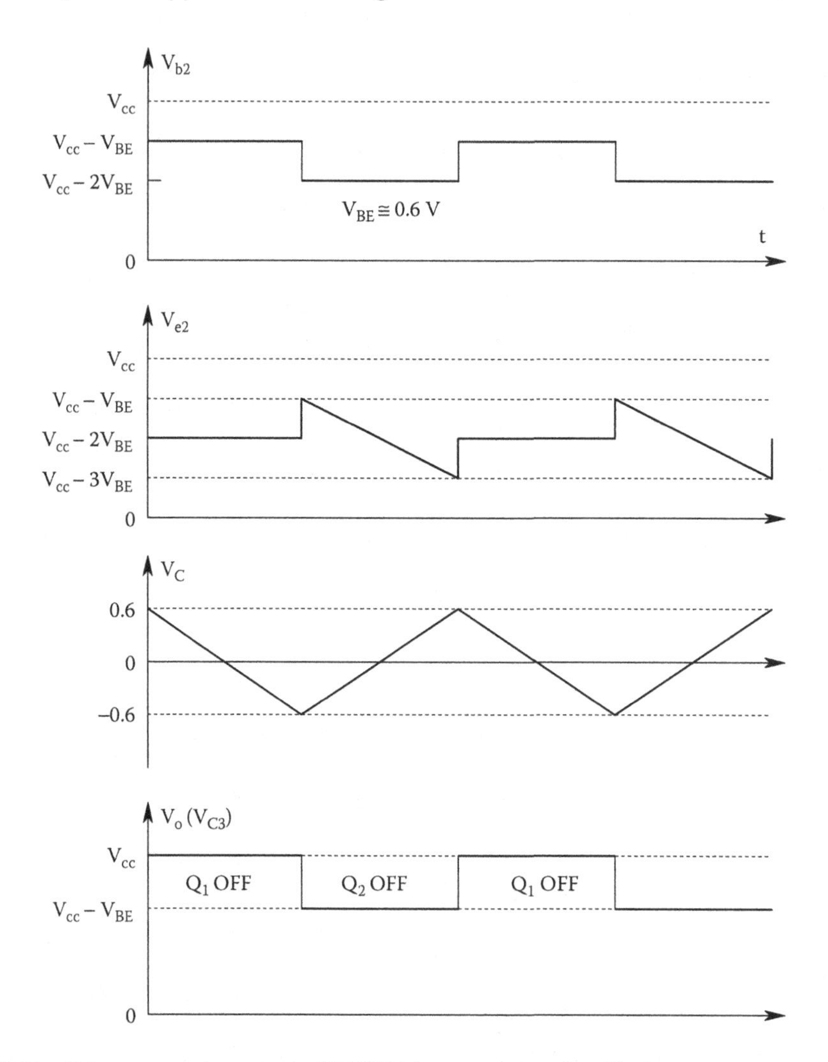

FIGURE 15.21 Relevant waveforms in the VCECM for two cycles of oscillation.

15.4.5 Voltage-to-Period Converter and Applications

The *voltage-to-period converter* (VPC) is a variable frequency oscillator in which the *period of the oscillation,* T, *is directly proportional to the controlling voltage,* $\mathbf{V_c}$. Mathematically, this is stated simply as

$$T = K_P V_c + b \text{ seconds} \tag{15.32}$$

where b is a positive constant, and K_P is the VPC constant in seconds/volt.

Practical considerations dictate lower and upper bounds to T. Obviously, the VPC's output frequency is 1/T Hz. The conventional voltage-to-frequency converter (VFC) has its output frequency directly proportional to its input voltage (or current), sic:

$$f_o = K_V V_c + d \tag{15.33}$$

where K_V is the VCO constant in Hz/V, and d is a constant (Hz).

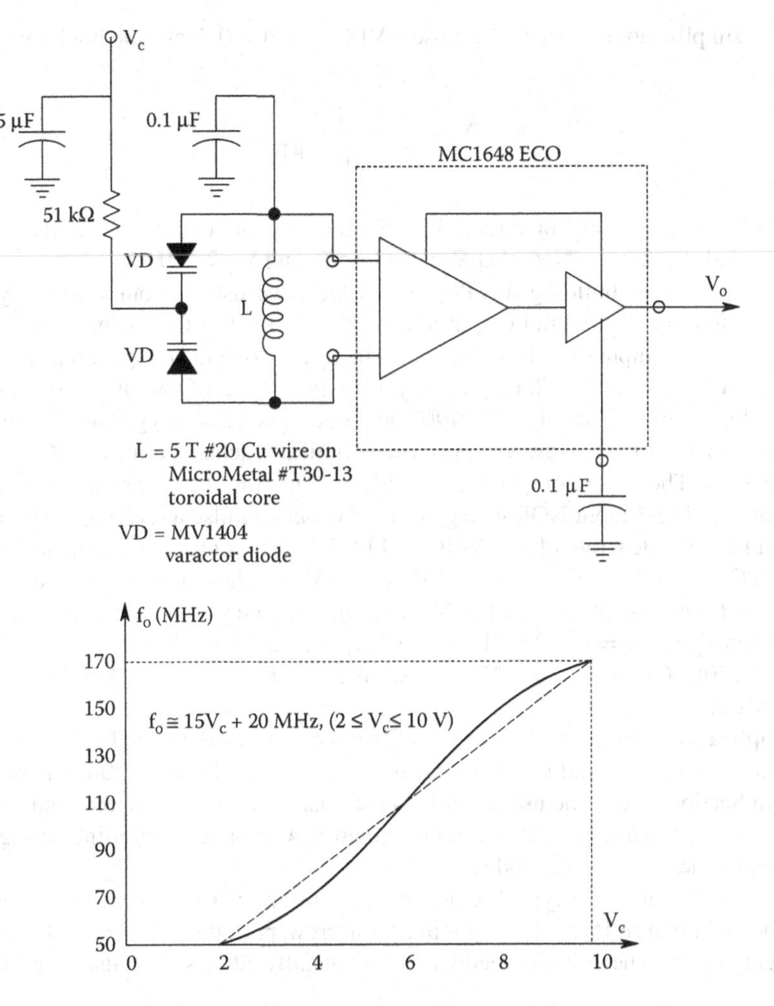

FIGURE 15.22 *Top*: A VCO that uses the voltage-variable capacitance of two varactor diodes to set its output frequency. *Bottom*: The frequency vs DC control voltage characteristic of this varactor VCO.

In several important instrumentation applications, it is found that use of a VPC (rather than a VFC) linearizes the measurement system output; several examples are described below.

Realization of VPCs: As we have seen, many IC manufacturers make VFC VCOs. Some have TTL outputs, others generate sine, triangle, and TTL outputs. No one, to this writer's knowledge, markets a VPC IC. One obvious way to make a VPC is to take a VFC in which $f_o = K_V V_c + d$, and use a nonlinear analog circuit to process the input, V_1, so that the net result is a VPC. Mathematically, it is desired to have

$$T = K_P V_1 + b = \frac{1}{K_V V_2 + d} \tag{15.34}$$

To find the required nonlinearity, solve Equation 15.34 for $V_2 = f(\mathbf{V_1})$. This gives

$$V_2 = \frac{1 - bd - d\,K_P V_1}{K_V (K_P V_1 + b)} \tag{15.35}$$

Considerable simplification accrues if we use a VFC with d = 0. Now, the nonlinearity needs to be

$$V_2 = \frac{1}{K_V(K_P V_1 + b)} \tag{15.36}$$

Figure 15.23 illustrates an op amp circuit that will generate the requisite V_2 for the VFC to produce voltage-to-period conversion. Note that V_3 must be >0, and $V_R = +0.1$ V.

Another approach to building a VPC, which we have used in our laboratory, is shown in Figure 15.24. Here the differential output of a NOR gate RS flip-flop is integrated by a high slew rate op amp. Assume output C of the FF is high. The op amp output voltage ramps up at a slope fixed by the voltage difference at the FF outputs (say 4 V) times 1/RC of the integrator. When V_o reaches the variable threshold, V_C, the upper AD790 comparator goes low, triggering the upper one-shot to reset the FF output C to low. Now V_o ramps down until it reaches the fixed, –10V threshold of the lower comparator. The lower comparator goes high, triggering the lower one-shot to set FF output C high again, etc. The 2-input NOR gate gives a VPC output pulse at every FF state transition. The AD840 op amp has a slew rate of 400 V/μs, or 4.E8 V/s. It is connected as a differential integrator.

In this VPC design, V_C varies over $-9 \leq V_c \leq +10$ V. We chose R = 1 k, C = 850 pF, and let the FF's ΔV = 4 V. From this data, we see that V_o ramps up or down with a slope of m = ΔV/RC = 4.71E6 V/s. Now, when $V_c = 0$, T = b = 2.125E–6 s, and K_P = 2.125E–7. It is easy to see that the T_{max} = 20 V/4.71E6 = 4.250E–6 s and f_{min} = 2.353E5 Hz. Likewise, the T_{min} = 1 V/4.71E6 = 2.125E–7 s, and f_{max} = 4.71 MHz.

VPC Applications: Either a VFC or a VPC can be used as the signal source in a closed-loop, constant phase velocimeter and ranging system (Nelson 1999; Northrop 2002). However, as shown below and in Section 15.8.3, the use of a VPC produces a *linear* range output and a velocity signal independent of range, while the use of a conventional VFC produces a nonlinear range output and a velocity signal which is range dependent.

The basic architecture of a type 1, closed-loop, constant-phase, laser velocimeter, and ranging system is shown in Figure 15.25. This system uses narrow, periodic pulses of IR laser light reflected from a moving target. The system's feedback automatically adjusts the pulse repetition rate so that

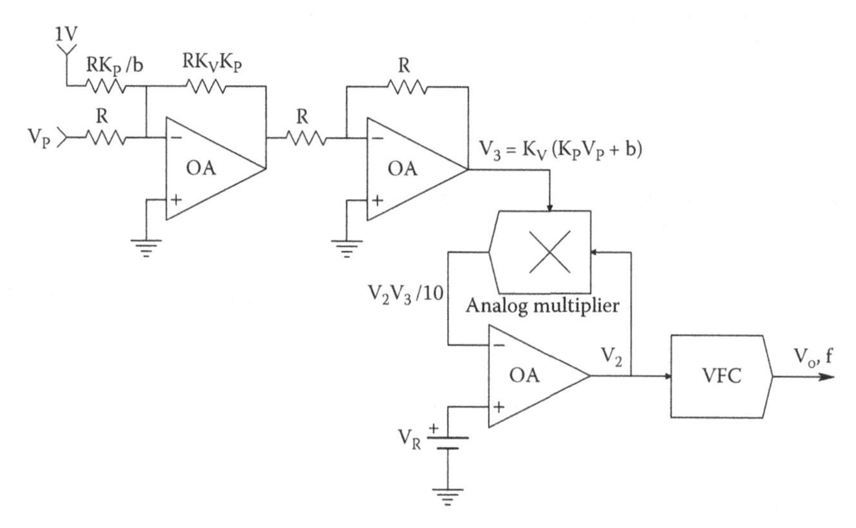

FIGURE 15.23 Schematic of a nonlinear op amp circuit used to make a *voltage-to-period converter* from a conventional voltage-to-frequency converter. See text for analysis.

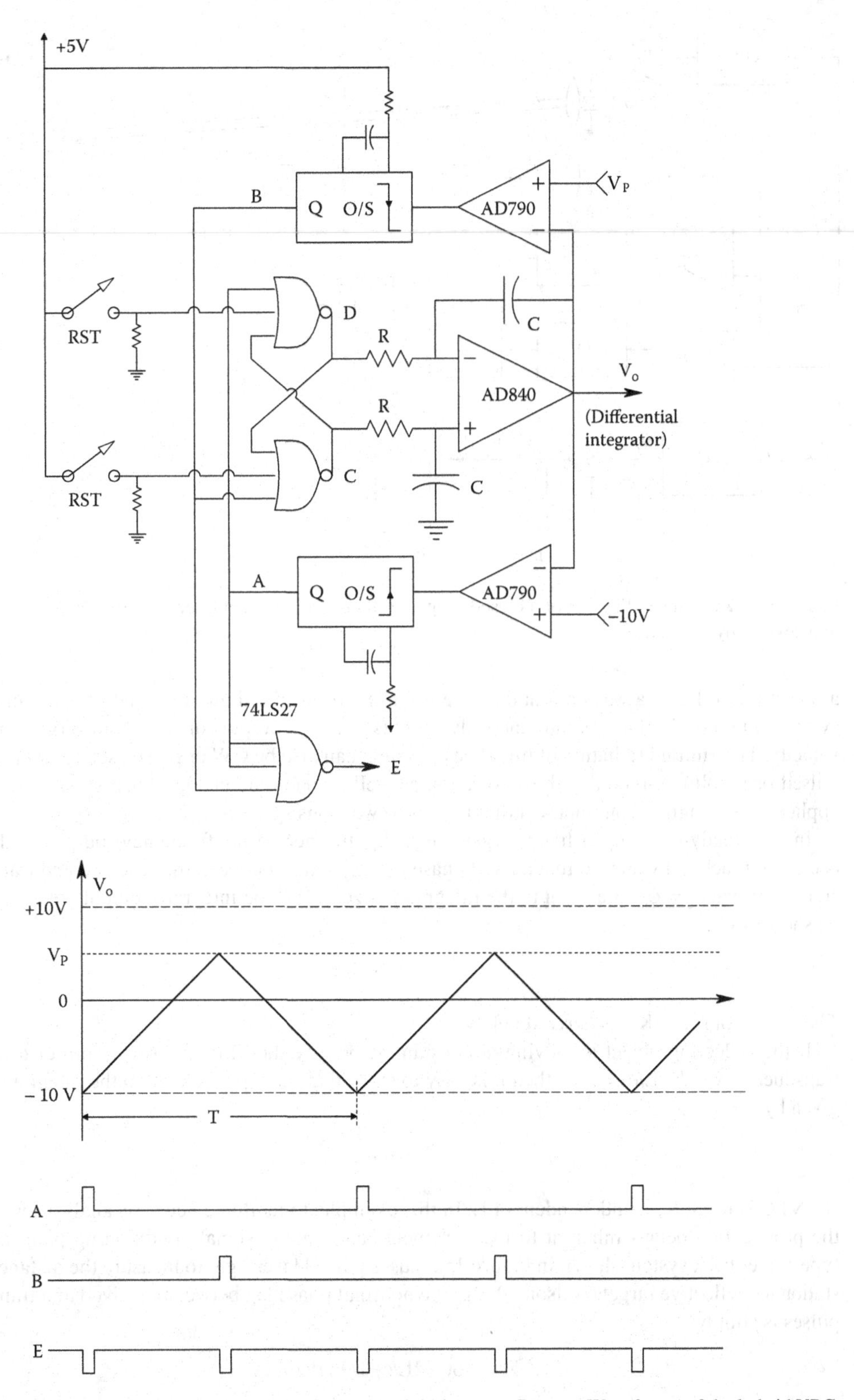

FIGURE 15.24 *Top*: Schematic of a hybrid VPC with digital output. *Bottom*: Waveforms of the hybrid VPC.

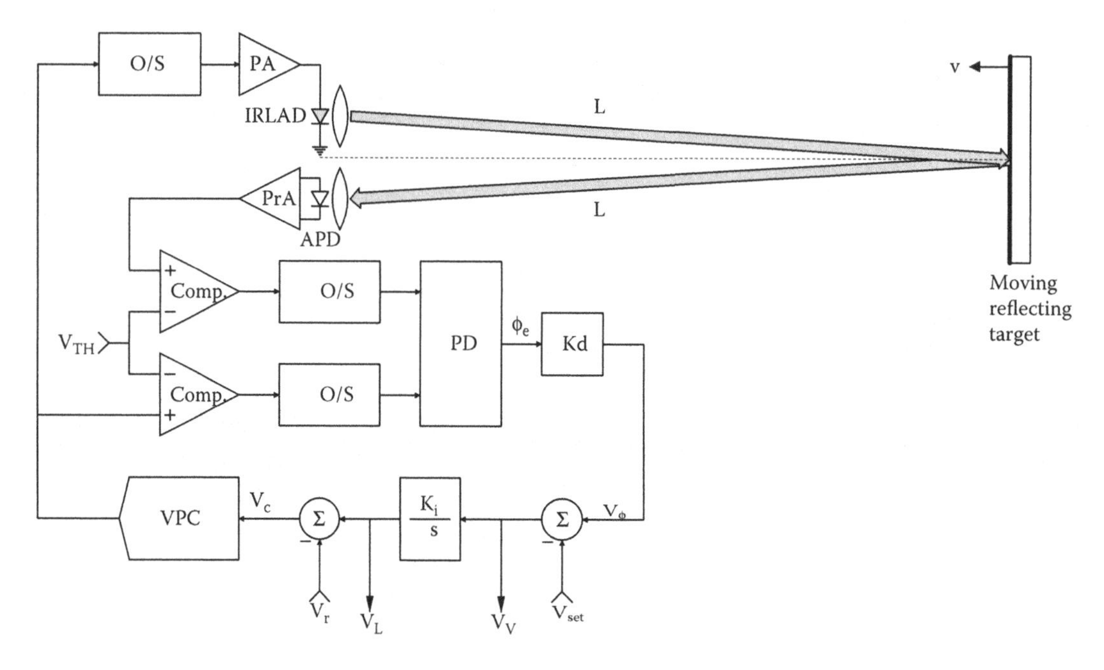

FIGURE 15.25 Block diagram of a closed-loop, constant-phase, pulsed laser velocimeter and ranging system devised by the author.

a preset phase lag is always maintained between the transmitted and received optical pulses. The system is unique in that it simultaneously outputs voltages proportional to both target range *and* velocity. The emitted radiation of this type of system can also be CW or pulsed sound or ultrasound, pulsed or amplitude-modulated microwaves, as well as photonic energy. Such systems have wide applications, ranging from medical diagnostics to weapons systems.

In the steady-state, for a fixed target range, L_o, the period (or frequency) output of the VPC oscillator reaches a value, so that a fixed phase lag, ϕ_m, exists between the received and transmitted signals. When $\phi_e = \phi_m$, the input to the integrator is zero, and the integrator output voltage, V_L, can be shown to be

$$V_L = K_R L_o \tag{15.37}$$

The range constant, K_R, is derived below.

If the reflecting object is moving at constant velocity, either directly away from or toward the transducers, $v = \pm dL/dt = \pm L$, then it is easy to show that the input voltage to the integrator, V_V, is given by

$$V_V = K_S v \tag{15.38}$$

If a VPC is used, K_S is independent of L. In this example, to facilitate heuristic analysis, we neglect the propagation delays inherent to logic elements and analog signal conditioning pathways. The type 1, feedback system shown in Figure 15.25 uses pulsed laser light to measure the distance L to a stationary reflective target (Nelson 1999). The nominal phase lag between received and transmitted pulses is simply

$$\phi_e = 360\ (2L/c)(1/T)\ \text{degrees} \tag{15.39}$$

where **c** is the velocity of light in m/s, T is the VPC output period, and (2L/c) is the round-trip time for a pulse reflected from the target.

The phase detector module produces an output voltage whose average value is

$$V_\phi = K_d\ \phi_e \tag{15.40}$$

K_d has the dimensions of volts/degree. A DC voltage, V_{set}, is subtracted from V_ϕ, so

$$V_V = V_\phi - V_{set} \tag{15.41}$$

V_V is the input to the integrator whose output, V_L, is added to $-V_r$ to give the input to the VPC, V_C. Because the closed-loop system is *type 1,* in the steady-state, $V_V \rightarrow 0$. Thus,

$$V_{set} = K_d\phi_m = K_d[360(2L/c)(1/T)] = K_d[360(2L/c)f] \tag{15.42}$$

Thus, the steady-state phase lag is simply

$$\phi_e = \phi_m = V_{set}/K_d \text{ degrees} \tag{15.43}$$

The VPC steady-state period is found from Equation 15.42 to be

$$T_{SS} = K_P V_C + b = \frac{720\ L}{c\ \phi_{mss}} \text{ seconds} \tag{15.44}$$

From Equation 15.44 above, the VPC input voltage is

$$V_C = \frac{720\ L}{c\ \phi_{mss}\ K_P} - b/K_P \text{ volts} \tag{15.45}$$

If we make $V_r = b/K_P$, then V_L is directly proportional to the range, L:

$$V_L = \frac{720}{c\ K_P(V_{set}/K_d)} L \text{ volts} \tag{15.46}$$

Now consider the situation where the reflecting target is approaching the transducers at constant velocity, **v** << **c**. Because $V_L = (K_i/s)\ V_V$, and $v = \dot{L}$, we can write in the time domain:

$$V_V = \dot{V}_o/K_i = v\frac{720\ K_d}{c\ K_P\ V_{set}\ K_i} \text{ volts} \tag{15.47}$$

Thus, a simple type 1, closed-loop, constant phase, feedback system can provide simultaneous voltage outputs that estimate target range and velocity in a linear manner.

Examine the system design with practical numbers: Let $\phi_m \equiv 10^\circ$, $K_i = 1$, and $K_P = 8.0E{-}6$ s/V, and 720/**c** = 2.40E−6. These numbers give a reasonable range sensitivity:

$$K_R = \frac{720}{c\ K_P\ \phi_{mss}} = 3.0E-2 \text{ volts/meter} \tag{15.48}$$

From Equation 15.47, the velocity sensitivity is also useful:

$$K_S = 2.40E-6\frac{1}{K_P\ \phi_{mss}\ K_i} = 3.0E-2 \text{ volts/m/s} \tag{15.49}$$

The steady-state output frequency of this VPC at a 1 m range is 4.17 MHz; when L = 100 m, it is 41.7 kHz.

15.4.6 Summary

We have seen that there are a variety of architectures for voltage-controlled oscillators, including "linear" VCOs using variable gain elements, switched integrating capacitor VCOs, and emitter-coupled, astable multivibrators. Versions of the latter architecture have been made to oscillate in the low GHz range. Another VHF-UHF VCO architecture (not shown here) makes use of the *varactor diode* (VD). The VD is a reverse biased, *pn* junction diode in which the diode depletion capacitance is controlled by the reverse bias voltage. This voltage-variable capacitance can be used to tune oscillators such as the familiar Hartley design, and to generate NBFM by adding the modulating signal to the reverse diode bias voltage.

VCOs are used in all phase-lock loops, and in FM communications applications, as well as many instrumentation systems.

The voltage-to-period converter (VPC) was introduced; this is a VCO in which the output oscillation's *period* is linearly proportional to the input voltage. The VPC was shown to be a useful circuit component in a closed-loop, constant phase, laser velocimeter, and ranging system. The same closed-loop, constant phase architecture can also be used with sound or ultrasound to simultaneously measure object range and velocity.

15.5 PHASE-LOCK LOOPS

15.5.1 Introduction

A phase-lock loop (PLL) (also called a phase-locked loop) is a closed-loop feedback system in which the phase of the PLL's periodic output is made to follow the phase of a periodic input signal. The closed-loop PLL system's natural frequencies are, in general, several orders of magnitude lower than the frequency of the input signal. Phase-lock loops have many applications in communications, control systems, and instrumentation systems. They can be used to modulate and demodulate narrow-band FM (NBFM) signals, demodulate double-sideband/suppressed carrier (DSBSC) signals, demodulate AM signals, generate a frequency-independent phase shift, measure frequencies including heart rate, synthesize signals used in digital communications systems, detect touch-tone frequencies and status signals used in telephony, control motor speed, etc.

The basic architecture of a PLL is shown in Figure 15.26a. It includes a phase (difference) detector (PD), a loop filter, a VCO (VFC), and sometimes a frequency divider in between the VCO and the PD. (Phase detectors were described in Section 15.3 of this text.) A phase detector returns an *average* voltage proportional to the phase difference between the input signal and the VCO output.

Analysis of PLL dynamics is done assuming lock, i.e., the input and VCO frequencies are equal. When a PLL first acquires its input signal, $f_1 \neq f_o$, and the loop must attain lock through a nonlinear process known as *acquisition*. The time required for acquisition is important in such PLL applications as telephone touch-tone decoding and the demodulation of FSK signals. Empirical formulas for acquisition times can be found in Northrop (1990) and in Gardiner (2005).

15.5.2 PLL Components

As mentioned earlier, phase detectors such as those used in PLLs were considered in Section 15.3. Most IC PLLs use PDs in which the analog input signal is effectively multiplied by a ±1 square wave derived from the VCO. This type of PD is a quadrature detector; the zero phase error condition requires that $\theta_1 - \theta_o = \pi/2$. Analog multiplier and exclusive OR PDs are also quadrature detectors. Only the RSFF PD and the MC 4044 PD are in-phase detectors. All PDs produce an analog output whose average value, V_ϕ, is either proportional to $\sin(\theta_e)$ or θ_e. When $|\theta_e| < 15°$, $\sin(\theta_e)$ can be replaced with θ_e in radians. Thus, for small-signal errors at lock, one can model the PLL by the linear block diagram in Figure 15.26b. Note that the VCO is modeled in the frequency domain by K_v/s. This is because $\omega_o = \mathbf{V}_c K_v$ r/s, and its output phase is the integral of its output frequency,

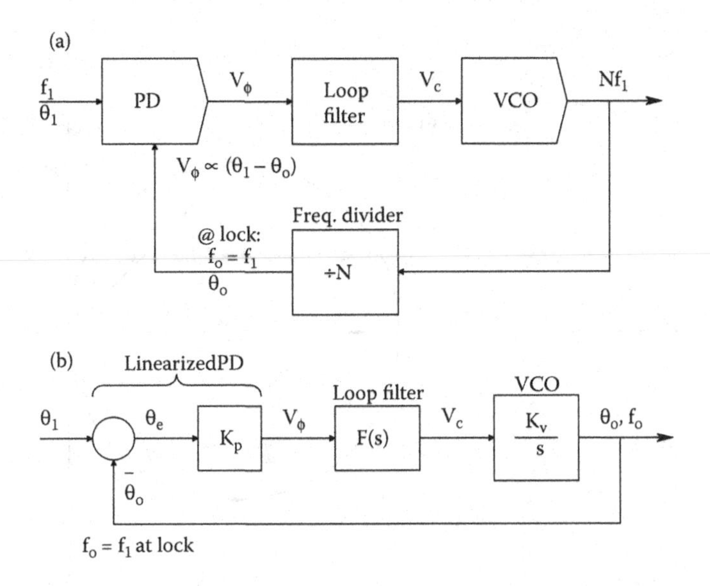

FIGURE 15.26 (a) Basic architecture of a phase-locked loop (PLL). (b) Systems block diagram of a PLL.

i.e., $\theta_o = \int \omega_o \, dt$. The PLL's dynamics in response to changes in θ_1 are determined in part by its closed-loop poles, which can be found from its linear loop gain using root locus techniques. The PLL's loop gain can be written as

$$A_L(s) = -\frac{K_P K_V F(s)}{s} \tag{15.50}$$

If $F(s) = K_f(s + a)/s$, then the loop gain function has a zero at $\mathbf{s} = -a$, and two poles at the origin. Its root locus is the well-known circle, shown in Figure 15.27. Effective design of this PLL wants the closed-loop poles at $\mathbf{s} = -a \pm ja$. This gives a damping factor of $\xi = 0.707$, and an undamped natural frequency of $\omega_n = a\sqrt{2}$ r/s. The scalar gain product, $K_p K_f K_v$, is adjusted to obtain these closed-loop parameters. It can be shown that $K_p K_f K_v = 2a$ will put the closed-loop poles at $\mathbf{s} = -a \pm ja$ (Northrop 1990).

The PLL's loop filter is generally low-pass, and can be of the form: $F(s) = K_f/(s/b + 1)$, $= K_f (s + a)/s$, $= K_f(s/a + 1)/(s/b + 1)$, etc. The loop filter is generally chosen to give the PLL the desired dynamic response in tracking changes in the input phase, θ_1.

The PLL's VCO can have a digital (TTL) or sinusoidal output. The VCO used on IC PLLs often uses the voltage-controlled, emitter-coupled, astable multivibrator architecture (see above).

15.5.3 PLL Applications in Biomedicine

One application of a PLL is to measure heart rate (f_H). Figure 15.28 illustrates the block diagram of a 4046 CMOS PLL used as a *cardiotachometer* (Northrop 1990). The loop filter's transfer function is found from the voltage-divider relation:

$$\frac{V_c}{V_\phi} = \frac{R_2 + 1/sC}{R_1 + R_2 + 1/sC} = \frac{sCR_2 + 1}{sC(R_1 + R_2) + 1} \tag{15.51}$$

Similarly, the output transfer function is

$$\frac{V_o}{V_\phi} = \frac{1/sC}{R_1 + R_2 + 1/sC} = \frac{1}{sC(R_1 + R_2) + 1} \tag{15.52}$$

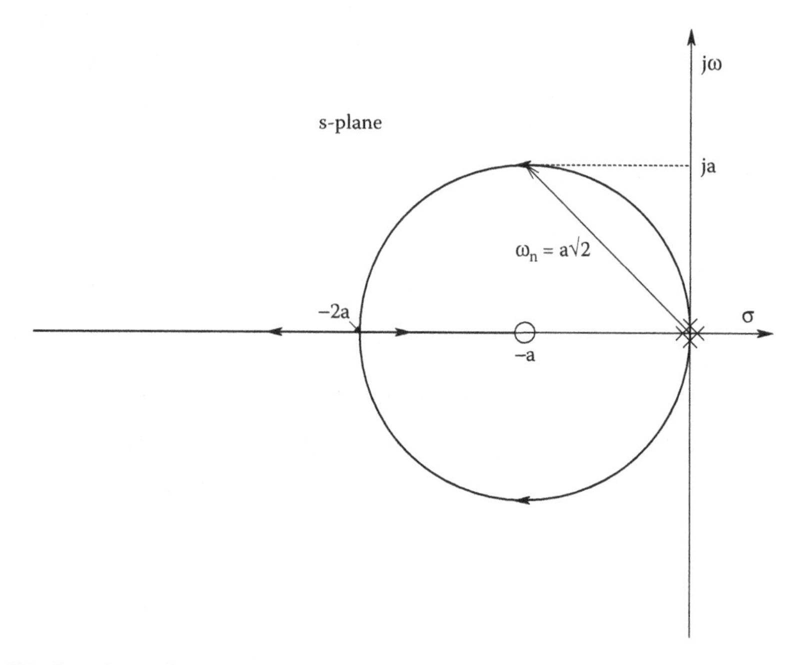

FIGURE 15.27 Root locus diagram of a PLL having a loop filter of the form, $F(s) = K_f (s + a)/s$.

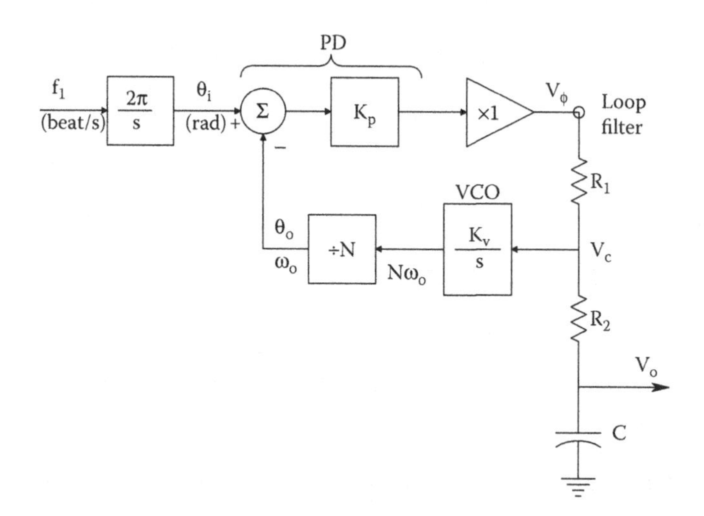

FIGURE 15.28 Block diagram of a PLL used as a heart rate monitor. The analog V_o is proportional to the average heart rate.

The PLL's loop gain is

$$A_L(s) = -\frac{K_pK_v(sCR_2 + 1)}{N\, s[sC(R_1 + R_2) + 1]} = -\frac{K_pK_vCR_2(s + 1/CR_2)}{NC(R_1 + R_2)\; s\; [s + 1/C(R_1 + R_2)]} \tag{15.53}$$

The PLL's transfer function is thus

$$\frac{V_o}{f_H} = \frac{(2\pi/s)\, K_p/C(R_1 + R_2)}{[1 - A_L(s)][s + 1/C(R_1 + R_2)]} = \frac{2\pi N/K_v}{s^2NC(R_1 + R_2)/K_pK_v + s[N + K_pK_vCR_2]/K_pK_v + 1} \tag{15.54}$$

The denominator of Equation 15.54 is of the standard quadratic form: $s^2/\omega_n^2 + s\,2\xi/\omega_n + 1$. Thus,

$$\omega_n = \sqrt{\frac{K_pK_v}{NC(R_1+R_2)}}\ \text{r/s and}\ \xi = \frac{N+K_pK_vR_2C}{2\sqrt{NC(R_1+R_2)K_pK_v}} \tag{15.55}$$

Examine the system's ω_n, ξ, and DC gain, given the typical circuit parameters: $K_p = 8.33$, $K_v = 3.14$, $N = 4$, $C = 1.$ E–5, $R_1 = 62k$, $R_2 = 150k$. These values yield the following: $\omega_n = 1.76$ r/s, $\xi = 1.45$ (overdamped), DC gain $V_o/f_H = 8.00$ volts/beat/s = 0.133 volts/beat/min. Note that ω_n and the damping ξ are measures of the PLL's response dynamics to *changes* in the heart rate, f_H beats/s.

In a second example of PLL applications, Figure 15.29 illustrates the block diagram of a PLL used to generate a *frequency-independent phase shift* between the input signal and the VCO output. This application is important in maximizing the output of a phase-sensitive rectifier or lock-in amplifier. The PLL's loop gain is

$$A_L(s) = -\frac{K_pK_fK_v(s+a)}{s^2} \tag{15.56}$$

If the reference phase input, $\theta_1 = 0$, we can write the transfer function between θ_o and V_p:

$$\frac{\theta_o}{V_p} = \frac{K_fK_v(s+a)}{s^2 + sK_pK_fK_v + aK_pK_fK_v} \tag{15.57}$$

The undamped natural frequency of this PLL is $\omega_n = \sqrt{a\,K_pK_fK_v}$ r/s and its damping factor is $\xi = \sqrt{K_pK_fK_v}/(2\sqrt{a})$. These parameters relate to the system's response to changes in the phase-shifting voltage, V_p, and have nothing to do with the input carrier frequency, ω_1. The steady-state phase-shift at lock is simply: $\theta_{oss} = V_p/K_p$.

In a third example of PLL applications, a *tone decoder* is examined, such as used in telephony. This is a PLL-based system that outputs a logic HI when a sinusoidal signal is present at its input having a frequency f_1 within some $\pm\Delta f_c$. Tone decoders are used in emergency response radios (for first responders; EMTs, firemen) to gate transmission of alert messages, as well as in digital telephony.

Note that $f_1/\Delta f_c$ defines a "capture Q" for the tone decoder. Figure 15.30 illustrates the block diagram of a tone decoder PLL. Note that this system uses two phase detectors of the quadrature (multiplicative) type. In the absence of a sinusoidal input signal, x_1, $V_c \to 0$, and the VCO output frequency is by design $\omega_o = b = 2\pi(440)$ r/s. Also, x_6 = LO. The PLL acquires lock if the input sinusoid, $x_1 = A\sin(\omega_1 t)$, lies within the capture range of $\pm\Delta\omega_c$ around ω_1. Once the loop acquires lock, and $x_2 = B\cos(\omega_1 t)$. $x_3 = B\sin(\omega_1 t)$, and $x_4 = x_3 x_1 = (AB/2)[\cos(0) - \cos(2\omega_1 t)]$. After the LPF, $x_5 = AB/2$, and $x_6 = 1$ (HI). It can be shown that lock occurs when the input frequency ω_1 lies in the capture range, given by

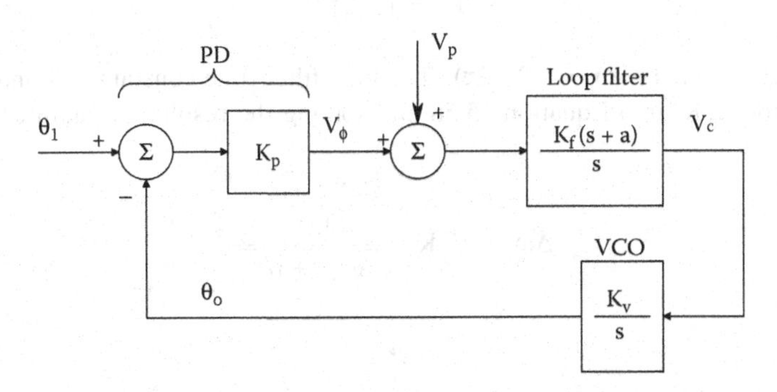

FIGURE 15.29 Block diagram of a PLL used to generate a frequency-independent phase shift. $(\theta_i - \theta_o) \propto V_p$.

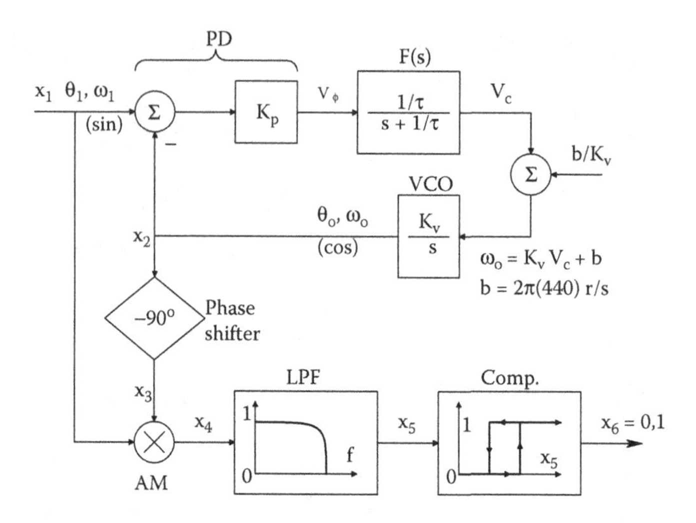

FIGURE 15.30 Block diagram of a (tuned or frequency-selective) audio tone decoder PLL.

$$\Delta\omega_c = 2\pi\Delta f_c \equiv K_T |F(j\Delta\omega_c)| \tag{15.58}$$

where $|\mathbf{F}(j\Delta\omega_c)|$ is the loop filter's gain magnitude at $\omega = \Delta\omega_c$ r/s, $F(s) = (1/\tau)/(s + 1/\tau)$, and $K_T \equiv K_p K_v \mathbf{F}(0)$.

The lock range of input frequency over which the PLL will maintain lock is given by $\Delta\omega_L = K_T > \Delta\omega_c$. Thus, the tone decoder PLL behaves like a nonlinear tuned filter.

To design the system to respond to A_{440} to within ±1%, the PLL must acquire $f_1 = 440 \pm 4.4$ Hz. Thus, $\Delta f_c = 8.8$ Hz. It is also necessary that the loop damping factor be $\xi = 0.707$. The PLL's loop gain is simply

$$A_L(s) = -\frac{K_p K_v/\tau}{s(s + 1/\tau)} \tag{15.59}$$

From $A_L(s)$, using the *root locus* technique, the value of the gain product $K_p K_v$ required to put the PLL's closed loop poles at $\mathbf{s}^* = -1/2\tau \pm j/2\tau$ can be found (see Figure 15.31). The RL magnitude criterion tells us

$$K_p K_v/\tau = [\sqrt{2}/(2\tau)]^2$$
$$\downarrow \tag{15.60}$$
$$K_p K_v = 1/(2\tau)$$

Also, from the RL geometry, $\omega_n = \sqrt{2}/(2\tau)$. The loop filter time constant is found by substituting Equation 12.60 for $K_p K_v$ into Equation 15.58 and solving the resultant quadratic equation for τ^2, hence τ. Thus,

$$\Delta\omega_c = K_p K_v \frac{1/\tau}{\sqrt{\Delta\omega_c^2 + 1/\tau^2}} \tag{15.61}$$

$$\downarrow$$

$$\tau^4 + \tau^2/\Delta\omega_c^2 - 1/(4\Delta\omega_c^4) = 0 \tag{15.62}$$

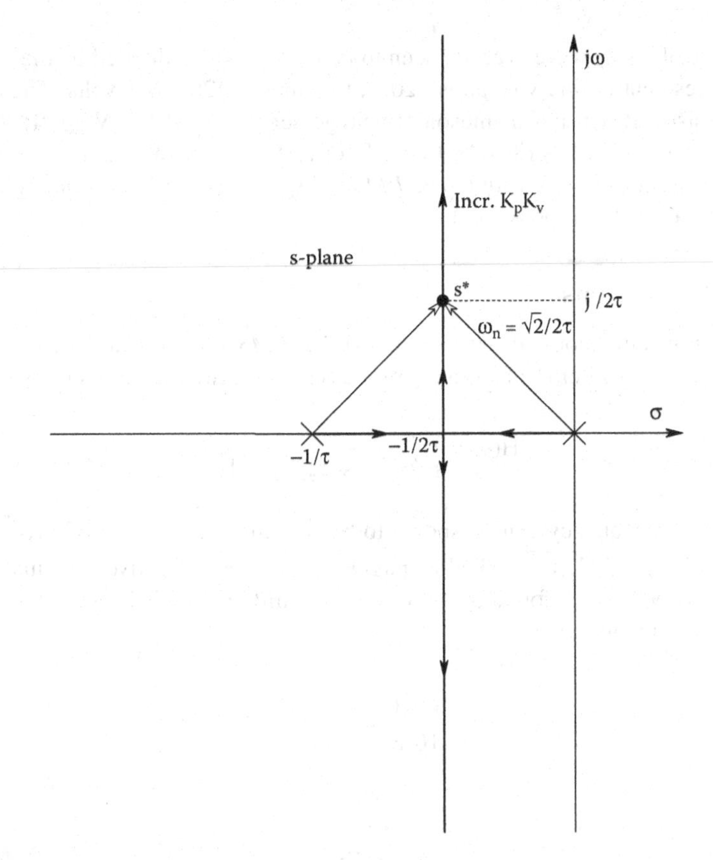

FIGURE 15.31 Root locus diagram for the PLL tone decoder.

When $\Delta\omega_c = 2\pi(8.8) = 55.292$ r/s is substituted into Equation 15.62, one finds $\tau = 8.231 \times 10^{-3}$ s, $\omega_n = 85.91$ r/s, and $K_p K_v = K_T = 60.75$ r/s.

The NE/SE567 tone decoder PLL IC (by Philips Semiconductors Linear Products) data sheets contain a wealth of design and operating information in graphical form, including the greatest number of input cycles in a tone burst before the PLL acquires the input and goes high.

15.5.4 Discussion

PLLs are versatile systems with wide applications in communications, control, and instrumentation. We have only scratched the surface of this topic in this section. The interested reader is encouraged to examine the many texts dealing with the design and applications of this ubiquitous IC. See for example the texts by Egan (2007), Gardner (2005), Northrop (1990, Chapter 11), Gray and Meyer (1984, Chapter 10), and Blanchard (1976).

15.6 TRUE RMS CONVERTERS

15.6.1 Introduction

The analog true RMS converter is a system that provides a DC output proportional to the *root-mean-square* of the input signal, $v_1(t)$. An analog RMS operation first squares $v_1(t)$ then estimates the mean value of $v_1^2(t)$, generally by time averaging by low-pass filtering. Finally, the square root of the mean squared value, $\sqrt{\overline{v_1^2(t)}}$, is taken.

The RMS value of a sine wave is easily seen to be its peak value divided by the $\sqrt{2}$. When one says that the US residential line voltage is 120 V, this means 120 RMS volts. The average power dissipated in a resistor R that has a sinusoidal voltage across it is $P_{av} = (V_{rms})^2/R$ Watts. Random signals and noise can also be described by their MS or RMS values. In fact, noise voltages are often characterized by measuring them with a *true RMS voltmeter.* In fact, it is meaningless to measure random noise with a rectifier-type AC meter.

15.6.2 True RMS Circuits

Figure 15.32 illustrates the block diagram of an *explicit RMS system* using analog multipliers and op amp ICs. The low-pass filter (LPF) is a quadratic Sallen & Key design. Its transfer function is

$$H(s) = \frac{1}{s^2/\omega_n^2 + s(2\xi)/\omega_n + 1} \quad (15.63)$$

Its undamped natural frequency can be shown to be (Northrop 2005) $\omega_n = 1/(R\sqrt{C_1C_2})$ r/s, and its damping factor is $\xi = \sqrt{(C_2/C_1)}$. The low-pass filtering action effectively estimates the mean of $v_1^2(t)/10$. The output, V_o, can be found by assuming the third op amp is ideal, and writing the node equation for its summing junction:

$$\frac{\overline{v_1^2(t)}}{10\,R} = \frac{V_o^2}{10\,R} \quad (15.64)$$

Thus, V_o is simply

$$V_o = \sqrt{\overline{v_1^2(t)}}, \quad (15.65)$$

the RMS value of $v_1(t)$. Note that this analog square root circuit requires that $\overline{v_1^2(t)} \geq 0$, which it is.

Another (implicit) true RMS (TRMS) circuit can be made from an analog IC known as a *multifunction converter* (MFC). A MFC, such as the Burr-Brown 4302, computes the analog function,

$$V_2 = V_Y(V_Z/V_X)m, \;\; 5 \geq m \geq 1, \; 0 \leq (V_x,\; V_y,\; V_Z) \leq 10\text{ V}. \quad (15.66)$$

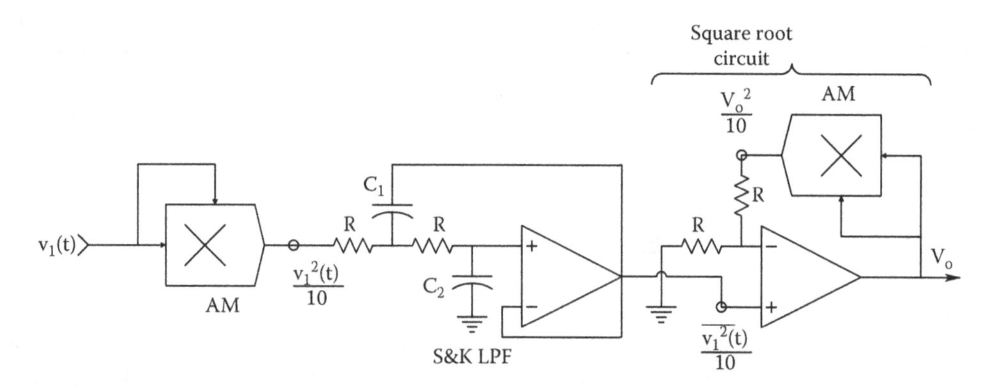

FIGURE 15.32 An analog circuit that finds the true RMS value of the input voltage, $v_1(t)$. Two analog multipliers (AMs) are used.

From the circuit of Figure 15.33, note that the R-C LPF acts as an averager of $V_2 = V_1^2/V_o$. Thus, we can write the identity:

$$V_o = \overline{V_1^2/V_o} \tag{15.67}$$

From which, it is clear that

$$V_o^2 = \overline{V_1^2} \ \text{MSV} \tag{15.68}$$

and V_o is the RMS value of V_1.

The RMS voltage of a signal can also be found using *vacuum thermocouple* (VTC) elements, as shown in Figure 15.34. The vacuum thermocouple consists of a thin heater wire of resistance R_{Ho} at a reference temperature, T_A (say 25°C) inside of an evacuated glass envelope. Electrically insulated from, but thermally intimate with R_H is a *thermocouple junction* (TJ) (Lion 1959; Pallàs-Areny and Webster 2001; Northrop 2005). For example, the venerable Western Electric model 20D VTC has $R_H = 35\Omega$ at room temperature, the nominal thermocouple resistance (Fe and constantan wires) is 12 Ω. The maximum heater current is 16 mA RMS (exceed this and the heater melts). The 20D VTC

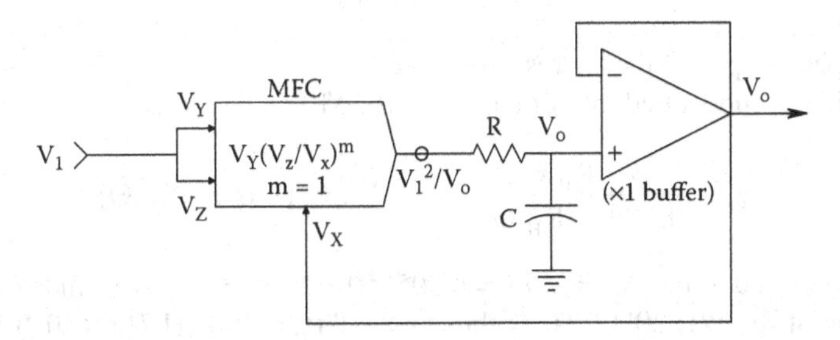

FIGURE 15.33 A true RMS conversion circuit using a multifunction converter (MFC).

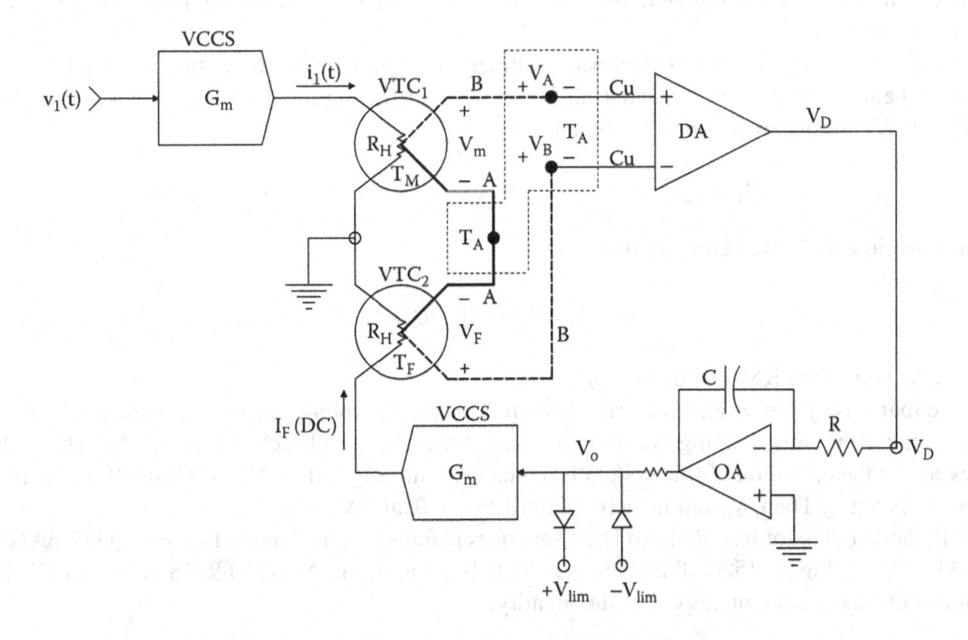

FIGURE 15.34 A feedback, vacuum thermocouple, true RMS voltmeter (or ammeter). The integrator in the feedback loop ensures zero steady-state error between V_F and V_m (a type 1 feedback system).

has an open-circuit, DC output voltage $V_o = 0.005$ V when $I_H = 0.007$ A RMS. Because the heater temperature is proportional to the average power dissipated in the heater, or the *mean squared current* × R_H, this VTC produces $K_T = 0.005/[(0.007)^2 \times 35] = 2.915$ Volts/Watt, or mV/mW. The EMF of the TJ is given in general by the truncated power series:

$$V_J = A(\Delta T) + B(\Delta T)^2/2 + C(\Delta T)^3/3 \cong S\,\Delta T \tag{15.69}$$

where ΔT is the difference in junction temperature above the *ambient temperature,* T_A. S for an iron/constant (Fe/CN) TC = 50×10^{-6} V/°C. In a VTC, $\Delta T = T_H - T_A$. T_H is the heater resistor temperature as the result of Joule's law heating. The steady-state DT can be described by

$$T = \overline{i_h^2} R_H \Theta \tag{15.70}$$

The electrical power dissipated in the heater element is given by the mean-squared current in the heater times the heater resistance. Q is the thermal resistance of the heater *in vacuo;* its units are degrees C/Watt. This relation is not that simple because R_H increases with increasing temperature. This effect can be approximated by

$$R_H = R_{Ho}(1 + \alpha \Delta T) \tag{15.71}$$

where α is the alpha tempco of the R_H resistance wire.

If Equation 15.71 is substituted into Equation 15.70, ΔT can be solved for

$$\Delta T = \frac{\overline{i_1^2}\, R_{Ho}\Theta}{1 - \alpha[\overline{i_1^2}\, R_{Ho}\Theta]} \cong \overline{i_1^2}\, R_{Ho}\Theta[1 + \alpha\, \overline{i_1^2}\, R_{Ho}\Theta] \tag{15.72}$$

Assuming R_H remains constant, $\Delta T = V_J/S = 0.005/(50 \times 10^{-6}) = 100$°C from Equation 15.69. The thermal resistance of the WE 20D VTC is thus $\Theta = \Delta T/P_H = 100^o/(1.715 \times 10^{-3})$ W = 5.831×10^4 °C/W. This thermal resistance is large because of the vacuum. Note that high Θ gives increased VTC sensitivity.

In the feedback TRMS meter, the TC EMF is found by substituting Equation 15.72 into Equation 15.69.

Examination of the TRMS TC feedback voltmeter of Figure 15.34 shows that it is a self-nulling system. At equilibrium, $V_F = V_m$, and it can be shown from the thermoelectric laws that $V_A - V_B = 0$, so $V_D = 0$. V_F and V_m are given approximately by

$$V_F \cong A[I_F^2 R_{Ho}\Theta] = A[(V_o G_m)^2 R_{Ho}\Theta] = V_m \cong A[\overline{(v_1(t) G_m)^2} R_{Ho}\Theta] \tag{15.73}$$

From Equation 15.73, we can write that

$$V_o(DC) = \sqrt{\overline{[v_1^2(t)]}} \tag{15.74}$$

That is, V_o equals the RMS value of $v_1(t)$.

Note that this system is an even-error system. That is, the voltage V_F is independent of the sign of V_o because the same heating occurs regardless if the sign (or phase) of I_F in R_H. Not shown but necessary to the operation of this system is a means of initially setting $V_o \to 0$ just before the measurement is made. Then, V_o and I_F increase until $V_D \to 0$, and $V_m = V_F$.

Still another class of true RMS to DC converters is found in the Analog Devices' AD536A/ 636 and AD637 ICs. Figure 15.35 illustrates the block diagram of the AD637 TRMS converter IC. The front end of this system makes use of the identity:

$$v_1^2 = |v_1|^2 \geq 0 \tag{15.75}$$

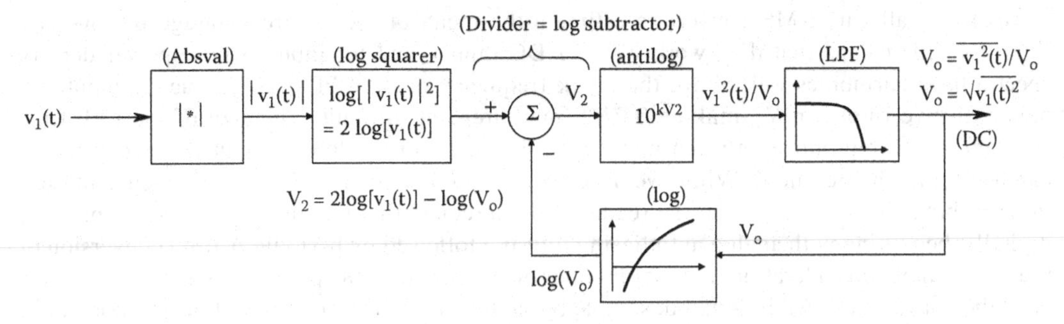

FIGURE 15.35 Simplified block diagram of the Analog Devices' AD637 true analog RMS conversion IC.

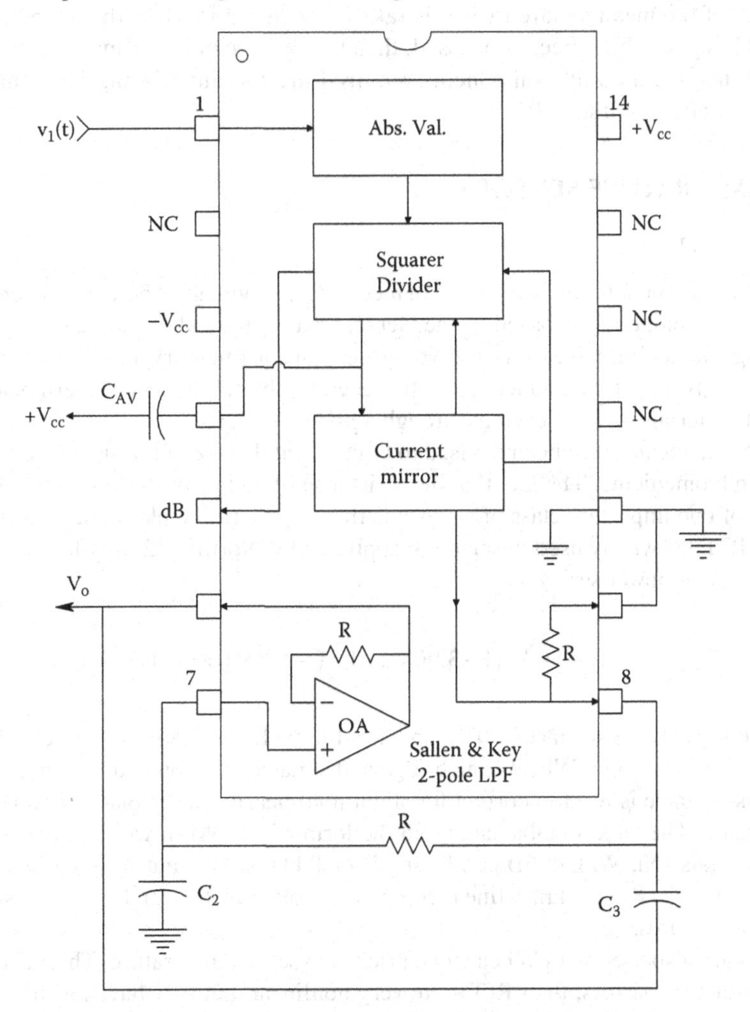

FIGURE 15.36 Block diagram of functions on the AD536 true RMS converter chip.

Squaring is done by taking the logarithm of $|v_1|$ and doubling it. Division by V_o is accomplished by subtracting the log of the DC output voltage, V_o, from $2\log(v_1)$ giving V_2, which is antilogged to recover $v_1^2(t)/V_o$. $v_1^2(t)/V_o$ is low-pass filtered to produce the implicitly derived, DC, RMS output voltage from $v_1(t)$. Figure 15.36 illustrates the organization of the TRMS subsystems in the AD536 TRMS converter. A two-pole, Sallen & Key low-pass filter is used to give a smooth DC output in this configuration (Kitchin and Counts 1983).

Note that all true RMS converters estimate the mean of the squared voltage by low-pass filtering. This means that they work well for DC inputs, and for inputs whose power density spectra have harmonics well above the break frequency of the LPF. Low-frequency input signals will give ripple on V_o, making TRMS measurement difficult. The size of the LPF time constant is a compromise between meter settling time and the lowest input frequency which can be accurately measured. While we have concentrated on analog electronic systems and ICs in describing TRMS conversion, the reader will appreciate that the entire process can be done digitally, beginning with analog antialiasing filtering followed by periodic A-to-D conversion of the signal under consideration. A finite number of samples (a data epoch) are stored in an array. Next the converted signal is squared, sample by sample, and the results stored in a second array. The squared samples are then numerically low-pass filtered to estimate their mean. The numerical square root of the mean squared value is taken and stored for the kth epoch. The process is repeated until M epochs have been processed, then the average of M estimates of the RMS signal is finally calculated. The only components required are the antialiasing LPF, an ADC, some interface chips, and of course, a PC.

15.7 IC TEMPERATURE SENSORS

15.7.1 Introduction

Temperature measurement is very important in medicine and biology. There have been many means devised to measure temperature, based on the fact that many physical phenomena vary with temperature, including, but not limited to: physical volume expansion (mercury and alcohol thermometers), resistance of metals and semiconductors, EMF generated by the Seebeck (thermoelectric) effect, permittivity of materials, reverse current through a *pn* junction, etc.

Many electronic means have been devised to circumvent the use of the slow (and toxic) mercury thermometer in biomedicine. The fact that the resistance of metals *increases* with temperature has been the basis of one important class of electronic thermometer. The platinum *resistance temperature detector* (RTD) is widely used in scientific applications (Northrop 2005). Its resistance is modeled by the truncated power series:

$$R(T) = R_o[1 + 3.908 \times 10^{-3} T - 5.8 \times 10^{-7} T^2] \tag{15.76}$$

where R_o is the Pt RTD's resistance at 0°C, and T is the RTD's temperature in °C. RTD resistance changes are sensed by using a Wheatstone bridge and suitable electronic amplification.

Often a look-up table is used to correct for slight nonlinearity in the platinum RTD's resistance vs T characteristic. The look-up table can be in the form of a ROM in which correction values are stored. Other metals (Ni, W, Cu, Si) can be used for RTD design, but Pt is the one most widely encountered because its R(T) is fairly linear compared to other metals, and it can be used at elevated (industrial) temperatures.

Thermistors are also used with Wheatstone bridges to sense temperature. Thermistors are amorphous semiconductor resistors; their R(T)s are very nonlinear, but they have much greater thermal sensitivity compared to metal RTDs. The resistance of a *negative temperature coefficient* (NTC) *thermistor* is modeled by the relation (Northrop 2005):

$$R(T) = R_o \exp[\beta(1/T - 1/T_o)] \tag{15.77}$$

where R_o is the thermistor's resistance at temperature T_o, and the reference temperature T_o in degrees Kelvin is generally equal to 273 + 25 = 298°K. T is also in °K (Pallás-Areny and Webster 1991).

The alpha temperature coefficient of a resistor is defined by

$$\alpha \equiv \frac{dR(T)/dT}{R(T)} \tag{15.78}$$

Applying Equations 15.78 to 15.77, an expression for the alpha tempco of a NTC thermistor is found:

$$\alpha = -\beta/T^2 \tag{15.79}$$

β is typically 4000°K, and for T = 300°K, $\alpha = -0.044$. By contrast, the α tempco of Pt is +0.00392. It should be remarked that there are also PTC thermistors. The author has used NTC thermistors to measure ΔTs on the order of 0.0005°C in *in vitro* chemical assays of blood glucose using the enzyme glucose oxidase.

Other electrical/electronic means of temperature measurement use the minute DC voltages generated by thermocouples, and thermocouple arrays called *thermopiles* used for photonic radiation power measurements. The interested reader should consult texts by Northrop (2005), Pallàs-Areny and Webster (2001), and Lion (1959), for further details on thermocouples and thermopiles.

Still other temperature measurement devices have been invented that measure the long-wave, infrared (LIR) blackbody radiation from the eardrum. This class of fever thermometer is characterized by a fast response time (seconds), a minimally invasive implementation (inserted in the ear canal), and reasonable expense. The primary sensor is either a thermopile, or a *pyroelectric material* (PYM) (such as triglicine sulfate or barium titanate) that responds to changes in the long-wave IR emitted from the eardrum by generating a small voltage change. Further details on the operation of the Thermo-scanÔ ear thermometers can be found in Northrop (2002).

15.7.2 IC Temperature Sensors

Figure 15.37 illustrates a simplified schematic of the Analog Devices' AD590 *temperature-controlled current source* (TCCS). AD also makes the AD592 precision TCCS, which uses basically the same circuit. These ICs behave as two-terminal, 1 μA/°K current sources using supply voltages between $+4 \leq V_{cc} \leq +30$ V. Analog Devices (1994) gave the following circuit description for the AD590:

> The AD590 uses a fundamental property of the silicon transistors from which it is made to realize its temperature proportional characteristic: If two identical transistors are operated at a constant ratio of collector current densities, r, then the difference in their base-emitter voltages will be (kT/q)ln(r). Since both k, Boltzmann's constant and q, the charge of an electron, are constant, the resulting voltage is directly proportional to absolute temperature (PTAT). In the AD590, this PTAT voltage is converted to a PTAT current by low temperature coefficient thin film resistors. The total current of the device is then forced to be a multiple of this PTAT current. Referring to Figure 15.37, the schematic diagram of the AD590, Q8 and Q11 are the transistors that produce the PTAT voltage. R5 and R6 convert the voltage to current. Q10, whose collector current tracks the collector currents in Q9 and Q11, supplies all the bias and substrate leakage current for the rest of the circuit, forcing the total current to be PTAT. R5 and R6 are laser trimmed on the wafer to calibrate the device at +25°C.

The AD590 temperature-to-current transducer can operate over a –55 to + 150°C range, and the AD592 operates over a –25 to + 105°C range. There are many applications for these electronic TCCSs. Figure 15.38 illustrates a simple op amp circuit that converts 1 μA/°K to 100 mV/°C. A *chopper-stabilized op amp* (CHSOA) is used for a low DC drift tempco. The trim pots are used to exactly calibrate the amplifier so it has zero gain and offset error at the design temperature, e.g., 37°C.

Note that National Semiconductor also makes IC temperature sensors. The National LM135 series of sensors behave as temperature-controlled voltage drops (much like a Zener diode). They give 10 mV/°K drop with ca. 1 Ω dynamic resistance for DC currents ranging from 400 μA to 5 mA.

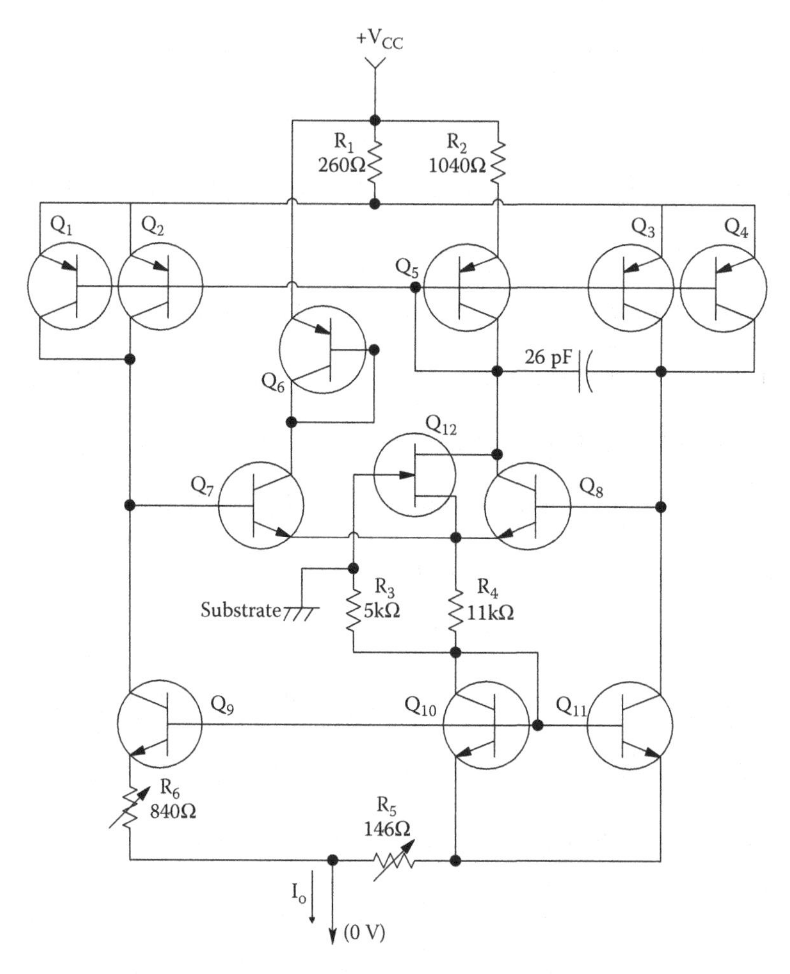

FIGURE 15.37 A simplified schematic of the Analog Devices' AD590 analog temperature-controlled current source (TCCS) temperature sensor.

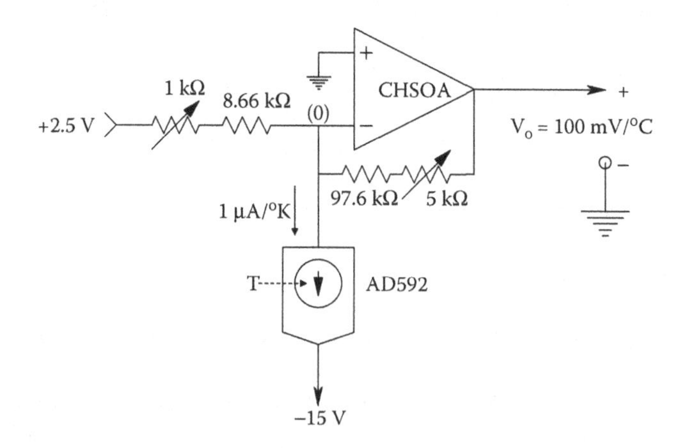

FIGURE 15.38 A simple op amp current-to-voltage converter that converts the current output of an AD592 temperature sensor to 100 mV/°C analog voltage output.

They cover a wide, –55 to +150°C range. The National LM135 precision Celsius temperature sensor is a three terminal device that outputs an EMF of 10 mV/°C over a –55 to + 150°C range, given a supply voltage from 4 to 30 VDC.

15.8 THREE EXAMPLES OF MEDICAL INSTRUMENTATION SYSTEMS

15.8.1 Introduction

The previous sections of this chapter have described and analyzed the characteristics of selected, specialized ICs useful in designing biomedical instrumentation systems. In this section, three examples of biomedical instrumentation systems taken from the author's research and that of some of his graduate students are examined. In each system, the extensive use will be found of op amps for various linear and nonlinear subsystems.

15.8.2 Self-Nulling, Microdegree Polarimeter

A *polarimeter* is an instrument used to measure the change in the angle of rotation of *linearly polarized light* when it is passed through an *optically active material.* There are many types of polarimeters, and there are a number of optically active substances found in living systems; probably, the most important physiologically is dissolved D-glucose. Clear biological liquids such as urine, blood plasma, fresh saliva, and the aqueous humor of the eyes contain dissolved D-glucose whose molar concentration is proportional to the blood glucose concentration (Northrop 2002). Using polarimetry, the d-glucose concentration can be measured using the simple relation:

$$\phi = [\alpha]_\lambda{}^T CL \text{ degrees} \tag{15.80}$$

where ϕ is the measured optical rotation of *linearly polarized light* (LPL) of wavelength λ passed through a sample chamber of length L containing the optically active analyte at concentration C and temperature T.

The constant $[\alpha]_\lambda{}^T$ is called the *specific optical rotation* parameter of the analyte; its units are generally in degrees per (optical path length unit × concentration unit). $[\alpha]_\lambda{}^T$ for d-glucose in 25°C water and at 512 nm is 0.0695 millidegrees/(cm × g/deciliter). Thus, the optical rotation of a 1 g/liter solution of D-glucose in a 10 cm cell is 69.5 millidegrees. Note that $[\alpha]_\lambda{}^T$ can have either sign, depending on the analyte, and if N optically active substances are present in the sample chamber, the *net optical rotation* is given by superposition:

$$\phi = L \sum_{k=1}^{N} [\alpha_k]_\lambda{}^T C_k \tag{15.81}$$

To describe how a polarimeter works, it is necessary to first describe what is meant by linearly polarized light. When light from an incoherent source such as a tungsten lamp is treated as an electromagnetic wave phenomenon (rather than photons), we observe that the propagating radiation is composed of a broad spectrum of wavelengths and polarization states. To facilitate the description of LPL, let us examine a monochromatic ray propagating in the z-direction (at the speed of light v_z in the medium in which it is traveling). This velocity in the z-direction is $v_z = c/n$ m/s. c is the velocity of light *in vacuo,* and n is the *refractive index* of the propagation medium (generally > 1.0). A beam of monochromatic light can have a variety of polarization states, including *random* (unpolarized), *circular* (CW or CCW), *elliptical,* and *linear* (Balanis 1989). Figure 15.39 illustrates a LPL ray in which the **E**-vector propagates entirely in the x-z plane, and its orthogonal $\mathbf{B}_y$-vector lies in the y-z plane. **E** and **B** are in-phase. Both vectors are functions of time and distance. For the $\mathbf{E}_x(t, z)$ vector,

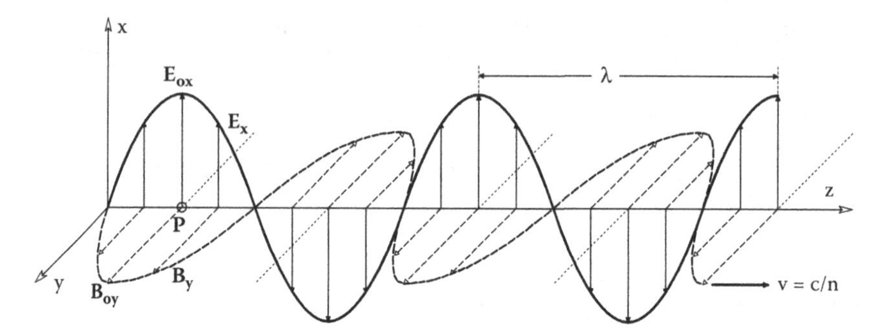

FIGURE 15.39 Diagram of a linearly polarized electromagnetic wave (e.g., light) propagating in the +z direction. $\mathbf{B}_y(t)$ is orthogonal in space to $\mathbf{E}_x(t)$.

$$E_x(t, z) = E_{ox} \cos\left[\frac{2\pi v_z}{\lambda} t - \frac{2\pi}{\lambda} z\right] \tag{15.82}$$

Note that the **E**-vector need not lie in the x–z plane; its plane of propagation can be tilted some angle θ with respect to the x-axis, and still propagate in the z-direction (the orthogonal **B** vector is also rotated θ with respect to the y-axis). When describing LPL, we examine the positive maximums of the **E**-vector and make a vector with this maximum and at an angle θ with the x-axis in the x–y plane.

Figure 15.40 illustrates what happens when LPL of wavelength λ passes though a sample chamber containing an optically active analyte. Polarizer P_1 converts the input light to a linearly polarized beam, which is passed through the sample chamber. As the result of the interaction of the light with the optically active solute, the emergent LPL ray is rotated by an angle, θ. In this figure, the analyte is *dextrorotary,* that is, the emergent **E**-vector, $\mathbf{E_2}$, is *rotated clockwise* when *viewed in the direction of photon propagation* (along the +z-axis) (Sears 1949). Note that D-glucose is dextrorotary. To measure the optical rotation of the sample, a second polarizer, P_2, is rotated until a null in the light intensity striking the photosensor is noted (in its simplest form, the photosensor can be a human eye). This null is when P_2's pass axis is orthogonal to $E_2 \angle \theta$. Since polarizer P_1 is set with its pass axis aligned with the x-axis (i.e., at 0°) it is easy to find θ, thence the concentration of the optically active analyte, [G]. In the simple polarimeter of Figure 15.40, and other polarimeters, the polarizers are generally made from calcite crystals (Glan calcite), and have an *extinction ratio* of ca. 10^4. (Extinction ratio is the ratio of LPL intensity passing through the polarizer when the LPL's polarization axis is aligned with the polarizer's pass axis, to the intensity of the emergent beam when the polarization axis is made 90° (is orthogonal) to the polarizer's axis.)

To make an electronic polarimeter, we need an electrical means of nulling the polarimeter output, as opposed to physically rotating P_2 around the z-axis. One means of generating an electrically controlled optical rotation is to use the *Faraday magneto-optical effect.* Figure 15.41 illustrates a *Faraday Rotator* (FR). A FR has two major components: (1) A magneto-optically (M-O) active medium. Many transparent gasses, liquids and solids exhibit magneto-optical activity, e.g., a lead glass rod with optically flat ends, or a glass test chamber with optically flat ends containing an M-O gas or liquid can be used. (2) A solenoidal coil wound around the rod or test chamber that generates an axial magnetic field, $\mathbf{B_z}$, inside the rod or chamber collinear with the entering LPL beam. The exiting LPL beam undergoes optical rotation according to the simple Faraday relation (Hecht 1987):

$$\theta_m = V(\lambda, T)\, \overline{B_z}\, l \tag{15.83}$$

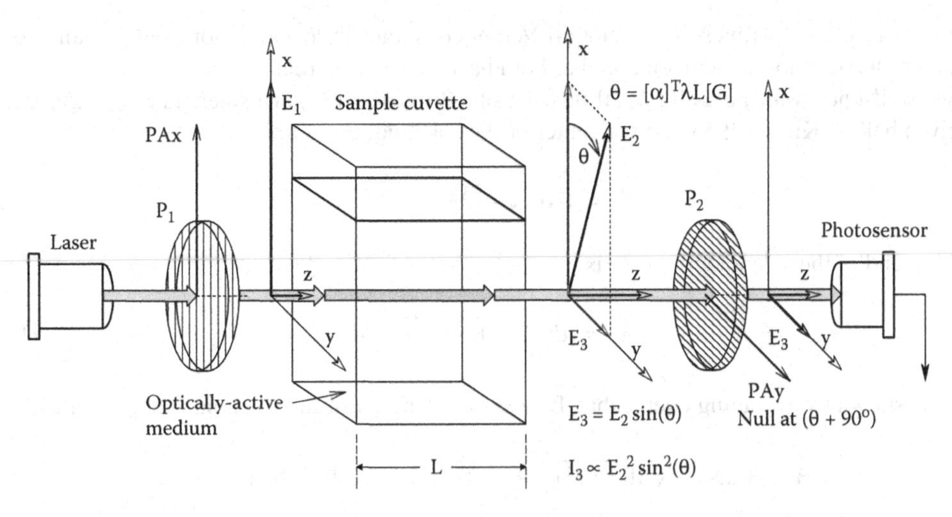

FIGURE 15.40 Diagram showing the rotation θ of the polarization axis of the incident $\mathbf{E}_1$ vector by passing the LPL through an optically active medium of length L. The system is a polarimeter: When the pass axis of linear polarizer P_2 is manually rotated by an angle θ + 90°, a null is observed in the output intensity, I_3. Thus, θ can be measured.

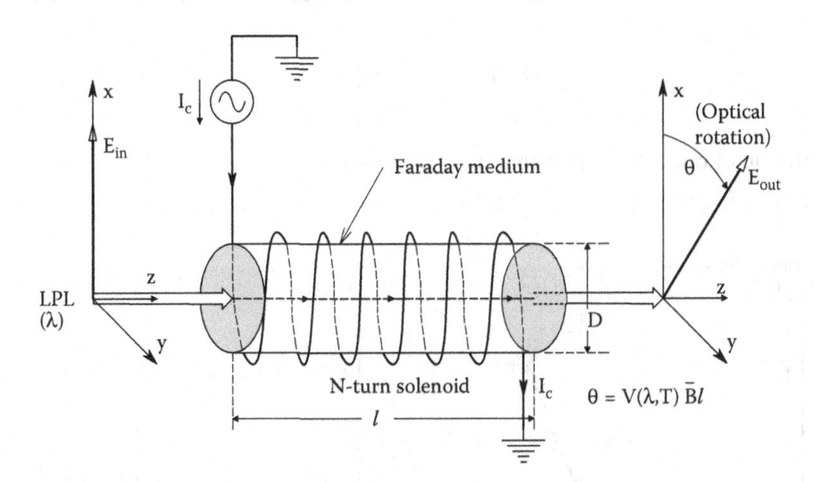

FIGURE 15.41 Diagram of a Faraday rotator (FR). The z-axis magnetic field component from the current-carrying solenoid interacts with the Faraday medium to cause optical rotation of LPL passing through the medium in the z-direction.

where θ_m is the Faraday optical rotation in degrees, V(λ, T) is the magneto-optically active material's *Verdet constant,* having units of degrees/(Tesla meter). Verdet constants are given in a variety of challenging units, such as 10^{-3} minutes of arc/(gauss.cm). $\overline{B}_z$ is the average axial flux density collinear with the optical path, and l is the length of the path where the LPL is exposed to the axial **B** field.

Generally, a material's Verdet constant *increases* with *decreasing* wavelength and also with *increasing* temperature. When a Verdet constant is specified, the wavelength and temperature at which it was measured must be given. For example, the Verdet constant of distilled water at 20°C and 578 nm is 218.3°/(Tesla m) (Hecht 1987, Chapter 8). This value may appear large, but the length of the test chamber on which the solenoid is wound is generally 10 cm = 10^{-1} m, and 1 Tesla = 10^4 gauss, so actual rotations tend to be < ±5°. The Verdet constant for lead glass under the same conditions is about six times larger. Not all Verdet constants are positive; for example, an aqueous solution of ferric chloride, and solid amber both have negative Verdet constants.

Two well-known formulas for axial flux density **B** inside an N-turn solenoid carrying current **I** are given below (Krauss 1953). At the center of the solenoid, on its axis:

$$B_z = \mu NI/(\sqrt{4R^2 + l^2}) \text{ Tesla} \tag{15.84}$$

At either end of the solenoid, on its axis:

$$B_z = \mu NI/(2\sqrt{R^2 + l^2}) \text{ Tesla} \tag{15.85}$$

It can be shown by averaging over l, that $\overline{B_z}$ over the length l of the solenoid is approximately

$$\overline{B_z} \cong 3\ \mu NI/(4\sqrt{4R^2 + l^2}) \rightarrow 3\ \mu NI/(4\ l) \text{ Tesla, when } l >> 2R \tag{15.86}$$

It should be clear that a Faraday rotator can be used to electrically null a simple polarimeter. See Figure 15.42 for an illustration of a simple, DC, electrically nulled polarimeter. The DC FR current is varied until the output photosensor registers a null ($E_4 = 0$). At null, the optical rotation from the FR is equal and opposite to the optical rotation from the optically active analyte. Thus,

$$V(\lambda, T)\frac{3\ \mu NI}{4\ l}\ l = [\alpha]_\lambda{}^T CL \tag{15.87}$$

The concentration of optically active analyte is thus found to be

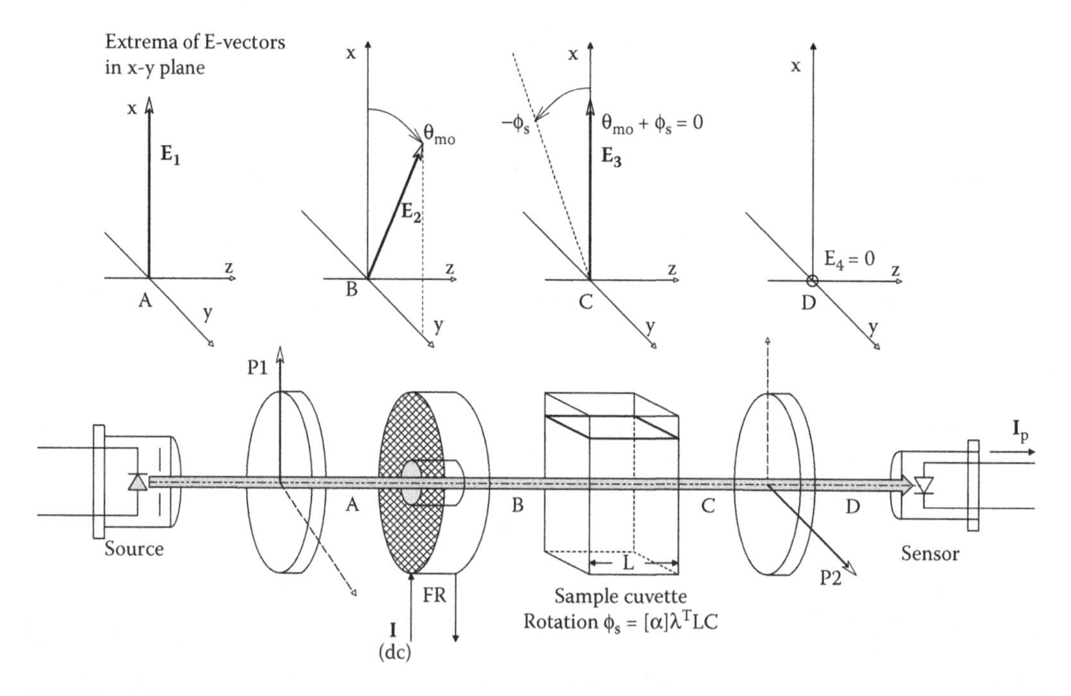

FIGURE 15.42 A simple electrically nulled polarimeter. The optical rotation from the FR is made equal and opposite to the optical rotation of the sample to get a null. Polarizer P2's pass axis is at right angles to that of P1.

$$C = \frac{3\,V\,\mu\,N\,I}{4\,[\alpha]\,L} \tag{15.88}$$

Note that C is dependent on three well-known physical parameters (N, I & L), and two that are less-well known and which are temperature- and wavelength-dependent (V and [α]). This type of operation yields accuracy in the tenths of a degree.

Figure 15.43 illustrates an improvement on the static polarimeter shown in Figure 15.42. Now an AC current is passed through the FR, causing the emergent polarization vector at point *B* to rock back and forth sinusoidally in the x–y plane at some audio frequency $f_m = \omega_m/2\pi$ Hz. The maximum rocking angle is θ_{mo}. This rocking $\mathbf{E_2}$ vector is next passed through the optically active sample where at any instant, the angle of $\mathbf{E_2}$ has the rotation ϕ_s added to it, as shown at point *C*. Next, the asymmetrically rocking $\mathbf{E_3}$ vector is passed through polarizer P_2, which only passes the y-components of $\mathbf{E_3}$, as $\mathbf{E_{4y}}$ at point *D*. Thus, $E_{4y}(t)$ can be written as

$$E_{4y}(t) = E_{4yo}\sin[\phi_s + \theta_{mo}\sin(\omega_m t)] \tag{15.89}$$

The sinusoidal component in the sin[*] argument is from the audio-frequency polarization angle modulation. The instantaneous intensity of the light at *D*, $i_4(t)$ is proportional to $E_{4y}{}^2(t)$:

$$i_4(t) = E_{4yo}{}^2\,[v_z\varepsilon/2]\sin^2[\phi_s + \theta_{mo}\sin(\omega_m t)]\ \text{Watts/m}^2 \tag{15.90}$$

Now by trig. identity, $\sin^2(x) = ½\,[1 - \cos(2x)]$, and we have

$$i_4(t) = E_{4yo}{}^2\,[v_z\varepsilon/2]\,1/2\,\{1 - \cos[2\phi_s + 2\theta_{mo}\sin(\omega_m t)]\} \tag{15.91}$$

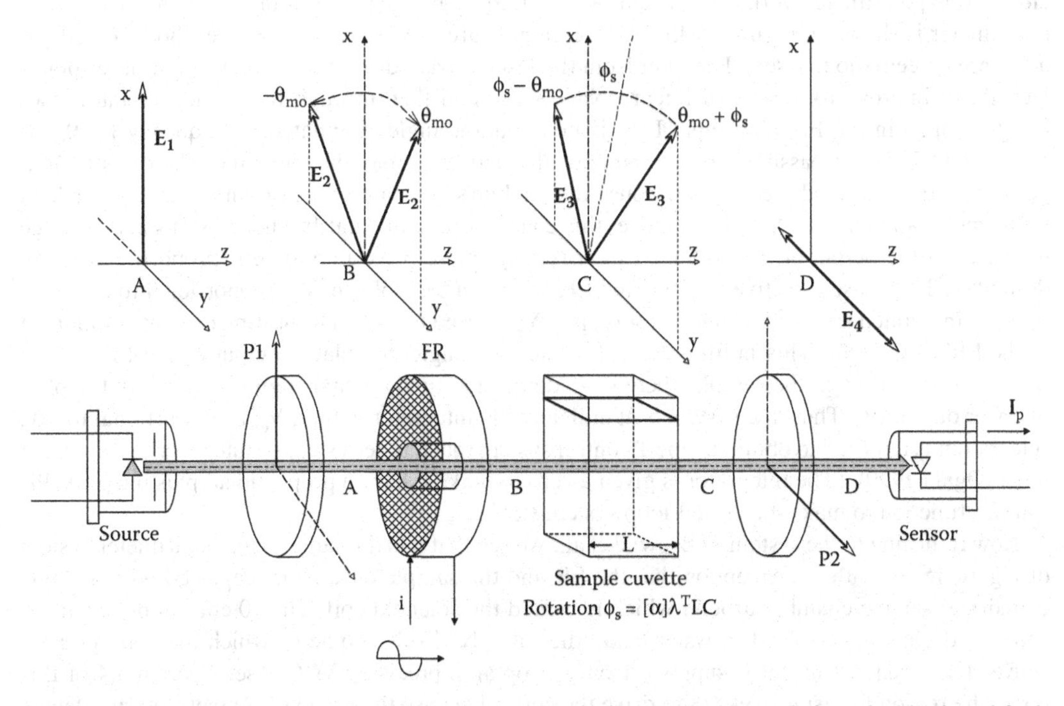

FIGURE 15.43 An open-loop Gilham polarimeter. The input polarization angle is rocked back and forth (modulated) by $\pm\,\theta_{mo}$ degrees by passing AC current through the FR coil. See Text for analysis.

Since the angle argument of the cosine is small, i.e., $|2(\phi_s + \theta_{mo})| < 3°$, we may use the approximation, $\cos(x) \cong (1 - x^2/2)$. Assume the instantaneous photosensor output voltage, $v_p(t)$, is proportional to $i_4(t)$, so we can finally write

$$v_p(t) = K_P i_4(t) \cong K_P\{E_{4yo}{}^2(v_z\varepsilon/2)\ 1/2 \left\{1 - \left[1 - \frac{4\phi_s{}^2 + 4\theta_{mo}{}^2 \sin^2(\omega_m t) + 8\phi_s\theta_{mo}\sin(\omega_m t)}{2}\right]\right\} \quad (15.92)$$

$$\downarrow$$

$$v_p(t) = K_v[\ \phi_s{}^2 + \theta_{mo}{}^2 1/2(1 - \cos(2\omega_m t)) + 2\phi_s\ \theta_{mo}\sin(\omega_m t)] \quad (15.93)$$

where $K_V = K_P E_{4yo}{}^2 (v_z\, \varepsilon/2)$. v_z is the velocity of propagation of light in the medium, and ε is its permittivity. (The permittivity of empty space is 8.85×10^{-12} coulomb^2/Nm^2.)

Thus, the photosensor output voltage contains three components: (1) A DC component which is not of interest, (2) A double-frequency component which has no information on ϕ_s, and (3) a fundamental frequency sinusoidal term whose peak amplitude is proportional to ϕ_s. By using a high-pass filter, the DC components can be blocked, and by using a phase-sensitive rectifier synchronized to the FR modulating current sinusoid at ω_m, one can recover a DC signal proportional to ϕ_s while rejecting the $2\omega_m$ sinusoidal term.

By feeding back a DC current proportional to ϕ_s into the FR, the system can be made closed-loop and self-nulling. The first such feedback polarimeter was invented by Gilham (1957); it has been improved and modified by various workers since then (Rabinovitch, March, and Adams 1982; Coté et al. 1992; Cameron and Coté 1997; Northrop 2002). Instruments of this sort can resolve ϕ_s to better than ± 12 μ-degrees.

Browne et al. (1997) devised a feedback polarimetry system that has microdegree resolution, designed to measure glucose in bioreactors. The system is illustrated in Figure 15.44. Before describing its design and operation, it is necessary to understand how a conventional, Gilham-type, closed-loop polarimeter works. A conventional, closed-loop, polarization-angle modulated, Gilham polarimeter is shown in Figure 15.45. The DC light source can be a laser or laser diode. (We used a 512 nm (green) diode laser.) The light from the laser is passed through a calcite Glan-laser polarizer, P_1, to improve its degree of linear polarization, and then through the Faraday rotator. Two things happen in the FR: The input LPL is polarization angle-modulated at frequency f_m. θ_{mo} is made about 2°. After passing through the optically active sample, the angle modulation is no longer symmetrical around the y-axis because the analyte's constant optical rotation has been added to the modulation angle. As shown above, this causes a fundamental frequency sinusoidal voltage to appear at the output of the high-pass filter (HPF) whose peak amplitude is proportional to the desired ϕ_s. The phase-sensitive rectifier and LPF output a DC voltage, V_L, proportional to ϕ_s.

V_L is integrated and the DC integrator output, V_o, is used to add a DC nulling current component to the FR's AC input. This nulling current rotates the angle-modulated output of the FR so that when it passes through the sample, there is no detectable fundamental frequency term in the photosensor output, V_d. Thus, the system is at null, and the integrator output, V_o, is proportional to $-\phi_s$. Integration is required to obtain a type 1 control system that has zero steady-state error to a constant input (Ogata 1990). (The integrator is given a zero to make it have a proportional plus integral (PI) transfer function to make the closed-loop system stable.)

Now returning to the system of Browne et al., we see that it is the same as the polarimeter system of Figure 15.45, with the exception that the FR and the sample cuvette are replaced with a single cylindrical sample chamber around which is wound the solenoid coil. The 10 cm sample chamber contains d-glucose dissolved in water, and other dissolved salts, some of which may be optically active. The solenoid current is supplied from a 3-op amp precision VCCS (see Section 4.4 of this text). The reason for using a VCCS to drive the coil is because the Faraday magnetorotary effect is proportional to the axial **B** field, which in turn depends on the current through the coil. Because the

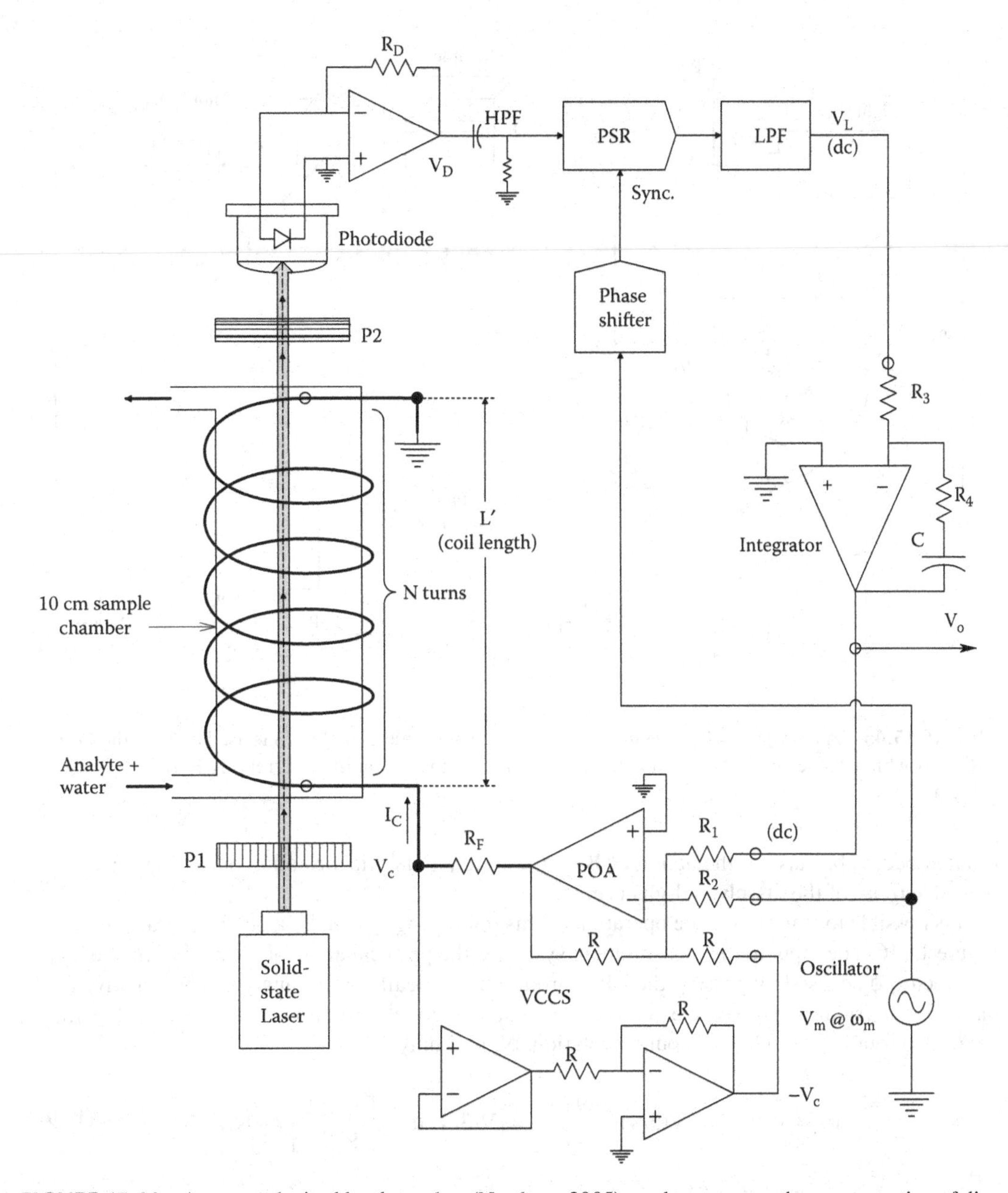

FIGURE 15.44 A system devised by the author (Northrop 2005) used to measure the concentration of dissolved glucose. It is a self-nulling, Gilham-type polarimeter in which the external FR has been replaced by the Faraday magneto optical effect of the water solvent in the test chamber. Glucose is the optically active medium (analyte) dissolved in the water. The system is self-nulling. See text for description.

coil is lossy, it gradually heats from the power dissipated by the AC modulation excitation and the DC nulling current. As the coil wire temperature increases, its resistance increases. Thus, if a voltage source (op amp) were used to drive the coil, **B** would be a function of temperature as well as the input voltage, V_c. The **B** (coil) temperature dependence is eliminated by using the VCCS.

The FR can be eliminated because the water solvent in the chamber has a Verdet constant, and when subject to AC and DC axial magnetic fields, causes optical rotation of the transmitted LPL. The glucose solute is optically active, so we find that in the same optical path length, Faraday

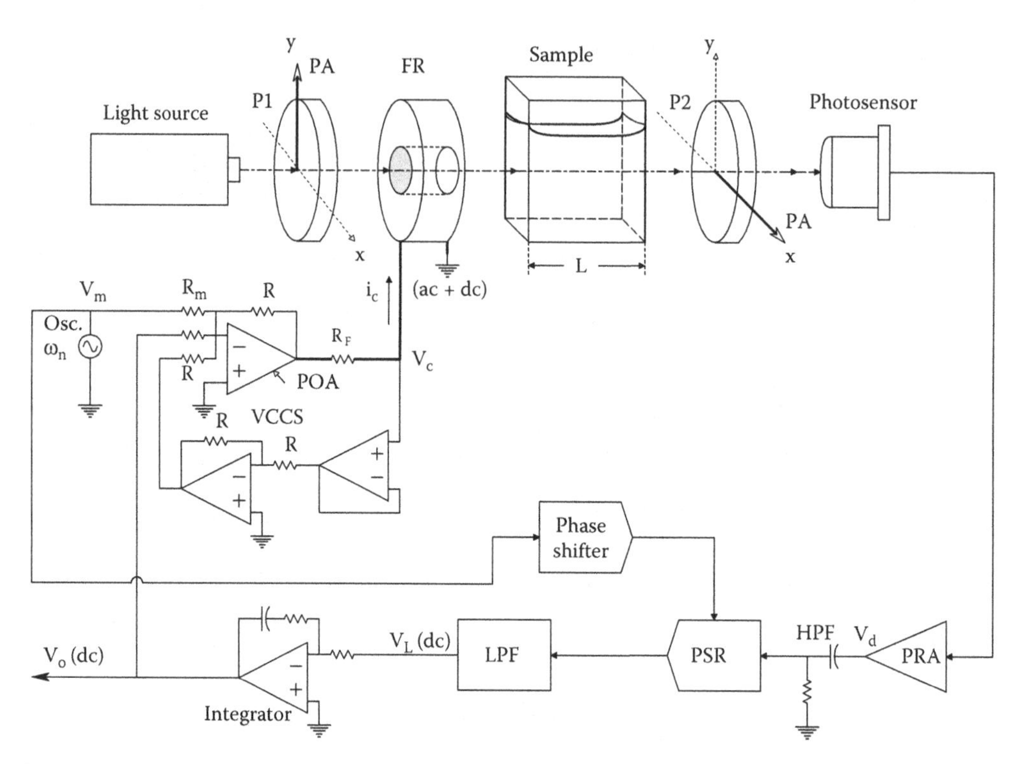

FIGURE 15.45 A conventional, self-nulling Gilham-type polarimeter. A VCCS is used to drive the external FR's coil which carries both the AC modulation signal, and the DC nulling current. A PSR/LPF is used to sense null.

rotation occurs because of the action of **B** on the water, and optical rotation occurs because of the optical activity of the dissolved d-glucose.

It is possible to summarize the operation of this interesting system by a block diagram, shown in Figure 15.46. The input to the measurement system is the physical angle of rotation of the polarization vector, ϕ_s, caused by passing the LPL through the optically active analyte. The negative feedback of the system output voltage, V_o leads to a Faraday counter-rotation of the LPL, ϕ_F, forming a net (error) rotation, ϕ_e. The DC counter-rotation, ϕ_F, is simply

$$\phi_F = V\,\bar{B}\,L' = V(3/4)\frac{\mu\,N}{L'}L'I_c = [V(3/4)\,\mu\,N]\left[\frac{-V_oR}{R_1R_F}\right] = -K_{FR}V_o \tag{15.94}$$

Clearly, $K_{FR} = V\,(3/4)\,\mu\,N\,R/(R_1R_F)$ degrees/volt. The closed-loop response of the system is found from the block diagram:

$$\frac{V_o}{\phi_s}(s) = \frac{-I_4\theta_{mo}K_PK_LK_i(\tau_is+1)}{s^2\tau_L + s[1+\tau_iI_4\theta_{mo}K_PK_LK_iK_{FR}] + I_4\theta_{mo}K_PK_LK_iK_{FR}} \tag{15.95}$$

It is of interest to consider the DC or steady-state response of this closed-loop polarimeter to a constant ϕ_s. This can be shown as

$$\frac{V_o}{\phi_s} = \frac{-1}{K_{FR}} \tag{15.96}$$

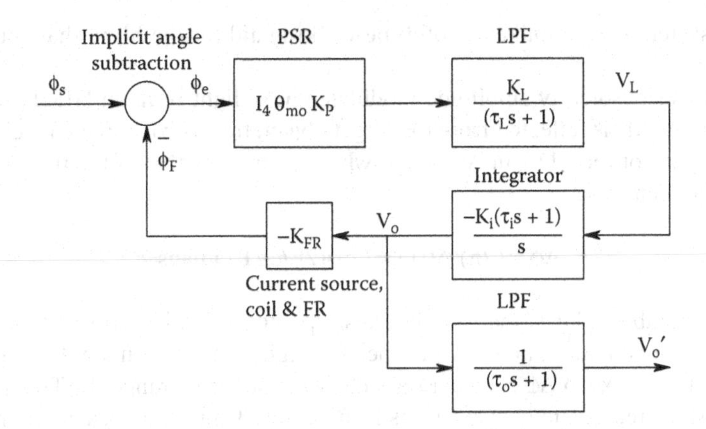

FIGURE 15.46 A block diagram describing the dynamics of the novel polarimeter of Figure 12.44.

Equation 15.96 is a rather serendipitous result. It tells us that the system's calibration depends only on K_{FR}, which depends on the transconductance of the VCCS, the dimensions and number of turns of the coil, the Verdet constant and the permeability (μ) of water. The DC gain *is independent* of the light intensity (I_4), the depth of polarization angle modulation (θ_{mo}), the frequency of modulation (ω_m), and the system's gain parameters (K_P, K_L, and K_i) and time constants (τ_L and τ_i).

The prototype system built and tested by Browne et al. (1997) was evaluated for d-glucose concentrations (**x**) from 60 to 140 mg/dl. By least mean-square error curve fitting, the output voltage (**y**) was found to follow the linear model

$$y = 0.0544\ x\ + 0.0846 \tag{15.97}$$

with $R^2 = 0.9986$. System resolution was 10.1 μ°/mV out, at 27°C with a 10 cm cell, and the glucose sensitivity was 55.4 mV/mg%. Noise in V_o was reduced by low-pass filtering (not shown in Figure 15.46).

Note that in this instrument, op amps were used exclusively for all active components, including: the photodiode current-to-voltage converter (transresistor) (cf. Section 2.6.4), the phase-sensitive rectifier (cf. Section 15.2.3), the low-pass filter (cf. Section 7.2), the PI integrator (cf. Section 6.6), the oscillator (cf. Section 5.5), and the VCCS (cf. Section 4.4).

15.8.3 Laser Velocimeter and Rangefinder

Many conventional laser-based velocimeters are based on a time-of-flight rangefinder principle in which laser pulses are reflected from a reflective (cooperative) target back to the source position and the range is found from the simple relation:

$$L = c\Delta t/2 \text{ meters} \tag{15.98}$$

If the target is moving toward or away from the laser/photosensor assembly, the relative velocity can be found by approximating v = L by numerically differentiating the sequence of return times for sequential output pulses, $Dt = \sum \Delta t_k$. In 1992, Laser Atlanta made a vehicular velocimeter for police use which used this principle.

The *laser velocimeter and rangefinder* (LAVERA) system we will describe in this section uses quite a different principle to provide simultaneous velocity and range output. The LAVERA system was developed by the author and reduced to practice by Todd Nelson (1999) for his MS research in Biomedical Engineering at the University of Connecticut. The motivation for developing the system was to make a prototype walking aid for the blind that could be incorporated into a cane.

The system uses sinusoidally amplitude-modulated, CW light from an NIR laser diode (LAD). The beam from the LAD is reflected from the target object, travels back to the receiver photosensor where its intensity is converted to an AC signal whose phase lags that of the transmitted light. The phase lag is easily seen to be

$$\Delta\phi = (2\pi)(\Delta t/T) = (2\pi)(2L/c)/T \text{ radians} \tag{15.99}$$

where, as discussed above, Dt is the time it takes a photon to make a round trip to the target, T is the period of the modulation, and c is the speed of light. The system we developed is a closed-loop system that tries to keep $\Delta\phi$ constant regardless of the target range, L. This means that as L decreases, T must decrease, and conversely, as L increases, T must increase to maintain a constant phase difference.

Figure 15.47 illustrates the functional architecture of the LAVERA system. We start the analysis by considering the *voltage-to-period converter* (VPC). The VPC is an oscillator in which the output period is proportional to V_P (see Section 15.4.5). Thus,

$$T = 1/f = K_{VPC}V_P + b \text{ seconds} \tag{15.100}$$

By way of contrast, the output from a conventional voltage-to-frequency oscillator is described by

$$f = K_{VCO}V_C + d \text{ Hz} \tag{15.101}$$

Next, consider the *phase detector*. This subsystem measures the phase difference between the transmitted, modulated signal intensity, and the delayed, reflected, modulated signal intensity. Although an analog multiplier can be used directly to measure this phase difference, in this system, the analog sine waves proportional to light intensity are passed through comparators to convert them to TTL waves whose phase difference is sensed by an exclusive or (EOR) gate phase detector

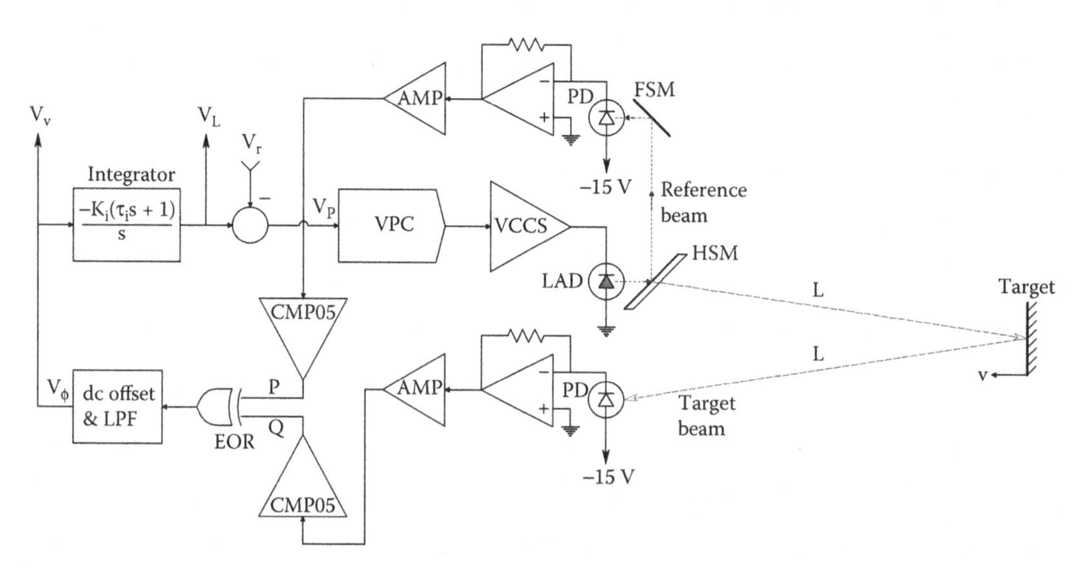

FIGURE 15.47 Block diagram of the LAVERA system developed by Nelson (1999). Sinusoidal modulation of the laser beam's intensity was used because less bandwidth is required for signal conditioning than for a pulsed system. The system simultaneously measures target range and velocity.

(PD). The EOR PD is a quadrature detector, i.e., its output duty cycle is 50% when one input lags (or leads) the other by odd multiples of π/2. Figure 15.48 illustrates the EOR PD's circuit and transfer function. The op amp inverts the TTL output of the EOR gate and subtracts a DC level so that V_z swings ± 1.7 V.

For a heuristic view of how the system works, we can write the PD output as

$$V_{\phi} = \overline{V_z} = V_v = -(3.4/\pi)\,\phi + 1.7 \text{ Volts} \tag{15.102}$$

In the steady-state with fixed L, $V_v = 0$ in a type 1 feedback loop. For $V_v = 0$, $\phi_{ss} = \pi/2$. However, it has already been established that the phase lag for a returning, modulated light beam is

$$\phi = (2\pi)(2L/c)(1/T) \text{ radians} \tag{15.103}$$

If Equation 15.103 for ϕ is solved for T, and T is substituted into the VPC equation, one has

$$T_{ss} = (2\pi)(2L/c)(1/\phi_{ss})\,K_{VPC}V_{Pss} + b \tag{15.104}$$

$$\downarrow$$

$$8L/c = K_{VPC}[V_{Lss} - V_r] + b \tag{15.105}$$

If one lets $V_r \equiv b/K_{VPC}$, the final expression for V_{Lss} is obtained:

$$V_{Lss} = 8L/(c\,K_{VPC}) \tag{15.106}$$

The steady-state V_L is indeed proportional to L. Going back to the VPC equation, one finds that for a stationary target, the steady-state VPC output frequency is given by

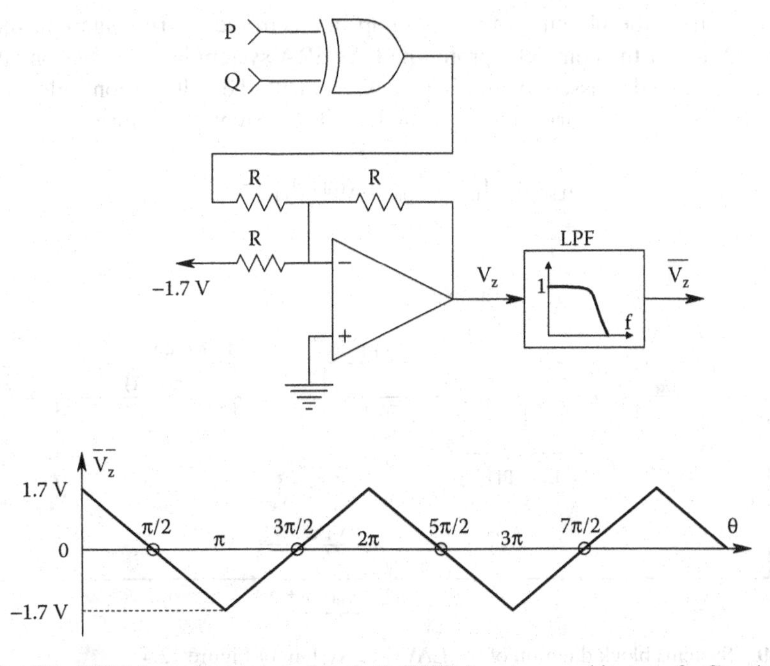

FIGURE 15.48 The EOR phase detector used in the LAVERA system, and its transfer function.

$$f_{ss} = 1/T_{ss} = c/(8L)\ \text{Hz} \tag{15.107}$$

At L = 1m, f_{ss} = 37.5 MHz; when L = 30 m, f_{ss} = 1.25 MHz, etc.

Now suppose the target is moving away from the transmitter/receiver at a *constant velocity*, v = L. V_v is no longer zero, but can be found from the integrator relation:

$$V_v = -V_L / K_i = \frac{-8L}{K_i K_{VPC} c} \tag{15.108}$$

Notice the sign of V_v is negative for a receding target, also as the target recedes, the VPC output frequency drops. Clearly, practical considerations set a maximum and a minimum for measuring L. The limit for near L is the upper modulation frequency possible in the system; the limit for far L is the diminishing intensity of the return signal, and noise.

To appreciate the closed-loop dynamics of the LAVERA system, it is possible to make a systems block diagram as shown in Figure 15.49. Note that this system is nonlinear in its closed-loop dynamics. It can be shown (Nelson 1999) that the closed-loop system's undamped natural frequency, ω_n, and damping factor are range-dependent, even though the steady-state range and velocity sensitivities are independent of L. The undamped natural frequency for the LAVERA system of Figure 15.49 can be shown as

$$\omega_n = \sqrt{\frac{4(3.4)\ c\ K_i K_{VPC}}{64\ \tau_1 L_o}}\ \text{r/s} \tag{15.109}$$

The closed-loop LAVERA system's damping factor can be shown as

$$\xi = 1/2\left[\frac{64\ L_o}{4(3.4)\ c\ K_i\ K_{VPC}} + \tau_i\right]\sqrt{4(4.3)\ c\ K_i K_{VPC}/(64\ \tau_1 L_o)} \tag{15.110}$$

Finally, to illustrate the ubiquity of the op amp in electronic instrumentation, refer to Figure 15.50 for a schematic of the complete, prototype LAVERA system built by Nelson (1999). The op amp subsystems will be discussed, beginning clockwise with the voltage-controlled current source (VCCS). The VCCS is used to drive the laser diode with a current of the form

$$i_{LD}(t) = I_{LDo} + I_{Dm}\sin(\omega t),\ I_{LDo} > I_{Dm} \tag{15.111}$$

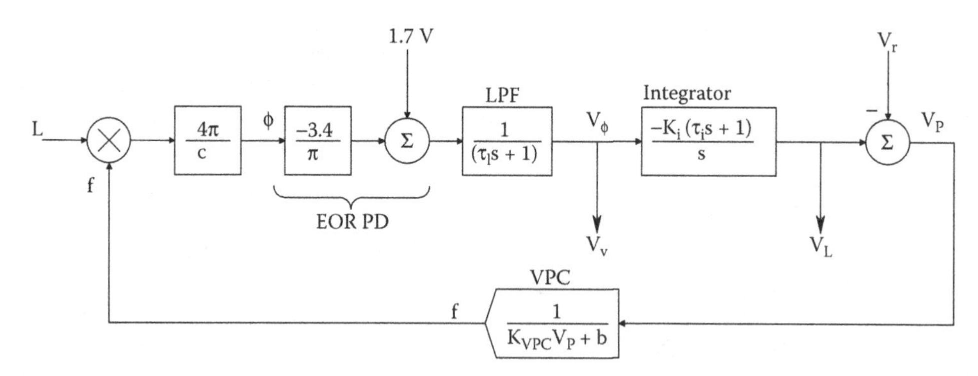

FIGURE 15.49 Systems block diagram of the LAVERA system of Figure 12.45.

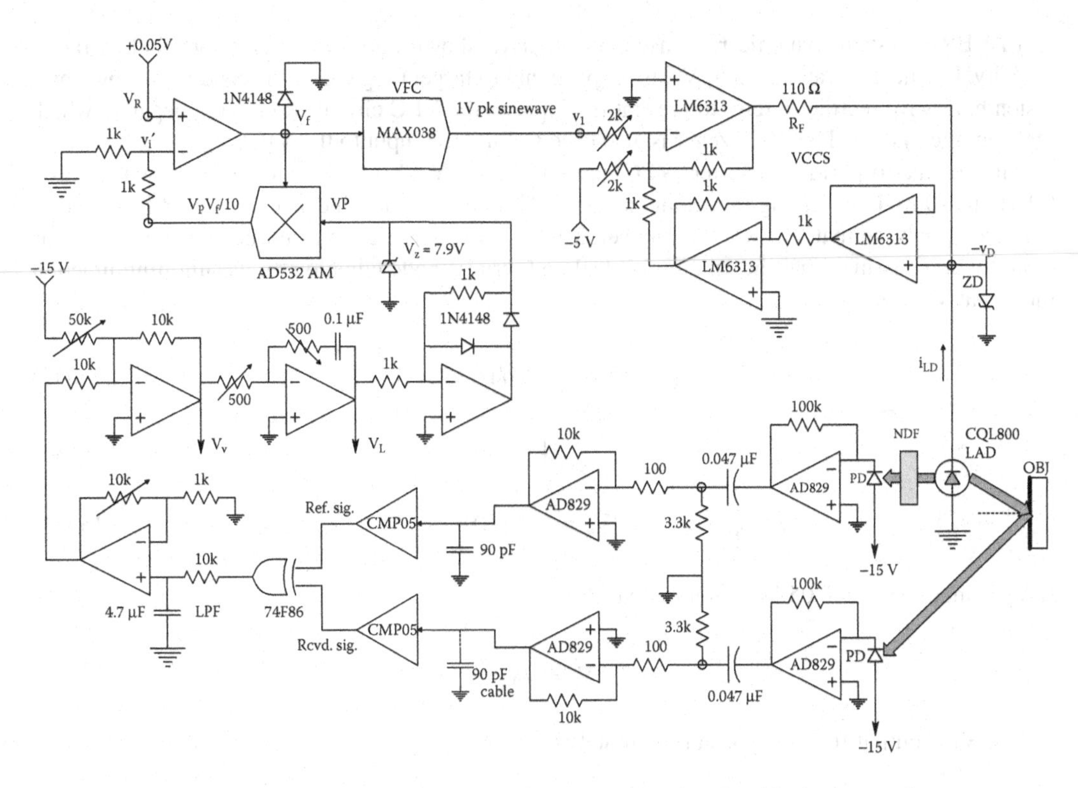

FIGURE 15.50 Simplified schematic of the LAVERA system showing the ubiquitous use of op amps.

This 3-op amp circuit was analyzed in detail in Section 4.4 of this text. At midfrequencies, it was shown that $i_{LD}(t) = -v_1(t)\,G_M = -v_1(t)/110$ amps. The zener diode is to protect the LAD from excess forward or reverse voltage.

A Philips CQL800, 675 nm, 5 mW laser diode (LAD) was used. A small fraction of its modulated light was directed in a very short path (ca. 1 cm) through a neutral density filter to the reference photodiode (PD). The PDs were Hammamatsu S2506-02, PIN photodiodes with spectral response from 320 to 1100 nm, with a peak at 960 nm. PD responsivity was ca. 0.4 A/W at 660 nm. Both the reference and received signal channels were made identical electronically to avoid a phase shift between channels. The receiver PD viewed the target through an inexpensive, collimated telescope. The photocurrents from the PDs were proportional to the light intensities striking their active areas. The photocurrents were amplified by AD829 high-frequency op amp transresistors. The AD829 has an $f_T = 120$ MHz, a slew rate of $\eta = 230$ V/µs, and low $e_{na} = 2$ nV/√Hz. The voltage outputs from the AD829 transresistors were passed through simple R-C high-pass filters to block DC. The HPF corner frequencies were 10 kHz. The high-pass filtered signals were then amplified by AD829 inverting amplifiers with gains of −100. A 90 pF capacitance to ground was placed at the input of the reference channel comparator to compensate for the measured 90 pF capacitance of the shielded cable coupling the receiver channel AD829 to its comparator. PMI CMP05 amplitude comparators were used to convert the sinusoidal signals at the outputs of the AD829 amplifiers to TTL digital signals which were then input to the exclusive OR gate used as a quadrature phase detector. The EOR output was low-pass filtered, and amplified, then a negative voltage of ca. 1.7 V was added to make $V_v = 0$ when the phase difference was 90° between the reference and received channels (cf. Figure 15.48). The nearly DC V_v is then integrated by the PI integrator. (The zero from the PI integrator is required for good closed-loop

LAVERA system dynamic response.) As we have shown above, V_v is proportional to target velocity, L. The integrator output, V_L, is proportional to target range, L. V_L is conditioned by a precision half-wave rectifier circuit to prevent the input to the VPC circuit from going negative which locks up the system. The 7.9 V zener is also used to limit the input to the VPC, V_P.

The voltage-to-period converter (VPC) used a Maxim MAX038, wide-range VFC which has a 0.1 Hz to 20 MHz operating range, and a sinusoidal output. A nonlinear op amp circuit is used to convert V_P to V_f so that $V_P \rightarrow v_1$ has an overall VPC characteristic. To examine how the non-linear circuit works, assume that the op amp is ideal and write a node equation on its summing junction (note that $V_i' = V_R$):

$$V_R G + (V_R - V_P V_f / 10)G = 0 \tag{15.112}$$

$$\downarrow$$

$$2V_R = V_P V_f / 10 \tag{15.113}$$

If V_R is made 1/20 = 0.05 V, then it is clear that

$$V_f = 1/V_P \tag{15.114}$$

The VFC output frequency is approximately

$$f = K_f V_f = K_f / V_P \text{ Hz} \tag{15.115}$$

or

$$T = 1/f = V_P / K_f = K_{VPC} V_P \tag{15.116}$$

The sinusoidal output of the MAX038 VFC, v_1, is a 1 V peak sine wave which is used to drive the LAD.

Nelson (1999) developed a prototype CW LAVERA system having a linear V_L vs L characteristic over $1 \text{ m} \leq L \leq 5 \text{ m}$ range with an $R^2 = 0.998$. A linear V_v vs L was observed over 0.5 to 2 m/s. Wider dynamic ranges were limited by practical considerations, not by the circuit.

A problem that remained to be solved in order to develop a practical system was how to use the velocity and range output voltages from the system to generate an audible or tactile signal that can warn a blind person of moving objects that may present a hazard. V_v goes positive for a moving target approaching the system, and negative for a receding target, and is zero for a stationary target. Thus, V_v might be used to control the pitch of an audio oscillator (not shown) around some zero-velocity frequency, say 550 Hz. An approaching target would raise the audio pitch to as high as 10 kHZ; a receding target might lower the velocity pitch to 30 Hz minimum. But how to code range? Range is always positive, and close objects should demand more attention, so we can use another VPC circuit (not shown) to generate "click" pulses which can be added to the velocity tone signal. Thus, a rapidly approaching, constant velocity vehicle would generate a high, steady sinusoidal tone plus a click rate of increasing frequency as the range decreases. If the vehicle stops nearby, as at a traffic light, the sinusoidal tone would drop to the zero-v frequency (550 Hz), but the click rate would remain high, say 20/sec f a 2 mL.

15.8.4 Self-Balancing, Admittance Plethysmograph

One way to measure volume changes in body tissues is by measuring the electrical impedance or admittance of the body part being studied. As blood is forced through arteries, veins, and capillaries by the heart, the tissue impedance is modulated. When used in conjunction with an external air pressure cuff that can gradually constrict blood flow, *impedance plethysmography* (IP) can provide noninvasive, diagnostic signs about abnormal venous and arterial blood flow. Also, by measuring the impedance of the chest, the relative depth and rate of a patient's breathing can be monitored noninvasively. As the lungs inflate and the chest expands, the admittance magnitude of the chest decreases; air is clearly a poorer conductor than tissues and blood.

IP is carried out using, for safety's sake, using a controlled AC current source of fixed frequency. The peak current is generally kept less than 1 mA, and the frequency used typically is between 30 and 75 kHz. The high frequency is used because the human susceptibility to electroshock, and the physiological effects on nerves and muscles from AC stimulation *decreases* with increasing frequency above 60 Hz (Webster 1992). The electrical impedance can be measured indirectly by measuring the AC voltage between two skin surface electrodes (generally ECG- or EEG-type, AgCl + conductive gel) placed between the two current electrodes. Thus, four electrodes are generally used, although the same two electrodes used for current injection can also be connected to the high input impedance, ac differential amplifier that measures the output voltage, $\mathbf{V_o}$. By Ohm's law, the body voltage is: $\mathbf{V_o} = \mathbf{I_s}\,\mathbf{Z_t} = \mathbf{I_s}\,[R_t + j\,B_t]$.

At a fixed frequency, the tissue impedance can be modeled by a single conductance in parallel with a capacitor. Thus, it is algebraically simpler to consider the tissue *admittance*, $\mathbf{Y_t} = \mathbf{Z_t}^{-1} = G_t + j\omega C_t$. Both G_t and C_t change as blood periodically flows into the tissue under measurement. The imposed AC current is carried in the tissue by moving ions, rather than electrons. Ions such as Cl^-, HCO_3^-, K^+, Na^+, Ca^{++}, etc., drift in the applied electric field (caused by the current-regulated source); they have three major pathways: A resistive path in the extracellular fluid electrolyte, a resistive path in blood, and a capacitive path caused by ions that charge the membranes of closely packed body cells. Ions can penetrate cell membranes and move inside cells, but not with the ease that they can travel in extracellular fluid space, and in blood. Of course, there are many, many cells effectively in series and parallel between the current electrodes. C_t represents the net equivalent capacitance of all the cell membranes. Each species of ion in solution has a different *mobility*. The mobility of an ion in solution, $\mu \equiv v/E$, where v is the mean drift velocity of the ion in a surrounding, uniform electric field, E. Ionic mobility also depends on the ionic concentration, and the other ions in solution. Ionic mobility has the units of $m^2\,s^{-1}\,V^{-1}$. Returning to Ohm's law, one can write in phasor notation:

$$V_o = I_s/Y_t = I_s \frac{G_t - j\omega C_t}{G_t^2 + \omega^2 C_t^2} = I_s[\mathrm{Re}\{Z_t\} - j\,\mathrm{Im}\{Z_t\}] \qquad (15.117)$$

where $\mathrm{Re}\{\mathbf{Z_t}\} = G_t/(G_t^2 + \omega^2 C_t^2)$ is the real part of the tissue impedance and $\mathrm{Im}\{\mathbf{Z_t}\} = B_t = -\omega C_t/(G_t^2 + \omega^2 C_t^2)$ is the imaginary part of the tissue impedance, Note that both $\mathrm{Re}\{\mathbf{Z_t}\}$ and $\mathrm{Im}\{\mathbf{Z_t}\}$ are frequency-dependent. Note that $\mathbf{V_o}$ *lags* $\mathbf{I_s}$.

There are several ways of measuring tissue $\mathbf{Z_t}$, both magnitude and angle. In the first method, described in detail below, an AC voltage, $\mathbf{V_s}$, is applied to the tissue. The amplitude is adjusted so that the resultant current, $\mathbf{I_o}$, remains less than 1 mA. $\mathbf{I_o}$ is converted to a proportional voltage, $\mathbf{V_o}$, by an op amp current-to-voltage converter circuit. In general $\mathbf{V_o}$ and $\mathbf{V_s}$ differ in phase and magnitude.

A self-nulling feedback circuit operates on $\mathbf{V_o}$ and $\mathbf{V_s}$. At null, its output voltage, V_c, is proportional to $|\mathbf{Z_t}|$. A second method uses the AC current source excitation, $\mathbf{I_s}$, and the output voltage described above, $\mathbf{V_o}$, is fed into a servo-tracking, two-phase, lock-in amplifier which produces an output voltage, $V_z \propto |\mathbf{Z_t}|$, and another voltage, $V_\theta \propto \angle\mathbf{Z_t}$. A self-nulling admittance plethysmograph designed by the author is illustrated in Figure 15.51. A 75 kHz, sinusoidal voltage, $\mathbf{V_s}$, is applied to

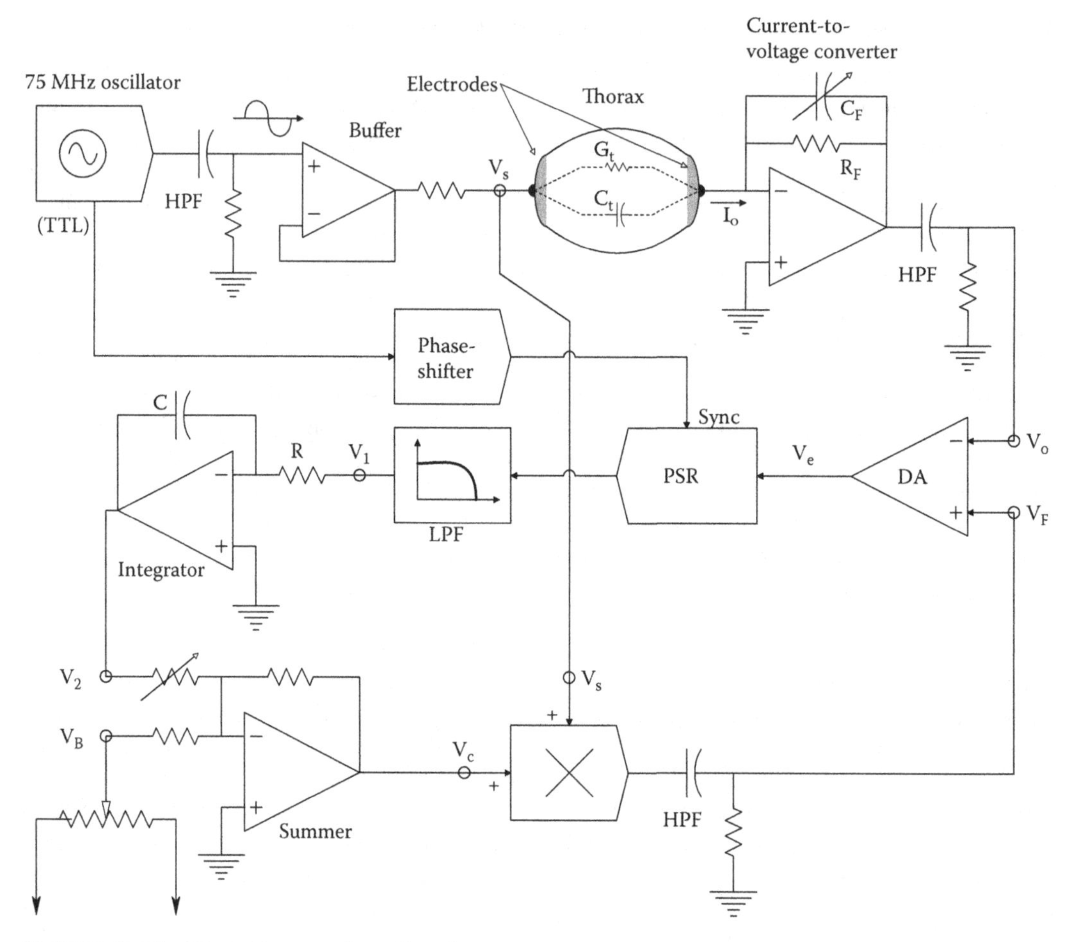

FIGURE 15.51 Block diagram of a self-nulling admittance plethysmograph designed by the author.

a chest electrode. An AC current phasor, $\mathbf{I_o}$, flows through the chest to virtual ground, and is given by Ohm's law:

$$I_o = V_s[G_t + j\omega C_t] \tag{15.118}$$

This current is converted to an AC voltage, $\mathbf{V_o}$, by the current-to-voltage op amp:

$$V_o = -\frac{I_o}{G_F + j\omega C_F} \tag{15.119}$$

$$\downarrow$$

$$V_o = -I_o \frac{G_F - j\omega C_F}{G_F^2 + \omega^2 C_F^2} = -V_s[G_t + j\omega C_t]\frac{G_F - j\omega C_F}{G_F^2 + \omega^2 C_F^2} \tag{15.120}$$

$$\downarrow$$

$$V_o = -V_s \frac{G_t G_F - j\omega C_F G_t + j\omega C_t C_F + \omega^2 C_t C_F}{G_F^2 + \omega^2 C_F^2} \tag{15.121}$$

With the patient having exhaled and holding his breath, C_F is adjusted so that $\mathbf{V_o}$ is in phase with $\mathbf{V_s}$. That is, C_F is set so that the imaginary terms in Equation 15.121 → 0. This gives

$$C_F = C_{Fo} \equiv C_{to}/(R_F G_{to}) \tag{15.122}$$

Then, there results

$$V_o = -V_s \frac{G_{to}G_F + \omega^2 C_{to} C_{Fo}}{G_F^2 + \omega^2 C_{Fo}^2} \rightarrow -V_s(R_F/R_{to}) \tag{15.123}$$

Now when the patient inhales, the lungs expand and the air displaces conductive tissue, causing the parallel conductance of the chest, G_t, to *decrease* from G_{to}. Substitute $G_t = G_{to} + \delta G_t$ and $C_t = C_{to} + \delta C_t$ into Equation 15.121, and also let $R_F C_F = C_{to} R_{to}$ from the initial phase nulling. After a considerable amount of algebra:

$$\frac{V_o}{V_s}(j\omega) = \frac{-R_F}{[1+\omega^2(R_F C_F)^2]}[G_{to}(1+\delta G_t/G_{to}) + \omega^2(R_F C_F)^2 G_{to}(1+\delta C_t/C_{to}) \\ + j\omega C_{to}(\delta C_t/C_{to} - \delta G_t/G_{to})] \tag{15.124}$$

This relation reduces to Equation 15.123 for $\delta C_t = \delta G_t \rightarrow 0$. Assuming that only $\delta C_t \rightarrow 0$, then Equation 15.124 can be written as

$$\frac{V_o + \delta V_o}{V_s}(j\omega) \cong -R_F G_{to} - \frac{\delta G_t\ R_F}{[1+\omega^2(R_F C_F)^2]} \tag{15.125a}$$

where

$$V_o = (-R_F G_{to})V_s \tag{15.125b}$$

$$\delta V_o = -\frac{(\delta G_t)\ R_F}{[1+\omega^2(R_F C_F)^2]} V_s \tag{15.125c}$$

Note that $\delta G_t < 0$ for an inhaled breath.

Figure 15.52 illustrates a systems block diagram for the author's self-balancing plethysmograph, configured for the condition where $\delta C_t \rightarrow 0$. Three, R-C high-pass filters shown in Figure 15.51 are used to block unwanted DC components from $\mathbf{V_s}$, $\mathbf{V_o}$, and $\mathbf{V_F}$. In the first case, $\delta G_t \rightarrow 0$. In the steady-state, $\mathbf{V_e} \rightarrow 0$, so

$$V_s V_c/10 = -V_s R_F G_{to} \tag{15.126}$$

Thus,

$$V_c = -10\ R_F G_{to} = -(V_B + \beta V_2) \tag{15.127}$$

and the DC integrator output, V_2, is proportional to G_{to}:

$$V_2 = (10\ R_F G_{to} - V_B)/\beta \tag{15.128}$$

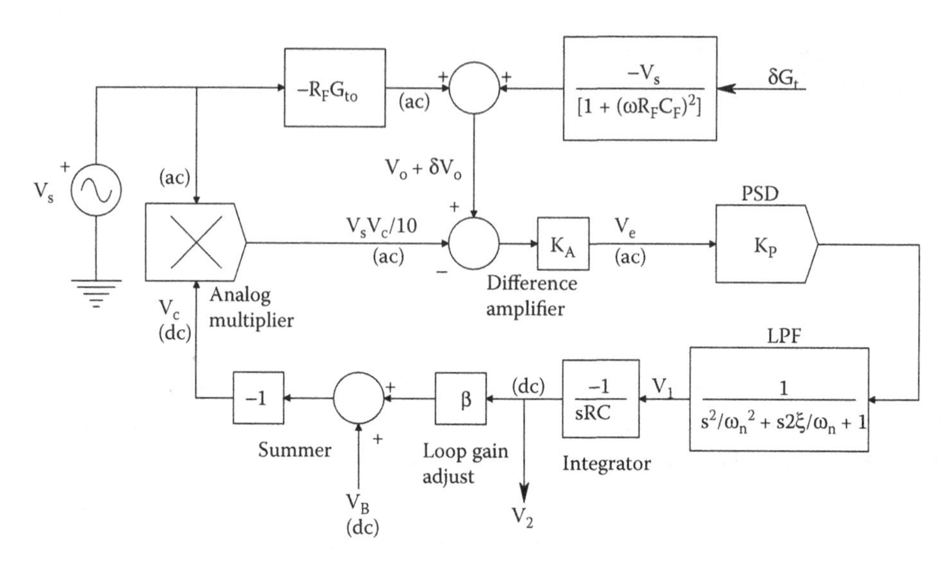

FIGURE 15.52 Systems block diagram describing the dynamics of the self-nulling plethysmograph.

V_B, G_{to}, and $\mathbf{V}_s$ do not change in time, so the steady-state analysis above is valid. Using superposition, we can examine the system's response to a time-varying, δG_t. The transfer function, $\delta V_2/\delta G_t$ can be written as

$$\frac{\delta V_2}{\delta G_t}(s) = \frac{V_s K_A K_P/\{RC[1+(\omega\ R_F C_F)^2]\}}{s(s^2/\omega_n^2 + s2\zeta/\omega_n + 1) + V_s \beta K_A K_P/(10RC)} \tag{15.129}$$

The damping of the *cubic* closed-loop system is adjusted with the attenuation, β. The DC steady-state, incremental gain is

$$\frac{\delta V_2}{\delta G_t} = \frac{10}{[(1+(\omega R_F C_F)^2]\ \beta} \tag{15.130}$$

A prototype of this system was run at 75 kHz and tested on the chests of several volunteers after informed consent was obtained. Both $\delta V_2 \propto \delta G_t$ and $V_1 \propto \delta G_t$ were recorded, as well as a spirometer output. System outputs followed the subjects' respiratory volumes, as expected.

15.9 CHAPTER SUMMARY

In this chapter, the characteristics and applications of several, special analog electronic signal processing modules, including the phase-sensitive rectifier/detector, the phase detector, voltage- and current-controlled oscillators, phase lock loops, true RMS converters, and IC temperature sensors have been examined.

To illustrate the use of analog electronic circuit ICs in biomedical instrumentation system design, three diverse examples were chosen:

The microdegree polarimeter represents an instrument that has evolved from a manually nulled instrument with limited sensitivity to the optical rotation angle caused by polarized light passing through an optically active medium, to a closed-loop optoelectronic system with microdegree sensitivity. The optical rotation is used to measure d-glucose concentration in clear liquids. In our design, we were able to eliminate an expensive Faraday rotator, and instead use the water solvent of the test solution for the Faraday medium.

Also described was a closed-loop laser velocimeter and ranging (LAVERA) system developed by the author and his students. In the LAVERA system, a CW laser beam was sinusoidally amplitude-modulated (instead of using pulsed laser light and measuring nanosecond delays in the return reflection). The frequency of the amplitude modulations was automatically adjusted so that the phase difference between the transmitted and received modulations was held constant. This LAVERA system gave two, simultaneous analog outputs proportional to target range and velocity. The system was designed as a prototype aid for blind persons.

A third system described was a self-balancing impedance plethysmograph, designed to measure small changes in volume as changes in admittance in certain anatomical regions, such as the chest or legs. This system operated at a constant 75 kHz, and used feedback to null an error voltage between the applied voltage and a voltage proportional to the body part's admittance at a standard condition. It was used to simultaneously detect respiration and heartbeat in an experimental context.

Appendix

SIGNAL FLOW GRAPHS AND MASON'S RULE

Signal flow graphs (SFGs) are an LTI systems tool that enables one to take a set of ODEs describing a dynamic, LTI system, put them in graphical form (with nodes and branches), and then using *Mason's gain formula,* easily find the I/O transfer function for the system. The SFG approach is ideally suited for quick, pencil-and-paper work because it replaces tedious, error-prone matrix inversion algebra as a necessary step in finding the state system's transfer function. SFGs were developed in 1953 by S. J. Mason; he published his gain formula in 1956. SFGs were developed in an era before desktop PCs running systems analysis applications such MATLAB™ and Simulink™. They have had application in electronic circuit analysis and, of course, the analysis of linear feedback systems.

An SFG has two components: *signal nodes* and *unidirectional branches* that condition the signals at the nodes. Signals from branches sum algebraically at nodes. The signal at a node is multiplied by the *transmission* or *gain* of a branch leaving it; i.e., the input at node from a branch is the product of the branch's transmission times the source node's signal. The signal at a node is unaffected by the directed branches leaving it. All signals are assumed to be in the frequency domain. As a first example of signal manipulation in SFGs, consider Figure A1a. Here, $y_1 = T_1 x_1$, $y_2 = T_2 x_1$, and $y_3 = T_3 x_1$. In Figure A1b, $y_1 = x_1 T_1 + x_2 T_2 + x_3 T_3$. When several branches are in series as in Figure A1c, $x_4 = T_1 T_2 T_3 x_1$. When they are in parallel as in Figure A1d, $y_1 = x_1(T_1 + T_2 + T_3)$.

The systematic gain formula for SFGs developed by Mason in 1956 is deceptively simple. However, it does require some interpretation. It is written as

$$\frac{V_{ok}}{V_{ij}} = H_{jk} = \frac{\sum_{n=1}^{N} F_n \Delta_n}{\Delta_D} \tag{A-1}$$

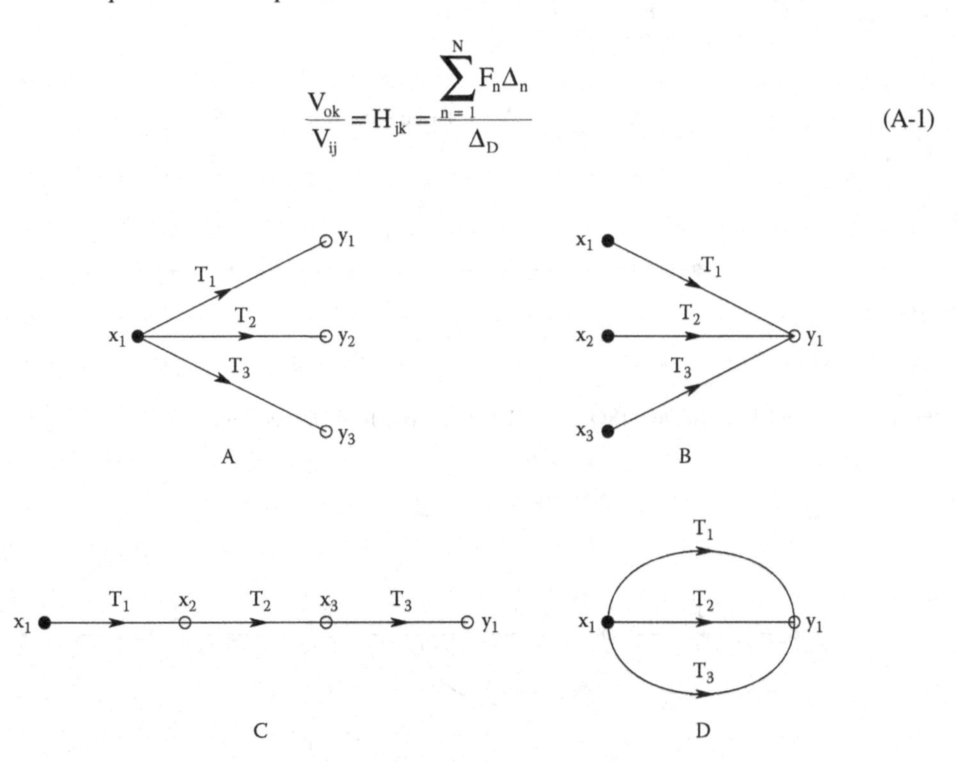

Figure A1 Four examples of simple, linear signal flow graph (SFG) architectures. See Text for descriptions.

where H_{jk} is the net transmission from the jth (input) node to the kth (output) node.

F_n is the transmission of the nth *forward path*. The nth forward path is a connected path of branches beginning on the jth (input) node and ending on the kth (output) node along which no node is passed through more than once. An SFG can have several forward paths which can share common nodes.

Δ_D is the SFG denominator or determinant. $\Delta_D \equiv 1$ – [sum of all individual loop gains] + [sum of products of pairs of all nontouching loop gains] – [sum of products of nontouching loop gains taken 3 at a time] + · · · .

The loop gain is the net gain around a closed loop one or more branches. The loop must start and finish on a common node. *Nontouching* loops share no nodes in common.

Δ_n is the *cofactor* for the nth forward path. $\Delta_n \equiv \Delta_D$ evaluated for nodes that do not touch the nth forward path.

The best way to learn how to use Mason's rule on systems SFGs is by example. *In the first example,* Figure A2 is a simple SISO system. There is only one forward path. The loop touches two of its nodes, so $\Delta_1 = 1$. F_1 is seen to be $1 \times K_v/(s + a) \times a$, and

$$\Delta_D = 1 - \left[\frac{-K_v\beta}{s(s+a)}\right] \tag{A-2}$$

The overall transfer function is put in Laplace form. Thus,

$$\frac{V_o}{V_1} = \frac{s\,K_v a}{s^2 + sa + K_v\beta} \tag{A-3}$$

In the second example, the SFG is shown in Figure A3. Now n = 1, $F_1 = ab$, $\Delta_D = 1 - [-ac - e - d] + 0$, and $\Delta_1 = 1$. From which we have,

$$\frac{V_o}{V_1} = \frac{ac}{1 + ac + e + d} \tag{A-4}$$

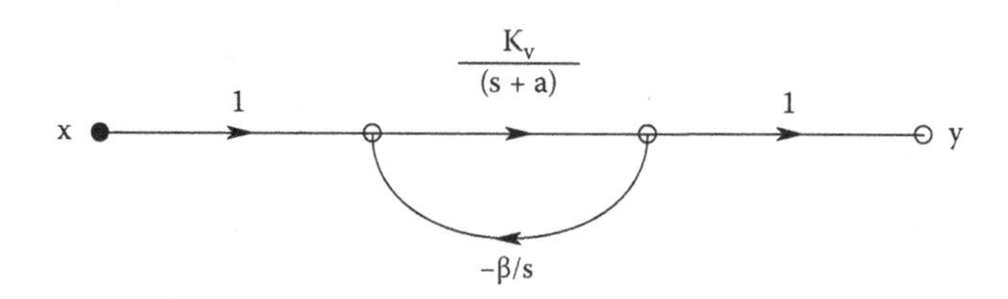

Figure A2 SFG for a simple, SISO, single-loop, negative feedback system.

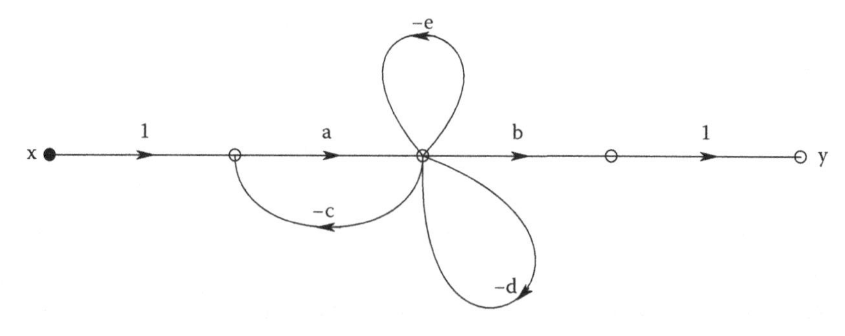

Figure A3 SFG for the 3-loop negative feedback system of Example 2.

In the third example shown in Figure A4, the SFG is more complicated: n = 3, F_1 = abc, F_2 = def, F_3 = −akf, $\Delta_D = 1 - [-bh - ge] + [(-bh)(-ge)] - 0$, $\Delta_1 = 1 + ge$, $\Delta_2 = 1 + bh$, $\Delta_3 = 1$. The transfer function is thus

$$\frac{V_o}{V_1} = \frac{abc(1+ge)+def(1+bh)-akf}{1+bh+ge+bhge} \tag{A-5}$$

In a fourth example, Figure A5 illustrates a state-variable form SFG: Here, n = 4, $F_1 = b_3$, $F_2 = b_2/s$, $F_3 = b_1/s^2$,

$F_4 = b_0/s^3$, and all $\Delta_k = 1$, $\Delta_D = 1 - [-a_1/s - a_2/s^2 - a_3/s^3] + 0$. The SFG's transfer function is easily seen to have a cubic polynomial in the numerator and denominator:

$$\frac{V_o}{V_1} = \frac{b_3\,s^3 + b_2\,s^2 + b_1 s^1 + b_0}{s^3 + a_1 s^2 + a_2\,s^1 + a_3} \tag{A-6}$$

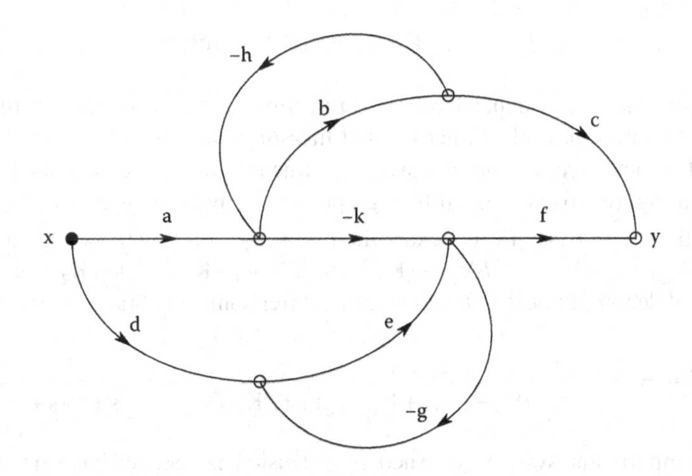

Figure A4 SFG for the system of Example 3 having 3 forward paths and 2 negative feedback loops.

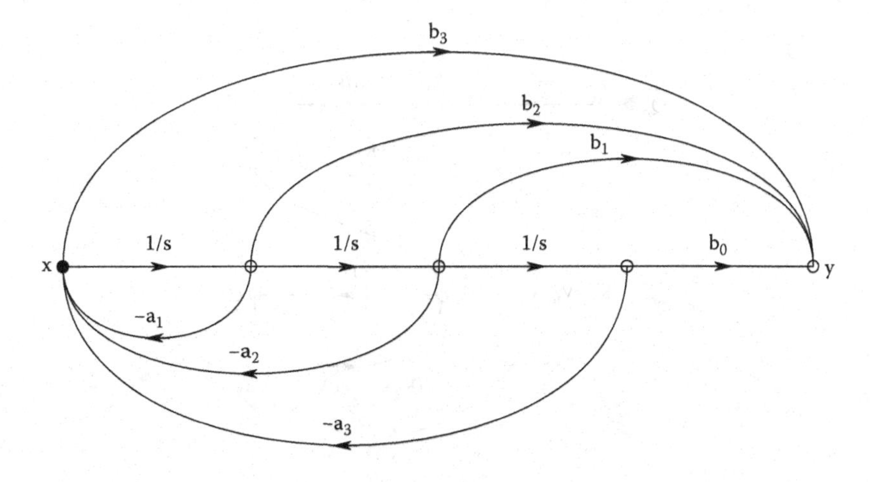

Figure A5 State-variable geometry linear SFG for Example 4. It has 4 forward paths and 3 negative feedback loops.

In a fifth and final example, a chemical, C, is synthesized in the mitochondria of a cell at a rate $\dot{Q}_o$. Its concentration is C_m μg/l in the mitochondria. It diffuses out of the mitochondria into the cytoplasm where its concentration is C_c. It next diffuses through the cell membrane to what is basically zero concentration outside of the cell. The two compartments are (1) the mitochondria and (2) the cytoplasm around the mitochondria. The compartmental state equations are based on simple diffusion (Fick's first law). V_m and V_c are compartment volumes:

$$V_m\dot{C}_m = \dot{Q}_o - K_{12}(C_m - C_c) \quad \mu g/min \tag{A-7A}$$

$$V_c\dot{C}_c = K_{12}(C_m - C_c) - K_2C_c \quad \mu g/min \tag{A-7B}$$

Written in state form, we have

$$\dot{C}_m = -C_m(K_{12}/V_m) + C_c(K_{12}/V_m) + \dot{Q}_o/V_m \quad \mu g/(liter\ min.) \tag{A-8A}$$

$$\dot{C}_c = C_m(K_{12}/V_c) - C_c(K_2 + K_{12})/V_c \quad \mu g/(liter\ min.) \tag{A-8B}$$

Note that mass diffusion rates depend on *concentrations* or mass/volume, so the diffusion rate constants, K_{12} and K_2 must have the dimensions of liters/minute.

From the ODEs above, we see that the system is linear, and can be described by a signal flow graph as shown in Figure A6. The signal flow graph can easily be reduced by Mason's rule to find the transfer function, $C_c/\dot{Q}_o(s)$: In this example, $n = 1$, $F_1 = (1/V_m)(1/s)(K_{12}/V_c)(1/s)$, $\Delta_1 = 1$, and $\Delta_D = 1 - [(-K_{12}/sV_m) + (-(K_2 + K_{12})/sV_c) + (K_{12}^2/s^2V_mV_c)] + [(-K_{12}/sV_m)(-(K_2 + K_{12})/sV_c)] - 0$. This somewhat involved denominator is only a quadratic. After some algebra,

$$\frac{C_c}{\dot{Q}_o} = \frac{K_{12}/V_mV_c}{s^2 + s[K_{12}/V_m + (K_{12} + K_2)/V_c] + K_2K_{12}/V_mV_c} = \frac{K}{(s+a)(s+b)} \tag{A-9}$$

Thus, the two-compartment system governed by diffusion is seen to have linear, second-order dynamics with two real poles after factoring. MATLAB's *Roots* utility can be used to numerically factor the denominator.

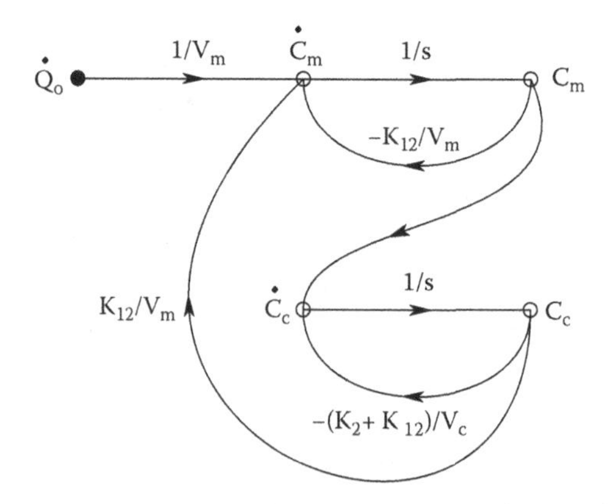

Figure A6 Linear SFG for a simple metabolic diffusion system with 2 compartments (states), one positive feedback loop, 2 negative feedback loops, and 1 forward path to outputs Cm and Cc.

Glossary

A. ABBREVIATIONS AND ACRONYMS USED IN THE TEXT

AC:	alternating current
ADC:	analog-to-digital converter
A/Dd:	analog-to-digital converted
ADM:	adaptive delta modulator
AECMV:	astable, emitter-coupled multivibrator
AF:	active filter
AIC:	analog integrated circuit
AMV:	astable (emitter-coupled) multivibrator
AP:	action potential
AR:	amplitude response (in a Bode plot); antireflection coating (in optics)
a-Se:	amorphous selenium
BDBPSR:	balanced diode bridge phase-sensitive rectifier
BPF:	band-pass filter
B-E:	base-emitter (junction)
BJT:	bipolar junction transistor
BW:	bandwidth
ca:	abbreviation for *circa* (Latin): approximately, around, or about
Cb:	Coulomb
C-B:	collector-base (junction)
C-C:	complex-conjugate
CCW:	counterclockwise
C-E:	common-emitter (transistor amplifier)
CHSOA:	chopper-stabilized op amp
CI:	coherent interference
CL:	closed-loop
CM:	common-mode
CMRR:	common-mode rejection ratio
CP:	clock pulse
CS:	complimentary symmetry
CW:	clockwise
D*:	1/NEP of a photodiode
DA:	differential amplifier
DAC:	digital-to-analog converter
DC:	direct current (zero frequency)
d-c:	direct-coupled
DCA:	digitally controlled attenuator
DCP:	digitally controlled potentiometer
DCVGE:	digitally controlled variable gain element
DFF:	D flip-flop
DGPS:	differential global positioning system
DM:	difference-mode or delta modulator
DSBSCM:	double-sideband, suppressed-carrier modulation
DUT:	device under test

EA: electrometer amplifier
ECG: electrocardiogram
ECL: emitter-coupled logic
ECoG: electrocochleogram
EEG: electroencephalogram
EF: emitter-follower
EFGB: emitter-follower grounded base (amplifier)
EM: electromagnetic
EMG: electromyogram
EMI: electromagnetic interference
$\mathbf{e_{na}}$: amplifier equivalent short circuit input noise voltage root power spectrum: Units = rms V/√Hz
EOA: electrometer op amp
EOC: end of conversion
EOG: electrooculogram
EPP: end-plate potential
ER: emergency room
ERG: electroretinogram
FA: fractal antenna
FBP: feedback pair (amplifier)
FET: field-effect transistor
FIR: finite impulse response
FM: frequency modulation
FR: Faraday rotator
GB: grounded-base
GBWP: gain-bandwidth product
GE: grounded-emitter
GF: generator function (of fractal)
G-G: grounded-gate (FET amplifier)
GME: glass (micropipette) microelectrode
GPS: global positioning system
HF: high frequency
IA: jnstrumentation amplifier
$\mathbf{I_B}$: DC bias current at amplifier input
IC: jntegrated circuit
ICE: Immigration and Customs Enforcement (US)
ICU: intensive care unit (of a hospital)
ID: ideal diode; identification; inside diameter
IIR: infinite impulse response
$\mathbf{i_{na}}$: amplifier equivalent input noise current root power spectrum: Units = rms A/√Hz
IOA: ideal operational amplifier
IP: internet protocol
IPFD: instantaneous pulse frequency demodulation
ISM: industrial, scientific. and medical (RF bands) (see ISM below for bands)
IT: ideal transformer
JFET: junction field-effect transistor
KVL: Kirchoff's voltage law
LAD: laser diode
LAVERA: laser velocity and ranging (system)
LED: light-emitting diode

LFID: low-frequency identification (tag)
LIA: lock-in amplifier
LIR: longwave infrared radiation
LNA: low-noise amplifier
LPF: low-pass filter
LPL: linearly polarized light
LSB: least significant bit
LTI: linear, time-invariant (system)
LVDT: linear variable differential transformer
MDAC: multiplying digital-to-analog converter
MFC: multifunction converter
mg%: milligrams/deciliter, a concentration often used for glucose
MIA: medical isolation amplifier
MOSFET: metal-oxide, semiconductor, field-effect transistor
MS: mean-squared
MRI: magnetic resonance imaging
MSB: most significant bit
NBFM: narrow-band frequency modulation
NCF: negative current feedback
NMR: nuclear magnetic resonance
NEP: noise-equivalent power [the NEP is the incident optical P_i @ λ required to generate a short-circuit response current, I_P, equal to the RMS noise current of the photodetector system (unity output signal-to-noise ratio)]
NTC: negative temperature coefficient
NVF: negative voltage feedback
OA: operational amplifier; optically active
OCV: open-circuit voltage
OR: operating region (of a transistor); operating room (hospital)
OS: operating system
PC: printed circuit; personal computer
PCB: printed circuit board
PCR: polymerase chain reaction (in DNA analysis)
PD: phase detector
PDA: personal digital assistant
PDS: power density spectrum
PhD: phase detector
PI: proportional plus integral
PIN: *p*-doped, intrinsic, *n*-doped photodiode
PLL: phase-locked loop
PMT: photomultiplier tube
PO: pulse oximeter
POC: photo-optic coupler
PSK: phase-shift keying (modulation)
PSR: phase-sensitive rectifier; power supply rejection
PTAT: proportional to absolute temperature
PTC: positive temperature coefficient
PTT: platform terminal transmitter (to satellite)
PYM: pyroelectric material
QN: quantization noise
QUM: quantity under measurement
RAM: random-access memory

r-c: reactively coupled (amplifier)
R-C: resistor-capacitor (coupled filter)
RD: return difference
RF: radio frequency
RFC: radio-frequency choke
RFI: radio-frequency interference
RFID: radio-frequency identification (tag)
RL: root locus
RMS (or rms): root-mean-square
ROM: read-only memory
RR: recovery room (of a hospital)
RTD: resistance temperature detector (sensor).
S: Siemens (unit of conductance)
SAW: surface acoustic wave (filter)
SBD: Schottky barrier diode
SCC: short-circuit current
SCF: switched capacitor filter
SCR: silicon controlled rectifier
SD: standard deviation
SF, S-F: source-follower
SHF: super high frequency (GHz)
SISO: single-input, single-output (system)
SJ: op amp summing junction
SNF: spot noise figure
SNR: signal-to-noise ratio
SS: steady state
s-s: small-signal
SSM: small-signal model (of a transistor)
HFSSM: high-frequency SSM
MFSSM: midfrequency SSM
SV: satellite vehicle
TCCS: temperature-controlled current source
TCXO: temperature-controlled crystal oscillator
THD: total harmonic distortion
TJ: thermocouple junction
TTL: transistor–transistor logic
UHF: ultrahigh frequency
USB: universal serial bus
VCCS: voltage-controlled current source
VCO: voltage-controlled oscillator
VCVS: voltage-controlled voltage source
VD: varactor diode
VFC: voltage-to-frequency converter
VGE: variable gain element
VHF: very high frequency
$\mathbf{V_{OS}}$: amplifier's input DC offset voltage
VPC: voltage-to-period converter
VTC: vacuum thermocouple
WAAS: wide-area augmentation system (GPS)
WPM: wireless patient monitoring
XO: crystal-controlled oscillator

B. GLOSSARY TERMS

Active Circuit: An electronic circuit that contains active, controlled, voltage and/or current sources (VCVS, CCVS, VCCS, and CCCS). All amplifiers are active circuits.

Antenna Resonance Frequency: The frequency (there may be more than one) at which an antenna (and its feed line) appears as a real load to the RF power amplifier driving it. The shortest resonant wire is $L = \lambda/2$ in length, or $L = 150/f_r$ m, where f_r is the resonant frequency in MHz. A center-fed dipole antenna has two elements each $\lambda/4$ in length. Element size reduction in antennas that are resonant at some f_r has made use of various interesting designs; helices, helical arrays, discones, various fractal designs, etc.

ARGOS Satellite Telemetry System: Used principally for wildlife tracking. Data from mobile transmitter platforms (tags) is uplinked in the 401.618–401.680 MHz band to nongeostationary, low **p**olar-**o**rbiting, **e**nvironmental **s**atellites (POES). These satellites are put in orbit and maintained by NOAA and MetOp of the European Organization for the Exploitation of Meteorological Satellites (Eumetsat). Orbital altitude is 850 km; orbital period is ca. 100 min. ARGOS-received messages are (1) stored on the onboard recorder and then retransmitted to the ground each time the SV passes over the main receiving stations located at Wallops Island, VA, Fairbanks, AK, and Svalbard, Norway. 2) The messages can also be retransmitted to other regional reception stations in range. At any given moment, each satellite in the system "sees" all ARGOS transmitters within a circle on the Earth's surface with ca. 5,000 km diameter. As a satellite orbits, the visibility circle sweeps a 5,000 km wide swath around the Earth, covering both poles. Because of the Earth's rotation, the swath shifts 25° west (2,800 km at the equator) around the polar axis at each revolution. This causes an overlap between successive swaths. Since overlap increases with latitude, the number of daily passes over a given transmitter or receiver also increases with their latitude. At the poles, each SV sees each polar transmitter on every pass, approximately 14 times/day.

The ARGOS system is widely used to track marine animals tagged with pop-up archival tags (PAT), platform terminal transmitters (PTT), or GPS data-logging tags.

ARGOS satellite transmitters suitable for fixed and mobile terrestrial applications, such remote weather stations, are offered by Campbell Scientific, Inc., Logan, UT (www.campbell.com).

Bisection Theorem: The bisection theorem (BT) is used to simplify the pencil-and-paper analysis of bilaterally symmetrical circuits, such as differential amplifiers. (It is described in detail in Northrop, 1990.) First, an *axis of symmetry* is defined for a *symmetrical linear active circuit* (SLAC). Difference- and common-mode input signals are defined. Components split by the axis of symmetry must be divided as in Figure 3.5. GL.BT. For pure common-mode excitation, it can be shown by superposition that zero currents flow on the cross-links of the bisected circuit, and therefore, the cross-links can be cut on the axis of symmetry (made open-circuit). For pure difference-mode excitation, all small-signal voltages on the axis of symmetry can be shown by superposition to be zero; thus, all cross-links can be shorted to ground on the axis of symmetry, simplifying analysis of the symmetrical circuit.

Chipping Rate (aka ChiP Rate): In direct-sequence, spread-spectrum technologies such as code division multiple access (CDMA), it is the number of bits (chips) per second used in the spreading signal. A different spreading signal is added to the data signal to uniquely code each transmission. The number of chips (bits) in the spreading signal is significantly greater than the data bits. Chip rate is generally measured in megachips per second (Mcps).

Cramer's Rule: *(In linear algebra)* Given a set of N, linear, simultaneous equations of the form

$$Y_1 = x_1\, a_{11} + x_2\, a_{12} + \ldots + x_N\, a_{1N}$$
$$Y_2 = x_1\, a_{21} + x_2\, a_{22} + \ldots + x_N\, a_{2N}$$
$$Y_N = x_1\, a_{N1} + x_2\, a_{N2} + \ldots + x_N\, a_{NN}$$

This system has an A matrix:

$$\mathbf{A} = \begin{matrix} a_{11}\ a_{12} \ldots a_{1k} \ldots a_{1N} \\ a_{21}\ a_{22} \ldots a_{2k} \ldots a_{2N} \\ a_{31}\ a_{32} \ldots a_{3k} \ldots a_{3N} \\ a_{N1}\ a_{N2} \ldots a_{Nk} \ldots a_{NN} \end{matrix}$$

Cramer's rule allows one to solve for x_k by dividing the determinant below by Det{**A**} = Δ:

$$x_k = \text{Det} \begin{vmatrix} a_{11} & a_{12} & \ldots & Y_1 & \ldots & a_{1N} \\ a_{21} & a_{22} & \ldots & Y_2 & \ldots & a_{2N} \\ a_{31} & a_{32} & \ldots & Y_3 & \ldots & a_{3N} \\ a_{N1} & a_{N2} & \ldots & Y_N & \ldots & a_{NN} \end{vmatrix} \div \text{Det}\{A\}$$

(The NYs are in the kth column of the A matrix.)

Cytosol: The interior fluid contents of a cell (excluding such organelles as mitochondria and ribosomes).

Diastolic Blood Pressure: BP defined by the cuff pressure when the last Korotkoff sound is heard as the sphygmomanometer cuff is slowly deflated. (Also see *Systolic BP.*)

Ergodic Noise: One sample record from a random process is assumed to be equivalent to any other record taken from the random process.

Fractal Antenna: A fractal antenna uses a fractal or self-similar element design to maximize its effective length and/or area and achieve broadband operation. Many fractal antennas use a space-filling strategy that repeats a basic geometric motif at progressively smaller levels of scale. Fractal antennas permit the compact construction of cellphones, GPS systems, and other wireless communication devices that operate in the UHF and SHF RF frequency bands.

f_T: Frequency at which a transistor's small-signal current gain = 1. That is: $|\mathbf{h_{fe}}(j2\pi f_T)| \equiv 1$. With op amps, f_T is used as the frequency at which the open-loop, DM gain is down by −3 dB.

Half-Cell Potential: In electrochemistry, a pair of half-cells make an electrochemical cell (e.g., a battery) whose EMF is the sum of the EMFs of the two half-cells. Redox reactions take place in the cell at the two half-cells. At one half-cell, there is change of thermodynamic free energy, ΔF, given by the Gibbs–Helmholtz equation (Maron and Prutton 1958). The fundamental relation between EMF and free energy is ΔF = −n**FE**. It can be shown that, using chemical thermodynamics, the half-cell EMF is

$$E = E_0 - \frac{RT}{nF} \ln \frac{a_C^c a_D^d \ldots}{a_A^a a_B^b \ldots}$$

where E0 is the half-cell's standard potential: the axX in the numerator are the chemical activities of the reaction products; those in the denominator are the activities of the reactants, R is the gas constant, T is the Kelvin temperature, n is the number of electrons in the reaction stoichiometry.

For example, the familiar silver: silver chloride half-cell has the oxidation reaction:

$$Ag(s) + Cl- = AgCl(s) + e-.$$

The standard electrode potential for this reaction is $E_0 = -0.2225$ V @ 25°C. Thus, the calculated half-cell EMF is

$$E_{Ag\text{-}AgCl} = -0.223 + 0.060 \log_{10}(a_{Cl-}) \text{ @ } 25°C$$

In practice, electrode half-cell EMFs must always be measured with a standard half-cell, such as the hydrogen + platinized platinum foil electrode half-cell, or a well-defined calomel half-cell electrode (Plonsey and Fleming 1969).

Headstage: The first (input) stage of a multistage amplifier.

Hodgkin–Huxley Model: A mathematical model based on chemical kinetics describing the initiation of a nerve impulse in active neuron membrane. Basically, a unit area "patch" of active nerve membrane is considered. The total ionic current density through the membrane is J_{in}:

$$J_{in} = C_m \dot{v} + J_K + J_{Na} + J_L \quad \mu A/cm^2$$

The leakage current density J_L is

$$J_L = g_{Lo}(v - V_L) \quad \mu A/cm^2$$

The net potassium current density, J_K, is

$$J_K = g_{Ko}\, n^4 (v - V_K) \quad \mu A/cm^2$$

The K^+ *activation parameter* n is given by the ODE

$$\dot{n} = -n(\alpha_n + \beta_n) + \alpha_n$$

The sodium current density, J_{Na}, is given by

$$J_{Na} = g_{Nao}\, \mathbf{m}^3\, \mathbf{h}\, (\mathbf{v} - \mathrm{VNa})$$

Sodium gate *activation parameter* is modeled by the m ODE:

$$\dot{m} = -m(\alpha_m + \beta_m) + \alpha_m.$$

The sodium deactivation parameter is modeled by the **h** ODE

$$\dot{h} = -h(\alpha_h + \beta_h) + \alpha_h,$$

where v(t) is the transmembrane voltage change: $v(t) = V_{m0} - V_m(t)$. $V_m(t)$ is the instantaneous membrane voltage; V_{m0} is the *resting* membrane voltage, −70 mV. The parameters are $\alpha_n = 0.01(v + 10)/[\exp(0.1v) - 1]$, $\beta_n = 0.125 \exp(v/80)$, $\alpha_m = 0.1(v + 25)/[\exp(0.1v + 2.5) - 1]$, $\beta_m = 4 \exp(v/18)$, $\alpha_h = 0.07 \exp(v/20)$, $\beta_h = 1/[\exp(0.1v + 3) + 1]$. C_m is the nerve membrane capacitance per unit area. V_K and V_{Na} are the equilibrium Nernst potentials for potassium and sodium ions, respectively. V_L is the equivalent Nernst potential for anions.

(See Section 4.5.4 in Northrop (2008) and Section 1.4.1 in Northrop (2001) for details and parameter values.)

Hold Circuit: A zero-order hold circuit has a continuous, stepwise analog output voltage. It converts a digital sample of an analog signal, x*(nT), to an analog voltage, x(nT), at its output which it holds constant until the next sample, x*[(n + 1)T], is ready for conversion.

Inmarsat™ Satellite System: The Inmarsat system became operational in 1982. Its primary focus was to provide communications for ships at sea, including distress, urgency, and safety messages (e.g., storms), and for routine, two-way communications between ships and ships and shore. There are four, active, Inmarsat SVs in equatorial, geostationary orbits ca. 36,000 km over the Earth's center; each "sees" about one-third of the Earth's surface, so there is overlap in SV coverage. On the ground, there are 34 Land Earth Stations (LESs) that provide links between the satellites and the terrestrial telecommunications networks. A Satellite Control Center located in London is responsible in looking after the satellites themselves (orbits, electronic performance, etc.).

The four geostationary Inmarsat satellites cover the four oceanic regions: Atlantic Ocean Region-East (AOR-E), Atlantic Ocean Region-West (AOR-W), Indian Ocean Region (IOR), and Pacific Ocean Region (POR). In addition, these four ORs are divided into a total of 15 NAVAREAs.

The transmission frequency (Tx) band (ship to satellite) is 1.6265–1.6465 GHz; the satellite to ship (Rx) band is 1.5250–1.5450 GHz; channel spacing is only 20 kHz. Inmarsat messages are prefaced by a two-digit code (00-99) to identify message category and priority. For example, a "38" message is one sent when there is a medical emergency aboard ship.

The Inmarsat system has several subsystems: Inmarsat-A supports two-way telephone, telex, fax, email, and with the high speed data option, can support 64 kbps data transmission. The A system requires a parabolic dish antenna that is actively kept pointed at the SV. It is housed in a dome of ca. 1.5 m diameter. Inmarsat-B is an all-digital version of the A system. Inmarsat- C supports only data transmission, not voice. It uses a small, fixed antenna, and includes the following services: *Two-way text messages. Polling and data reporting*—shore to ship requests for navigation data, etc. *Position reporting*—ship can send automatically data from its GPS, etc. *Distress Alerting*—sends SOS message with ship coordinates. *Enhanced Group Calling*—allows messages to be sent to groups of vessels via SafetyNET or FleetNET. Inmarsat-E—for emergencies at sea, such as flooding, engine failure, etc.; sends an EPIRB message to an Inmarsat SV, which sends it to one of three land stations: Niles Canyon, USA (AOR-W, POR), Perth, Australia (IOR), and Raisting, Germany (AOR-E).

Inmarsat offers three fleet broadband enhanced connectivity options: For example, the FB500 option has standard IP up to 432 kbps, ISDN at 64 kbps, vox at 3.1 kHz, standard 3G SMS (text messages up to 160 characters), and uses a dish antenna as small as 0.6 m diameter.

For more details, see: Services (2004), SafetyNET (2004)

Iridium™ Satellite System: The Iridium system, introduced to the market in 2008, has a 66-satellite network in low Earth orbits (LEOs), ca. 780 km above the Earth. Orbital velocity of the satellites is ca. 26,804 km/h, giving an orbital period of 100 min, 28 s. The 66 SVs are arranged in six planes in near circular orbits; each plane is inclined at 86.4° and contains 11 SVs. Coverage on the Earth's surface from a single satellite has a footprint radius of 2,209 km, and an area of 15.3×10^6 km^2.

Iridium handset channels are spaced at 41.666 kHz and each channel occupies a bandwidth of 31.5 kHz; this allows space for Doppler shifts. The system delivers two-way, UHF radio coverage anywhere in the world, including the extreme polar regions on the 1.616–1.6265 GHz L-band (handset to and from satellites). Intersatellite communication (to four other SVs) is at 25 Mbps in the 23.18–23.38 GHz Ka-band. Downlinks to Iridium Gateway ground stations (there are 13) are at 19.4–19.6 GHz;

uplinks from the Gateways are on the 29.1–29.3 GHz Ka-band. Gateways are located in: Tempe, Arizona; Wahiawa, Hawaii; and Avezzano, Italy. Gateways link the satellite radio communications to earth-side cellphone systems and landlines, etc.

The Iridium company's OpenPortä service, developed specifically for maritime users, offers multiple data links and bandwidth connections of up to 128 kbps via the satellites. The OpenPort shipboard unit can handle three simultaneous two-way phone channels as well as data channels. See Wiki (2010h) Iridium_Communications_Inc. and Jabbar (2004) for more details on the Iridium communication system.

ISM: The industrial, scientific, and medical radio bands defined by the ITU-R are as follows:

Frequency range (Hz)	Center frequency (Hz)	Availability/comment
6.765–6.795 MHz	6.780 MHz	Subject to local acceptance
13.553–13.567 MHz	13.560 MHz	
26.957–27.283 MHz	27.120 MHz	
40.66–40.70 MHz	40.68 MHz	
433.05–434.79 MHz	433.92 MHz	
902–928 MHz	915 MHz	Region 2 only*
2.400–2.500 GHz	2.450 GHz	
5.725–5.875 GHz	5.800 GHz	
24.000–24.250 GHz	24.125 GHz	
61.00–61.50 GHz	61.25 GHz	Subject to local acceptance
122–123 GHz	122.5 GHz	Subject to local acceptance
244–246 GHz	245 GHz	Subject to local acceptance

Isobestic Wavelength *(in spectrophotometry):* The wavelength where absorption of photons is equal for two different analytes.

Mason's Rule: (See Appendix C in Northrop (2010), and the Appendix of this text for a detailed description of signal flow graphs and Mason's rule.) Mason's rule (gain formula), given a system's representation by a linear *signal flow graph* (SFG), is

$$\frac{V_{ok}}{V_{ij}} = H_{jk} \frac{\sum_{n=1}^{N} F_n \Delta_n}{\Delta_D}$$

where H_{jk} = net transmission from jth (input) node to kth (output) node. F_n = transmission of the nth *forward path.* The nth forward path (FP) is a connected path of branches beginning on the jth node and ending on the kth node, along which no node is passed through more than once. A SFG can have several FPs that can share common nodes. Δ_D = SFG denominator or determinant. $\Delta_D \equiv 1 -$ [sum of all individual *loop gains*] + [sum of products of pairs of all *nontouching loop* gains] – [sum of products of nontouching loop gains taken 3 at a time] + · · · · *Loop gain* is the net gain around a closed loop of one or more branches. The loop must start and finish on a common node. *Nontouching loops* share no nodes in common. Δ_n = cofactor for the nth FP. Simply, $\Delta_n = \Delta_D$ calculated for nodes that do not touch the nth FP.

Application of Mason's formula gives Hjk as a rational polynomial in powers of the complex variable, s, if the SFG branch gains are constants and/or functions of s.

Maximum Power Transfer *(to a resistive load coupled by an ideal transformer):* Assume a power device can be represented by a Thevenin open-circuit voltage, V_{1OC}, and a Thevenin series resistance, R_1. This Thevenin model is coupled to a resistive load, R_L, by an ideal transformer with primary-to-secondary turns ratio (n_1/n_2). We have shown that the equivalent resistance looking into the primary is $R_L' = R_L (n_1/n_2)^2$. Thus we can attach the equivalent load resistor to the Thevenin circuit for the PA; the current through R_L' is simply: $I_1 = V_{1OC}/(R_1 + R_L')$, and the power delivered to the apparent load is $P_L' = I_1^2 R_L'$ Watts. It is easy to show by differentiation that P_L' is maximum when $R_1 = R_L' = R_L(n_1/n_2)^2$; hence, the optimum turns ratio for maximum power to the load is $(n_1/n_2) = \sqrt{(h_{oe}^{-1}/R_L)}$ for a grounded emitter BJT amplifier.

Nondispersive Spectrophotometry: Spectrophotometry that eliminates the use of an expensive grating or prism. Generally, two different wavelengths of light are used: from LEDs or LADs. One LED emits at the isobestic wavelength of the analyte, and the other emits at a wavelength where absorbance is proportional to the analyte's concentration. The common finger pulse oximeter (used to measure the hemoglobin % O_2 saturation) is an example of a nondispersive spectrophotometer.

Passband *(of a filter):* The frequency region(s) in a filter's output frequency response where the input signal's power spectrum is minimally attenuated (see *Stopband*).

Perveance: A high-perveance transistor or vacuum tube is a power device; that is, its collector, drain, or plate current has a substantially higher range than for a low-power, voltage amplifier device. For example, for a FET, $I_D = \mathbf{P}\, f(V_{GE}^{3/2}, V_{CE})$. **P** is the perveance factor.

***Phasor*:** A complex function of time, i.e., a time-varying quantity that, at any instant, has a real and imaginary part, and thus can be represented in the complex plane as a two-dimensional vector (Kraus 1953).

Poles *(of transfer functions):* When a linear transfer function (TF) is written as a rational polynomial in the complex variable, **s**, the poles are the complex locations of the roots of the TF denominator in the s-plane. That is, they are the complex **s** values that when substituted into the denominator polynomial, make it ≡ 0.

***Q-Point* (of a transistor):** The Q-point is the quiescent operating point (quiescent biasing point) around which an input signal causes voltages and currents to change. That is, I_{CQ}, I_{BQ}, V_{CEQ}. A BJT has a nominal set of small-signal parameters (e.g., h_{fe}, h_{re}, h_{oe}, h_{ie}) at any Q-point.

Radio Frequency Bands: The table below lists the US radio frequency bands. Note that the RF bands defined by the ITU differ slightly from IEEE bands.

Band name	Abbrev.	Freq. range	Uses
Extremely low frequency	ELF	3–30 Hz	Communication with submarines
Super low frequency	SLF	30–300 Hz	Communication with submarines
Ultralow frequency	ULF	300–3,000 Hz	Communication within mines
Very low frequency	VLF	3–30 kHz	Submarine communication, avalanche beacons, geophysics, wireless heart rate monitors
Low frequency	LF	30–300 kHz	Navigation, time signals, AM longwave broadcasting, RFID, over-the-horizon radio communication
Medium frequency	MF	300–3,000 kHz	AM broadcasting
High frequency	HF	3–30 MHz	Shortwave radio, amateur radio, aviation radio, RFID
Very high frequency	VHF	30–300 MHz	FM radio, TV, line-of-sight aircraft to aircraft, and aircraft to ground radio, maritime mobile, ground mobile radio
Ultrahigh frequency	UHF	300–3,000 MHz	TV, microwave ovens, mobile phones, RFID, WPM, GPS, Bluetooth, Wi-Fi, Zigbee
Super high frequency	SHF	3–30 GHz	Microwave devices, wireless LAN, radars
Extremely high frequency	EHF	30–300 GHz	Radio astronomy, High-freq. microwave radio relay
Terahertz	THz	300–3,000 GHz	THz imaging, THz time-domain spectroscopy, THz computing/communications

In addition to the designations in the preceding table, the UHF, SHF, and EHF bands have been further subdivided by the US IEEE, and named as follows:

Band	Freq. range
UHF	300–1,000 MHz
L band	1–2 GHz
S band	2–4 GHz
C band	4–8 GHz
X band	8–12 GHz
K_u band	12–18 GHz
K band	18–27 GHz
K_a band	27–40 GHz
V band	40–75 GHz
W band	75–110 GHz
mm band	110–300 GHz

QRS Spike: Largest electrical feature of the electrocardiogram, caused by the depolarization–repolarization of ventricular muscle fibers during cardiac systole.

Stationary Noise: Noise whose statistical properties do not change in time. The noise-generating parameters in the random process are constant and do not change with time.

Stopband *(of a filter):* The frequency region(s) of a filter's frequency response in which the input signal's spectrum is most heavily attenuated.

Systolic Blood Pressure: The peak (arterial) blood pressure (BP) that occurs during or slightly after left ventricular contraction (systole) of the heart. It can be measured in a variety of locations. Brachial BP is most widely measured using a sphygmomanometer cuff on the upper arm and an aneroid or mercury manometer to measure the cuff air pressure. The pressure at the first Korotkoff sound heard through a stethoscope over the lower brachial artery defines the systolic BP.

Tank Coil: The inductor in a resonant RF, RLC circuit.

Telehealth *(aka telemedicine):* The transfer of electronic medical data (sounds, physiological measurements, images, live video, and patient records) from one location to another. It includes the use of electronic information and telecommunication technologies to support long distance clinical care, emergency medicine, patient and professional health-related education, public health and health administration. *e-health* is telehealth specifically using the internet (email, Skype, image transfer, etc.). Telehealth communications can also be by RF links, including by satellite networks (such as Iridium and Inmarsat).

Tempco: Acronym for temperature coefficient. The tempco of a parameter **P** at temperature $\mathbf{T_o}$ is defined as $\alpha = [d\mathbf{P}(\mathbf{T_o})/dT]/\mathbf{P}(\mathbf{T_o})$.

Triphasic potential spike: Triphasic spikes are recorded, for example, from the surface of a nerve axon or muscle fiber. First, the potential goes briefly positive, then a large negative spike occurs, followed directly by a smaller positive spike; the entire duration is ca. 1 ms.

Very Small Aperture Terminal (VSAT): A two-way, satellite ground or shipboard microwave (SHF) communication station. Shipboard VSAT antennas are generally gyrostabilized to track the target satellite in spite of ship motion. VSAT antennas are generally parabolic dishes ranging from 0.75 m to 2.5 m diameter (depending on RF frequency). They are commonly used to transmit narrowband data generated by credit card sales, polling, or RFID data. Importantly, they are used for on-the-move, mobile maritime communications (to *Inmarsat* or *Iridium* satellite systems). Ka (27–40 GHz) or Ku (12–18 GHz) band frequencies are used. A large VSAT network (more than 12,000 stations) is used by the

US Postal Service. Other VSAT users include car dealerships (Ford, GM), store chains (Wal-Mart, Walgreen Pharmacies, CVS, Yum! Brands (Taco Bell, Pizza Hut, Long John Silver's, etc.)).

Window circuit: A circuit used to select pulses in a certain amplitude range (e.g., from metal microelectrodes recording nerve spikes, or the QRS complex in an ECG). The input waveform is compared to two analog voltage threshold voltages; analog comparators and logic gates are used. A window output pulse is generated when a narrow input voltage pulse crosses the lower threshold voltage while increasing in amplitude and *does not cross* the upper threshold before it recrosses the lower threshold while decreasing in amplitude. Rising input pulses that cross the lower threshold and then the upper threshold before falling below the upper and lower thresholds do not give an output, nor do pulses with peak amplitudes below the lower threshold.

Bibliography and Recommended Reading

Ali, S.M., Raut, R., and Sawan, M. 2006. Digital encoders for high speed flash-ADCs: Modeling and comparison. *Proceedings of the Northeast Workshop on Circuits and Systems,* Concordia University, Montreal, Canada, pp. 69–72.

Allen, P.E. and Holberg, D.R. 2002. *CMOS Analog Circuit Design.* Oxford University Press, New York.

AN928. 2010. *Understanding High Speed DAC Testing and Evaluation.* Available at: www.analog.com/static/imported-files/application_notes/an_928.pdf (Last accessed 22 September 2010).

Analog Devices. 1994. *Design-In Reference Manual.* Analog Devices. One Technology Way. Norwood, MA.

Angelo, E.J., Jr. 1969. *Electronics: BJTs, FETs and Microcircuits.* McGraw-Hill, New York.

Anscombe, D.L. 2010. Healthcare delivery for oil rig workers: Telemedicine plays a vital role. *Telemedicine and e-Health.* 16(6): 759–663.

Arizona. 2010. *Fish Tagging and Marking Techniques.* Arizona Game and Fish Dept. 7 pp. Available at: www.azgfd.gov/w_c/Fish_Tagging_Marking_Techniques.shtml (Last accessed 15 November 2010).

ARRL Staff. 1953. *The Radio Amateur's Handbook.* American Radio Relay League, W. Hartford, CT.

ARRL Staff. 1974. *The ARRL Antenna Book.* American Radio Relay League, Newington, CT.

Aseltine, J.A. 1958. *Transform Method in Linear System Analysis.* McGraw-Hill, New York.

Ayers, J.E. 2009. *Digital Integrated Circuits,* 2nd ed. CRC Press, Boca Raton, FL.

Azaro, R., Zeni, E., Rocca P., and Massa, A. 2007. Innovative design of a planar fractal-shaped GPS/GSM/Wi-Fi antenna. *Microwave and Optical Technology Letters.* 50(3): 825–839.

Balanis, C.A. 1989. *Advanced Engineering Electromagnetics.* Wiley, New York.

Baisa, N. 2005. Designing wireless interfaces for patient monitoring equipment. *RF Design.* 1 April 2005. Accessed 11/03/11 at: http://rfdesign.com/mag/504rfdf4b.pdf.

Barkhordarian, V. 2010. *Power MOSFET Basics.* International Rectifier. *App. Note AN1084.* Available at: http://www.irf.com/technical-info/appnotes/mosfet.pdf (Last accessed 13 May 2010)

Barnes, J.R. 1987. *Electronic System Design: Interference and Noise Control Techniques.* Prentice-Hall, Englewood Cliffs, NJ.

Beihold, F. and Wang, J. 2002. Packing more antenna into available space. *Applied Microwave & Wireless.* October. 56–61. Accessed 11/03/11 at: www.cst.com/Content/Documents/Journals/applied_cover_10_02.pdf

Beis, U. 2008. *An Introduction to Sigma Delta Converters.* Web tutorial. Available at: www.beis.de/Electronik/DeltaSigma/DeltaSigma.html (Last accessed 2 May 2011)

Berglund, B., Johannson, J., and Lejon, T. 2006. High efficiency power amplifiers. *Ericsson Review.* 3: 92–96.

Berry, E. *et al.* 2004. Multispectral classification techniques for terahertz pulsed imaging: An example in histopathology. *Medical Engineering & Physics.* 26: 423–430.

Blanchard, A. 1976. *Phase-Locked Loops.* Wiley, New York.

Boylstead, R. and Nashelsky, L. 1987. *Electronic Devices and Circuit Theory,* 4th ed. Prentice-Hall, Englewood Cliffs, NJ.

Browne, A.F., Nelson, T.R., and Northrop, R.B. 1997. Microdegree polarimetric measurement of glucose concentrations for biotechnology applications. *Proceedings of the 23rd Annual Northeast Bioengineering Conference.* J.R. Lacourse, Ed. UNH/Durham. pp. 9–10.

Cameron, B.D. and Coté, G.L. 1997. Noninvasive glucose sensing utilizing a digital closed-loop polarimetric approach. *IEEE Transactions on Biomedical Engineering.* 44(12): 1221–1227.

Chalasani, S., Boppana, R.V., and Sounderpandian, J. 2005. RFID tag reader designs for retail store applications. *Proceedings of American Conference on Information Systems (AMCIS).* pp. 2219–2228.

Chen, W.-K. 1986. *Passive and Active Filters: Theory and Implementation.* Wiley, New York.

Chirlian, P.M. 1981. *Analysis and Design of Integrated Electronic Circuits.* Harper & Row, New York.

Clarke, K.K. and Hess, D.T. 1971. *Communication Circuits: Analysis and Design.* Addison-Wesley, Reading, MA.

Cohen, N. 1997. Fractal antenna applications in wireless telecommunications. *IEEE Electronic Industries Forum of New England.* 43–49. Accessed 11/03/11 at: http://ieeexplore.ieee.org/stamp/stamp.jsp?arnumber=00605374.

Copeland, J., Yates, R., and Ruggiero, L. 2004. *Wolverine Population Assessment in Glacier National Park.* Progress Report, US Forest Service. 18 pp. Available at: www.wolverinefoundation.org/research/glacier04.pdf (Last accessed 15 November 2010).

Costa, D. et al. 2010. Accuracy of ARGOS locations of pinnipeds at-sea estimated using Fastloc GPS. *PLoS ONE.* 5(1): e8677.

Coté, G.L., Fox, M.D., and Northrop, R.B. 1992. Noninvasive optical polarimetric glucose sensing using a true phase measurement technique. *IEEE Transactions on Biomedical Engineering.* 39(7): 752–756.

Curtis, D.W. *et al.* 2008. SMART—An integrated wireless system for monitoring unattended patients. *Journal* of the *American Medical Informatics Association.* 15: 44–53.

Dorf, R.C. 1967. *Modern Control Systems.* Addison-Wesley, Reading, MA.

Du, Z. 1993. *A Frequency-Independent, High Resolution Phase Meter.* MS dissertation in Biomedical Engineering, University of Connecticut, Storrs. (R.B. Northrop, major adviser.)

Dudenbostel, D., Krieger, K-L., Candler, C., and Laur, R. 1997. A new passive CMOS telemetry chip to receive power and transmit data for a wide range of sensor applications. *Proc. 1997 Int'l. Conf. on Solid-State Sensors and Actuators.* Chicago. June 16–19. 995–998.

Egan, W.F. 2007. *Phase-Lock Basics.* Wiley-IEEE Press, New York.

Ehrenberg, J.E. and Steig, T.W. 2003. Improved techniques for studying the temporal and spatial behavior of fish in a fixed location. *ICES Journal of Marine Science.* 60: 700–706.

Eisner, L., Brown, R.M., and Modi, D. 2004. Leakage current standards simplified. *MDDI Magazine* (online). Available at: www.mddionline.com/print/957 (Last accessed 15 July 2010).

Eisner Safety Consultants. 2010. *Overview of IEC 60601-1 Medical Electrical Equipment.* Available at: www.EisnerSafety.com (Last accessed 15 July 2010).

Felber, P. 2001. *Fractal Antennas.* Class Project for ECE 576, Illinois Institute of Technology. 15 pp.

Fitzgerald, A.J. et al. 2006. Terahertz pulsed imaging of human breast tumors. *Radiology.* 239(2): 533–540.

Franco, S. 1988. *Design with Operational Amplifiers and Integrated Circuits.* McGraw-Hill, New York.

Gaalaas, E. 2006. Class D audio amplifiers: What, why and how. *Analog Dialog.* 40–06: 1–7.

Gardner, F.M. 2005. *Phaselock Techniques.* 3rd ed. Wiley-Interscience, New York.

Gaubert, C. et al. 2004. THz fractal antennas for electrical and optical semiconductor emitters and receptors. *Physics Status Solidi C.* 1(6): 1439–1444.

GE Healthcare. 2009. *GE Healthcare Introduces CARESCAPE Telemetry Platform for Wireless Patient Monitoring.* Business Wire. Available at: www.gehealthcare.com/euen/patient_monitoring/index.html (Last accessed 8 June 2011)

Geddes, L.A. 1998. *Medical Device Accidents.* CRC Press, Boca Raton, FL.

Ghaussi, M.S. 1971. *Electronic Circuits.* D. Van Nostrand Co., New York.

Ghaussi, M.S. and Laker, K.R. 2003. *Modern Filter Design: Active RC and Switched Capacitor.* Noble Publishing Co. Cranbrook, TN.

Gilham, E.J. 1957. A high-precision photoelectric polarimeter. *Journal of Scientific Instruments.* 34: 435–439.

Gray, P.R. and Meyer, R.G. 1984. *Analysis and Design of Analog Integrated Circuits.* Wiley, New York.

Guyton, A.C. 1991. *Textbook of Medical Physiology,* 8th ed. W.B. Saunders Co., Philadelphia.

Hannaford, B. and Lehman, S. 1986. Short-time Fourier analysis of the electromyogram: fast movements and constant contraction. *IEEE Transactions on Biomedical Engineering.* 33(12): 1173–1181.

Harrington, D. 2010. *Tracking the Wolverine.* 9 pp web post. Available at: http://danielharrington.wordpress.com/2010/01/31/tracking-the-wolverine/ (Last accessed 4 May 2011).

Hashemi, K. 2009. *Subcutaneous Transmitter.* Open Source Instruments, Inc. Web paper. Available at: www.opensourceinstruments.com/Electronics/A3013/M3013.html (Last accessed 17 June 2010).

Hay, C.E., Harrell, M.E., and Kansy, R.L. 2004. 2.4 and 2.5 GHz miniature, low-noise oscillators using surface transverse wave resonators and a SiGe sustaining amplifier. *Proceedings of the 2004 IEEE International Ultrasonics, Ferroelectrics, and Frequency Control Joint 50th Anniversary Conference.* pp. 174–179.

Hecht, E. 1987. *Optics,* 2nd ed. Addison-Wesley, Reading, MA.

Herzel, F., Erzgräber, H., and Weger, P. 2001. Integrated CMOS wideband oscillator for RF applications. *Electronics Letters.* 37(6): 330–331.

Hitachi. 2011. *Hitachi RFID Solutions: The mu Chip.* Available at: www.hitachi-eu.com/mu/ Products/Mu%20 Chip.htm (Last accessed 2 May 2011).

Hobby. 2010. *170W Audio Power Amplifier.* 3 pp. Available at: www.hobby-hour.com/electronics/ 170w-audio-power-amplifier.php (Last accessed 6 May 2010).

Hodgkin, A.L. and Huxley, A.F. 1952. A quantitative description of membrane current and its application to conduction and excitation in nerve. *Journal of Physiology* (London) 117: 500–544.

Holejšovská, P., Peroutka, Z., and Čengery, J. 2003. Non-invasive monitoring of the human blood pressure. *Proceedings of the 16th IEEE Symposium on Computer-Based Medical Systems (CMBS'03)*. 6 pp.

Ibrahhiem, A. et al. 2006. Bi-band fractal antenna design for RFID applications at UHF. *Proceedings of EuCAP 2006*, Nice, France. 6–10 November 2006. 3 pp.

Irons, F. 2005. *Active Filters for Integrated-Circuit Applications.* Artech House, Norwood, MA. 426 pp.

Iyriboz, Y. 1990. Oscillometric finger blood pressure versus brachial auscultative blood pressure recording. *Journal of Family Practice*. Available at: http://findarticles.com/p/mi_m0689/is_n4_v31/ai_13084613/ (Last accessed 2 May 2011)

Jabbar, M.A. 2004. *Multi-Link Iridium Satellite Data Communication System.* MS Dissertation, The University of Kansas. (V.S. Frost, major adviser.) Available at: citeseerx.ist.psu/viewdoc/download?doi=10.1.1.129.3230.pdf/ (Last accessed 16 September 2010)

James, H.J., Nichols, N.B., and Philips, R.S. 1947. *Theory of Servomechanisms.* McGraw-Hill, New York.

Jones, I. et al. 2008. Wireless RF communication in biomedical applications. *Smart Materials and Structures.* 17: 1–10.

Kalorama. 2010. *Remote & Wireless Patient Monitoring Markets.* Kalorama Information. R566-530. 8 pp. Available at: www.mindbranch.com/catalog/print_product_page.jsp?code=R566-530 (Last accessed 17 June 2010).

Kanai, H., Noma, K., and Hong, J. 2001. Advanced spin-valve GMR-head. *Fujitsu Scientific and Technical Journal.* 37(2): 174–182.

Kandel, E.R., Schwartz, J.H., and Jessel, T.M. 1991. *Principles of Neural Science,* 3rd ed. Appleton and Lange, Norwalk, CT.

Karim, M.N.A. et al. 2010. Log periodic fractal Koch antenna for UHF band applications. *Progress in Electromagnetics Research.* 100: 201–218.

Katz, B. 1966. *Nerve, Muscle and Synapse.* McGraw-Hill, New York.

Kaye & Laby. 2008. 2.4 Acoustics, 2.4.1 The speed and attenuation of sound. *Tables of Physical & Chemical Constants.* Available at: www.kayelaby.npl.co.uk/general_physics/2_4/2_4_1.html (Last accessed: 19 October 2010).

Kennedy, L. 2009. *Problem Solving in Hypertension.* Atlas Medical Publishing, Ltd., Oxford.

Kester, W. 2008. *ADC Architectures I: The Flash Converter.* Analog Devices MT-020 Tutorial. 15 pp.

Kiger, P.J. 2010. *Migration Science: Mali Elephant.* 3 pp National Geographic web post. Available at: http://channel.nationalgeographic.com/channel/great-migrations-science-mali-elephant (Last accessed 2 May 2011).

Kitchin, C. and Counts, L. 1983. *RMS to DC Conversion Application Guide.* Analog Devices Inc., Norwood, MA.

Kollár, I. 1986. The noise model of quantization. *Proceedings of the IMEKO TC4 Symposium, "Noise in Electrical Measurements."* Como, Italy. 19–21 June 1986. OMIKK-Technoinform, Budapest. 1987. pp. 125–129.

Krauss, J.D. 1953. *Electromagnetics.* McGraw-Hill, New York.

Kulkarni, M., Sridhar, V., and Kulkarni, G.H. 2010. The quantized differential comparator in flash analog to digital converter design. *International Journal of Computer Networks & Communications (IJCNC).* 2(4): 37–45.

Kumar, R. and Malathi, P. 2009. On the design of wheel shape fractal antenna. *International Journal of Recent Trends in Engineering.* 2(6): 98–100.

Kuo, B.C. 1982. *Automatic Control Systems,* 4th ed. Prentice-Hall, Englewood Cliffs, NJ.

Lai, P.W., Dobos, L., and Long, S. 2003. A 2.4 GHz low phase-noise VCO using on chip tapped inductor. *Proceedings of the 29th European Solid-State Circuits Conference (ESSCIRC'03).* pp. 505–508. Available at: http://ieeexplore.ieee.org/xpls/abs_all.jsp?arnumber=1257183 (Last accessed 8 June 2011).

Landolsi, T., Al-Ali, A.R., and Al-Assaf, Y. 2007. Wireless stand-alone portable patient monitoring and logging system. *Journal of Communications.* 2(4): 65–70.

Lavallée, M., Schanne, O.F., and Hébert, N.C. 1969. *Glass Microelectrodes.* Wiley, New York.

Leister, W. et al. 2008. Threat assessment of wireless patient monitoring systems. *Proceedings of the 3rd Conference on Infomation and Communication Technologies: From Theory to Applications.* 7–11 April 2008. Damascus, Syria. pp. 1–6.

Lemson, J. et al. 2009. The reliability of continuous noninvasive finger blood pressure measurement in critically ill children. *Anesthesia & Analgesia.* 108(9): 814–821.

Lewis, S.B., Flynn, R., and Barten, N. 2008. *Wolverine Population Ecology in Berners Bay, Alaska.* Wildlife research progress report. 23 pp. Alaska Department of Fish & Game, Division of Wildlife Conservation. Available at: www.wolverinefoundation.org/research/BBAKProgress2008.pdf (Last accessed 15 November 2010).

Lion, K.S. 1959. Instrumentation in Scientific Research: Electrical Input Transducers. McGraw-Hill, New York.

Liu, J.-C. et al. 2006. Modified Sierpinski fractal monopole antenna with Descartes circle theorem. *Microwave and Optical Technology Letters.* 48(5): 909–911.

Locher, R. 1998. Introduction to Power MOSFETs and their Applications. *Fairchild Semiconductor Application Note 558.*

LT. 2010. Ultralow voltage energy harvester uses thermoelectric generator for battery-free wireless sensors. *Linear Technology Journal of Analog Innovation.* 20(3): 1–11.

Maron, S.H. and Prutton, C.F. 1958. *Principles of Physical Chemistry.* Macmillan, New York.

Maxim. 2007. *Class D Amplifiers: Fundamentals of Operation and Recent Developments.* Application Note 3977. Available at: www.maxim-ic.com/an3977 (Last accessed 1 July 2010).

McDonald, B.M. and Northrop, R.B. 1993. Two-phase lock-in amplifier with phase-locked loop vector tracking. *Proceedings of the European Conference on Circuit Theory and Design.* Davos, Switzerland, 30 Aug.–3 Sept. 6 pp.

Mentelos, R.A. 2003. *Electrical Safety in PC Based Medical Products.* Application Note AN-10. RAM Technologies LLC, Guilford, CT. Available at: www.ramtechno.com

Mentelos, R.A. 2010. *Medical-Grade Power Supplies: Safety and Reliability Set Them Apart.* Available at: www.ramtechno.com/medsafety.php (Last accessed 20 September 2010).

Merck Manual of Diagnosis and Therapy. 2010. M.H. Beers, and Berkow, R., eds. *Electrical Injury.* Available at: www.merck.com/mmpe/section21/ch316/ch316b.html (Last accessed 15 July 2010).

Millman, J. 1979. *Microelectronics.* McGraw-Hill, New York.

Mitchell, K. 2001. *Tutorial: Hilbert Curve Coloring.* Available at: http://www.fractalus.com/kerry/tutorials/hilbert/hilbert-tutorial.html (Last accessed 28 July 2010)

Nanavati, R.P. 1975. *Semiconductor Devices: BJTs, JFETs, MOSFETs, and Integrated Circuits.* Intext Educational Publishers, New York.

Navon, D.H. 1975. *Electronic Materials and Devices.* Houghton-Mifflin, Boston.

Nelson, T.R. 1999. *Development of a Type 1 Nonlinear Feedback System for Laser Velocimetry and Ranging.* MS Dissertation in Biomedical Engineering, University of Connecticut, Storrs. (R.B. Northrop, major adviser.)

Newport Photonics. 2011. *Laser Diode Technology: Tutorial.* Available at: www.newport.com/Tutorial-Laser-Diode-Technology/852182/1033/content.aspx (Last accessed 8 June 2011).

Nise, N.S. 1995. *Control Systems Engineering.* Benjamin Cummings, Redwood City, CA.

NOAA. 2010. *Draft Environmental Assessment. Gulf of the Farallones National Marine Sanctuary White Shark Research Permit Application for Project Entitled: Fine Scale, Long-Term Tracking of Adult White Sharks.* Web document. Available at: http://farallones.noaa.gov/eco/sharks/pdf/mcsi_draft_ea_sept_24_2010.pdf (Last accessed 11 November 2010).

Northrop, R.B. 1966. An instantaneous pulse frequency demodulator for neurophysiological applications. Proceedings of the Symposium on Biomedical Engineering. Milwaukee, WI. Vol. 1, pp. 5–8.

Northrop, R.B. 1990. *Analog Electronic Circuits: Analysis and Applications.* Addison-Wesley, Reading, MA.

Northrop, R.B., Wu, J.M., and Horowitz, H.M. 1967. An instantaneous frequency cardiotachometer. *Digest 7th International Conference on Engineering in Medicine and Biology.* Stockholm. p. 417.

Northrop, R.B. and Guignon, E.F. 1970. Information processing in the optic lobes of the lubber grasshopper. *Journal of Insect Physiology.* 16: 691–713.

Northrop, R.B. and Grossman, H.J. 1974. An integrated-circuit pulse-height discriminator with multiplexed display. *Journal of Applied Physiology.* 37(6): 946–950.

Northrop, R.B. 2000. *Endogenous and Exogenous Regulation and Control of Physiological Systems.* CRC Press, Boca Raton, FL.

———2001. *Introduction to Dynamic Modeling of Neuro-Sensory Systems.* CRC Press, Boca Raton, FL.

———2002. *Non-Invasive Instrumentation and Measurements in Medical Diagnosis.* CRC Press, Boca Raton, FL.

———2005. *Introduction to Instrumentation and Measurements,* 2nd ed. CRC Press, Boca Raton, FL.

———2010. *Signals and Systems Analysis in Biomedical Engineering,* 2nd ed. CRC Press, Boca Raton, FL.

———2011. *Introduction to Complexity and Complex Systems.* CRC Press, Boca Raton, FL, 531 pp.

NuPhysicia. 2008. The Telemedicine Cart (T-Cart®) (2pp), *also*, The B3ZERO Telemedicine Suitcase System (2 pp). Available at: www.nuphysicia.com (Last accessed 2 May 2011).

Ogata, K.1990. *Modern Control Engineering,* 2nd ed. Prentice-Hall, Englewood Cliffs, NJ.

Olson, H.F. 1940. *Elements of Acoustical Engineering.* D. Van Nostrand Co. Inc., New York.

Ott, H.W. 1976. *Noise Reduction Techniques in Electronic Systems.* Wiley, New York.

Pactitis, S.A. 2007. *Active filters: Theory and Design.* CRC Press, Boca Raton, FL.

Pallás-Areny, R. and Webster, J.G. 1991. *Sensors and Signal Conditioning.* Wiley, New York.

Pallás-Areny, R. and Webster, J.G. 2001. *Sensors and Signal Conditioning*. 2nd ed. Wiley, New York.

Pasta, M., La Mantia, F., and Cui, Y. 2010. A new approach to glucose sensing at gold electrodes. *Electrochemistry Communications*. 12: 1407–1410.

Perkin-Elmer. 2010. *Avalanche Photodiodes: A User Guide*. Accessed 11/03/11 at: http://www.perkinelmer.com/CMSResources/Images/44-6538APP_AvalanchePhotodiodeUsersGuide.pdf

Phillips, C.L. and Nagle, H.T. 1984. *Digital Control System Analysis and Design*. 3rd ed. Prentice-Hall, Englewood Cliffs, NJ.

Plonsey, R. and Fleming, D.G. 1969. *Bioelectric Phenomena*. McGraw-Hill, New York.

Praxmayer, C. 2010. *Great White Sharks Tracked by Satellite*. Web note. Available at: www.shark-tracker.com/en/Tagging/Pop-up-archival-tags/index.php (Last accessed 10 November 2010).

Proakis, J.G. and Manolakis, D.G. 1989. *Introduction to Digital Signal Processing*. Macmillan Publishing Co., New York.

Puente-Baliarda, C. et al. 1998. On the behavior of the Sierpinski multiband antenna. *IEEE Transactions on Antennas and Propagation*. 46(4): 517–524.

Raamat, R., Jagomagi, K., and Talts, J. 2000. Different responses of Finapres and the oscillometric finger blood pressure monitor during intensive vasomotion. *Journal of Medical Engineering & Technology*. 24(3): 95–101.

Raamat, R. et al. 2003. Beat-to-beat measurement of the finger arterial pressure pulse shape index at rest and during exercise. *Clinical Physiology and Functional Imaging*. 23: 87–91.

Rabinovitch, B., March, W.F., and Adams, R.L. 1982. Noninvasive glucose monitoring of the aqueous humor of the eye. Part I. Measurements of very small optical rotations. *Diabetes Care*. 5(3): 254–258.

Richards, J. 2010. *Medical Electronics: Ensuring Compliance with Product Safety Tests*. 6 pp Web paper. Available at: www.ce-mag.com/archive/02/Spring/richards.html (Last accessed 20 September 2010).

SafetyNET. 2004. *The SafetyNET Users Handbook*, 4th ed. Available at: www.inmarsat.com/Maritimesafety/snet.pdf?language=EN&textonly=False (Last accessed 15 September 2010).

Sandner, C. et al. 2005. A 6 bit, 1.2 GSps, low-power flash-ADC in 1.13 μm digital CMOS. *IEEE J. Solid-State Circuits*. 40(7): 1499–1505.

Scharfeld, T.A. 2001. *An Analysis of the Fundamental Constraints on Low Cost Passive Radio-Frequency Identification System Design*. MS Dissertation in Mechanical Engineering, M.I.T., Cambridge, MA. 115 pp.

Schaumann, R., Xiao, H., and Van Valkenburg, M.E. 2009. *Design of Analog Filters*, 2nd ed. Oxford University Press.

Schilling, D.L. and Belove, C. 1989. *Electronic Circuits: Discrete and Integrated*, 3rd ed. McGraw-Hill, New York.

Sears, F.W. 1949. *Optics*. Addison-Wesley, Cambridge, MA.

Seaturtle 2010. *Wildlife Tracking*. Web paper. Available at: www.wildlifetracking.org/faq.shtml (also see: www.seaturtle.org) (Last accessed 11 November 2010).

Services. 2004. *The Inmarsat Services: [A], [B], [C], [E], [Mini-M]*. Available at: www.marinetelecom.net/Inmarsat-Satellite-System.html (Last accessed 15 September 2010).

Sexton, J., Tauqueer, T., Mohiuddin, M., and Missous, M. 2008. *GHz Class Low-Power Flash ADC for Broadband Communications*. Web paper. Available at: www.skads-eu.org/PDF/GHz Class Low-Power Flash ADC for Broadband Communications-ASDAM08_Sextonj.pdf (Last accessed 22 November 2010).

Shahid, S.M. 2005. Use of RFID technology in libraries: A new approach to circulation, tracking, inventorying, and security of library materials. *Library Philosophy and Practice*. 8(1): 10 pp. Available at: http://unllib.unl.edu/LPP/shahid.htm (Last accessed 7 June 2010).

Siakavara, K. 2007. A compact fractal microstrip antenna for GPS and terrestrial radio services. *International Journal of Electronics*. 94(3): 277–283.

Sims, D.W. *et al.* 2009. Long-term GPS tracking of ocean sunfish *Mola mola* offers a new direction in fish monitoring. *PLoS One*. 4(10): 1–6. Available at: www.plosone.org (Last accessed 10 November 2010).

Soltani, P.K., Wysnewski, D., and Swartz, K. 1999. Amorphous selenium direct radiography for industrial imaging. *Paper 22. Proceedings of the Conference on Computerized Tomography for Industrial Applications and Image Processing in Radiology*. 15–17 March. Berlin. pp. 123–132.

Soora, S. 2005. *A Comparison of Two and Three Dimensional Wire Antennas for Biomedical Applications*. MS Dissertation in EE, North Carolina State University, 95 pp. Available at: http://www.lib.ncsu.edu/theses/available/etd-11292005-125256/unrestricted/etd.pdf (Last accessed 26 May 2010).

Sorrells, P. 1998. Passive RFID Basics. *Application note AN680*, Microchip Technology, Inc., Chandler, AZ.

Stapleton, H. and O'Grady, A. 2001. Isolation techniques for high-resolution data acquisition systems. *EDN.* 1 Feb. 2001. 113–118. Accessed 11/03/11 at: www.edn.com/article/501267-Isolation_techniques_for_high-resolution_data_acquisition_systems.php

Stark, L. 1988. *Neurological Control Systems.* Plenum Press, New York.

Stark, H., Tuteur, F.B., and Anderson, J.B. 1988. *Modern Electrical Communications,* 2nd ed. Prentice-Hall, Englewood Cliffs, NJ.

Stefanovska, A. 2007. Coupled oscillations. *IEEE Engineering in Medicine and Biology Magazine.* 26(6): 25–29.

St. Onge, J. 2007. *Leakage-Current Testing for Patient Monitoring Devices. MDDI Magazine.* Available at: www.mdonline.com/print/1825 (Last accessed 20 September 2010).

Thorson, T., Esterberg, G., and Johnson, J. 1969. *Ultrasonic Shark Tag Monitoring System Technical Report.* Faculty Publications in the Biological Sciences, University of Nebraska, Lincoln. Available at: http://digitalcommons.unl.edu/cgi/viewcontent.cgi?article=1006&context=bioscifacpub&sei-redir=1#search=%22Thorson,+Esterberg+1969+%22Ultrasonic+Shark+Tag+Monitoring+ System%22%22 (Last accessed 8 June 2011).

Townsend, P. 2008. *Terahertz Radiation.* Web paper. Available at: www.paultownsend.co.uk/research/fundamentals/terahertz-radiation/ (Last accessed 20 November 2010).

Tremblay, Y., Robinson, P.W., and Costa, D.P. 2009. A parsimonious approach to modeling animal movement data. *PLoS ONE.* 4(3): e4711.

ublox. 2009a. *GPS: Essentials of Satellite Navigation.* (Tutorial on GPS technology.) Document No. GPS-X-02007-D. 174 pp. μ-blox AG, Thalwil, Switzerland. Available at: www.u-blox.com (Last accessed 1 June 2010).

ublox. 2009b. *GPS Antennas.* Application Note GPS-X-08014-A1. Available at: www.u-blox.com (Last accessed 1 June 2010).

Ukkonen, L., Sydänheimo, L., and Kivikoski, M. 2007. Read range performance comparison of compact reader antennas for a handheld UHF RFID reader. *Proceedings of the 2007 IEEE International Conference on RFID.* 26–28 March, Grapevine, TX, TuB1.2: 63–70.

van der Ziel, A. 1974. *Introductory Electronics.* Prentice-Hall, Englewood Cliffs, NJ.

Webster, J.G., Ed. 1992. *Medical Instrumentation,* 2nd ed. Houghton-Mifflin, Boston.

Webster, J.G. 2009. *Medical Instrumentation, Application and Design,* 4th ed. Wiley, New York.

Werner, D.H. and Ganguly, S. 2003. An overview of fractal antenna engineering research. *IEEE Antennas & Propagation Magazine.* 45(1): 38–57.

Wesseling, K.H. et al. 1995. Physiocal calibrating finger vascular physiology for Finapress. *Homeostasis.* 36: 67–82..

West, J.B., Ed. 1985. *Best and Taylor's Physiological Basis of Medical Practice,* 11th ed. Williams & Wilkins, Baltimore.

Wiki. 2010a. Bluetooth. Available at: http://en.wikipedia.org/wiki/Bluetooth (Last accessed 15 June 2010).

Wiki. 2010b. ZigBee. Available at: http://en.wikipedia.org/wiki/ZigBee (Last accessed 15 June 2010).

Wiki. 2010c. IEEE 802.11b-1999. Available at: http://en.wikipedia.org/wiki/IEEE_802.11b-1999 (Last accessed 15 June 2010).

Wiki. 2010d. Wi-Fi. Available at: http://en.wikipedia.org/wiki/Wi-Fi (Last accessed 15 June 2010).

Wiki. 2010e. Hilbert curve. Available at: http://en.wikipedia.org/wiki/Hilbert_curve (Last accessed 28 July 2010).

Wiki. 2010f. Sterling (program). Available at: http://en.wikipedia.org/wiki/Sterling_(program) (Last accessed 15 September 2010).

Wiki. 2010g. Fractal antenna. Available at: http://en.wikipedia.org/wiki/Fractal_antenna (Last accessed 15 September 2010).

Williams, A. and Taylor, F. 2006. *Electronic Filter Design Handbook,* 4th ed. McGraw-Hill, New York.

Wilson, W.L., Jr. 1996. *A Sensitive Magnetoresistive MEMS Acoustic Sensor.* Final Report. Contract #961004. Rice University, Houston, TX. 28 pp.

Wolfram. 2010. *Hilbert Curve.* Available at: http://mathworld.wolfram.com/HilbertCurve.html (Last accessed 28 July 2010).

Xu, L., Lindfors, S., and Stadius, K. 2009. A digitally controlled 2.4-GHz oscillator in 65-nm CMOS. Analog Integrated Circuits and Signal Processing. 58(1): 35–42. Accessed 11/03/11 at: www.springerlink.com/content/a8q1t353365ut165/fulltext.pdf

Yang, E.S. 1988. *Microelectronic Devices.* McGraw-Hill, New York.

Zainud-Deen, S.H., Malhat, H.A., and Adwalla, K.W. 2009. Fractal antenna for passive UHF RFID applications. *Progress in Electromagnetics Research B.* 16: 209–228.

Zhu, Z. 2005. *Low Phase Noise Voltage-Controlled Oscillator Design.* PhD Dissertation. University of Texas, Arlington.

Ziemer, R.E. and Tranter, W.H. 1990. *Principles of Communications: Systems, Modulation, and Noise,* 3rd ed. Houghton-Mifflin Co., Boston.

Zigbee. 2010. Zigbee Tutorial. Available at: www.tutorial-reports.com/print/152 (Last accessed 15 June 2010).

Index

H

I

J

K

L

M

Printed in the United States
by Baker & Taylor Publisher Services